CORONARY STENTING
A Companion to Topol's Textbook of Interventional Cardiology

CORONARY STENTING

A Companion to Topol's Textbook of Interventional Cardiology

MATTHEW J. PRICE, MD

Director, Cardiac Catheterization Laboratory
Scripps Green Hospital;
Division of Cardiovascular Diseases
Scripps Clinic;
Assistant Professor
Scripps Translational Science Institute
La Jolla, California

ELSEVIER
SAUNDERS

ELSEVIER
SAUNDERS

1600 John F. Kennedy Blvd.
Ste 1800
Philadelphia, PA 19103-2899

CORONARY STENTING: A COMPANION TO TOPOL'S TEXTBOOK   ISBN: 978-1-4557-0764-5
OF INTERVENTIONAL CARDIOLOGY
Copyright © 2014 by Saunders, an imprint of Elsevier Inc.

NOTICES

Knowledge and best practice in this field are constantly changing. As new research and experience broaden our understanding, changes in research methods, professional practices, or medical treatment may become necessary.

Practitioners and researchers must always rely on their own experience and knowledge in evaluating and using any information, methods, compounds, or experiments described herein. In using such information or methods, they should be mindful of their own safety and the safety of others, including parties for whom they have a professional responsibility.

With respect to any drug or pharmaceutical products identified, readers are advised to check the most current information provided (i) on procedures featured or (ii) by the manufacturer of each product to be administered to verify the recommended dose or formula, the method and duration of administration, and contraindications. It is the responsibility of practitioners, relying on their own experience and knowledge of their patients, to make diagnoses, to determine dosages and the best treatment for each individual patient, and to take all appropriate safety precautions.

To the fullest extent of the law, neither the Publisher nor the authors, contributors, or editors assume any liability for any injury and/or damage to persons or property as a matter of products liability, negligence or otherwise, or from any use or operation of any methods, products, instructions, or ideas contained in the material herein.

Library of Congress Cataloging-in-Publication Data
Coronary stenting : a companion to Topol's Textbook of interventional cardiology / [edited by] Matthew J. Price.—1st ed.
    p. ; cm.
  Includes index.
  Companion to: Textbook of interventional cardiology / edited by Eric J. Topol, Paul S. Teirstein. 6th ed. c2012.
  ISBN 978-1-4557-0764-5 (hardcover)
  I. Price, Matthew J., 1969- II. Topol, Eric J., 1954- Textbook of interventional cardiology.
  [DNLM: 1. Coronary Artery Disease. 2. Stents. 3. Cardiac Surgical Procedures. 4. Coronary Restenosis. 5. Drug-Eluting Stents. WG 300]
  RD598
  617.4′12059–dc23

                2013003641

Executive Content Strategist: Dolores Meloni
Senior Content Development Specialist: Joan Ryan
Publishing Services Manager: Pat Joiner
Project Manager: Nisha Selvaraj
Design Direction: Ellen Zanolle

Printed in China

Last digit is the print number: 9 8 7 6 5 4 3 2 1

To my wife, Martha, for her patience, support, and love; and to my children, Alexander and Gabriella.

Christina Adams, MD
Chief Fellow, Cardiovascular Division
Scripps Clinic/Scripps Green Hospital
La Jolla, California

Dominick J. Angiolillo, MD, PhD, FACC, FESC, FSCAI
Director, Cardiovascular Research
Associate Professor of Medicine
University of Florida College of Medicine–Jacksonville.
Jacksonville, Florida

Gill Louise Buchanan, MBChB
Invasive Cardiology Unit
San Raffaele Scientific Institute
Milan, Italy

Alaide Chieffo, MD
Invasive Cardiology Unit
San Raffaele Scientific Institute
Milan, Italy

Marco A. Costa MD, PhD
Harrington Heart and Vascular Institute
University Hospitals of Cleveland
Case Western Reserve University
Cleveland, Ohio

Ricardo A. Costa, MD
Chief
Clinical Research
Department of Invasive Cardiology
Institute Dante Pazzanese of Cardiology;
Director
Angiographic Core Laboratory
Cardiovascular Research Center
São Paulo, Brazil

David Daniels, MD
Palo Alto Medical Foundation
Woodside, California

Andrejs Ērglis, MD
Professor
University of Latvia;
Chief
Latvian Centre of Cardiology
Pauls Stradins Clinical University Hospital
Riga, Latvia

William F. Fearon, MD
Associate Professor
Director, Interventional Cardiology
Division of Cardiovascular Medicine
Stanford University Medical Center
Stanford, California

Aloke V. Finn, MD
Assistant Professor
Division of Cardiology
Emory University School of Medicine
Atlanta, Georgia

Juan F. Granada, MD, FACC
Executive Director and Chief Scientific Officer
Skirball Center for Cardiovascular Research
The Cardiovascular Research Foundation;
Assistant Professor
Columbia University Medical Center
New York, New York

J. Aaron Grantham, MD
Associate Professor of Medicine
University of Missouri—Kansas City
Saint Luke's Mid America Heart Institute
Kansas City, Missouri

Karthik Gujja, MD, MPH
Interventional Cardiology
Division of Cardiovascular Diseases
Beth Israel Medical Center
New York, New York

Greg L. Kaluza, MD, PhD, FACC
Director of Research
Skirball Center for Cardiovascular Research
The Cardiovascular Research Foundation
New York, New York

Ajay J. Kirtane, MD, SM
Chief Academic Officer
Center for Interventional Vascular Therapy;
Director, Interventional Cardiology Fellowship Program
Columbia University Medical Center/New York-Presbyterian
   Hospital
New York, New York

Frank D. Kolodgie, PhD
Associate Director
CVPath Institute, Inc.
Gaithersburg, Maryland

Lawrence D. Lazar, MD
Clinical Instructor of Medicine
Division of Cardiology
School of Medicine
University of California, Los Angeles
Los Angeles, California

Michael S. Lee, MD
Assistant Clinical Professor of Medicine
Division of Cardiology
School of Medicine
University of California, Los Angeles
Los Angeles, California

William L. Lombardi, MD, FACC, FSCAI
Medical Director
Cardiac Catheterization Laboratories
PeaceHealth St. Joseph Medical Center
Bellingham, Washington

Roxana Mehran, MD
Professor of Medicine
Department of Cardiology
Mount Sinai School of Medicine
Mount Sinai Medical Center
New York, New York

William J. Mosley II, MD
Division of Cardiovascular Diseases
Scripps Clinic
La Jolla, California

Masataka Nakano, MD
CVPath Institute, Inc.
Gaithersburg, Maryland

Amar Narula, MD
Division of Cardiology
New York University Medical Center
New York, New York

Yoshinobu Onuma, MD
Thoraxcenter
Erasmus Medical Center
Rotterdam, The Netherlands

John A. Ormiston, MBChB
Mercy Angiography, Mercy Hospital
Auckland City Hospital
Auckland, New Zealand

Fumiyuki Otsuka, MD, PhD
CVPath Institute, Inc.
Gaithersburg, Maryland

Matthew J. Price, MD
Director, Cardiac Catheterization Laboratory
Scripps Green Hospital;
Division of Cardiovascular Diseases
Scripps Clinic;
Assistant Professor
Scripps Translational Science Institute
La Jolla, California

Richard A. Schatz, MD
Director of Research, Cardiovascular Interventions
Scripps Clinic
La Jolla, California

Patrick W. Serruys, MD, PhD
Thoraxcenter
Erasmus Medical Center
Rotterdam, The Netherlands

Gregg W. Stone, MD
Professor of Medicine
Columbia University;
Director of Cardiovascular Research and Education
Center for Interventional Vascular Therapy
Columbia University Medical Center/New York-Presbyterian
    Hospital;
Co-Director of Medical Research and Education
The Cardiovascular Research Foundation
New York, New York

Armando Tellez, MD
Assistant Director, Pathology
Skirball Center for Cardiovascular Research
The Cardiovascular Research Foundation
New York, New York

Marco Valgimigli, MD, PhD, FESC
Director, Catheterization Laboratory
University Hospital of Ferrara
Ferrara, Italy

Renu Virmani, MD
President and Medical Director
CVPath Institute, Inc.
Gaithersburg, Maryland

Georgios J. Vlachojannis, MD, PhD
Interventional Cardiovascular Research
Mount Sinai Medical Center
New York, New York

Mark W. I. Webster, MBChB
Auckland City Hospital
Auckland, New Zealand

Neil J. Wimmer, MD
Division of Cardiovascular Medicine
Brigham and Women's Hospital
Harvard Medical School
Boston, Massachusetts

Hirosada Yamamoto, MD
Harrington Heart and Vascular Institute
University Hospitals of Cleveland
Case Western Reserve University
Cleveland, Ohio

Robert W. Yeh, MD, MBA
Medical Director of Clinical Trial Design
Harvard Clinical Research Institute;
Assistant Professor
Cardiology Division, Department of Medicine
Massachusetts General Hospital
Harvard Medical School
Boston, Massachusetts

Jennifer Yu, MD
Interventional Cardiology Fellow
Mount Sinai Medical Center
New York, New York

PREFACE

The procedure first performed by Andreas Gruntzig on September 16, 1977—dilating a coronary stenosis with a semicompliant balloon on a catheter—was revolutionary. Yet the coronary stent, in combination with advances in adjunctive pharmacology, overcame the substantial limitations of coronary angioplasty (e.g., acute vessel closure and poor long-term patency) and is responsible for successfully transforming the management of patients with obstructive coronary artery disease. This paradigm shift in patient care from surgical to percutaneous coronary revascularization was consolidated further by the development of the drug-eluting stent, which substantially reduced neointimal proliferation and the need for repeat revascularization that were observed with bare metal stents. To the neophyte interventional cardiology fellow, the acute efficacy of the coronary stent to treat a severe dissection caused by balloon angioplasty appears self-evident, an observation that reminds me of an aphorism that William Ganz once shared with me while I was in training, as he leaned into my ear and spoke softly, as if sharing a secret: "You don't need fancy statistics to tell you when something really works."

However, the introduction and rapid adoption of the stent into clinical practice raised a host of scientific and clinical questions that led to the establishment and maturation of a new field of research and clinical inquiry. Appropriate preclinical models were developed to assess stent safety; the investigation of the vascular response to injury and the biology of platelet activation and aggregation unraveled the mechanisms of neointimal proliferation and stent thrombosis; a workable framework to measure angiographic efficacy outcomes was developed (e.g., quantitative coronary angiography and the endpoints of acute gain and late luminal loss); and the design of randomized clinical trials was standardized to definitively assess safety and the angiographic and clinical efficacy of different stent types. The development of drug-eluting stents added further layers of complexity in device development, required the expansion of preclinical models, and after the observation of the phenomenon of late stent thrombosis, necessitated studies with longer-term clinical follow-up to better assess safety. The coronary stent has therefore become one of the most intensively studied devices in medical history and certainly deserves a textbook that is specifically dedicated to it.

The goal of Coronary Stenting is to provide the reader with a broad and deep understanding of the field of coronary stenting that can be applied in the research setting and in clinical practice in particular. I have divided the text into four sections. The prologue discusses the development and history of stents. The second section, "Basic Principles," focuses on the fundamentals of stent design, the ways in which stent safety is validated in preclinical models, the design and biology of bioresorbable scaffolds, and the methods used to assess safety and clinical efficacy. The third, "Clinical Use," examines the adjunctive devices and pharmacologic measures that can optimize clinical outcomes during and after stent implantation and discusses the clinical differences between bare metal and drug-eluting stents that may guide operator decision-making. The last section, "Specific Lesion Subsets," provides a detailed focus on the role, techniques, and outcomes of stenting in particular types of coronary anatomies and patient populations, incorporating the most recent randomized clinical trials that can inform patient management.

Coronary Stenting will be especially useful for interventional and invasive cardiologists in training or in practice. It will also serve as a valuable resource for medical trainees with an interest in cardiology and for the ever-growing number of providers of patient care before, during, and after percutaneous coronary intervention, including physician assistants, nurse practitioners, and cardiac catheterization laboratory staff.

I am indebted to my colleagues who have contributed their time and expertise to this volume, to Joan Ryan at Elsevier, and to Eric Topol, the editor of the seminal Textbook of Interventional Cardiology, to which this text serves as a companion. I have been lucky to have Paul Teirstein as a mentor and colleague and can only hope to emulate his ability to push the boundaries of our field with such energy and wit. I am especially grateful to the many patients whom I have treated in the cardiac catheterization laboratory; if the care of a single such patient is improved through this text, then the efforts of this endeavor will have proved worthwhile.

Matthew J. Price, MD
La Jolla, California
January, 2013

CONTENTS

Prologue

CHAPTER 1

Development of Coronary Stents: A Historical Perspective

RICHARD A. SCHATZ | CHRISTINA ADAMS

KEY POINTS

- Angioplasty was a very important milestone in cardiology; however, results were limited by abrupt closure and restenosis.

- Many investigators recognized these limitations in the 1960s and 1970s and attempted to overcome them with self-expanding metal coils in experimental animal models.

- Palmaz, inspired by Grüntzig, conceived of the first balloon expandable stainless steel stent in the late 1970s.

- The first stents were rigid slotted tubes, 30 mm in length and 3 mm in diameter.

- In 1985, Palmaz teamed up with Schatz and placed the first stents in dog coronaries. These were smaller but still rigid.

- As the U.S. trials began in the late 1980s, several competing devices appeared, including a self-expanding spring and a balloon expandable coil.

- The Palmaz-Schatz stent underwent several changes to make it more flexible and more deliverable and was released outside the United States in 1988.

- After many years of trials, the Gianturco-Roubin stent was approved in the United States, followed by the Palmaz-Schatz stent in 1994.

- By 1998, two more stents were approved, the Multilink and the Advanced Vascular Engineering Microstent, followed by the Crown stent, a modification of the Palmaz-Schatz stent, and later the GFX stent.

- Since the introduction of stents, millions of patients have been treated with coronary stents, virtually eliminating abrupt closure and reducing restenosis compared with angioplasty.

- Despite their limitations, stents are the cornerstone of interventional therapy for the treatment of coronary artery disease worldwide.

No discipline in the history of medicine has seen the explosion of growth and innovation that has occurred in interventional cardiology. This explosion was due to a combination of a driving need for better results for the treatment of a deadly and prevalent disease and the unique personality of individuals attracted to the specialty of cardiology. In the early 1970s, the treatment of coronary disease was fairly pedestrian, with a few drugs (nitroglycerin and propranolol), a few diagnostic tests, no randomized trials, and little understanding of the more acute phases of myocardial infarction. Diagnostic angiography was a relatively new procedure with crude equipment by today's standards and strict rules about when a patient could be offered angiography. Bypass surgery was reserved strictly for patients who had severe angina despite maximal medical therapy. Even angiography was strongly discouraged unless the patient had refractory symptoms and a strongly positive stress test. Noninvasive testing as we now know it did not exist. Echocardiography and nuclear medicine did not become widely available as adjuncts to the basic treadmill until the late 1970s.

The treatment for myocardial infarction was even more alarming by today's standards. Patients were admitted to the intensive care unit and given only oxygen and morphine and observed for weeks at a time in the hospital. Furosemide and aminophylline were added if the patient developed congestive heart failure as determined by physical examination. It was not unusual for a patient to be hospitalized for 4 to 6 weeks during this observation period. Nitroglycerin was strictly forbidden for fear of hypotension and worsening ischemia from a "steal" phenomenon. There was much consternation and anxiety during this period for both the patient and the physician because options were very limited.

Angioplasty: The Beginnings

In September 1977, a daring young physician in Zurich, Switzerland, performed the first angioplasty on a conscious patient with a tight lesion of the left anterior descending (LAD) artery. Andreas Grüntzig had been quietly working on a concept that he had conceived while studying under one of the great mentors of radiology, Charles Dotter. Grüntzig had watched Dotter's procedure of dilating peripheral arterial stenoses with progressively larger, tapered tubes. From these observations, he had the idea of adding a balloon to the catheter tip and a central lumen inside the catheter to fill the balloon with contrast material. On expansion of the balloon at the target site, the plaque would give way (like "crushed snow") and, it was hoped, remain open. Grüntzig struggled to get support from many sources to build a workable prototype and to test it in animal models. He eventually was able to build a catheter suitable for human use and after much difficulty received permission to try the first case in a human. The case was a success, and the 37-year-old patient walked out of the hospital angina free without bypass surgery. The world would never be the same.[1]

Word of Grüntzig's work spread quickly. Physicians from all over the world traveled to Zurich to see live case demonstrations of this new procedure, which was coined "coronary angioplasty." Although many were mesmerized by the possibilities of such a paradigm-shifting approach to obstructive coronary artery disease (CAD), others were skeptical and dismissed it as a passing fancy. Eventually, after meeting resistance at home, Grüntzig moved to the United States in 1980 and built the first laboratory for teaching his new procedure at Emory University. This soon became the epicenter for this new discipline of "interventional" cardiology. Hundreds of physicians made the pilgrimage to Emory to watch, learn, and then return home to start angioplasty programs at their respective institutions. Grüntzig was meticulous at collecting data and painfully honest regarding his new procedure, and he encouraged registries, randomized trials, and the sharing of information to understand the limitations of what he was proposing. To say the participants in his courses were in awe of his performance and results would be an understatement, myself included. The tension in the room was palpable as Grüntzig would cannulate the coronaries, pass crude balloons with fixed wire tips down the vessels, and then expand the balloons. ST segment elevation and ventricular arrhythmias were common and routinely prompted panicked shouts from the crowd to deflate the balloon; when the balloon would deflate, an audible gasp of relief could be heard from the crowd, followed by applause and sometimes standing ovations as the final angiogram showed a widely patent vessel and brisk flow down the artery. Not all cases went smoothly, and abrupt closure, dissection, and cardiac arrest were common occurrences. At least once or twice during these demonstrations, patients would experience cardiac arrest and would be whisked off to the waiting operating room with a physician performing cardiopulmonary resuscitation while straddled on top of the patient.

Genesis of the Metal Graft

Although we all witnessed these crashes and prayed for a successful save by our surgical colleagues, one observer in particular, Julio Palmaz, saw things differently: as an opportunity. This "flash of genius" is what frequently separates the brilliant inventors from the rest of us. Palmaz was technically gifted, and he saw the failure of angioplasty as a *mechanical* problem of recoil or collapse in need of a *mechanical* solution. By 1978, he developed the concept of a metal sleeve that could be placed on top of the balloon, carried to the site, and deployed by balloon expansion to support the walls of the artery, preventing mechanical collapse. This concept was not new; several investigators had similar ideas and published widely on the topic in the 1960s.[2-6] Palmaz noted that although these proposed devices were all different, their common characteristic was that they were all variations of springs and coils and were self-expanding. He saw the limitations of these devices as imprecise expansion and unpredictable delivery, both of which could be solved with a balloon expandable piece of metal. The challenge became *what* stent design and which metal.

A trip to Radio Shack resulted in a shopping bag filled with wire, solder, and a soldering gun. His kitchen table converted to a laboratory, Palmaz set out to wrap the wire around a pencil, first in one spiral direction then the other so the wire crossed itself at 90 degrees at many points. The points were soldered to keep them from sliding against each other uncontrollably. When cooled, the device could be slipped off the pencil, ready for use. Palmaz threaded the device over a balloon catheter and crimped it by rolling it with his hands until it fit snugly on the balloon (Figure 1-1). Between 1980 and 1985, Palmaz placed dozens of these "grafts" (he did not call them stents) in dog arteries successfully.[7] His meticulous attention to study design ensured a methodical assessment of the graft tissue interaction with careful long-term follow-up and pathology (thanks to Fermin Tio) to ensure that the device was biocompatible and not toxic to the animal. Because of its size, he was restricted to testing the device in large, straight vessels such as iliac arteries and the descending aorta. It worked very well in these areas, but he knew that the real challenge would be to deliver the device into the smaller and more precarious coronary arteries, where the risks of clotting and restenosis would be amplified.

By 1980, Palmaz moved from northern California to the University of Texas at San Antonio with his chief and mentor, Stewart Reuter,

who was instrumental in supporting his early research. Palmaz published his first paper in 1985 after presenting the data for the first time at the Radiological Society of North America meeting the year before. On arrival in San Antonio and with some minimal funding from the University and a functional laboratory, Palmaz set out to accelerate his efforts. While watching some construction workers at his house, the plasterers caught his eye as he saw them working with a metal lathe that could be easily expanded by pulling on its ends. He grabbed a piece and noticed that the metal was cut in a diamond configuration, which allowed for stretching without recoil. By curling this flat metal into a circle, Palmaz now had a tube that could be expanded radially. This was the spark he needed to conceive of a smaller version suitable for blood vessels. His imagination took him to several experts in thin metals, and soon he identified the right metal and the appropriate technology to construct such a device. His first prototypes were made of 316L stainless steel, a metal commonly used for sutures and needles; it already had a track record for human use with the U.S. Food and Drug Administration (FDA) and was readily available in many different sizes and lengths. He used hypodermic needle tubing that could be easily cut by a well-known technology called *electromagnetic discharge*, which uses tiny graphite electrodes and spark erosion to cut shapes into metal. However, only rectangles could be cut because the technology was limited to rectolinear shapes; Palmaz instructed the technicians to configure the rectangles in a staggered fashion so that on expansion they stretched into diamond shapes (Figure 1-2). By heating the grafts, Palmaz was able to take the spring out of the metal so that once expanded, the tube resisted recoil.

The first of these devices were placed in large arteries and proved to be much easier to deliver than the original devices because of their low profile, although their size (30 mm × 3 mm) and rigid configuration made them suitable only for large, straight vessels. Nonetheless, the technology was easily transferrable to smaller tubes, and by 1985, Palmaz produced a smaller prototype (15 mm × 1.5 mm) (Figure 1-3) that could be placed in vessels ranging in size from 2.5 to 5 mm.

When I met Palmaz in 1985, he was ready to test the grafts in coronary arteries. Because we were now working as a team and had new private funding, the pace of work increased dramatically. Within months, we had placed scores of grafts into rabbit iliacs, dog coronaries, and pig renal arteries. The results in these smaller arteries confirmed that delivery was possible in straight arteries, and clotting did not occur if the animals were pretreated with a combination of aspirin, dipyridamole, and dextran. A randomized trial in dogs showed that this combination was essential to prevent thrombosis.[8] Although we never saw a case of stent thrombosis in treated animals, we recognized

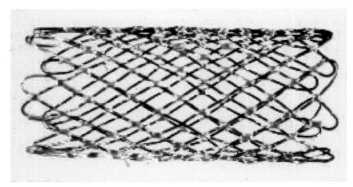

Figure 1-1 The first balloon expandable stent was made of 316L wire wrapped around a mandril. Each crosspoint was soldered with silver solder to prevent sliding of the wires against each other.

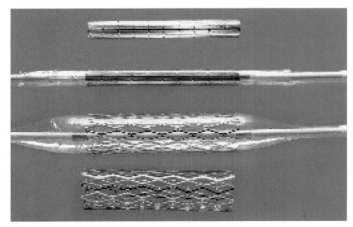

Figure 1-2 The first slotted tube balloon expandable stent measured 3 mm in diameter and 30 mm in length. It was cut from a hollow tube using electromagnetic discharge and could be expanded to 18 mm in diameter.

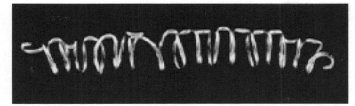

Figure 1-5 The Gianturco-Roubin stent was the first stent placed in humans in the United States. It was made of round wire wrapped around a balloon.

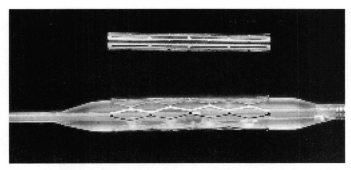

Figure 1-3 The smaller version of the slotted tube stent was designed for vessels 3 to 5 mm in diameter. It was 1.5 mm in diameter and 15 mm in length.

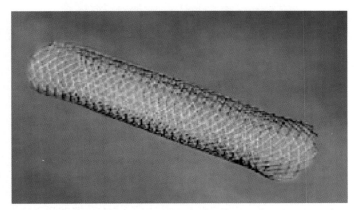

Figure 1-4 The Wallstent was the first self-expanding stent used in humans.

that these were normal arteries and that greater challenges lay ahead of us in diseased human vessels.

Early on, we recognized the need for a more flexible device. It was clear that the slotted tube would not be able to go through standard coronary guide catheters, much less go down human coronaries. Meanwhile, unbeknownst to us, several investigators in Europe were working on a springlike device—the Wallstent, (Medinvent, Lausanne, Switzerland)—with some early successes (Figure 1-4).[9] We received word in March 1986 of the first patients being treated for abrupt closure, long before we were ready to proceed with our first human case. Puel, Marco, and Sigwart placed Wallstents in two patients with excellent results.[10] Gary Roubin, who had abandoned further development of a springlike device that he worked on with Grüntzig, collaborated with Gianturco to develop a wire coil that was balloon expandable (Figure 1-5). He filed for a trial with the FDA to test this wire coil for the treatment of acute closure, in which the protocol required the patient to undergo coronary artery bypass graft (CABG) surgery after the coil was placed. Roubin placed the first such stent in the United States in September 1986.

By now, Palmaz and I had signed a licensing agreement with Johnson & Johnson (New Brunswick, New Jersey) and were working diligently on the iliac protocol. We had already submitted the first draft to the FDA in May 1986, even before we had first met with Johnson & Johnson. Once we signed our licensing agreement with them in August 1986, they took over all regulatory tasks, which freed us to focus on the submission of a proposed coronary artery study. By now, we had completed the first 30 dog coronary implants plus a large series of renal implants, all of which were successful, so we thought acquiring an investigational device exemption for a coronary study would be easy. To our surprise, the FDA informed us we would have

to complete a peripheral trial before we could start implanting within the coronaries. In my earliest discussions with the agency, the FDA had indicated we would have to complete only 75 cases in the coronaries and then would be able submit for premarket approval. We were also specifically told that we would not have to perform a randomized trial—unheard of by today's standards. No other stents required a peripheral artery study before being granted permission to implant devices into the coronaries.

In May 1987, Palmaz traveled to Freiburg, Germany, and with Dr. Goetz Richter placed the first iliac stent in a human. The procedure was successful. Several months later, we received FDA approval to begin the iliac trial in the United States, and the trial launched successfully with multiple centers across the United States. Despite some early skepticism, the trial was completed quickly and led to FDA approval in 1991.

With the Gianturco-Roubin stent (Cook, Inc., Indianapolis, Indiana) gaining traction in the coronaries, we felt we were suddenly behind in the race, so we pushed harder and harder for Johnson & Johnson to accelerate the coronary protocol, which had languished in favor of the iliac launch. Disappointed at how long the FDA was taking to give approval in the United States, we received permission to start placing stents internationally. This made everyone nervous at Johnson & Johnson because this was not the usual method for launching products at that company. However, we believed we had clinical quality coronary stents ready by November 1987 and put the word out worldwide that we were ready to move forward in humans.

Because we had only the rigid 15-mm stent, I knew it would not go through the usual guiding catheters easily, so we had to select our patients wisely to ensure success. The protocol was written to include only short, focal, large right coronary arteries with excellent collaterals and good left ventricular function. I wanted to make sure that if the worst thing happened and the stent clotted, it would have a minimal clinical impact on the patient. Further, I wanted to use the straightest catheter to avoid any issues with curves, so we proscribed (1) the use of the 8F multipurpose or 8.3F Stertzer catheter and (2) an approach (usually a cutdown) from the right brachial artery. This approach allowed us to place the guide wire into the distal coronary first and then remove the guiding catheter with the wire in place. Next, the balloon was advanced through the guide outside the patient. Once the balloon was through the guide, we would then hand crimp the stent on the balloon and backload it into the guide. The entire apparatus was slipped over the wire and tracked to the right coronary artery (RCA) ostium where the balloon and stent could be pushed out across the lesion.

🔹 First Human Case

It did not take long to find our first patient. Dr. Eduardo D'Souza, a prolific cardiologist from Sao Paulo, Brazil, sent me a film that showed the perfect patient. He was a young man with classic angina and a tight lesion involving a down-going RCA with good collaterals and normal left ventricular function. I approved the case immediately, and we traveled to Brazil in December 1987. The entourage consisted of

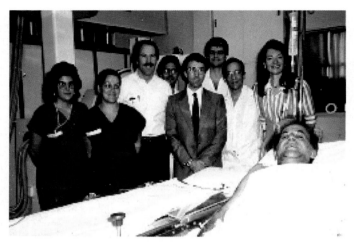

Figure 1-6 The Sao Paolo team and the first patient to receive a Palmaz stent.

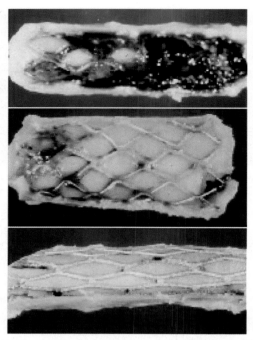

Figure 1-7 Three stents from dogs treated with different anticoagulation regimens. The top stent came from a dog that did not receive any medication before placement. The middle stent was from a dog treated with aspirin, heparin, and dipyridamole. The bottom stent shows the difference when dextran was added to aspirin, heparin, and dipyridamole.

Palmaz, engineers and clinical specialists from Johnson & Johnson, and myself (Figure 1-6).

When we performed our first diagnostic angiogram of the RCA, we found a total occlusion, a clot no doubt, but without an infarct, so we presumed it had closed silently without incident as a result of the patient's brisk collaterals. The protocol did not permit enrollment of patients with total occlusions, but we had come 6000 miles, so we were not going home without performing the procedure. We had never seen stent thrombosis in any of our animals pretreated with antiplatelet agents. Grüntzig had insisted early on that aspirin, dipyridamole, sulfinpyrazone, dextran, and warfarin should be given to all patients for prevention of thrombosis. Warfarin and dextran were later eliminated. Our animal work showed benefit with dextran alone, and I did not want to prescribe warfarin in all patients for fear that once we did so, we would never be able to stop giving it without data from a huge trial (Figure 1-7). Suddenly we were faced with the prospect of placing a metal stent in a fresh clot. We expanded the lesion with a balloon and obtained a good result without further clotting, then placed a 3.0-mm stent and dilated it with a 3.5-mm balloon. The final result was excellent. The patient had an uneventful night and was discharged on aspirin and dipyridamole but no warfarin after a follow-up angiogram the next morning showed the stent widely patent. The patient remained asymptomatic for many years and had several follow-up angiograms that showed only mild intimal hyperplasia (Figure 1-8).

After this success, we rapidly visited many other sites around the world to introduce the procedure to anyone who would listen. Back home, we were working on a more flexible version that consisted of two or three 7-mm slotted tube segments connected with a short flexible strut (Figure 1-9). The animal testing went better than expected, proving that this articulated version could navigate through all conventional guides and into all the coronaries. However, the stents still required hand crimping; this made us nervous because the balloons we were using were off-the-shelf products that were low in profile and slippery, the exact opposite of what we needed. Meanwhile, both the Wallstent and the Gianturco-Roubin stent were gaining popularity worldwide because they were very flexible and easier to deliver than the eventual, articulated Palmaz-Schatz stent. This situation would prove to be a nagging setback for us for quite some time.

Although the iliac investigational device exemption took more than a year to get approved, the coronary protocol was approved in about 8 weeks. By January 1988, we finally were ready to do our first cases using the rigid prototype in the United States. In February 1988, I found what looked like a perfect patient while at the Arizona Heart Institute in Phoenix. However, everything went wrong during the procedure: I could not deliver the stent to a not-so-straight vessel. The stent would not pass to the lesion, and I was not sure I could retrieve it without stripping it from the balloon, so I deployed it proximal to the target lesion. The patient later underwent bypass surgery for restenosis. This was another wake-up call that we had to get the flexible stent released as soon as possible.

Finally, in May 1988, we received permission from Johnson & Johnson to implant the first articulated stent, the Palmaz-Schatz stent, in humans. We quickly set out to Mainz, Germany, where, with Dr. Raimund Erbel, a single Palmaz-Schatz stent was placed in the proximal LAD artery of a patient. The procedure was a great success and proved that the new design was flexible enough to go through a Judkins curve and down the LAD artery (Figure 1-10).[11]

🔹 Stent Thrombosis

The rest of the year was spent opening new centers all over the world with the flexible stent. Despite encouraging early results, reports of stent embolization, thrombosis, and major bleeding became increasingly prevalent. In the United States, more and more patients were being enrolled in the coronary protocol, and similar concerns were being voiced. Although subacute stent thrombosis did not occur in the first 10 to 15 patients, this serious complication increased to almost 2.8% once the protocol was opened to the new centers.[12] We also noted that, in contrast to angioplasty, early thrombosis (occurring in <24 hours, which we called "acute" thrombosis) did not occur.

By December 1988, as a result of concerns from the investigators, Johnson & Johnson (now Johnson and Johnson Interventional Systems) decided to recommend warfarin, in addition to aspirin and dipyridamole, in all patients receiving a coronary stent in the U.S. protocol. After reviewing many of the subacute stent thrombosis cases, I believed that the cause of subacute stent thrombosis was more operator error and incomplete stent expansion than not enough anticoagulation. Nonetheless, warfarin was added, and as predicted, bleeding complications increased from adding warfarin, usually from

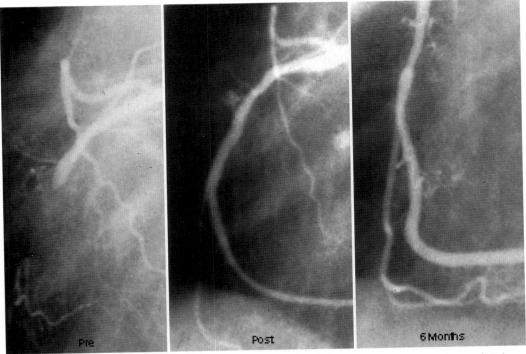

Figure 1-8   First rigid stent placed in a human. *Left,* Before the procedure. *Center,* After the procedure. *Right,* Six months after the procedure. There was moderate intimal hyperplasia by intravascular ultrasound at follow-up. The patient remained asymptomatic for 13 years.

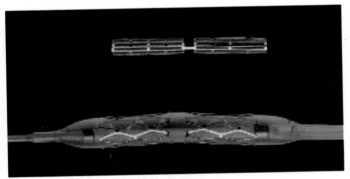

Figure 1-9   First articulated stent, the Palmaz-Schatz stent.

groin hematomas.[13] Years later, when Colombo and colleagues[14] reconfirmed the importance of full stent expansion and newer antiplatelet agents such as ticlopidine and later clopidogrel became available as the hedge against stent thrombosis, the prevalence of subacute stent thrombosis decreased from approximately 5% to a more acceptable 1% to 2% without warfarin.

In 1987, Sigwart and colleagues[10] published the first paper summarizing both the preclinical and the nonrandomized clinical data with the Wallstent, showing encouraging early outcomes. Without regulatory barriers, all three of the available stents (Wallstent, Gianturco-Roubin coil, Palmaz-Schatz) were being sold and used widely outside the United States. However, only anecdotal data for the most part were published about their outcomes.[15-19] In general, it was agreed that both the Wallstent and the Gianturco-Roubin stent were more flexible and more deliverable than the Palmaz-Schatz stent, but all three stents were associated with subacute stent thrombosis and restenosis. Embolization was never well accounted for; however, it appeared to be a serious problem with both the Gianturco-Roubin stent and the Palmaz-Schatz stent.

Solving Embolization

Our first solution to solve the flexibility problem was to construct a sheath system (Figure 1-11) to prevent the stent from contacting the vessel wall. This sheath system worked reasonably well but was still difficult to deliver to tortuous or distal parts of the vessel. Eventually, a custom sheath system was developed by PAS Systems (Menlo Park, California) and named the Stent Delivery System (SDS) (Figure 1-12). This system was provided to all U.S. investigators as well and became the clinical grade quality product eventually released on FDA approval. Although an improvement overall, delivery was challenging because of the bulky size of the outer sheath. It was not until several years later when Johnson & Johnson Interventional Systems, now named Cordis Corporation (Lakewood, Florida), developed the Crown stent with a nesting technique that secured the stent to the balloon well enough that the sheath could be eliminated (Figure 1-13). This stent was an improvement over the Palmaz-Schatz stent in regard to flexibility; however, it never quite caught on enough to compete with other devices. Later, the Palmaz-Schatz stent evolved into another stent called the Velocity (Figure 1-14), which was also a slotted tube but replaced the straight connector between the slots with an S-shaped connector. This connector improved flexibility further and later became the platform for the Cypher, the first drug-eluting stent.

Embolization was not as much an issue for the Wallstent, yet widespread use was hampered by both stent thrombosis and restenosis.[20,21] These two complications proved fatal to the success of both the Wallstent and the Gianturco-Roubin stent, and over time they gradually disappeared from the market.

Randomized Clinical Trials

Now that a safer delivery system was in place, two large randomized trials were conducted in the United States (Stent Restenosis Study [STRESS], n = 410) and Europe (BENESTENT, n = 520); both were designed to test whether coronary stenting reduced restenosis

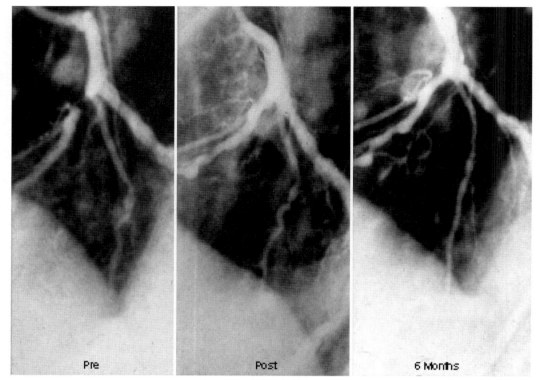

Figure 1-10   First Palmaz-Schatz stent placed in the proximal LAD artery in a patient in Mainz, Germany. *Left,* Before the procedure. *Center,* After the procedure. *Right,* Six months after the procedure.

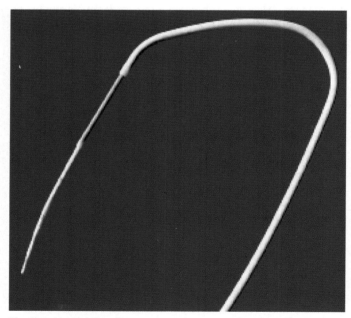

Figure 1-11   Our first attempt to prevent stent embolization. This was a 5F custom-guiding catheter inside a 7F guiding catheter that was placed across the target lesion first. The stent was advanced inside the 5F sheath until it was at the lesion, after which the sheath was withdrawn.

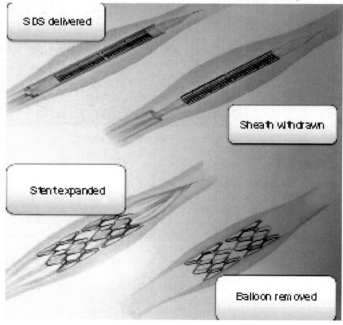

Figure 1-12   Stent Delivery System (SDS), the commercial version of the delivery system used in the United States after FDA approval.

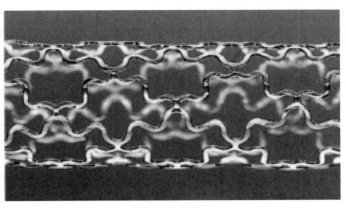

Figure 1-13 Crown stent. This modification of the Palmaz-Schatz stent incorporated a wavy design in the metal struts to improve flexibility.

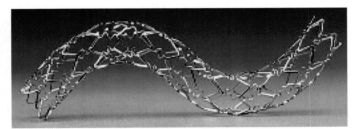

Figure 1-14 Velocity stent. This further modification of the Palmaz-Schatz stent included an S-shaped connector between the slotted tube members instead of a straight strut.

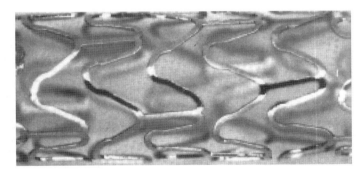

Figure 1-15 The Multilink stent was the first "open" design slotted tube stent developed and released by Advanced Cardiac Sciences in 1998.

compared with balloon angioplasty in de novo, single, native coronary lesions. No such large randomized trial had ever been performed, and much was riding on the outcome of these two studies. Both studies showed very similar outcomes with a significant reduction in restenosis in the stent group compared with angioplasty (42% vs. 31% for STRESS, $P = .046$, and 32% vs. 22% for BENESTENT, $P = .02$).[22,23] These two landmark trials led the way for FDA approval in the United States in 1994. Once approved, sales increased briskly both in the United States and abroad.

Other Slotted Tube Stents

In 1998, Advanced Cardiac Sciences (Indianapolis, Indiana) released the Multilink design, another slotted tube design but with alternating open slots (Figure 1-15). Initial nonrandomized data appeared to show clinical outcomes comparable with the Palmaz-Schatz stent.

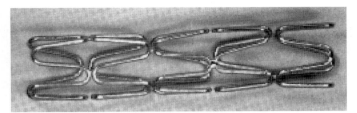

Figure 1-16 Microstent. This slotted tube stent was released by Advanced Vascular Engineering in 2000. It incorporated rounded edges of the slots instead of rectangles and a welded connector between the slotted tube members.

The Multilink had thinner struts, was more flexible than the Palmaz-Schatz and Crown stents, and quickly took over the bulk of the market share. Around this time, another company called Advanced Vascular Engineering (Santa Rosa, California) released the Microstent and later the GFX stent, another closed slotted tube design made of smooth round wire and welded connectors (Figure 1-16). No randomized data were available comparing the GFX stent with the Multilink and Crown stents; however, registry data showed it to appear comparable. Soon both of these stents shared the bulk of the market, with the Crown a distant third. Advanced Cardiac Sciences was soon acquired by Guidant, then Lilly (Indianapolis, Indiana), and Advanced Vascular Engineering was acquired by Medtronic (Minneapolis, Minnesota). Stents enjoyed enormous success once warfarin was eliminated and intravascular ultrasound (IVUS) showed the importance of full stent expansion; this, along with newer antiplatelet agents, made coronary stents the most successful launch of a medical device in history.

Limitations of the Bare Metal Stent

At this time, market share was based purely on deliverability because restenosis rates for all the available stents remained around 15% to 20% and subacute thrombosis rates around 1% for routine cases. No stent improved on the success of the Palmaz-Schatz stent in that regard. More interesting, however, was the rapid expansion of use far beyond the narrow FDA indication of single de novo lesions in 3.0- to 3.5-mm-diameter native vessels. With no data at all, stents were quickly used "off-label" for every possible indication, such as acute myocardial infarction, saphenous vein bypass grafts, chronic total occlusions, bifurcations, long lesions, and short lesions. Eventually, the data caught up with this exuberance and revealed that restenosis rates in these more complicated patients were not 15% to 20% but much higher. The rate of subacute stent thrombosis also was higher than expected, especially in unstable patients with angiographic thrombus or acute myocardial infarction.[24] Design changes in the fundamental stainless steel platform had peaked, so it became clear that the answer to the nagging problems of restenosis and subacute stent thrombosis would have to be pharmacologic, in the form of a surface coating and a drug-delivery system.

First "Drug-Coated" Stent

Palmaz and I had predicted this, and as such our earliest patents claimed the use of a coating of the stent surface with anticoagulants such as heparin to prevent clotting. In the early 1990s, we started working with Cordis on the first heparin-coated stent; after encouraging animal work, around 1995, we treated the first patients after FDA approval. This product was released worldwide shortly thereafter and was used for the first time in a major trial, BENESTENT II.[25] In this important trial, resumption of heparin was progressively delayed after stenting, and in the final group, aspirin and ticlopidine were used instead of heparin and warfarin. There were no episodes of subacute thrombosis in any of the enrolled patients, and the bleeding complication rates were reduced from 7.9% to 0% in the final group. This study showed that the heparin coating appeared to reduce both subacute thrombosis and bleeding complications.

Now we needed to address restenosis with a pharmacologic approach to reduce intimal hyperplasia. Without a substantial reduction in restenosis, CABG would remain a superior strategy for multivessel disease.

Modern Drug-Eluting Stents

Restenosis was understood to be the result of exuberant smooth muscle tissue growth inside the stent. Our earliest publications from animal studies noted this predictable tissue growth inside the stent at various intervals of sampling.[26] Early thick cellular proliferation at 4 to 8 weeks gave way to an acellular matrix by 32 weeks and longer. Isner's group and others confirmed that the predominant cause of in-stent restenosis was smooth muscle cell proliferation.[27] Once the molecular pathways of this process were understood, various drugs targeting the cell cycle were studied to see which were most suitable for a stent coating. Cordis developed the first such system by using a static cell inhibitor, rapamycin (sirolimus). By inhibiting the mTOR (mammalian target of rapamycin) protein kinase of the cell cycle, sirolimus interrupted cellular proliferation, limiting cell growth and restenosis. The first in human trials were very exciting, showing no restenosis in the first patients treated.[28] Larger trials followed, showing an impressively low restenosis rate of 5% to 7% in simple de novo lesions of native coronary arteries. The Cypher stent was launched in 2003 on a new slotted tube platform called the Velocity, which was designed to be more flexible than the past Crown and Palmaz-Schatz stents.

Soon after, in 2005, Boston Scientific (Natick, Massachusetts) launched a stent with a cytotoxic agent, paclitaxel, which was a commonly used cancer drug, on their NIR and then Liberté slotted tube platform, called the Taxus stent. Early data compared with non–drug-coated stents showed an impressive reduction in restenosis to less than 10% despite a higher late loss than Cypher.[29]

As more data became available, it became evident that a new phenomenon of late and very late thrombosis was present with drug-eluting stents. Autopsy data from Vermani and colleagues[30,31] demonstrated an inflammatory reaction in patients with late stent thrombosis, thought to be a result of the polymer coating used to control the release of the antiproliferative drug. This inflammatory reaction prompted interest in more potent antiplatelet agents and the empiric use of prolonged dual antiplatelet therapy for up to 1 year or longer—an extension of the brachytherapy experience.[32] Newer, more biocompatible polymers, nonpolymeric stents, bioabsorbable stents, cobalt and platinum chromium alloys, and nanotechnology surface treatments illustrate the spectrum of approaches to solve, it is hoped, the elusive problems of both thrombosis and restenosis.[33-37]

Conclusion

In retrospect, it is impossible to have foreseen the impact of our work so many years ago. Many individuals predicted that stents would be a passing fancy, but some 25 years after the first stents were placed in humans, the basic slotted tube metal platform remains the fundamental approach of modern mechanical therapies for the treatment of obstructive CAD. The challenge now is to develop the right combination of drugs and coatings to eliminate, and not just reduce, thrombosis and restenosis. Stents have fulfilled Grüntzig's dream of routinely dilating coronary arteries in the conscious human patient and have allowed hopes of one day eliminating the need for CABG. We were given a wonderful gift by Andreas Grüntzig: if he were he alive today, he would be very proud of what we have accomplished with the coronary stent and excited by the future it has heralded.

REFERENCES

1. Grüntzig AR, Senning A, Siegenthaler WE. Non-operative dilatation of coronary-artery stenosis: percutaneous transluminal coronary angioplasty. *N Engl J Med* 1979;301:61-68.
2. Dotter CT. Transluminally placed coil-spring endarterial tube grafts, long-term patency in canine popliteal artery. *Invest Radiol* 1969;4:329-332.
3. Dotter CT, Buschmann RW, McKinney MK, et al. Transluminal expandable nitinol coil stent grafting: preliminary report. *Radiology* 1983;147:259-260.
4. Cragg A, Lund G, Rysavy J, et al. Nonsurgical placement of arterial endoprothesis: a new technique using nitinol wire. *Radiology* 1983;147(1):261-263.
5. Cragg A, Lung G, Rysavy JA, et al. Percutaneous arterial grafting. *Radiology* 1984;150:45-49.
6. Maass D, Zollikofer ChL, Largiader F, et al. Radiological follow-up of transluminally inserted endoprotheses: an experimental study using expandable spirals. *Radiology* 1984;152:659-663.
7. Palmaz JC, Sibbitt RR, Reuter SR, et al. Expandable intraluminal graft: a preliminary study. Work in progress. *Radiology* 1985;156:73-77.
8. Palmaz JC, Garcia O, Kopp DB, et al. Balloon-expandable intra-arterial stents: effect of antithrombotic medication on thrombus formation. In: Seither C, Seyferth W, eds. *Pros and Cons in PTA and Auxillary Methods.* Berlin: Springer-Verlag; 1989.
9. Rousseau H, Puel J, Joffre F, et al. Self-expanding endovascular prosthesis: an experimental study. *Radiology* 1987;164:709-714.
10. Sigwart U, Puel J, Mirkovitch V, et al. Intravascular stents to prevent occlusion and restenosis after transluminal angioplasty. *N Engl J Med* 1987;316:701-706.
11. Schatz RA, Palmaz JC, Tio F, et al. Report of a new articulated balloon expandable intravascular stent (abstract). *Circulation* 1988;78(suppl II):449.
12. Schatz RA, Goldberg S, Leon M, et al. Clinical experience with the Palmaz-Schatz coronary stent. *J Am Coll Cardiol* 1991;17:155B-159B.
13. Schatz RA, Baim DS, Leon M, et al. Clinical experience with the Palmaz-Schatz coronary stent: initial results of a multicenter study. *Circulation* 1991;83:148-161.
14. Colombo A, Hall P, Nakamura S, et al. Intracoronary stenting without anticoagulation accomplished with intravascular ultrasound guidance. *Circulation* 1995;91:1676.
15. Roubin GS, Douglas JS, Lembo NJ, et al. Intracoronary stenting for acute closure following percutaneous transluminal coronary angioplasty (PTCA) (abstract). *Circulation* 1988;78(suppl II):407.

16. Sigwart U, Urban P, Gold S, et al. Emergency stenting for acute occlusion after coronary balloon angioplasty. *Circulation* 1988;79:1121.
17. Urban P, Sigwart U, Gold S, et al. Intravascular stenting for stenosis of aortocoronary venous bypass grafts. *J Am Coll Cardiol* 1989;13:1085-1091.
18. Sigwart U, Urban P, Sadeghi H, et al. Implantation of 100 coronary artery stents: learning curve for the incidence of acute early complications (abstract). *J Am Coll Cardiol* 1989;13:107A.
19. Sigwart U, Gold S, Kaufman U, et al. Analysis of complications associated with coronary stenting (abstract). *J Am Coll Cardiol* 1988;11:66A.
20. Sigwart U, Puel J, Mirkovitch V, et al. Intravascular stents to prevent occlusions and restenosis after transluminal angioplasty. *N Engl J Med* 1987;316:701-706.
21. Lansky AJ, Roubin GS, O'Shaughnessy CD, et al. Randomized comparison of GR-II stent and Palmaz-Schatz stent for elective treatment of coronary stenoses. *Circulation* 2000;102:1364-1368.
22. Fischman DL, Leon M, Baim DS, et al. A randomized comparison of coronary stent placement and balloon angioplasty in the treatment of coronary artery disease. *N Engl J Med* 1994;27:255.
23. Serruys PW, de Jaegere P, Kiemeneij F, et al. Benestent Study Group. A comparison of balloon-expandable stent implantation with balloon angioplasty in patients with coronary artery disease. *N Engl J Med* 1994;331:489-495.
24. Grines CL. Off-label use of drug-eluting stents: putting it in perspective. *J Am Coll Cardiol* 2008;51:615-617.
25. Serruys PW, Emanuelsson H, van der Giessen W, et al. Benestent II Study Group. Heparin-coated stents in human coronary arteries: early outcome of Benestent II pilot study. *Circulation* 1996;93:412-422.
26. Schatz RA, Palmaz JC, Tio FO, et al. Balloon-expandable intracoronary stents in the adult dog. *Circulation* 1987;76:450-457.
27. Kearney M, Pieczek A, Haley L, et al. Histopathology of in-stent restenosis in patients with peripheral artery disease. *Circulation* 1997;95:1998-2002.
28. Morice MC, Colombo A, Meier B, et al. Sirolimus- vs paclitaxel-eluting stents in de novo coronary artery lesions. The REALITY trial: a randomized controlled trial. *JAMA* 2006;295:895-904.
29. Dawkins KD, Grube E, Guagliumi G, et al. TAXUS VI investigators. Clinical efficacy of polymer-based paclitaxel-eluting stents in the treatment of complex, long coronary artery lesions from a multicenter, randomized, trial: support for the use of drug-eluting stents in contemporary clinical practice. *Circulation* 2005;112:3306-3313.

30. Virmani R, Guagliumi G, Farb A, et al. Localized hypersensitivity and late coronary thrombosis secondary to a sirolimus-eluting stent: should we be cautious? *Circulation* 2004;109(6):701-705.
31. Joner M, Finn AV, Farb A, et al. Pathology of drug-eluting stents in humans: delayed healing and late thrombotic risk. *J Am Coll Cardiol* 2006;48(1):193-202.
32. Wilson GJ, Nakazawa G, Schwartz RS, et al. Comparison of inflammatory response after implantation of sirolimus- and paclitaxel-eluting stents in porcine coronary arteries. *Circulation* 2009;120:141-149.
33. Kim JW, Kang WC, Kim KS, et al. Outcome of non-surgical procedure and brief interruption of dual anti-platelet therapy in patients within 12 months following Endeavor (zotarolimus-eluting stent) stent implantation (SENS): a multicenter study. *J Am Coll Cardiol* 2009;53(Suppl):A16.
34. Hamilos M, Sarma J, Ostojic M, et al. Interference of drug-eluting stents with endothelium-dependent coronary vasomotion: evidence for device-specific responses. *Circ Cardiovasc Interv* 2008;1:193-200.
35. Garg S, Serruys P, Onuma Y, et al. 3-year clinical follow-up of the XIENCE V Everolimus-eluting coronary stent system in the treatment of patients with de novo coronary artery lesions. The SPIRIT II Trial (Clinical Evaluation of the Xience V Everolimus Eluting Coronary Stent System in the Treatment of Patients with de novo Native Coronary Artery Lesions). *JACC Cardiol Interv* 2009;2:1190-1198.
36. Park DW, Kim YH, Yun SC, et al. Comparison of Zotarolimus-Eluting Stents with Sirolimus- and Paclitaxel-Eluting Stents for Coronary Revascularization. The ZEST (Comparison of the Efficacy and Safety of Zotarolimus-Eluting Stent with Sirolimus-Eluting and PacliTaxel-Eluting Stents for Coronary Lesions) randomized trial. *J Am Coll Cardiol* 2010;56:1187-1195.
37. Morice MC, Serruys PW, Kappetein AP, et al. Outcomes in patients with de novo left main disease treated with either percutaneous coronary intervention using paclitaxel-eluting stents or coronary artery bypass graft treatment in the Synergy Between Percutaneous Coronary Intervention with TAXUS and Cardiac Surgery (SYNTAX) trial. *Circulation* 2010;121:2645-2653.

SECTION **TWO**

Basic Principles

CHAPTER 2

Fundamentals of Drug-Eluting Stent Design

MATTHEW J. PRICE | WILLIAM J. MOSLEY II

KEY POINTS

- Neointimal proliferation is the primary determinant of restenosis and luminal renarrowing after stent implantation.
- Key pathways that contribute to neointimal formation include thrombosis, inflammation, smooth muscle cell proliferation and migration into the intima, and secretion of the extracellular matrix; these occur with a defined temporal pattern after stent implantation that dictates the optimal release kinetics of antiproliferative agents from drug-eluting stents.
- The most commonly used alloys for coronary stents are 316L stainless steel, cobalt chromium, and platinum chromium; these latter alloys enable the use of thinner struts while maintaining the other performance characteristics of 316L stainless steel (e.g., radial strength, radiopacity).
- Paclitaxel interferes with microtubule dynamics, stabilizing the microtubules and preventing depolymerization, inhibiting human arterial smooth muscle cell proliferation and migration in a dose-dependent manner.
- Rapamycin (also known as sirolimus) and its analogues, including everolimus and zotarolimus, bind FK506 binding protein-12 (FKB12), which in turn blocks the activation of the cell cycle–specific kinase, mammalian target of rapamycin (mTOR), thereby halting cell cycle progression at the juncture of the G1 and S phases.
- Polymers, which consist of long-chain molecules made up of small repeating units, enable the delivery of antiproliferative agents to the vessel intima at a sufficient dose and temporal pattern to achieve a therapeutic antirestenotic effect.
- Several drug-eluting stent platforms, which combine different bare metal scaffolds, nonerodible polymers, and antiproliferative agents (either paclitaxel or rapamycin analogues), have been approved for use in the United States.

As of 2010, approximately 15 million adults in the United States suffered from ischemic heart disease or angina. The concept of percutaneous therapy for the relief of obstructive coronary artery disease began with balloon angioplasty, first performed by Dr. Andreas Grüntzig in 1977.[1] The success of stand-alone balloon angioplasty was limited by acute closure and poor longer term outcomes, with high rates of vessel closure and 6-month restenosis rates as high as 30% to 40%. Apart from dissection, luminal narrowing after angioplasty results from a combination of elastic recoil, negative arterial remodeling, and neointimal hyperplasia (Figure 2-1). The metallic coronary stent acts as a scaffold that prevents acute closure and provides greater acute luminal gain at the time of the procedure, in turn improving early and late angiographic and clinical outcomes (Figure 2-2). By minimizing elastic recoil and negative remodeling, stent implantation isolates neointimal hyperplasia as the primary determinant of restenosis and subsequent luminal renarrowing. Key pathways that contribute to neointimal formation include thrombosis, inflammation, smooth muscle cell proliferation and migration into the intima, and secretion of the extracellular matrix. These occur with a defined temporal pattern that dictates the optimal dosing and timing of antirestenotic therapies, such as brachytherapy or

drug elution (Figure 2-3). This chapter discusses the basic parameters that describe stent design and performance, the design of drug-eluting stents, in particular polymer technology and the mechanisms of the antiproliferative agents used, and the results of the pivotal trials of the drug-eluting stents that are commonly used in clinical practice.

Scaffold Design Parameters

To achieve acute and long-term success, a coronary stent must be able to do the following:
1. Be successfully delivered to the target lesion, often distally in the coronary tree through tortuous anatomy
2. Provide and maintain adequate scaffolding after balloon expansion and retraction of the stent delivery system to maximize poststent luminal diameter and minimize plaque prolapse
3. Conform to the vessel architecture and thereby prevent hinge points or other anatomic distortion
4. Have adequate fluoroscopic visibility radiopacity so that stent edges can be seen by the operator in cases of post-dilation or stent overlap
5. Minimize vascular trauma, which results in an injury response that stimulates neointimal proliferation and may result in restenosis
6. Minimize mechanical obstruction of side branches, which can compromise flow and result in periprocedural myocardial infarction
7. Not corrode or otherwise lose structural integrity
8. Be at low risk for fracture
9. In the case of drug-eluting stents, deliver the antiproliferative agent at a tissue dose and over a time course that sufficiently prevents neointimal hyperplasia without vascular toxicity (Figure 2-4).

In the case of metallic stents, these goals are achieved through a combination of alloys, structural design (i.e., scaffold architecture), biocompatible polymers, and drugs.

SCAFFOLD CHARACTERISTICS

The performance characteristics of a scaffold can be quantified by flexibility and trackability, conformability, radial strength, longitudinal strength, recoil, and radiopacity.[2]

Flexibility and Trackability

Flexibility is the force required to bend a stent to a specific radius—that is, a stent with low flexibility requires greater force, whereas a stent with high flexibility requires less force.[2] Flexibility contributes to trackability, which describes the ease with which the stent system can be advanced distally through the coronary anatomy to the target lesion. Trackability can be quantified on the bench top by measuring the work required to maneuver a stent through a tortuous artery model. High flexibility enhances trackability, facilitating the delivery of the stent system, particularly through tortuous vessels and/or complex anatomy.

13

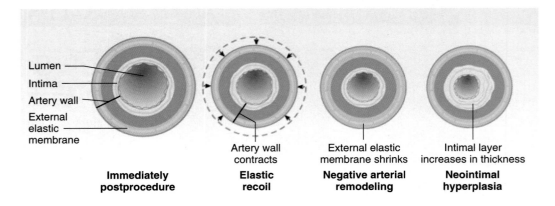

Figure 2-1 Mechanisms of luminal renarrowing after balloon angioplasty. Restenosis occurs through elastic recoil, negative arterial remodeling, and neointimal hyperplasia. Because metal stent implantation eliminates elastic recoil and negative remodeling, for the most part, neointimal hyperplasia is the primary determinant of in-stent restenosis and is therefore the target of antirestenotic therapies, such as brachytherapy and local drug elution.

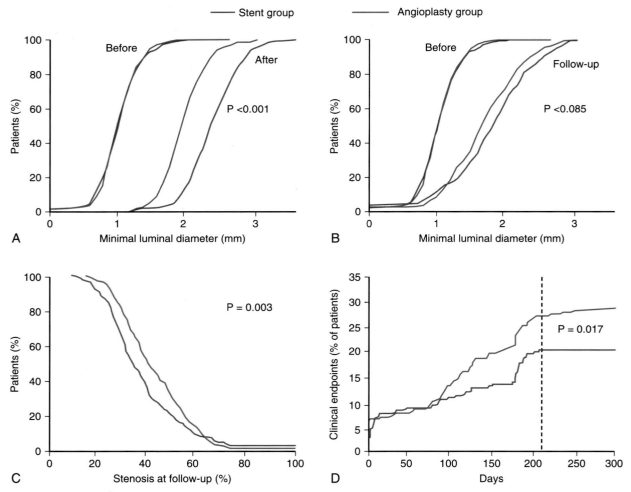

Figure 2-2 Cumulative frequency distribution curves for early and late angiographic outcomes for stand-alone balloon angioplasty compared with stenting in the Benestent trial. Compared with angioplasty, stenting increased the minimal luminal diameter at intervention **(A)** and follow-up **(B)**, decreased the percentage of angiographic stenosis at follow-up **(C)**, and reduced the incidence of major clinical events **(D)**. (Adapted from Serruys PW, de Jaegere P, Kiemeneij F, et al. A comparison of balloon-expandable-stent implantation with balloon angioplasty in patients with coronary artery disease: Benestent Study Group. *N Engl J Med* 1994;331:489-495.)

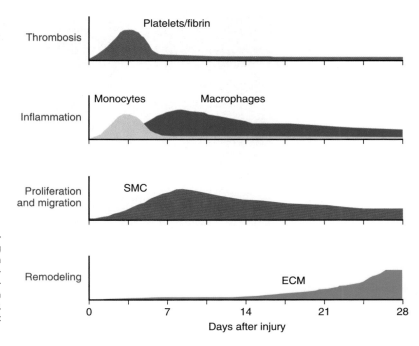

Figure 2-3   Time course of vascular healing after stent-induced injury. Phases of healing include thrombosis, involving platelets and fibrin, inflammation, involving monoctyes and then macrophages, smooth muscle cell *(SMC)* proliferation and migration, and extracellular matrix *(ECM)* production and luminal narrowing. (Adapted from Garasic J, Rogers C, Edelman ER. Stent design and the biologic response. In: Beyar R, Keren G, Leon MB, et al., eds. *Frontiers in Interventional Cardiology.* London: Martin Dunitz; 1997: 95-100.)

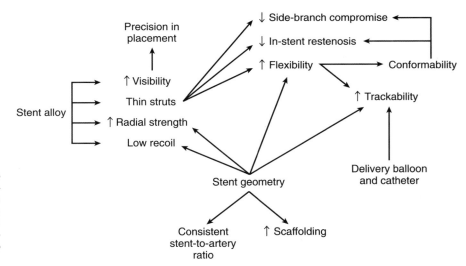

Figure 2-4   Relationship among stent design, acute procedural outcomes, and longer term clinical outcomes. The stent alloy, geometry, and delivery system all influence stent characteristics that can have an impact on early and late outcomes. (Adapted from Menown IB, Noad R, Garcia EJ, et al. The platinum chromium element stent platform: from alloy, to design, to clinical practice. *Adv Ther* 2010;27:129-141.)

Conformability

Conformability describes the ability of the stent to adapt to the natural curvature of the artery in which it is implanted. A very rigid stent will straighten out tortuosity or bends, possibly resulting in hinge points at its edges.

Radial Strength

Radial strength, or compression resistance, is a quantitative measure of stent scaffolding strength and the ability of the stent to maintain the vessel lumen after implantation.[2] Radial strength is critical in the treatment of fibrocalcific and ostial lesions. Design characteristics that influence radial strength include the metallic alloy, strut thickness, and stent geometry. Lack of scaffolding strength can contribute to late luminal loss. For example, in Cohort A of the ABSORB trial of a poly-L-lactic acid bioresorbable vascular scaffold that eluted everolimus, a substantial proportion of late luminal loss was the result of scaffold shrinkage (i.e., reduction in scaffold area) rather than

neointimal hyperplasia. This led to structural redesign to increase radial strength, which in turn improved angiographic outcomes.[3]

Longitudinal Strength

Longitudinal strength describes the resistance of the stent to compression or elongation along its long axis when exposed to pushing or pulling forces, respectively. Stents with weaker longitudinal strength suffer greater longitudinal shortening and/or elongation in response to a standardized amount of force. In vivo, recrossing of an implanted stent with equipment such as post-dilation balloons, another stent delivery system, or intravascular imaging catheters may exert force along the longitudinal axis of the stent, particularly in the setting of ostial lesions and proximal stent underexpansion or malapposition, resulting in longitudinal compression. Longitudinal strength is likely influenced by stent geometry. A bench top model has demonstrated that stent designs with the least longitudinal strength are those with fewer connectors between segments, particularly when the

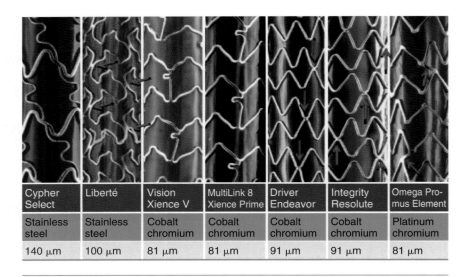

Figure 2-5   Various stent designs. Listed below each stent is the stent name, metal composition, and strut thickness. The Cypher stent is cut from a stainless steel tube, has struts 140 μm thick, and consists of out-of-phase sinusoidal hoops linked by six sinusoidal bridges oriented about 30 degrees from the stent long axis. The Liberté and its repective drug-eluting stent, Taxus Liberté, are cut from a stainless steel tube, have struts 100 μm thick, and consist of out-of-phase hoops joined directly by three links. The Vision, MultiLink 8, and their respective drug-eluting stents, Xience V and Xience Prime, are cut from a CoCr tube, have struts 81 μm thick, and consist of in-phase sinusoidal hoops linked by three connectors aligned with the stent long axis that are U-shaped to improve flexibility. The Driver and Endeavor drug-eluting stent have sinusoidal, largely out-of-phase hoops made of CoCr, linked by two welds. The Integrity and drug-eluting Resolute stents consist of a single sinusoidal CoCr component, 91 μm thick, that winds helically from one end of the stent to the other, with two welds between adjacent arcs. The Omega and drug-eluting Promus Element, Ion, and Synergy stents have sinusoidal hoops made of PtCr, linked by two straight bridges per hoop that are aligned at an angle of about 45 degrees from the stent long axis. *Red arrows,* Links and connectors; *yellow line,* stent "hoop." (Adapted from Ormiston JA, Webber B, Webster MW. Stent longitudinal integrity bench insights into a clinical problem. *JACC Cardiovasc Interv* 2011;4:1310-1317.)

connectors are offset and angled away from the longitudinal axis of the stent (Figure 2-5).[4]

Recoil

Recoil describes the ability of a stent to maintain its initial diameter after expansion. Low recoil is desirable to maximize acute gain, which influences restenosis, and prevent early malapposition, although the clinical sequelae of this phenomenon are unclear beyond potentially insufficient drug delivery to the intima.

Radiopacity

Radiopacity describes the fluoroscopic visibility of the implanted stent. Radiopacity depends on the thickness and density of the metallic alloy. Therefore, although thinner stent struts are advantageous (see later, "Impact of Strut Thickness"), radiopacity is inferior compared with thicker struts of the same alloy. The visibility of 316L stainless steel can be improved by using markers or plating with radiopaque alloys. However, incorporation of stent coatings or markers (e.g., gold) to increase radiopacity resulted in significantly increased rates of neointimal hyperplasia and restenosis and was subsequently abandoned.[5,6] More recently, platinum chromium (PtCr) and cobalt chromium (CoCr) have been used for the metal scaffold because they have greater density but similar strength as 316L stainless steel.

Impact of Strut Thickness

Strut thickness is a critical element of the stent scaffold. Thicker struts enhance radiopacity and radial strength. However, thicker struts reduce the deliverability of the stent and may obstruct side branches after implantation, compromising flow and increasing the risk of periprocedural myocardial infarction. Thinner struts have also been associated with reduced late loss and restenosis, likely resulting from reduced vascular injury. In the Intracoronary Stenting and Angiographic Results: Strut Thickness Effect on Restenosis Outcome (ISAR-STEREO) trial, a thin-strut stent of interconnected ring design (strut thickness of 50 μm) significantly reduced the risk of angiographic restenosis at 1 year compared with a thick-strut stent of

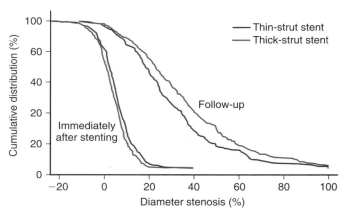

Figure 2-6   Cumulative distribution curves of diameter stenosis immediately after procedure and at 6-month follow-up angiography in the ISAR-STERO trial. Diameter stenosis was significantly reduced at follow-up in the thin-strut versus the thick-strut group (leftward displacement of respective curve, *P* = .002). (Adapted from Kastrati A, Mehilli J, Dirschinger J, et al. Intracoronary stenting and angiographic results: strut thickness effect on restenosis outcome [ISAR-STEREO] trial. *Circulation* 2001;103:2816-2821.)

otherwise comparable design (strut thickness of 140 μm; 15% vs. 25.8%; relative risk [RR], 0.58; 95% confidence interval [CI], 0.39-0.87; *P* = .003; Figure 2-6).[7] Similarly, the thin-strut stent was associated with a lower incidence of target vessel revascularization (8.6% vs. 13.8%; RR, 0.62; 95% CI, 0.39-0.99). A reduction in the risk of angiographic and clinical restenosis was also observed with a thin-strut interconnected ring design stent (strut thickness of 50 μm) compared with a thick-strut, closed cell design stent.[8,9]

Stent Alloys

The struggle to reduce strut thickness while preserving radiopacity and strength has led to the incorporation of newer alloys in place of the traditional 316L stainless steel. These include MP35N CoCr (used in the Driver bare metal and Endeavor and Resolute drug-eluting stents), L605 CoCr (used in the Vision bare metal and Xience drug-eluting stents), and PtCr (used in the Omega bare metal and Promus Element and Ion/Taxus Element drug-eluting stents). The introduction of these alloys has enabled a substantial reduction in strut thickness, from approximately 0.10 to 0.14 mm to 0.081 to 0.090 mm, while maintaining the other performance characteristics of 316L stainless steel. For example, PtCr has a higher density compared with 316L stainless steel or L605 CoCr (9.9 g/cm³, 8.0 g/cm³, and 9.1 g/cm³, respectively), thereby enabling a decrease in strut width and thickness while maintaining radiopacity.[2]

Cellular Architecture: Open and Closed Cell Designs

A closed cell design consists of sequential rings in which all internal inflection points are connected by bridging elements with regular peak-to-peak connections.[10] This provides uniform cell expansion, minimal change in cell size, optimal scaffolding, and, ideally, uniformity in drug elution, regardless of the degree of vessel curvature. The disadvantage of the closed cell design is its rigidity, thereby limiting deliverability through tortuous vessels. Examples of closed cell stents include the Cypher sirolimus-eluting stent and its bare metal stent platform, the Bx Velocity. In an open cell design, a portion of the internal inflection points of the structural members are not connected by bridging elements. This allows for better longitudinal flexibility, conformability, side branch access, and deliverability. Improved conformability may lead to opening of the cells along the arc of vessel curvature, potentially leading to heterogeneous drug distribution within a particular cell. This may result in inadequate dosing at sites at which struts are far apart, although this is less of a concern with the sirolimus analogues, which display a wide toxic to therapeutic window, allowing for higher dosing adequate for sufficient distribution across the cell.[11] Modern stents have different numbers of connectors or bridging elements, varying along the continuum between open and closed cell designs (see Figure 2-5).

🔲 Antiproliferative Agents

In-stent restenosis results primarily from neointimal hyperplasia that occurs in response to local arterial injury from percutaneous coronary intervention (PCI). Neointimal formation involves the activation, proliferation, and migration of vascular smooth muscle cells, as well as increased production of extracellular matrix components. Therefore, antiproliferative agents that safely inhibit vascular smooth muscle cell proliferation form the basis of drug-eluting stents currently used in clinical practice. Two classes of antiproliferative agents have proven successful in preventing neointimal hyperplasia and, in turn, in-stent restenosis—paclitaxel and the rapamycin analogues (including sirolimus, everolimus, zotarolimus, and biolimus). In addition to their antiproliferative properties, these agents have different characteristics (e.g., hydrophilicity) that may have an impact on their clinical efficacy.

PACLITAXEL

Paclitaxel is a diterpenoid compound isolated from the Pacific Yew tree (*Taxus brevifolia*; Figure 2-7). It is a widely used chemotherapeutic agent.[12] It is highly lipophilic, which promotes rapid cellular uptake when delivered locally via a drug-eluting stent. Paclitaxel interferes with microtubule dynamics, stabilizing the microtubules and preventing depolymerization.[13,14] Microtubules are important parts of the cytoskeleton, in particular the mitotic spindle. Therefore paclitaxel inhibits mitotic progression and cell proliferation, primarily in the G0-G1 and G2-M phases of the cell cycle (Figure 2-8). Paclitaxel inhibits human arterial smooth muscle cell proliferation and migration in a dose-dependent manner (Figure 2-9).[15] Paclitaxel is also capable of inhibiting cellular division, motility, activation, secretory processes, and signal transduction.[12] Although it is cytostatic at low

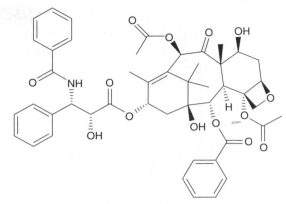

Figure 2-7 Chemical structure of paclitaxel. Paclitaxel, isolated from the Pacific Yew tree, interferes with microtubule dynamics and inhibits human arterial smooth muscle cell proliferation and migration in a dose-dependent manner.

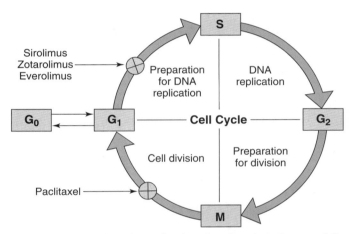

Figure 2-8 Cell cycle and site of action of paclitaxel, sirolimus, and the sirolimus analogues everolimus and zotarolimus. (Adapted from Martin DM, Boyle FJ. Drug-eluting stents for coronary artery disease: a review. *Med Eng Phys* 2011;33:148-163.)

doses, paclitaxel has a relatively narrow therapeutic window and can cause local vascular toxicity in the form of focal medial necrosis at higher levels of exposure.[16] Stent-based elution of paclitaxel significantly reduces neointimal hyperplasia, angiographic restenosis, and the need for repeat revascularization in patients undergoing PCI.[17,18]

RAPAMYCIN AND ITS ANALOGUES

Rapamycin (also known as sirolimus) and its analogues, including everolimus, zotarolimus, and biolimus, share a similar mechanism of action that interferes with the cell cycle.

Sirolimus

Sirolimus is a macrolide antibiotic produced by *Streptomyces hygroscopicus*, an actinomycete isolated in 1975 from a soil sample collected from Rapa Nui, commonly known as Easter Island (Figure 2-10, A).[19] It was first noted to have antifungal properties, but subsequent studies have demonstrated significant immunosuppressive and antitumor activities. Sirolimus forms a complex with the cytosolic immunophilin, FK506 binding protein-12 (FKB12), which in turn blocks the activation of the cell cycle–specific kinase, mammalian target of rapamycin (mTOR).[19-21] mTOR has different functions, depending on whether it binds to the regulatory-associated protein of mTOR

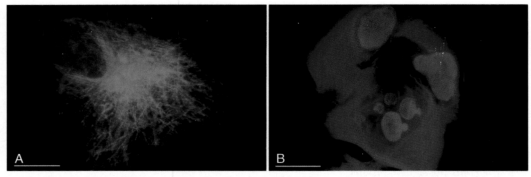

Figure 2-9   Immunofluorescence micrographs showing the effect of paclitaxel on cytoplasmic microtubule distribution within human arterial smooth muscle cells. Suppression of microtubule dynamics is responsible for the ability of paclitaxel to inhibit mitotic progression and cell proliferation. **A,** Nontreated human arterial smooth muscle cells stained with a monoclonal anti–β-tubulin antibody (nuclear counterstaining with DAPI). Microtubules are densely packed in a microtubule organizing center near the nucleus and form a network through the entire cytoplasm that reaches to the cell periphery. **B,** Paclitaxel-treated human arterial smooth muscle cells (haSMCs) are smaller and ellipsoid and show an unorganized, decentralized tubulin distribution, with densely packed tubulin rings in the cell periphery. Scale bars represent 5 μm. (Adapted from Axel DI, Kunert W, Goggelmann C, et al. Paclitaxel inhibits arterial smooth muscle cell proliferation and migration in vitro and in vivo using local drug delivery. *Circulation* 1997;96:636-645.)

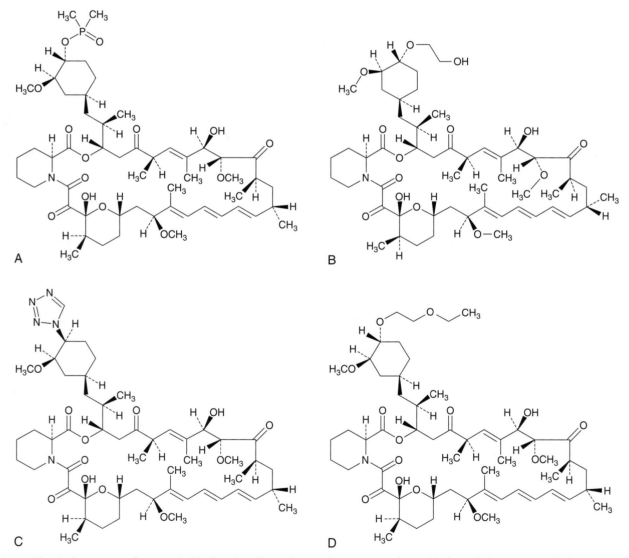

Figure 2-10   Chemical structures of rapamycin (sirolimus) and its analogues that are currently used in drug-eluting stents. A, Sirolimus (rapamycin) is a macrolide antibiotic produced by *Streptomyces hygroscopicus,* an actinomycete isolated from a soil sample collected from Rapa Nui (Easter Island). The rapamycin analogues differ from the parent molecule in substitutions at position 40 of the rapamycin ring. **B,** Everolimus is a hydroxyethyl ether derivative of sirolimus. **C,** Zotarolimus contains a tetrazole ring substituted for the hydroxyl group, resulting in substantially greater lipophilicity. **D,** Umirolimus, or Biolimus A9, has an ethoxyl ethyl modification, which also results in roughly 10-fold greater lipophilicity compared with sirolimus.

(RAPTOR, mTOR complex 1 [mTORC1]) or rapamycin-insensitive companion of mTOR (RICTOR, mTOR complex 2 [mTORC2]). mTORC1 regulates translation, transcription, cell cycle progression, and survival through the phosphorylation of downstream substrates, most importantly p70 S6 kinase and 4E-BP1(Figure 2-11).[22] Inhibition of mTORc1 by sirolimus and its analogues results in the blockage of cell cycle progression at the juncture of the G1 and S phases (see Figure 2-8). This effect is cytostatic. Sirolimus is the antiproliferative agent incorporated into the Cypher drug-eluting stent, which has been shown to reduce restenosis and the need for repeat revascularization significantly compared with bare metal stents.[23]

Everolimus

Everolimus is a hydroxyethyl ether derivative of sirolimus, with a 2-hydroxyethyl group in position 40 of sirolimus (see Figure 2-10, B). Like sirolimus, everolimus binds the cytosolic immunophilin FKBP-12, and this complex binds mTOR when it associated with RAPTOR, thereby inhibiting downstream signaling.[20,24] It has also been used extensively in organ transplantation. It is the antiproliferative agent used in the Xience V, Xience Prime, and Promus Element drug-eluting stents.

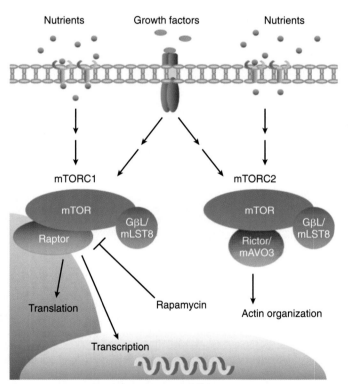

Figure 2-11 Mechanism of action of rapamycin (sirolimus) and its analogues. Sirolimus forms a complex with the cytosolic immunophilin FKBP-12, which in turn binds and inhibits the mammalian target of rapamycin (mTOR). There are two mTOR complexes. TORC1 regulates a variety of functions, including transcription, messenger ribonucleic acid turnover, protein turnover, and translation. All these TORC1 functions are rapamycin-sensitive. Through its interaction with mTORC1, sirolimus and its analogues inhibit the following: (1) the phosphorylation of 4E-BP1, preventing release of eIF-4E and initiation of translation; (2) P27-mediated activation of cdk2-cyclin E and synthesis of proteins important for cell cycle progression; and (3) p70S6 kinase activation, limiting ribosomal protein S6 phosphorylation and reducing synthesis of ribosomal-translational proteins. (Adapted from Saunders RN Metcalfe MS, Nicolson ML. Rapamycin in transplantation: a review of the evidence. *Kidney International* 2001;59:3-16; and Inoki K, Ouyang H, Li Y, et al. Signaling by target of rapamycin proteins in cell growth control. *Microbiol Mol Biol Rev* 2005;69:79-100.)

Zotarolimus

Zotarolimus was originally developed in 1997 as an immunosuppressant for the treatment of rheumatoid arthritis. It is a semisynthetic analogue of sirolimus in which a hydrophilic hydroxyl group has been replaced with a lipophilic tetrazole group (see Figure 2-10, C). As a result, zotarolimus is substantially more lipophilic than sirolimus, increasing its tissue retention time and potentially enhancing absorption of drug across the cellular membranes of target cells.[25] Zotarolimus is the antiproliferative agent used in the Endeavor and Resolute drug-eluting stents.

Biolimus A9

Biolimus A9, also known as umirolimus, is a semisynthetic derivative of sirolimus, with an ethoxyl ethyl modification at position 40 of the sirolimus ring (see Figure 2-10, D). It is roughly 10 times more lipophilic than sirolimus or everolimus. It is the active agent of the Biomatrix/Nobori drug-eluting stent.

Polymers

Drug delivery in drug-eluting stents can be achieved by three primary mechanisms: (1) a nonerodible polymer coating that can be loaded with drug and provide controlled elution of an antiproliferative agent; (2) a bioabsorbable, erodible, or degradable polymer coating or stent that is loaded with drug and liberates drug over time through degradation; and (3) apolymeric stents with drug bound to their surface or embedded in macroscopic fenestrations or nanopores (Figure 2-12).[10,26]

Polymers enable the delivery of antiproliferative agents at a sufficient dose and temporal pattern to achieve a therapeutic antirestenotic effect. They consist of long-chain molecules made up of small repeating units.[27] They differ in regard to porosity, texture, and surface charge and in the ability of drugs to diffuse in and out of the matrix.[26] Ideally, a polymer should be noninflammatory, should be nontoxic, should not elicit a thrombotic response, and should be able to deliver a drug at a sustained and controlled rate. Nonbiodegradable polymers remain with the implanted stent indefinitely after drug elution is complete. Nonbiodegradable, inert synthetic polymers are the predominant mode of drug delivery in currently used drug-eluting stents, particularly in the United States. Some nonbioerodible polymers have been associated with delayed vascular healing, incomplete endothelialization, and hypersensitivity reactions that may contribute to an increased risk of late and very late stent thrombosis compared with bare metal stents.[28-30]

Biodegradable carriers undergo hydrolytic or enzymatic degradation into molecules that are eventually eliminated through metabolic pathways. For example, the biodegradable polymer poly-L-lactic acid (PLLA) undergoes hydrolysis into lactic acid, which is in turn converted by the Krebs cycle into water and carbon dioxide. PLLA has been incorporated into several drug-eluting metallic stents and bioresorbable vascular scaffolds.[31,32] Other biodegradable or bioabsorbable polymers being evaluated for drug delivery via coronary stents include polylactic-co-glycolic acid (PGLA), D-lactic polylactic acid (DLPA), and polyhydroxybutyrate.[33] Drug release from biodegradable polymers can be achieved through degradation of the polymer chains, dissolution of drug, or diffusion of drug from the polymeric matrix.[26]

Appropriate drug release kinetics is critical to achieve antirestenotic efficacy without vascular injury. The carrier matrix forms interconnecting pores through which drug is eluted through diffusion (random molecular agitation) and/or solvent-driven flow (convection; Figure 2-13).[26] Factors affecting drug release include the polymer properties, coating design, and drug characteristics. Drug binding with the carrier matrix, drug-to-polymer ratio, dosing density, coating thickness, and partition coefficient of the drug all influence elution kinetics. A barrier top coat of polymer without drug can also prolong the duration of elution. Other factors beyond release kinetics can influence the safety and efficacy of the drug-polymer matrix. The

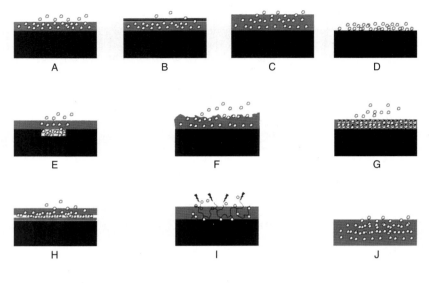

Figure 2-12   Schematic representation of different modalities of drug-eluting stent platforms. A, Drug-polymer blend, release by diffusion. **B,** Drug diffusion through additional polymer coating. **C,** Drug release by swelling of coating. **D,** Non–polymer-based drug release. **E,** Drug loaded in stent reservoir. **F,** Drug release by coating erosion. **G,** Drug loaded in nanoporous coating reservoirs. **H,** Drug loaded between coatings (coating sandwich). **I,** Polymer-drug conjugate cleaved by hydrolysis or enzymatic action. **J,** Bioerodible polymeric stent. *Black* represents the stent strut; *gray* represents the coating.

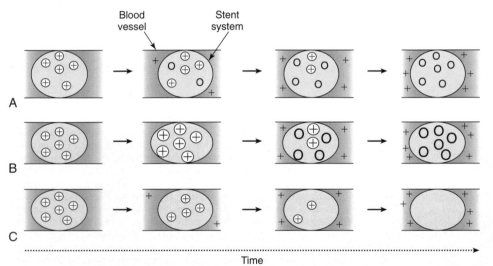

Figure 2-13   Mechanisms of drug release from a carrier vehicle matrix. A, Diffusion from a homogeneously mixed drug with a nonbiodegradable polymer. **B,** Diffusion from an absorbent hydrogel polymer matrix that increases the mesh size on hydration, enabling the drug to diffuse through the swollen matrix. **C,** Biodegradable polymer releases drug in proportion to the rate of polymer degradation. The rate of release generally declines with time because the drug has to travel a longer distance from the innermost layers. *Circle,* Polymer; *+,* released drug. (Adapted from Tesfamariam B. Drug release kinetics from stent device-based delivery systems. *J Cardiovasc Pharmacol* 2008;51:118-125.)

physical integrity of the polymer must be maintained during the rapid expansion and implantation of the balloon-expandable stent under high atmospheric pressure. Hydrophobic characteristics allow a polymer to adhere to the stent surface and assist drug distribution and controlled elution, whereas hydrophilic characteristics promote biocompatibility.[34] Release and retention of absorbed drug from the stent depends in part on solubility, because hydrophilic drugs are distributed across the blood vessel wall and remain within local arterial tissue for a shorter period of time than hydrophobic drugs, which have a longer elution time and are cleared more slowly from the local arterial tissue. In the case of sirolimus and its analogues, the persistence time of receptor saturation and therapeutic effect may be more sensitive to duration of elution than to the eluted amount. Dose escalation is inefficient at compensating for suboptimal elution duration, which may explain the inferior clinical outcomes with sirolimus-eluting polymer-free stents.[35]

NONERODABLE POLYMERS IN CLINICAL USE

Poly(styrene-b-isobutylene-b-styrene)

Poly(styrene-b-isobutylene-b-styrene), or SIBS, commercially known as Translute, is a hydrophobic triblock copolymer composed of styrene

and isobutylene units built on 1,3-di(2-methoxy-2-propyl)-5-tert-butylbenzene (Figure 2-14). It is a biostable elastomer with physical properties that overlap those of silicone rubber and polyurethane.[36] SIBS stent grafts and coatings on metallic stents demonstrate hemocompatability and biocompatibility.[37] The Taxus and Ion (also known as Taxus Element) drug-eluting stents use SIBS to deliver paclitaxel to reduce neointimal proliferation after implantation. Most loaded paclitaxel exists as discrete particles in the SIBS matrix. The Higuchi model for a drug dispersed in a solid matrix describes the paclitaxel-SIBS elution kinetics[38]—that is, the drug dissolves first from the surface layer of the device and when this layer is exhausted of drug, dissolution of drug from the next layer occurs via diffusion to the external surroundings through nanometer-sized pores of the inert SIBS carrier matrix (Figure 2-15).[37] Two formulations of the Translute polymer-paclitaxel blend, slow-release and moderate-release versions, were initially developed and clinically tested. With the slow-release version (8.8% formulation; i.e., percentage weight of paclitaxel in the polymer coating), approximately 10% of the loaded paclitaxel is eluted over the initial 10 days after implantation, but there is no detectable release of paclitaxel thereafter. That is, 90% of the loaded drug remains indefinitely within the polymer. The moderate-release formulation results in approximately threefold higher drug release

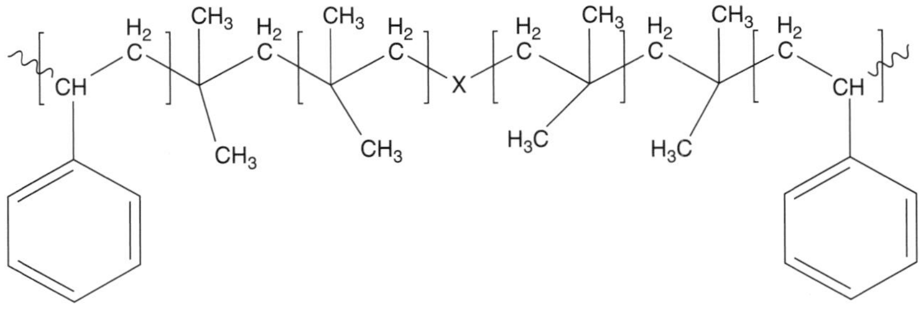

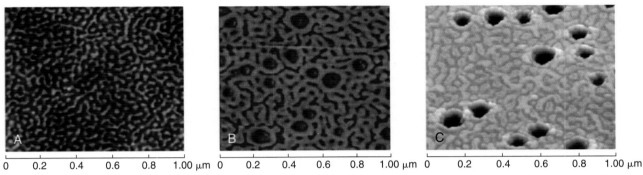

Figure 2-14 Chemical structure of poly(styrene-isobutylene-styrene) copolymer (SIBS). This copolymer is used to elute paclitaxel in the Taxus and Taxus Element/Ion stents.

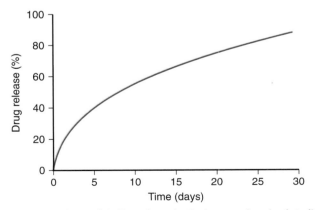

Figure 2-15 Topographic images of the subsurface morphology of styrene-isobutylene-styrene (SIBS) and paclitaxel-SIBS matrix using atomic force microscopy. **A,** SIBS-only matrix without paclitaxel. **B,** Paclitaxel-SIBS matrix. **C,** Paclitaxel-SIBS matrix after exposure to PBS-Tween solvent, demonstrating voids in the matrix previously occupied by paclitaxel. (Adapted from Kamath KR, Barry JJ, Miller KM. The taxus drug-eluting stent: a new paradigm in controlled drug delivery. *Adv Drug Deliv Rev* 2006;58:412-436.)

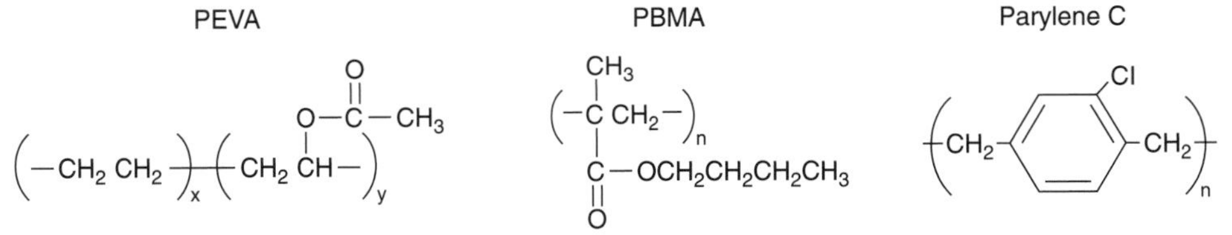

Figure 2-16   Chemical structures of poly(ethylene-co-vinyl acetate) (PEVA), poly(n-butyl methacrylate) (PBMA), and parylene C. A blend of PEVA and PBMA mixed with sirolimus make up the base coat formulation of the Cypher stent, which is applied to a parylene C–treated stent. A drug-free top coat of PBMA provides further control of the release kinetics of sirolimus.

than the slow-release version.[39] The slow-release formulation is the commercially available version.

Poly(ethylene-co-vinyl acetate) and Poly(n-butyl methacrylate) Blend

A 67% to 33% blend of poly(ethylene-co-vinyl acetate) and poly(n-butyl methacrylate) (PEVA-PBMA) is used to deliver the antiproliferative agent sirolimus as part of the Cypher drug-eluting stent (Figure 2-16). A drug-free top layer (top coat) of PBMA functions as a barrier through which drug elutes out under diffusion, thereby controlling the rate of release. A layer of parylene C is applied to the bare metal scaffold under the base coat. A total of 50% of the drug is eluted by 10 days and 90% by 60 days, and complete elution is achieved by 90 days (Figure 2-17).

Vinylidene Fluoride and Hexafluoropropylene Copolymer

Vinylidene fluoride and hexafluoropropylene (PVDF-HFP) copolymer is an acrylic and fluoro copolymer made from vinylidene fluoride (VF) and hexafluoropropylene (HFP) monomers; the HFP unit is perfluorinated (Figure 2-18). The copolymer contains no reactive functional groups. Solid drug is dispersed in a matrix of polymer saturated with

Figure 2-17   Release of sirolimus from the Cypher stent in animal studies. The Cypher stent elutes sirolimus from a 67% to 33% blend of PEVA and PBMA. A total of 50% of the drug is eluted by 10 days and 90% by 60 days, and complete elution is achieved by 90 days. (Adapted from Acharya G, Park K. Mechanisms of controlled drug release from drug-eluting stents. *Adv Drug Deliv Rev* 2006;58:387-401.)

drug, and the profile of drug elution is linear with the square root of time for a significant fraction of its release. A wide range of release rates can be achieved by varying the drug-to-polymer ratio and thickness of the coating.[25] VDF-HFP is the drug matrix polymer of the Xience series of everolimus-eluting stents (Xience V, Xience Prime, and Xience Expedition), as well as the Promus Element everolimus-eluting stents. The release kinetics of everolimus from the Xience V stent is displayed in Figure 2-19.

Phosphorylcholine Polymer

Phosphorylcholine (PC) is the major lipid head group component found in the outer surface of biologic cell membranes. The PC polymer consists of 2-methacryloyloxyethyl phosphorylcholine cross-linked with several different methacrylate comonomers (Figure 2-20).[34] The goal of this absorbent hydrogel polymer matrix is to increase the biocompatibility and hemocompatibility of implanted materials through biomembrane mimicry.[41] PC polymer has been used in the BiodivYsioTM PC-coated stent (which did not elute drug) and the Endeavor zotarolimus-eluting stent. Zotarolimus elutes from PC polymer through dissolution into the surrounding environment. To control the release kinetics, the Endeavor stent has a 1-μm-thick PC base coat, a 3-μm-thick coating loaded with drug (90% zotarolimus and 10% PC polymer), and a thin, less than 0.1-μm-thick drug-free PC overcoat. The Endeavor stent has rapid release kinetics, with substantial release of zotarolimus over the first few days after implantation and almost complete elution by 14 days (Figure 2-21).

BioLinx

The BioLinx polymer system is a blend of three polymers—water-soluble polyvinyl pyrrolidinone (PVP, 10%), hydrophobic C10 polymer (27%), and hydrophilic C19 polymer (63%; Figure 2-22). This system is used by the Resolute zotarolimus-eluting stent. Together, the unique characteristics of the individual components of the system

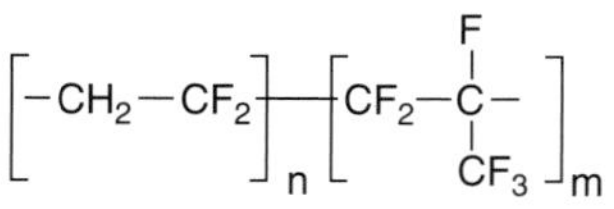

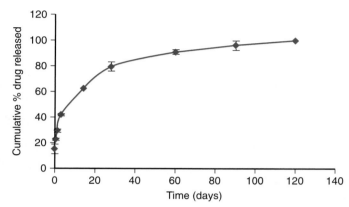

Figure 2-18 Chemical structure of vinylidene fluoride and hexafluoropropylene (PVF-HFP) copolymer. The PVF-HFP copolymer is loaded with everolimus in the Xience V, Xience Prime, and Promus Element everolimus-eluting stents.

Figure 2-19 Release of everolimus from the Xience V stent in animal pharmacokinetic studies. The Xience V stent uses vinylidene fluoride and hexafluoropropylene (PVF-HFP) copolymer loaded with everolimus at a concentration of 100 μg/cm². After an initial burst over the first 2 to 4 weeks after implantation, almost all the drug has been eluted after 120 days. (Adapted from Johnson GC. XIENCE Everolimus eluting coronary stent system (EECSS], 2007 (http://www.fda.gov/ohrms/dockets/ac/07/slides/2007-4333s1-03%20-%20XIENCE%20V%20Panel_Abbott%20Vascular%20Presentation.pdf.)

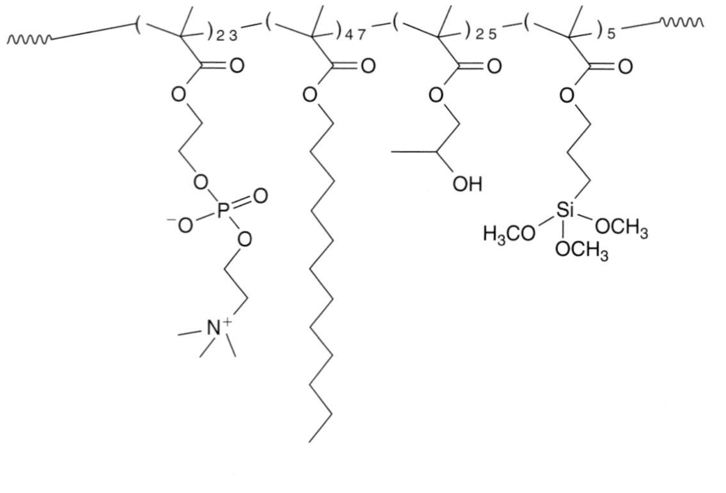

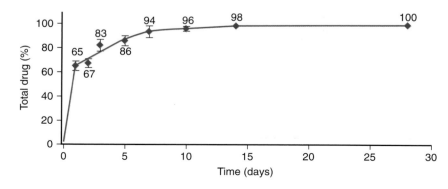

Figure 2-20 Chemical structure of phosphorylcholine (PC) polymer. The PC polymer is the delivery vehicle for zotarolimus in the Endeavor stent. Zotarolimus is released into the surrounding environment by dissolution.

Figure 2-21 Elution of zotarolimus from the Endeavor stent in animal studies. The Endeavor stent elutes zotarolimus from phosphorylcholine polymer. Elution is rapid, with most of the drug released within the first few days, and all drug released by approximately 2 weeks.

provide biocompatibility as well as specific elution characteristics. The vinyl pyrrolidinone units provide hydrophilicity analogous to the zwitterionic phosphoryl choline group found in the PC polymer. The hydrophobic C10 polymer holds and locks in zotarolimus, providing extended elution by diffusion; the C19 polymer elutes zotarolimus rapidly; and the PVP is responsible for the initial drug burst.[41] Approximately 50% of drug elution occurs within the first week after Resolute stent implantation; 85% of the zotarolimus content is eluted by 60 days, and the drug is eluted completely by 180 days (Figure 2-23). Compared with the Endeavor stent with PC coating, the Resolute

stent elutes zotarolimus more gradually, providing lower drug levels in the arterial tissue sustained over a longer duration, despite similar drug loads (1.6 µg/mm² of stent surface).

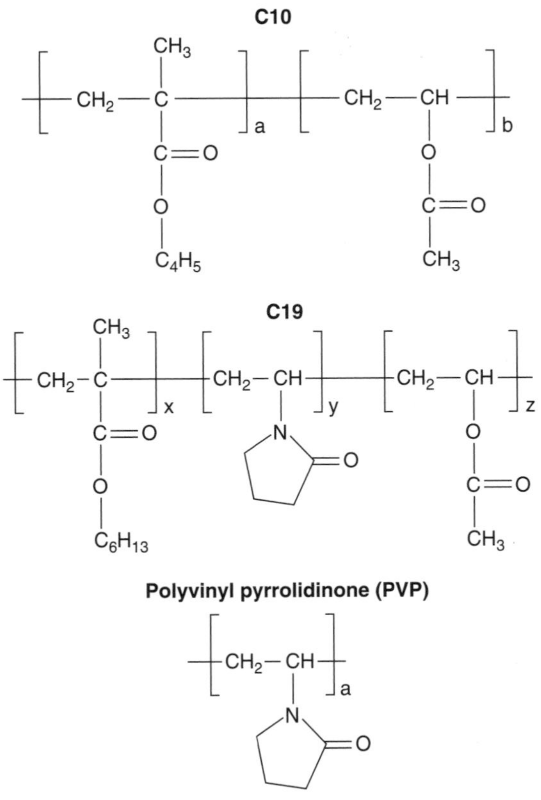

Drug-Eluting Stents

In general, drug-eluting stents consist of three components—a bare metal platform, polymer, and antiproliferative drug to inhibit the restenotic process. Although these types of stents are simply bare metal stents adapted for drug elution, newer drug-eluting stents have been developed or are being studied that are made completely of polymer (i.e., bioresorbable) or are polymer free, with the metal stent surface being specifically designed to bind and elute drug. The following section describes the components of the initial and newer drug-eluting stents with nonerodible polymers approved for use by the U.S. Food and Drug Administration (FDA; Table 2-1). Bioresorbable polymers and stents are discussed elsewhere in the text.

CYPHER

The Cypher stent was the first drug-eluting stent approved by the FDA. It consists of the closed cell, Bx Velocity 316L stainless steel bare metal stent (140 µm strut thickness) coated with a combination of PEVA and PBMA polymers (67% to 33%) mixed with the antiproliferative agent sirolimus, which inhibits mTOR and thereby prevents cell cycle progression from the G1 to the S phase.[19] A drug-free layer or top coat of PBMA is used to control sirolimus release kinetics (Figure 2-24). The drug dose is 1.0 µg/mm²; half of the sirolimus is eluted over the first 10 days and 90% by 60 days, and all drug is

C10

C19

Polyvinyl pyrrolidinone (PVP)

Figure 2-22   Chemical structure of the BioLinx polymer system. The BioLinx polymer system is a blend of three polymers with unique characteristics—polyvinyl pyrrolidinone (PVP), C10 polymer, and C19 polymer. It is used by the Resolute Integrity stent to elute zotarolimus. Each component of the polymer system has different characteristics. Compared with the PC polymer used in the Endeavor stent, the BioLinx polymer system provides more gradual elution of zotarolimus, resulting in lower drug levels in arterial tissue sustained over a longer duration of time.

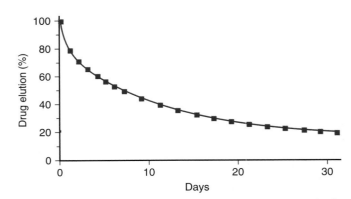

Figure 2-23   Elution of zotarolimus from the Resolute stent over the first 30 days after implantation. Approximately 50% of drug elution occurs within the first week after stent implantation; 85% of the content is eluted by 60 days, and the drug is eluted completely by 180 days. (Adapted from Udipi K, Melder RJ, Chen M, et al. The next generation Endeavor Resolute Stent: role of the Biolinx Polymer System. *EuroIntervention* 2007;3:137-139.)

TABLE 2-1	Drug-Eluting Stent Platforms: Scaffold Design, Polymer, and Eluted Drug					
Stent	*Bare Metal Platform*	*Material*	*Strut Thickness (µm)*	*Polymer*	*Drug*	*Pivotal Clinical Trial*
Cypher	Bx Velocity	316L stainless steel	140	PEVA-PBMA	Sirolimus	SIRIUS
Taxus	Liberté	316L stainless steel	100	SIBS	Paclitaxel	TAXUS IV
Xience V	MultiLink Vision	L605 cobalt chromium	81	PVDF-HFP fluoropolymer	Everolimus	SPIRIT IV
Endeavor	Driver	MP35N cobalt chromium	91	Phosphorylcholine polymer	Zotarolimus	ENDEAVOR IV
Resolute	Integrity	MP35N cobalt chromium	91	BioLinx (PVP/C10/C19)	Zotarolimus	RESOLUTE AC
Promus Element	Omega	Platinum chromium	81	PVDF-HFP fluoropolymer	Everolimus	PLATINUM
ION/Taxus Element	Omega	Platinum chromium	81	SIBS	Paclitaxel	PERSEUS

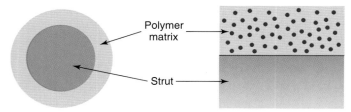

Figure 2-24 The Cypher stent. Shown are the cross-sectional view *(left)* and side view *(right)* of a strut. (Adapted from Acharya G, Park K. Mechanisms of controlled drug release from drug-eluting stents. *Adv Drug Deliv Rev* 2006;58:387-401.)

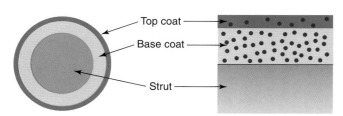

Figure 2-26 Taxus Express² and Taxus Liberté stents. Shown are the cross-sectional view *(left)* and side view *(right)* of a strut. (Adapted from Acharya G, Park K. Mechanisms of controlled drug release from drug-eluting stents. *Adv Drug Deliv Rev* 2006;58:387-401.)

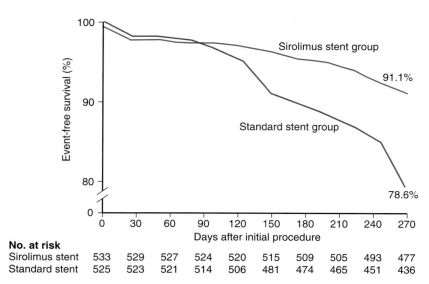

No. at risk									
Sirolimus stent	533	529	527	524	520	515	509	505	493	477
Standard stent	525	523	521	514	506	481	474	465	451	436

Figure 2-25 Survival free from target vessel failure in patients who received a sirolimus-eluting stent or bare metal stent in the SIRIUS randomized clinical trial. Target lesion failure was defined as the occurrence of any of the following within 270 days after the index procedure: death from cardiac causes, Q-wave or non–Q-wave myocardial infarction, or revascularization of the target vessel. The sirolimus-eluting stent also significantly reduced the rates of target vessel revascularization and major adverse events. (Adapted from Moses JW, Leon MB, Popma JJ, et al. Sirolimus-eluting stents vs. standard stents in patients with stenosis in a native coronary artery. *N Engl J Med* 2003;349:1315-1323.)

released by 90 days after implantation. The efficacy of the Cypher stent in reducing angiographic restenosis was first demonstrated in the RAVEL (Randomized Study with the Sirolimus-Coated Bx Velocity Balloon-Expandable Stent in the Treatment of Patients with de Novo Native Coronary Artery Lesions) study.[42] The safety and clinical efficacy of this sirolimus-eluting stent in reducing target vessel failure and target vessel revascularization compared with the Bx Velocity bare metal stent were demonstrated in the pivotal SIRIUS randomized clinical trial (Figure 2-25).[23] A pooled analysis of randomized trials has shown that the Cypher stent is associated with a small but significantly higher risk of late stent thrombosis compared with bare metal stents, potentially because of an inflammatory response to the durable polymer that delays the healing process.[29,43,44]

TAXUS EXPRESS AND TAXUS LIBERTÉ

The Taxus Express² and Taxus Liberté stents elute paclitaxel from SIBS triblock (Translute) copolymer from a 316L stainless steel stent.[37] There are no primer or top coat layers (Figure 2-26). The total drug dose is 1.0 μg/mm². The stents differ in the bare metal stent platform and in the thickness of the polymer coating. The Taxus Express² uses the Express² bare metal stent (strut thickness, 132 μm) with a 22-μm-thick polymer coat, whereas the Taxus Liberté uses the Liberté (Veriflex) bare metal stent design (strut thickness, 97 μm) with a 20-μm-thick polymer coat. The commercially available Taxus system uses a polymer-drug blend referred to as slow release. A total of 10% of the loaded paclitaxel is eluted over the initial 10 days after implantation, with the rest of the drug remaining in the polymer indefinitely. The efficacy of the Taxus slow-release stent in reducing

in-stent neointimal proliferation was first demonstrated in the Taxus II trial[45]; the Taxus IV[17] and Taxus V[46] trials demonstrated that the Taxus stent provided superior angiographic and clinical outcomes in simple and complex anatomies compared with its bare metal stent counterpart (Figure 2-27).

PROMUS ELEMENT

The Promus Element stent elutes everolimus from the PtCr Omega platform. This platform was designed to provide improved deliverability, vessel conformability, side branch access, radiopacity, radial strength, and fracture resistance.[47] As noted, PtCr has a higher density compared with 316L stainless steel or L605 CoCr, thereby enabling a decrease in strut width and thickness while maintaining radiopacity.[2] PtCr has similar low recoil and radial strength as 316L stainless steel and a lower nickel content. In terms of design, the Omega platform consists of a series of serpentine segments joined by two connectors, making a double helix configuration. There are eight crests per ring in diameter sizes 2.25 through 3.5 mm, and 10 crests per ring in the diameter size 4.0 mm. The segment peaks are offset to minimize strut-to-strut contact, thereby enhancing flexibility, and the peak to valley segment has been shortened for improved conformability (see Fig. 2-5).[2] In addition, the peaks have been widened to redirect expansion strain and improve radial strength. The radial strength of the Omega platform is similar to that of the thicker Liberté stent (0.26 N/mm vs. 0.24 N/mm) and greater than that of the MultiLink stent, the L605 CoCr platform of the Xience drug-eluting stent (0.11 N/mm).[2]

The Promus Element stent uses an identical polymer, antiproliferative agent, drug formulation, and dose density as the Promus/Xience

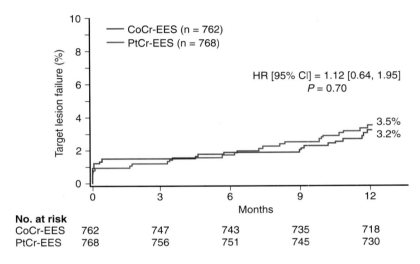

Figure 2-27 Cumulative distribution curves for percentage stenosis of the luminal diameter with the Taxus paclitaxel-eluting stent versus a bare metal stent in the pivotal Taxus IV trial. At 9 months, the mean degree of stenosis in the group that received a paclitaxel-eluting stent was 13.5 percentage points less than the value in the group that received a bare metal stent (95% CI, −16.3 to −10.7; P < .001). (Adapted from Stone GW, Ellis SG, Cox DA, et al. The TAXUS-IV Investigators: a polymer-based, paclitaxel-eluting stent in patients with coronary artery disease. *N Engl J Med* 2004;350:221-231.)

Figure 2-28   Primary results of the PLATINUM trial according to intention-to-treat analysis. The platinum chromium *(PtCr)* everolimus-eluting stent (EES; Promus Element) was noninferior to the cobalt chromium *(CoCr)* everolimus-eluting stent (Promus/Xience V) for the primary endpoint of target lesion failure at 1 year in patients undergoing percutaneous coronary intervention of one or two de novo lesions.

V cobalt-chromium everolimus-eluting stent and therefore has the same release kinetics.[47] Everolimus is blended in a 7-μm-thick layer of PVDF-HFP copolymer that adheres to the metal stent via a primer layer of drug-free PBMA. The drug-loading density is 10 μg/mm². Approximately 80% of the drug is released at 30 days after implantation, and no remaining drug is detectable at 120 days.

The Promus Element stent was first evaluated in the PLATINUM QCA trial, which assessed 9-month angiographic outcomes. In-stent late loss was 0.17 ± 0.25 mm, and the percentage volume obstruction with intravascular ultrasound was 7.2 ± 6.2%,[48] similar to that observed with the everolimus-eluting stent in the SPIRIT (A Clinical Evaluation of the Xience V Everolimus Eluting Coronary Stent System) trials. The clinical safety and efficacy of the Promus Element stent were assessed in the noninferiority PLATINUM (Prospective Randomized Multicenter Trial to Assess an Everolimus-Eluting Coronary Stent System [PROMUS Element] for the Treatment of up to Two De Novo Coronary Artery Lesions) trial.[47] In this study, the per-protocol rate of target lesion failure was 3.4% in patients randomly assigned to the Promus Element, compared with 2.9% in the patients randomly assigned to the CoCr everolimus-eluting stent, thereby satisfying the criteria for noninferiority (P = .001). There was no difference in the 1-year target lesion failure between groups, according to the intent to treat analysis (3.5% vs. 3.2%; noninferiority P = 0.0009; Figure 2-28).

In a bench top model, greater longitudinal compression compared with other stent platforms occurs with the Promus and Taxus Element

Omega–based stents at similar levels of force, likely because of offset connectors between hoops angled at 30 to 45 degrees off the long axis of the stent (see Figure 2-5).[4] These angled and offset connectors increase flexibility, thereby improving deliverability and conformability, but likely decrease longitudinal strength. In a quantitative coronary analysis of pooled data from the PERSEUS[49] and PLATINUM[47] trials, which evaluated the Taxus Element/Ion and Promus Element stents, respectively, there was no objective evidence of stent deformation between Taxus Element/Ion and Taxus Express or between Promus Element and Promus/Xience V CoCr stents.[50]

TAXUS ELEMENT (ION)

The Taxus Element (also known as Ion) stent elutes paclitaxel from the PtCr Omega bare metal stent platform. The Taxus Element/Ion uses the identical polymer, drug, and drug density as the 316L stainless steel–based Taxus Express and Taxus Liberté stents.[49] The antiproliferative agent paclitaxel is loaded onto SIBS polymer at a dose density of 1.0 μg of paclitaxel/mm² of stent surface area in an 8.8% formulation (percentage weight of paclitaxel in the polymer coating), providing similar release kinetics as the other Taxus stents. A total of 10% of the loaded paclitaxel is eluted over the first 10 days, and approximately 90% remains in the polymer indefinitely. As noted, the PtCr alloy used in the Taxus Element/Ion stent has increased bend fatigue resistance, greater conformability, and increased radial strength compared with the 316L stainless steel of the other Taxus platforms, as well as enhanced radiopacity, despite thinner struts (81 vs. 132 μm for the Taxus Express and 97 μm for the Taxus Liberté.)[2]

The clinical safety and efficacy of the Ion/Taxus Element stent were evaluated in the PERSEUS (Prospective Evaluation in a Randomized Trial of the Safety and Efficacy of the Use of the Taxus Element Paclitaxel-Eluting Coronary Stent System) trial.[49] In this randomized trial, in-stent late loss at 9-month angiographic follow-up was not significantly different between the Taxus Element/Ion and Taxus Express (0.24 ± 0.52 mm vs. 0.34 ± 0.55 mm; P = .33); 1-year target lesion failure (a composite of ischemia-driven target lesion revascularization, myocardial infarction related to the target vessel, and/or cardiac death related to the target vessel) occurred in 5.57% of patients randomly assigned to the Taxus Element and 6.14% of the patients randomly assigned to the Taxus Express, satisfying the criteria for noninferiority (Figure 2-29). The safety and efficacy of the Taxus Element/Ion stent have also been evaluated in small vessels (reference vessel diameters ≥ 2.25 to < 2.75 mm) in the PERSEUS Small Vessels trial.[51] In-stent late loss was significantly less with the Taxus Element compared with lesion-matched historical Express[2] bare metal control subjects from the Taxus V trial (0.38 ± 0.51 mm vs. 0.80 ± 0.53 mm; P < .001), as was target lesion failure (7.3% vs. 19.5%), supporting the clinical efficacy of this platform in small-diameter coronary vessels.

XIENCE SERIES

The Xience drug-eluting stent system elutes everolimus from a fluorinated copolymer coating a CoCr MultiLink Vision stent platform. This platform consists of serpentine rings connected by links formed from a single piece of L605 CoCr alloy (see Figure 2-5).[52] CoCr provides improved radial strength and radiopacity, despite thinner strut thickness (0.81 μm). In the diameters up to 3.0 mm, the stent is composed of six crests per ring, whereas in diameters of 3.5 mm or more, there are nine crests per ring. The antiproliferative agent everolimus is loaded at 100 μg/cm[2] onto the nonerodible biocompatible fluorinated copolymer, which is made of vinylidene fluoride and hexfluoropropylene at 83% to 17% by weight polymer-to-everolimus ratio. No drug-free top coat layer is used. Over the first 30 days after implantation, 80% of the everolimus is eluted; by 120 days after implantation, it is completely gone (see Figure 2-19).[40]

The safety and efficacy of the Xience drug-eluting stents have been evaluated in the SPIRIT (A Clinical Evaluation of the Xience V Everolimus Eluting Coronary Stent System) series of trials. SPIRIT FIRST demonstrated that the Xience everolimus-eluting stent significantly reduced late loss compared with its bare metal stent counterpart (0.10 vs. 0.87 mm; P < .01)[53]; SPIRIT II and III showed that the

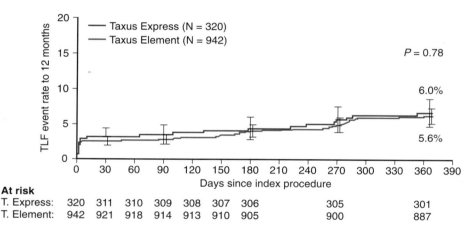

At risk

T. Express:	320	311	310	309	308	307	306		305	301
T. Element:	942	921	918	914	913	910	905		900	887

Figure 2-29 Primary results of the PERSEUS Workhorse trial according to intention to treat analysis. The platinum chromium paclitaxel-eluting stent (Taxus Element/Ion) was noninferior to the 316L stainless steel paclitaxel-eluting stent (Taxus Express[2]) for target lesion failure at 1 year in patients undergoing percutaneous coronary intervention of a single de novo lesion. *TLF*, Target lesion failure.

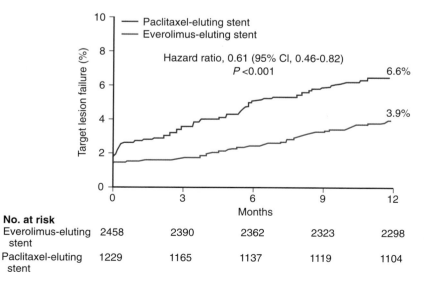

No. at risk

Everolimus-eluting stent	2458	2390	2362	2323	2298
Paclitaxel-eluting stent	1229	1165	1137	1119	1104

Figure 2-30 Primary outcome of the SPIRIT IV randomized clinical trial. This trial compared the Xience V everolimus-eluting stent with the Taxus Express[2] paclitaxel-eluting stent. Compared with the paclitaxel-eluting stent, the everolimus-eluting stent was associated with a significantly lower rate of the primary endpoint of ischemia-driven target lesion failure (defined as a composite of cardiac death, target-vessel myocardial infarction, and/or ischemia-driven target-lesion revascularization with the use of percutaneous coronary intervention or bypass graft surgery. (Adapted from Stone GW, Rizvi A, Newman W, et al. Everolimus-eluting versus paclitaxel-eluting stents in coronary artery disease. *N Engl J Med* 2010;362: 1663-1674.)

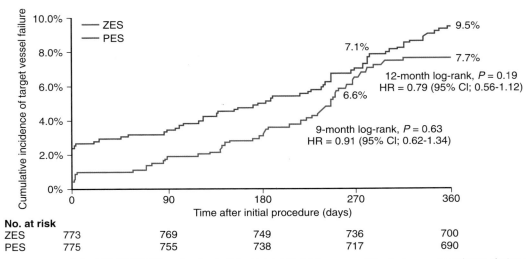

Figure 2-31   Primary outcome of the ENDEAVOR IV randomized clinical trial. This trial compared the Endeavor zotarolimus-eluting stent *(ZES)* with the Taxus Express[2] paclitaxel-eluting stent *(PES)*. The Endeavor stent was noninferior to the Taxus stent with respect to the primary endpoint of target lesion failure (a composite of cardiac death, myocardial infarction, and/or clinically driven target vessel revascularization 9 months after the procedure). (Adapted from Leon MB, Mauri L, Popma JJ, et al. ENDEAVOR IV Investigators. A randomized comparison of the ENDEAVOR zotarolimus-eluting stent versus the TAXUS paclitaxel-eluting stent in de novo native coronary lesions 12-month outcomes from the ENDEAVOR IV trial. *J Am Coll Cardiol* 2010;55:543-554.)

Xience everolimus-eluting stent reduced in-stent late loss compared with the Taxus Express[2] paclitaxel-eluting stent (0.14 ± 0.41 mm vs. 0.28 ± 0.48 mm; $P = .004$)[54]; and the SPIRIT IV large randomized clinical trial demonstrated that the rate of target lesion failure (defined as the composite of cardiac death, target vessel myocardial infarction, and/or ischemia-driven target lesion revascularization) was significantly lower with the Xience everolimus-eluting stent compared with the Taxus Express[2] paclitaxel-eluting stent (4.2% vs. 6.8%; RR, 0.62; 95% CI, 0.46-0.82; $P = .001$; Figure 2-30).[55]

ENDEAVOR

The Endeavor stent elutes zotarolimus from PC polymer applied to the MP35N CoCr Driver bare metal stent (strut thickness, 91 μm).[56] The Driver stent segments are created from a single ring formed into a repeating pattern of crowns and struts. The dose of zotarolimus is 10 μg/mm stent length (1.6 μg/mm²) and is eluted from a 2- to 3-μm-thick layer of the drug-polymer matrix (90% zotarolimus and 10% PC). This rests on a PC base coat (≈1 μm thick) and is covered by a thin, drug-free overspray of PC polymer (≈0.1 μm thick). The drug and polymer are asymmetrically distributed on the stent surface by a proprietary coating technique, so the drug is localized mainly on the abluminal arterial wall side of the stent. Zotarolimus is rapidly eluted from the stent in the first few days after implantation and is completely released by approximately 2 weeks after implantation (Figure 2-31).[25]

The safety and efficacy of the Endeavor zotarolimus-eluting stent were examined in the ENDEAVOR series of trials. ENDEAVOR I was a small, first in human series.[56] The ENDEAVOR II trial demonstrated that the Endeavor zotarolimus-eluting stent significantly reduced in-stent late loss compared with its bare metal counterpart, the Driver stent (1.03 ± 0.58 mm vs. 0.61 ± 0.46 mm; $P < .001$), as well as the primary clinical endpoint of target lesion failure.[57] However, in the ENDEAVOR III trial, the Endeavor stent had significantly worse angiographic outcomes at 9 months compared with the Cypher sirolimus-eluting stent (in-stent late luminal loss, 0.60 ± 0.48 mm vs. 0.15 ± 0.34 mm, respectively; $P < 0.01$),[58] although at 5-year follow-up, clinical outcomes favored the Endeavor zotarolimus-eluting stent.[59] The large randomized trial ENDEAVOR IV demonstrated that the Endeavor zotarolimus-eluting stent was noninferior to the Taxus Express[2] paclitaxel-eluting stent with respect to the clinical endpoint of target lesion failure.[60]

RESOLUTE INTEGRITY

The Resolute stent elutes zotarolimus from a BioLinx polymer coating an Integrity bare metal stent. The Integrity stent is manufactured from MP35N CoCr alloy and is formed from a single wire bent into a continuous sinusoid pattern and then laser-fused back onto itself. An earlier version of this stent, the Endeavor Resolute, used the same drug and polymer but on the Driver bare metal stent platform, which is formed from several laser-fused elements, whereas the Integrity bare metal stent is formed from a single wire. The drug-polymer formulation (35% zotarolimus–65% BioLinx) provides a zotarolimus dose of approximately 1.6 μg/mm². Despite a similar drug load, the elution kinetics of the Resolute stent differ dramatically compared with the Endeavor stent as a result of polymer characteristics.[41] Although zotarolimus is rapidly released from the Endeavor stent in the first few days after implantation, only 50% of drug elution occurs within the first week after Resolute stent implantation; 85% of the zotarolimus content is eluted by 60 days, and the drug is eluted completely by 180 days (see Figure 2-23). Differences in polymer formulation likely explain the relative amount of neointimal proliferation observed with these two zotarolimus-eluting stents.[61]

The bulk of the clinical data supporting the efficacy of the Resolute stent is derived from the Resolute All-Comers randomized trial, which enrolled patients with a broad range of clinical and anatomic complexity and randomly assigned them to the Endeavor Resolute or Xience V stent. The Resolute zotarolimus-eluting stent was noninferior to the Xience V everolimus-eluting stent with regard to target lesion failure, which was defined as a composite of death from cardiac causes, any myocardial infarction (not clearly attributable to a non-target vessel), and/or clinically indicated target lesion revascularization within 12 months (Figure 2-32).[62] In-stent late lumen loss was 0.27 ± 0.43 mm in the zotarolimus-stent group versus 0.19 ± 0.40 mm in the everolimus-stent group.[62]

◆ Conclusions

Coronary stents significantly reduce acute vessel closure and improve long-term outcomes compared with stand-alone balloon angioplasty. Procedural and long-term success, however, depend on specific characteristics of a given stent platform. Stent alloy, cell design, strut thickness, and the stent delivery system contribute to a given

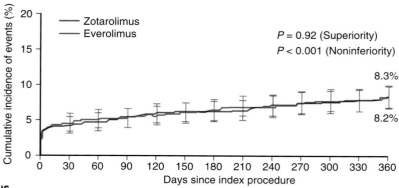

Figure 2-32   Primary outcome of the RESOLUTE All Comers trial. This trial compared the Resolute zotarolimus-eluting stent with the Xience V everolimus-eluting stent. The Resolute stent was noninferior to the Xience V stent with respect to the primary endpoint of target lesion failure (defined as the composite of death from cardiac causes, any myocardial infarction not clearly attributable to a nontarget vessel, or target vessel revascularization; $P < .001$ for noninferiority). (Adapted from Serruys PW, Silber S, Garg S, et al. Comparison of zotarolimus-eluting and everolimus-eluting coronary stents. N Engl J Med 2010;363:136-146.)

stent's flexibility, trackability, conformability, longitudinal and radial strength, acute recoil, extent of scaffolding, and radiopacity. Despite the technologic advance represented by the bare metal stent, long-term outcomes are limited by neointimal proliferation, restenosis, and subsequent target lesion revascularization. Current drug-eluting stents combine a bare metal stent scaffold with a polymer coating that allows for the elution of an antiproliferative agent, which can suppress vascular smooth muscle cell proliferation, migration, and extracellular matrix production. The antirestenotic efficacy of a drug-eluting stent is critically dependent on the complex interplay between elution kinetics and therapeutic efficacy of the eluted drug, which in turn depends on specific characteristics of the polymer, drug, dose formulation, and design of the polymer layers. Emerging and future drug-eluting stent designs use bioresorbable polymers or completely bioresorbable scaffolds, which could mitigate the negative impact of nonerodible polymers on long-term vascular healing.

REFERENCES

1. Grüntzig AR, Senning A, Siegenthaler WE. Nonoperative dilatation of coronary-artery stenosis: percutaneous transluminal coronary angioplasty. N Engl J Med 1979;301:61-68.
2. Menown IB, Noad R, Garcia EJ, et al. The platinum chromium element stent platform: from alloy, to design, to clinical practice. Adv Ther 2010;27:129-141.
3. Serruys PW, Onuma Y, Ormiston JA, et al. Evaluation of the second generation of a bioresorbable everolimus drug-eluting vascular scaffold for treatment of de novo coronary artery stenosis: six-month clinical and imaging outcomes. Circulation 2010; 122:2301-2312.
4. Ormiston JA, Webber B, Webster MW. Stent longitudinal integrity bench insights into a clinical problem. JACC Cardiovasc Interv 2011;4:1310-1317.
5. Kastrati A, Schomig A, Dirschinger J, et al. Increased risk of restenosis after placement of gold-coated stents: results of a randomized trial comparing gold-coated with uncoated steel stents in patients with coronary artery disease. Circulation 2000;101: 2478-2483.
6. Park SJ, Lee CW, Hong MK, et al. Comparison of gold-coated nir stents with uncoated nir stents in patients with coronary artery disease. Am J Cardiol 2002;89:872-875.
7. Kastrati A, Mehilli J, Dirschinger J, et al. Intracoronary stenting and angiographic results: strut thickness effect on restenosis outcome (ISAR-STEREO) trial. Circulation 2001;103: 2816-2821.
8. Pache J, Kastrati A, Mehilli J, et al. Intracoronary stenting and angiographic results: strut thickness effect on restenosis outcome (ISAR-STEREO-2) trial. J Am Coll Cardiol 2003;41: 1283-1288.
9. Morton AC, Crossman D, Gunn J. The influence of physical stent parameters upon restenosis. Pathologie-biologie 2004;52: 196-205.
10. Sangiorgi G, Melzi G, Agostoni P, et al. Engineering aspects of stents design and their translation into clinical practice. Ann Ist Super Sanita 2007;43:89-100.
11. Abizaid A. Sirolimus-eluting coronary stents: a review. Vasc Health Risk Manag 2007;3:191-201.
12. Rowinsky EK, Donehower RC. Paclitaxel (taxol). N Engl J Med 1995;332:1004-1014.
13. Yvon AM, Wadsworth P, Jordan MA. Taxol suppresses dynamics of individual microtubules in living human tumor cells. Molecular biology of the cell 1999;10:947-959.
14. Jordan MA, Toso RJ, Thrower D, et al. Mechanism of mitotic block and inhibition of cell proliferation by taxol at low concentrations. Proc Natl Acad Sci U S A 1993;90:9552-9556.

15. Axel DI, Kunert W, Goggelmann C, et al. Paclitaxel inhibits arterial smooth muscle cell proliferation and migration in vitro and in vivo using local drug delivery. Circulation 1997;96: 636-645.
16. Wessely R, Schomig A, Kastrati A. Sirolimus and paclitaxel on polymer-based drug-eluting stents: similar but different. J Am Coll Cardiol 2006;47:708-714.
17. Stone GW, Ellis SG, Cox DA, et al; TAXUS-IV Investigators. A polymer-baseD, paclitaxel-eluting stent in patients with coronary artery disease. N Engl J Med 2004;350:221-231.
18. Serruys PW, Sianos G, Abizaid A, et al. The effect of variable dose and release kinetics on neointimal hyperplasia using a novel paclitaxel-eluting stent platform: the Paclitaxel In-Stent Controlled Elution Study (PISCES). J Am Coll Cardiol 2005;46: 253-260.
19. Sehgal SN. Sirolimus: its discovery, biological properties, and mechanism of action. Transplantation proceedings 2003;35: 7S-14S.
20. Klumpen HJ, Beijnen JH, Gurney H, et al. Inhibitors of mtor. Oncologist 2010;15:1262-1269.
21. Huang S, Bjornsti MA, Houghton PJ. Rapamycins: mechanism of action and cellular resistance. Cancer biology & therapy 2003;2:222-232.
22. Inoki K, Ouyang H, Li Y, et al. Signaling by target of rapamycin proteins in cell growth control. Microbiol Mol Biol Rev 2005; 69:79-100.
23. Moses JW, Leon MB, Popma JJ, et al. Sirolimus-eluting stents versus standard stents in patients with stenosis in a native coronary artery. N Engl J Med 2003;349:1315-1323.
24. Houghton PJ. Everolimus. Clin Cancer Res 2010;16:1368-1372.
25. Johnson GC. XIENCE Everolimus eluting coronary stent system (EECSS), 2007 (http://www.fda.gov/ohrms/dockets/ac/07/slides/2007-4333s1-03%20-%20XIENCE%20V%20Panel_Abbott%20Vascular%20Presentation.pdf).
26. Tesfamariam B. Drug release kinetics from stent device-based delivery systems. J Cardiovasc Pharmacol 2008;51:118-125.
27. Bertrand OF, Sipehia R, Mongrain R, et al. Biocompatibility aspects of new stent technology. J Am Coll Cardiol 1998;32: 562-571.
28. Finn AV, Joner M, Nakazawa G, et al. Pathological correlates of late drug-eluting stent thrombosis: strut coverage as a marker of endothelialization. Circulation 2007;115:2435-2441.
29. Finn AV, Nakazawa G, Joner M, et al. Vascular responses to drug eluting stents: importance of delayed healing. Arterioscler Thromb Vasc Biol 2007;27:1500-1510.

30. Joner M, Finn AV, Farb A, et al. Pathology of drug-eluting stents in humans: delayed healing and late thrombotic risk. J Am Coll Cardiol 2006;48:193-202.
31. Onuma Y, Serruys PW. Bioresorbable scaffold: the advent of a new era in percutaneous coronary and peripheral revascularization? Circulation 2011;123:779-797.
32. Windecker S, Serruys PW, Wandel S, et al. Biolimus-eluting stent with biodegradable polymer versus sirolimus-eluting stent with durable polymer for coronary revascularisation (leaders): a randomised non-inferiority trial. Lancet 2008;372:1163-1173.
33. Meredith IT, Verheye S, Dubois CL, et al. Primary endpoint results of the evolve trial: a randomized evaluation of a novel bioabsorbable polymer-coateD, everolimus-eluting coronary stent. J Am Coll Cardiol 2012;59:1362-1370.
34. Hezi-Yamit A, Sullivan C, Wong J, et al. Impact of polymer hydrophilicity on biocompatibility: implication for des polymer design. J Biomed Mater Res A 2009;90:133-141.
35. Tzafriri AR, Groothuis A, Price GS, et al. Stent elution rate determines drug deposition and receptor-mediated effects. J Control Release 2012;161:918-926.
36. Pinchuk L, Wilson GJ, Barry JJ, et al. Medical applications of poly(styrene-block-isobutylene-block-styrene) ("sibs"). Biomaterials 2008;29:448-460.
37. Kamath KR, Barry JJ, Miller KM. The taxus drug-eluting stent: a new paradigm in controlled drug delivery. Advanced drug delivery reviews 2006;58:412-436.
38. Boden M, Richard R, Schwarz MC. In vitro and in vivo evaluation of the safety and stability of the TAXUS Paclitaxel-Eluting Coronary Stent. J Mater Sci Mater Med 2009;20: 1553-1562.
39. Dawkins KD, Grube E, Guagliumi G, et al. Clinical efficacy of polymer-based paclitaxel-eluting stents in the treatment of complex, long coronary artery lesions from a multicenter, randomized trial: support for the use of drug-eluting stents in contemporary clinical practice. Circulation 2005;112: 3306-3313.
40. Reference 40 deleted in proof.
41. Udipi K, Melder RJ, Chen M, et al. The next generation endeavor resolute stent: role of the biolinx polymer system. EuroIntervention 2007;3:137-139.
42. Morice MC, Serruys PW, Sousa JE, et al. A randomized comparison of a sirolimus-eluting stent with a standard stent for coronary revascularization. N Engl J Med 2002;346:1773-1780.
43. Stone GW, Moses JW, Ellis SG, et al. Safety and efficacy of sirolimus- and paclitaxel-eluting coronary stents. N Engl J Med 2007.

44. Finn AV, Kolodgie FD, Harnek J, et al. Differential response of delayed healing and persistent inflammation at sites of overlapping sirolimus- or paclitaxel-eluting stents. *Circulation* 2005; 112:270-278.

45. Colombo A, Drzewiecki J, Banning A, et al. Randomized study to assess the effectiveness of slow- and moderate-release polymer-based paclitaxel-eluting stents for coronary artery lesions. *Circulation* 2003;108:788-794.

46. Stone GW, Ellis SG, Cannon L, et al. Comparison of a polymer-based paclitaxel-eluting stent with a bare metal stent in patients with complex coronary artery disease: a randomized controlled trial. *JAMA* 2005;294:1215-1223.

47. Stone GW, Teirstein PS, Meredith IT, et al; PLATINUM Trial Investigators. A prospective, randomized evaluation of a novel everolimus-eluting coronary stent: the PLATINUM (a Prospective, RandomizeD, Multicenter Trial to Assess an Everolimus-Eluting Coronary Stent System [PROMUS Element] for the Treatment of Up to Two de Novo Coronary Artery Lesions) trial. *J Am Coll Cardiol* 2011;57:1700-1708.

48. Meredith IT, Whitbourn R, Scott D, et al. PLATINUM QCA: A prospective, multicentre study assessing clinical, angiographiC, and intravascular ultrasound outcomes with the novel platinum chromium thin-strut PROMUS Element everolimus-eluting stent in de novo coronary stenoses. *EuroIntervention* 2011;7:84-90.

49. Kereiakes DJ, Cannon LA, Feldman RL, et al. Clinical and angiographic outcomes after treatment of de novo coronary stenoses with a novel platinum chromium thin-strut stent: primary results of the PERSEUS (Prospective Evaluation in a Randomized Trial of the Safety and Efficacy of the Use of the TAXUS Element Paclitaxel-Eluting Coronary Stent System) trial. *J Am Coll Cardiol* 2010;56:264-271.

50. Kereiakes DJ, Popma JJ, Cannon LA, et al. Longitudinal stent deformation: quantitative coronary angiographic analysis from the PERSEUS and PLATINUM randomised controlled clinical trials. *EuroIntervention* 2012;8:187-195.

51. Cannon LA, Kereiakes DJ, Mann T, et al. A prospective evaluation of the safety and efficacy of TAXUS Element paclitaxel-eluting coronary stent implantation for the treatment of de novo coronary artery lesions in small vessels: the PERSEUS Small Vessel trial. *EuroIntervention* 2011;6:920-927, 921-922.

52. Kukreja N, Onuma Y, Serruys PW. Xience v everolimus-eluting coronary stent. *Expert Rev Med Devices* 2009;6:219-229.

53. Serruys PW, Ong AT, Piek JJ, et al. A randomized comparison of a durable polymer everolimus-eluting stent with a bare metal coronary stent: the SPIRIT first trial. *EuroIntervention* 2005;1: 58-65.

54. Stone GW, Midei M, Newman W, et al. SPIRIT III Investigators. Comparison of an everolimus-eluting stent and a paclitaxel-eluting stent in patients with coronary artery disease: a randomized trial. *JAMA* 2008;299:1903-1913.

55. Stone GW, Rizvi A, Newman W, et al. Everolimus-eluting versus paclitaxel-eluting stents in coronary artery disease. *N Engl J Med* 2010;362:1663-1674.

56. Meredith IT, Ormiston J, Whitbourn R, et al. First-in-human study of the Endeavor ABT-578-eluting phosphorylcholine-encapsulated stent system in de novo native coronary artery lesions: Endeavor I trial. *EuroIntervention* 2005;1:157-164.

57. Fajadet J, Wijns W, Laarman GJ, et al. ENDEAVOR II Investigators. RandomizeD, double-blinD, multicenter study of the Endeavor zotarolimus-eluting phosphorylcholine-encapsulated stent for treatment of native coronary artery lesions: clinical and angiographic results of the Endeavor II trial. *Circulation* 2006; 114:798-806.

58. Kandzari DE, Leon MB, Popma JJ, et al. ENDEAVOR III Investigators. Comparison of zotarolimus-eluting and sirolimus-eluting stents in patients with native coronary artery disease: a randomized controlled trial. *J Am Coll Cardiol* 2006;48: 2440-2447.

59. Kandzari DE, Mauri L, Popma JJ, et al. Late-term clinical outcomes with zotarolimus- and sirolimus-eluting stents. 5-year follow-up of the ENDEAVOR III (A Randomized Controlled Trial of the Medtronic Endeavor Drug [ABT-578] Eluting Coronary Stent System Versus the Cypher Sirolimus-Eluting Coronary Stent System in De Novo Native Coronary Artery Lesions). *JACC Cardiovasc Interv* 2011;4:543-550.

60. Leon MB, Mauri L, Popma JJ, et al. ENDEAVOR IV Investigators. A randomized comparison of the ENDEAVOR zotarolimus-eluting stent versus the TAXUS paclitaxel-eluting stent in de novo native coronary lesions 12-month outcomes from the ENDEAVOR IV trial. *J Am Coll Cardiol* 2010;55: 543-554.

61. Waseda K, Ako J, Yamasaki M, et al. Impact of polymer formulations on neointimal proliferation after zotarolimus-eluting stent with different polymers: insights from the resolute trial. *Circ Cardiovasc Interv* 2011;4:248-255.

62. Serruys PW, Silber S, Garg S, et al. Comparison of zotarolimus-eluting and everolimus-eluting coronary stents. *N Engl J Med* 2010;363:136-146.

CHAPTER 3

Preclinical Evaluation of Coronary Stents

JUAN F. GRANADA | ARMANDO TELLEZ | GREG L. KALUZA

KEY POINTS

- The amount of neointimal growth in response to stent placement is a linear function of the depth of mechanical injury and the degree of inflammatory reaction.

- The arterial response to a bare metal stent in an animal model, consisting of injury, inflammation, and neointimal proliferation, is predictable in its sequence and time course and differs little among different metallic stents, rendering a complete healing response and largely definitive amount of neointima at 4 to 6 weeks after implantation.

- The preclinical evaluation of drug-eluting stents is more challenging than evaluation of bare metal stents because the metallic stent platform of established biocompatibility is complicated by the presence of additional bioactive elements—drug and polymeric carrier.

- Preclinical validation of drug-eluting stents mandates (1) biocompatibility testing of the polymeric carrier, (2) biochemical compatibility testing of the carrier and the drug, (3) evaluation of the durability and stability of the coating after manufacturing and sterilization, and (4) assessment of the pharmacokinetics of the drug in the arterial wall when released from a particular carrier.

- A central focus of drug-eluting stent validation is the assessment of safety via histopathologic methods established originally for bare metal stents but expanded further to include not only metrics of efficacy (i.e., neointimal proliferation) but also details of the healing process.

- Development of a bioresorbable scaffold further increases the complexity and volume of multidisciplinary research required to develop and validate a functional device. The aspects to be addressed when validating a drug-eluting stent are still in place but are now complicated by the fact that the entire scaffold is made of a material biochemically active over its entire lifetime within the arterial wall.

Historical Background

Percutaneous coronary balloon angioplasty radically changed the treatment of obstructive coronary atherosclerotic disease but was initially limited in its safety and efficacy by various serious complications in a significant proportion of patients. Abrupt vessel closure, the most important acute failure of balloon angioplasty resulting from elastic recoil and plaque dissection, was effectively solved by the introduction of metallic stents.[1] The most important chronic form of failure of balloon angioplasty was restenosis after the initial procedure, requiring repeat intervention, often with coronary artery bypass surgery. Restenosis after balloon angioplasty is the result of the interaction of various mechanical and biologic processes starting immediately after balloon injury, including acute vessel recoil,[2,3] negative vascular remodeling,[4] and excessive neointimal proliferation.[4-6]

The introduction of stents resulted in a reduction in the incidence of restenosis by countering vascular recoil and negative remodeling. In 1969, Dotter[7] originally proposed the idea of introducing a vascular scaffold to overcome acute occlusion and vessel recoil induced by balloon dilation. The initial test of this concept consisted of the direct insertion of a stainless steel springlike tubular prosthesis in the peripheral arteries of dogs. Although this landmark study demonstrated that delivery of this device was feasible, acute occlusions and significant long-term lumen narrowing were observed, discouraging further development.[7] Nevertheless, the idea was revisited as new materials and technologies became available. In 1983, the same group of investigators tested the safety and short-term biocompatibility of a nitinol-based stent design in the peripheral arteries of dogs.[8,9] The initial results were more promising this time, and the vascular safety, healing, and compatibility of this device at 2-year follow-up were subsequently evaluated in canine iliofemoral arteries. Although long-term patency was demonstrated, significant luminal narrowing occurred.[10]

The concept of a fully percutaneous endovascular stent continued to evolve over time, alternating between the original coil-like design and a tubular structure, which in the end turned out to be more functional and successful. In 1984, Maass and colleagues[11] tested the long-term (24 months) vascular biocompatibility of a novel stainless steel double helix vascular endoprosthesis expanded by a dedicated catheter system in dogs and calves. Almost simultaneously, Wright and coworkers[12] introduced the concept of a self-expanding stainless steel stent using a zigzag design expandable by a dedicated delivery catheter. In 1985, an inflection point in stent development occurred by the introduction of two pioneering devices delivered via angioplasty balloon catheters, one based on stainless steel wire continuously woven to form an expandable coil (Gianturco) and another cut from a stainless steel tube to form a slotted, cylindrical, expandable mesh structure (Palmaz).[13] Both devices were tested in peripheral arteries of dogs and for the first time proved that long-term vascular patency and healing of a fully implantable stent delivered via an angioplasty balloon were viable. The concept of a self-expanding nitinol-based stent was similarly and contemporaneously tested in the peripheral and coronary territory of dogs.[14]

During early stent development, dogs were commonly used in cardiovascular research, and initial stent validation was also primarily conducted in the canine model. For safety and accessibility reasons, these experiments were initially restricted to the peripheral vasculature. As the devices in development started varying in size, design, materials, and mechanism of deployment, a need arose to explore additional vascular territories, including the coronary arteries, and animal models other than canine.[15] Standardization of the methods by which stent technologies were evaluated was required to ensure reliable safety and efficacy and provide valid comparisons among stent technologies.

Animal Models Used for Stent Validation Testing

NORMAL SWINE MODELS

As the development in stent designs and delivery systems continued to evolve from small-scale experimentation by individual physicians and engineers toward a more mature form of industry-based development programs, it became evident that universally reliable and reproducible animal models were required to test stent biocompatibility and safety. The porcine heart and vessels rapidly became the model of choice because of anatomy, histology, and physiology closely resembling that of humans and easy availability.[16-18] The domestic crossbred farm pig, *Sus scrofa domesticus*, is the most commonly used strain in cardiovascular research today.[19] Miniature swine such as the Yucatan, Hanford, Gottingen, and Sinclair Hormel are commonly chosen for long-term studies when significant growth in body mass over time is a problem. Swine achieve sexual maturity by 6 to 8 months and at that age weigh between 40 and 100 kg, according to the breed. The heart of the pig is anatomically similar to humans with the exception of having a left azygos vein that drains the intercostal system into the coronary sinus[20] and a right coronary artery ostium arising substantially higher than in humans. The heart of a 40-kg to 50-kg miniature pig is approximately the same size as an adult human heart, and the caliber of the coronary arteries is similar.[21] The blood supply to the conduction system is from the posterior septal artery and is predominantly right-dominant, similar to a human. The conduction system is also similar to that of humans, although the endocardium and epicardium are activated simultaneously.[22] The swine aorta has a comparable histopathologic anatomy and contains vasa vasorum. The coronary artery system is similar to 90% of the human population in anatomy and function, although it is more prone to vasospasm during manipulation. Similar to the human heart, and in contrast to the canine heart, the porcine heart has no preexisting collaterals between the coronary arteries and their branches.[23] Other animal species such as rabbits and sheep have been used less frequently in the validation phase of stent development for specific research needs (e.g., efficacy models) or anatomic requirements (e.g., bifurcations).

ATHEROSCLEROTIC ANIMAL MODELS AND STENT EFFICACY

The juvenile coronary swine model of restenosis, although well validated for the evaluation of stent safety, has been shown to be of limited utility in the evaluation of efficacy.[16] Alternatives have been explored, most of which use some form of atherosclerosis in the hopes of creating an environment that simulates human pathophysiology and that is capable of highlighting differences between treatments not evident in healthy animal models. The normal rabbit iliac injury model showed early promise in the evaluation of stent efficacy. It provides a straight elastic arterial segment with higher resistance to arterial tears and ruptures that has been suggested to provide a greater consistency in vascular injury.[24] The reproducible vascular response to injury[25,26] and slower healing response compared with swine[24] has encouraged the use of this model in the study of differences in efficacy and endothelialization among drug-eluting stents (DES).[25-27] However, the rabbit model has limitations in the assessment of efficacy because the arterial response elicited by newer and improved bare metal stents (BMS) is less pronounced; it is challenging to evaluate incremental improvement of DES on this control background.[28,29] In addition, initial differences between DES and BMS controls often disappear at later times in the normal model, making inferences about long-term efficacy difficult.[30] The combination of arterial injury and a high-cholesterol diet induces plaques that are rich in lipid-laden foamy macrophages and contain fewer smooth muscle cells with moderate levels of extracellular proteoglycan and collagen matrix.[24] This atherosclerotic rabbit model has proved useful for DES comparisons.[31-34]

Although models of coronary atherosclerosis in the swine model have been developed,[35] the diet-induced atherosclerosis model has limited added value for stent evaluation, in contrast to the rabbit model.[36] A model with diabetes can be induced with the use of intravenous streptozotocin, resulting in a metabolic profile that includes hyperglycemia, hypercholesterolemia, and increased platelet aggregation.[37] At 20 weeks after diabetes induction, atherosclerotic lesions can be identified with characteristics similar to lesions observed in humans, such as the presence of lipid pools, intraplaque hemorrhage,

and coronary calcifications. Paclitaxel-eluting stents implanted in the coronary arteries of this model showed less neointimal area, less strut endothelialization, and higher degrees of inflammation compared with identical BMS controls at 28 days and 90 days after implantation.[38] Another model, the familial hypercholesterolemic swine, displays spontaneous elevations in plasma cholesterol, low-density lipoprotein (LDL), and apolipoprotein B and reductions in high-density lipopoprotein and apolipoprotein A-I while fed a low-fat, low-cholesterol diet.[39] This phenotype is polygenic arising from a missense mutation of the LDL receptor and variations in the apolipoprotein B locus, including Lpb5, that result in LDL that binds defectively to the LDL receptor in vitro.[40] These swine naturally develop atherosclerosis[40,41]; early lesions can be identified between 6 and 8 months of age, and fully developed atherosclerotic lesions were demonstrated at 18 months.[41] The healing of BMS implanted in the coronary territory of familial hypercholesterolemic swine follows a different progression pattern compared with domestic juvenile swine under similar implantation conditions and appears to be more similar to what occurs in humans.[42] The efficacy of several DES platforms has been successfully evaluated in this model, including paclitaxel-eluting and everolimus-eluting stents (Figure 3-1) and paclitaxel-coated balloons in the ileofemoral arteries.[43,44] It is still unknown how reliably these diseased models mimic the natural history of human restenosis and predict future clinical safety and efficacy of DES. Nevertheless, the introduction of animal models of human-like coronary atherosclerosis has provided new opportunities to study the biology of restenosis and stent healing in a human-like environment.

Evaluation of Bare Metal Stents

One of the first attempts to study the vascular response of porcine coronary arteries to stent implantation was undertaken by Schwartz and colleagues.[45] Coronary coil-like stents were implanted in normal swine coronary arteries and followed for up to 70 days. This study was one of the first to demonstrate the potential of this model to reproduce the proliferative component of restenosis seen in humans.[46,47] Soon thereafter, van der Giessen and associates[48] studied the early vascular effects of a balloon expandable single tantalum helicoid stent (Wiktor stent) in porcine coronary arteries.

ARTERIAL OVERSTRETCH AND PORCINE MODEL OF STENT RESTENOSIS

In the seminal study by Schwartz and colleagues,[45] balloon-expandable BMS (tantalum and stainless steel coils) were implanted in normal swine coronary arteries and followed up to 70 days. For comparison, control arteries were subjected to oversized balloon dilation without coil placement to simulate arterial injury during balloon angioplasty. Oversized coil placement resulted in a far more robust neointimal response than balloon dilation alone. A more predictable porcine model of coronary restenosis was established than that previously achieved with oversized stand-alone balloon inflation. This study also made a preliminary observation that stents with diameters that were more mismatched to the artery caliber (i.e., overexpanded) caused rupture of the internal elastic lamina, medial lacerations, and extensive smooth muscle cell proliferation, whereas when stents closely matched the arterial diameter, injury and neointimal proliferation were minimal. This observation led to a hypothesis that the amount of neointimal proliferation is directly related to the extent and depth of arterial wall injury. This concept was subsequently confirmed and validated in a benchmark study, which demonstrated that the degree of arterial wall injury, quantified by a score, was linearly correlated with geometric measures of neointimal proliferation, such as neointimal thickness and percent area stenosis.[49] The methodology of characterizing arterial injury induced by stent struts used in that study is in principle still used today and relies on the fact that a programmed degree of injury, calculated by the percentage of arterial overstretch (stent-to-artery ratio) can be reliably

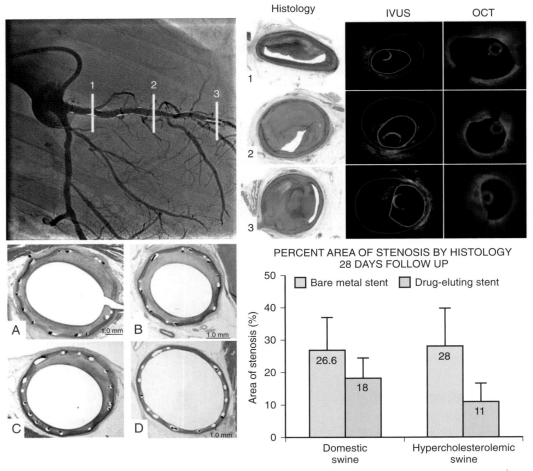

Figure 3-1   Familial hypercholesterolemic (FH) swine as a model for evaluation of stent efficacy. *Upper panel,* Native coronary atherosclerosis with three complex lesions *(1, 2, 3),* with varying degrees of stenosis on angiography and corresponding cross-sections of histology, intravascular ultrasound *(IVUS),* and optical coherence tomography *(OCT). Bottom panel,* Differential response to placement of BMS and drug-eluting stent *(DES)* in domestic swine and FH swine illustrated by histologic sections *(left)* and comparison of percent area stenosis *(right). A,* BMS in domestic swine. *B,* BMS in FH swine. *C,* DES in domestic swine. *D,* DES in FH swine. DES has a more profound inhibitory effect on restenosis in FH swine compared with domestic swine.

induced and results in a proportionate degree of neointimal formation measurable by histologic methods.[50] This experimental model, although lacking atherosclerotic components, adequately replicates the process of human coronary injury and subsequent neointimal formation[45,51] and became the standard porcine model of coronary in-stent restenosis by which stents are reliably and reproducibly characterized to this day.

INFLAMMATION AFTER BARE METAL STENT IMPLANTATION

In 1998, Kornowski and colleagues[52] expanded the understanding of the relationship between neointimal formation and the degree of injury after stent implantation by quantifying the inflammatory response to stenting observed after 1 month. The inflammatory reaction was found to be mainly composed of histiocytes, lymphocytes, granuloma formation, and neutrophils. The degree of neointimal proliferation was associated with the intensity of inflammatory response in a similarly linear manner because it is proportional to the severity of arterial injury. However, even with a mild injury score, a higher inflammatory response leads to greater neointimal formation. Kornowski and colleagues[52] suggested that the inflammatory reaction after coronary stenting played an equally important role in neointimal formation as did mechanical injury.

TEMPORAL RESPONSE AFTER BARE METAL STENT IMPLANTATION

The temporal sequence of events after BMS placement was also defined using the porcine model. By evaluating various time points (24 hours and 7, 14, and 28 days) after BMS placement, Carter and associates[53] demonstrated that early thrombus formation was minimal and accounted for a small portion of subsequent neointimal formation. Smooth muscle proliferation peaked at 7 days after implantation, and in-stent neointimal cell proliferation and matrix formation were largely complete after 28 days. Although the absolute amount of in-stent neointima varied, the process appeared complete at 28 days regardless of the stent design.[53a] This key observation allowed confident adaptation of the 4- to 6-week follow-up length as the standard duration for porcine studies of BMS.

METHODOLOGIES FOR PRECLINICAL TESTING OF BARE METAL STENTS

The validation process for BMS has been standardized in the porcine model using a comprehensive set of in vivo and ex vivo analytical tests (Table 3-1). Because of its anatomic similarity with humans, the porcine coronary model has also provided important information regarding device performance, such as deliverability, expansion, and

TABLE 3-1	Histologic and Histomorphometric Evaluation of Bare Metal Stents				
	Qualitative Score*				
	0	1	2	3	4
Injury	IEL intact, media compressed	IEL lacerated, media compressed	IEL and media lacerated, EEL compressed	IEL, media, and EEL lacerated; struts in adventitia	—
Peristrut inflammation	<25% of struts with <10 inflammatory cells	25% of struts with >10 inflammatory cells	25%-50% of struts with >10 inflammatory cells	>50% of struts with >10 inflammatory cells	>2 strut-associated granulomas
Adventitial inflammation	No inflammation	Mild inflammatory infiltration focally <25%	Moderate peripheral inflammatory infiltration 25%-50%	Severe peripheral inflammatory infiltration 25%-50% of adventitial area	Severe peripheral inflammatory infiltration >50%
Endothelialization	<25%	25%-75%	75%-95%	>95%	—
Adventitial fibrosis	None	Minimal thickening of adventitia	More pronounced segmental thickening of adventitia	Widespread fibrous thickening of adventitia	—
Quantitative Analysis†					
Area (mm²)	Lumen IEL EEL Media Intima/neointima				
Diameter (mm)	Lumen Original lumen/stent Neointimal thickness (mm) Percent area of stenosis (%)				

EEL, external elastic lamina; *IEL*, internal elastic lamina.
*Representative semiquantitative scoring system used to evaluate qualitative histologic parameters in bare metal stent sections by light microscopy.
†Histomorphometric evaluation provides quantitative measures of changes in arterial geometry and resultant stenosis in response to stent placement.

BOX 3-1 TIME COURSE OF STENT ASSESSMENT IN NORMAL PORCINE MODEL

Acute (<7 days): Stent-related injury, stent surface thrombogenicity
Midterm (14-42 days): Vessel healing, biocompatibility, neointimal proliferation
Long-term (up to 180 days): Completeness of healing

---

positioning. In addition, several analytical methods have been developed with the objective of testing the overall safety of the device. Such tests assume the stent as a foreign object, focusing objectives on the assessment of device biocompatibility.

After stent implantation, blood compatibility can be tested by measuring platelet activation and coagulation proteins. Tissue compatibility of an implanted stent is determined by a series of analytical methods based on histologic evaluation at different time intervals (Box 3-1).[54] Acute time points (<7 days) are used to assess the degree of device-induced injury and overall stent surface thrombogenicity by using conventional light microscopy and surface electron microscopy. Midterm time points (14 to 42 days) are used to determine biocompatibility and evolution of vessel healing and the amount of neointimal proliferation. Longer-term time points (up to 180 days) have been mandated by regulatory agencies to ensure the completeness of healing.[55,56]

Histologic samples obtained at multiple time points have served as the bases for the evaluation of stent safety. Standardized analytical tools exist to measure the biologic response to stent injury,[57] and histologic variables of injury and healing assessed in several cross-sections within the stent are used to quantify stent-related injury and healing.[49] Several of these histologic parameters are described in Table 3-1. The degree of vessel injury induced by the stent is measured by a semiqualitative score (Figure 3-2). The vascular injury should be assessed down to a single strut level for greater precision and better

capture of regional differences. A numeric value is assigned to each strut according to the degree of injury and averaged per histologic section and per stent to determine a mean injury score. Similarly, inflammation is measured by a semiquantitative score at the strut level, after which the score is averaged per slide and then per stent to determine an inflammatory score per stent group (Figure 3-3). Fibrin and thrombus formation after BMS implantation may be included as part of the analysis, especially at early time points after implantation (1, 3, and 7 days of follow-up). In this case, a semiquantitative score at the strut level may also be applied. However, at long-term follow-up, a BMS is not commonly expected to display residual peristrut fibrin deposition. Other aspects assessed in such a semiquantitative manner may include medial and adventitial fibrosis, calcification, and presence of giant cells. Quantitative geometric parameters to measure neointimal formation in histologic cross-sections have also been developed (see Figure 3-3). In the histologic analysis, the neointimal area is calculated by measuring the original lumen area (equal to the inner stent cross-sectional area immediately after implantation) compared with the resulting lumen area at follow-up. To normalize the obstruction to artery size, percent area stenosis is also calculated. These quantitative measures of neointimal formation are evaluated in the context of injury and inflammation scores. However, although the domestic juvenile swine model is a good predictor of device safety and material biocompatibility, it is not universally predictive of efficacy.

Overall arterial healing is another important variable evaluated after stent implantation. Commonly used metrics of healing are stent endothelialization, strut coverage by neointima, and the presence of a surface free of thrombus. Several methods have been used to determine the degree of surface coverage and strut endothelialization (Figure 3-4). Endothelialization can be grossly evaluated by light microscopy on a slide stained with hematoxylin and eosin using a semiquantitative score based on the percentage of luminal circumference covered by endothelial cells. Scanning electron microscopy is the "gold standard" for assessing endothelial cell morphology and

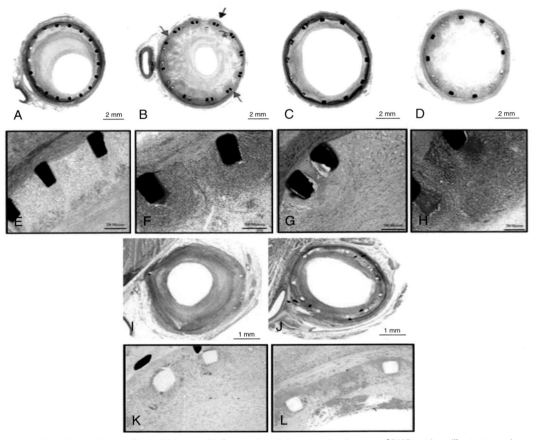

Figure 3-2   Histologic analysis of stent-induced vessel injury and inflammation. Representative images of BMS sections illustrate semiquantitative evaluation (scoring) of histologic parameters. **A,** Luminal stenosis, low injury score, and preserved internal and external elastic laminae with all stent struts residing inside the medial layer, which is compressed by the stent strut without laceration anywhere **(E)**. **B,** Example of a high injury score. Two *red arrows* indicate a ruptured external elastic lamina. There is complete rupture of the medial layer in almost half of the vascular circumference *(red asterisk)*. Multiple stent struts reside in adventitial layer **(F)**. **C,** Low inflammatory score. No inflammatory infiltration is observed in medial or adventitial vascular layers **(G)**. **D,** High inflammatory score with more than 75% of the circumference involved and inflammation extending to the media and adventitia. The inflammation is typically featuring lymphocytes and histiocytes **(H)**. Fibrin deposition. An example without fibrin deposition in neointima or around the strut **(I** and **K,** low and high magnification) compared with a histologic sample of a high score of fibrin deposition **(J** and **L).**

continuity of coverage. Immunohistochemistry detects the presence and arrangement of endothelial cell arrangement and may determine the viability of a functional endothelium, so it provides a more detailed evaluation of endothelial cell coverage. Significant advances have also been made in the assessment of endothelium by use of confocal laser scanning microscopy.[31]

The interdependence of neointimal proliferation, injury and inflammation, and the temporal sequence of the response to stent placement independent of stent type has allowed for the establishment of a standard method for BMS evaluation. From this perspective, a BMS is a simple device to test and validate. The BMS is built from a material that is nearly inert biologically (e.g., stainless steel or nitinol) whose biocompatibility has been long established in various human applications. The response of an artery to its placement, measured by cardinal metrics of neointimal growth, is a relatively simple (linear) function of the depth of mechanical injury and inflammatory reaction.[49,52] The time course of the arterial response to a BMS in an animal model is predictable and differs very little among different metallic stents, rendering a complete healing response and a largely definitive amount of neointima 4 to 6 weeks after placement.[53] With such predictable response, the major biologic differentiator between the BMS is the amount of neointimal formation, and this has been the chief parameter by which different BMS are compared with one another.

⬡ Evaluation of Drug-Eluting Stents

DES are more challenging to evaluate compared with BMS because the established biocompatibility of the metallic stent platform is complicated by the presence of additional bioactive elements: drug and polymeric carrier. The validation of such a combination device entails first the selection and validation of each component separately until a functional combination is identified and then testing of the resulting combination device as a whole. The principal elements of a DES are often distinctly different from one another with regard to the nature and time course of their interaction with the arterial wall. Consequently, the net arterial response to such a device arises not only from the initial, mechanical impact of metal struts penetrating the wall but also from the biochemical actions of the carrier and drug, which both actively alter, purposefully or inadvertently, the tissue reaction to the device. In such a dynamic and multifactorial milieu, even a small manipulation of one component may result in a disproportionately large change in the way the arterial wall reacts.[58]

KEY CONCEPTS OF DRUG-ELUTING STENT VALIDATION

Given the complexity of the DES platform, preclinical validation of DES requires techniques and models not necessary in the era of BMS

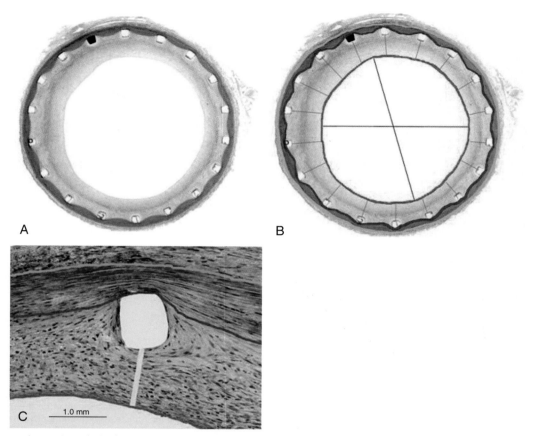

Figure 3-3 Histomorphometric analysis of an artery with stent. Representative image of an in-stent restenosis model. **A,** Original histologic cross-section of a stent. **B,** Same histologic cross-section with planimetric tracings of the key structures, allowing quantification of dimensions and areas. The *red line* delimits the luminal area. The minimum and maximum luminal diameters *(black lines)* render an average of the lumen diameter. The area behind the stent struts where the internal elastic lamina is compressed renders the stent area *(dark blue)*. The neointimal area is calculated as a difference between the stent and luminal areas. The neointimal thickness *(light blue)* is measured for each strut as perpendicular distance from the stent strut to the lumen surface and then averaged for the section. The outer border of the adventitia *(light green)* determines the vessel area. The medial area is calculated as a difference between the vessel and stent areas. **C,** Magnification of a single stent strut illustrating the three vessel layer tracings and the neointimal thickness measurement.

development, including biocompatibility testing of the polymeric carriers, biochemical compatibility testing of the combination of the carrier and the drug, analysis of the durability and stability of the coating after manufacturing and sterilization, and assessment of the pharmacokinetics of the drug in the arterial wall when released from a particular carrier. Only after these aspects are addressed adequately can a mature device be tested for overall biocompatibility and efficacy. However, as long as the device contains components that remain bioactive over time (e.g., polymer and drug), the conventional end-point of geometrically measured obstruction (stenosis) no longer suffices as the primary preclinical validation parameter. Instead, it is imperative to ascertain (1) the nature of arterial wall healing; (2) the stability and quiescence of active processes in the arterial wall, such as inflammation, fibrin resorption, and smooth muscle cell proliferation; and (3) the timing of complete neointimal response and whether it is associated with adequate endothelialization and mature extracellular matrix synthesis.[56,59]

In-stent restenosis, caused by the vascular response to injury that leads to excessive neointimal proliferation, is the most important mechanism of coronary stent failure.[60] DES effectively reduce in-stent restenosis by reducing neointimal proliferation and have become the mainstay of treatment for obstructive coronary atherosclerotic disease.[61] However, the demonstrated efficacy of DES is balanced by their negative effect on vascular healing as a result of either the antiproliferative effect of the drug (and associated late acquired incomplete stent apposition) or hypersensitivity reactions to drug,

polymer coating, or both.[62,63] A central piece in the process of DES validation is balancing stent efficacy (lack of neointimal proliferation) with safety (healing profile).

POLYMERS

Early DES delivered drugs by directly coating the surface of the stent with antiproliferative agents but without polymeric drug carriers.[64-66] However, the rapid washout of these pharmacologic agents because of short retention time limited stent efficacy, as a sustained and well-controlled tissue pharmacokinetic signature is required for the inhibition of vascular smooth muscle cell proliferation.[64,65,67-69] The use of nonabsorbable polymers as drug reservoirs made such sustained drug delivery after stent implantation feasible.[70] At the earliest stage of DES development, most research efforts focused on demonstrating polymer biocompatibility.[71] Early studies that aimed to test the biocompatibility of several nonabsorbable polymers demonstrated significant amounts of inflammation and neointimal proliferation.[72] However, most of these observations were related to polymer and coating manufacturing processes rather than true biologic incompatibility, and subsequent advances in stent coating technology have allowed the deposition of purer and more homogeneous polymeric coating layers at the micron scale, resolving these issues.

Stent polymer biocompatibility is assessed by analyzing the biologic response to the implant over time. The goal of histologic analysis of polymer biocompatibility is to determine the potential impact of the

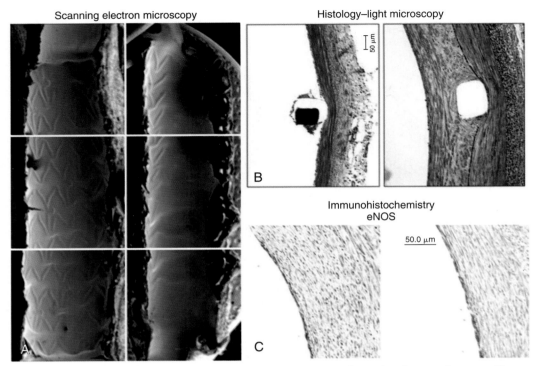

Scanning electron microscopy

Histology–light microscopy

Immunohistochemistry
eNOS

Figure 3-4 Assessment of strut coverage and endothelialization. **A,** Representative images of scanning electron microscopy. The vessel with a stent was sectioned longitudinally and separated in halves to provide an en face assessment of the stent's tissue coverage and endothelialization. The stent contours can be distinguished if the neointima is thin *(left)*. **B,** Stent coverage assessment can also be performed with regular or special stains under light microscopy. Stent struts can be assessed in early *(left)* or late *(right)* time points to determine coverage over time by determining the quantity and morphology of endothelial cells and the continuity of the lining. **C,** To add precision to endothelialization assessment by light microscopy, immunohistochemistry labeling may be used to target markers specific to endothelial cells, such as eNOS, CD34, and some lectins (magnified image shows a portion of the wall between the struts).

polymer on inflammation and neointimal proliferation (Figure 3-5). Analytical methods of stent morphometry similar to those for BMS testing are used (see Table 3-1). Compared with BMS surfaces, the inflammatory response to nonabsorbable polymeric coatings in porcine coronary arteries is dynamic over time, and several follow-up time points are required to assess fully the degree and stability of such inflammation, first to identify its initial magnitude and then later to demonstrate stabilization of this early response. The typical inflammatory reaction peaks from 28 to 90 days according to the coating and results in a variable extent of cellular infiltrates and neointimal hyperplasia.[73,74] After this peak, the inflammatory response and neointimal proliferation gradually stabilize by 180 days after implantation but may persist,[75,76] necessitating a much longer follow-up period than for BMS. Similarly, bioabsorbable polymers elicit various inflammatory responses, but the peak in inflammation is related to the degradation profile of the particular polymeric coating.[74]

DRUG-RELEASE KINETICS

The controlled drug release from the stent platform adds additional complexities to the DES validation process. Smooth muscle cell proliferation is the therapeutic target for modern DES.[77,78] A central challenge for a successful DES is to provide reproducible and adequate tissue levels of an antiproliferative drug within a specific therapeutic window over a specific time frame. Variables such as drug lipophilicity[79,80] and stent-polymer interaction with plaque components equally affect drug uptake and overall tissue pharmacokinetics.[81] The resulting pharmacokinetic profile of each individual DES platform depends on the type of drug and polymer coating.

The accurate quantification of the pharmacokinetics of antiproliferative agents on DES is performed following U.S. Food and Drug Administration guidance.[82] After DES implantation, pharmacologic compounds are released locally into surrounding tissue, so precise tissue harvesting and preservation are crucial for the proper analysis of the samples. High-performance liquid chromatography with tandem mass spectrometry detection is used to detect antiproliferative agents or other therapeutics within body fluids or tissue.[83,84] Tissue collection must avoid carryover, cross-contamination, or drug destruction that could lead to inconclusive or inaccurate data. Tissue drug concentration decreases significantly as the distance from the stent increases. Distal target organ samples must be evaluated to detect systemic effects; in particular, sampling from liver, kidney, spleen, and lung and distal muscle are normally required.[85] The assessment of the acute dynamics of drug delivery is performed immediately after stent implantation and 1 to 3 days after implantation. Assessment between 1 and 3 weeks after stent implantation is also required to evaluate subacute and maintenance drug levels and to monitor drug clearance. Assessment of long-term biodistribution may be required to determine the presence of the pharmacologic agent more than 6 months after stent implantation (Figure 3-6).

PRECLINICAL ASSESSMENT OF COMBINED DRUG-ELUTING STENT PLATFORM (POLYMER, DRUG, AND STENT)

Preclinical observations suggest that vascular response and morphology at 1 month after DES in the porcine model is comparable to the vascular response observed in humans after 6 months, and the findings of longer-term (3 and 6 months) studies with DES in animals are predictive of longer-term studies (24 to 30 months) in humans.[86] However, although some degree of neointimal inhibition is observed with the domestic swine model, it is a relatively poor predictor of

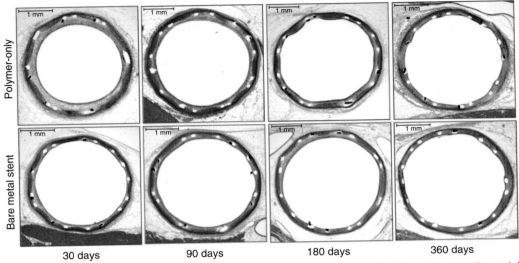

Figure 3-5   Long-term biocompatibility evaluation of the polymer carrier-only stent compared with the identical (alloy and design) BMS.

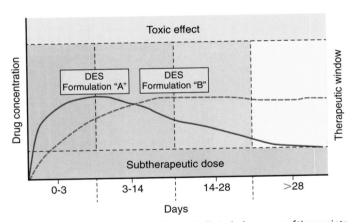

Figure 3-6   Pharmacokinetic studies typically include a range of time points to characterize the temporal course and the levels of drug in the arterial wall (e.g., 0 to 3 days, 3 to 14 days, 14 to 28 days, and >28 days). Formulation "A" exemplifies a rapid drug uptake, quickly peaking and slowly declining over time. Formulation "B" is characterized by a slower initial uptake, a long plateau phase, and persistent retention. *DES*, Drug-eluting stent.

overall efficacy. The suppression of neointimal hyperplasia observed at 28 days is lost at 90 days; by 180 days, there is "catch-up," and the magnitude of neointimal proliferation is similar compared with BMS controls.[30,87] Preclinical work is focused on the identification of signs of vascular toxicity and overall biocompatibility. A specific set of standardized histologic parameters is used for this safety assessment, which takes into consideration the potential vascular effects of multiple variables beyond the metal stent scaffold. The goal of this assessment is to identify signs of vascular toxicity, delayed healing, and profound inhibition of vascular response through the qualitative scoring of aneurysm formation, medial smooth muscle cell loss, calcification, collagen, unresorbed fibrin, thrombus, and angiogenesis (Table 3-2).[56]

PRECLINICAL ASSESSMENT OF SIROLIMUS-ELUTING AND PACLITAXEL-ELUTING STENTS

The type of drug eluted and its release kinetics play a critical role in the overall safety and efficacy profile of a particular DES. Antiproliferative drugs with a wide therapeutic window and low vascular toxicity profiles are preferred to maximize the antirestenotic effect without promoting vascular injury. Two classes of antiproliferative agents are currently used in DES: the sirolimus analogues and paclitaxel. Sirolimus is a macrocyclic lactone that binds to specific cytosolic proteins called immunophilins and blocks cell cycle progression from the G_1 to S phases by inhibiting the activation of the target protein, mammalian target of rapamycin (mTOR). Paclitaxel exerts its biologic effects by inhibiting the formation of cellular microtubules. Paclitaxel is highly lipophilic, which promotes rapid cellular uptake, and as a result of structural alteration of the cytoskeleton, it has a long-lasting cellular effect.[88,89]

The Cypher sirolimus-eluting stent (Johnson & Johnson, Miami Lakes, Florida) used a nonabsorbable polymeric blend with an additional top coat to delay drug release over time. Pharmacokinetics studies performed in normal porcine coronary arteries showed that sirolimus tissue levels peaked at 10 to 14 days[30] and remained detectable 28 days after implantation; at this time point, approximately one third of the initial drug load could still be recovered from the stent surface.[87] Systemic levels of sirolimus were detectable within 1 hour after stent implantation and became undetectable after 72 hours. In comparison, Taxus (Boston Scientific, Natick, Massachusetts), a first-generation paclitaxel-eluting stent, displayed a very slow pattern of release from its nonabsorbable polymer, achieving therapeutic levels at 28 days. Because of its molecular characteristics, paclitaxel is less homogeneously distributed and retained deeper into the vessel layers than sirolimus. Less than 10% of the overall drug loaded onto the polymer is eventually released into tissue.[79]

Compared with BMS, both Cypher and Taxus stents demonstrated a decrease in neointimal formation and acute inflammatory response on histologic analysis at 28 days after stent implantation. However, at later time points there were increased inflammation, more fibrin deposition, and less endothelial strut coverage.[90] Although the overall vascular response to the two DES systems appeared grossly similar, each resulted in a specific biologic signature in porcine coronary arteries. With the Cypher stent, neointimal inhibition was accompanied by short-term deposition of fibrin adjacent to the stent struts.[30] Long-term histology showed resolution of these fibrin deposits but persistence of a chronic inflammatory response featuring giant cell accumulation. Although the Taxus stent displayed a similar pattern of neointimal formation compared with the Cypher stent, smooth muscle cell loss and peristrut fibrin deposits were the biologic hallmark of this delivery system.[86]

The vascular response to paclitaxel is dose dependent; higher paclitaxel dosing results in decreased neointimal thickness, evidence of

TABLE 3-2	Histologic Evaluation of Drug-Eluting Stents*				
	Qualitative Score				
	0	**1**	**2**	**3**	**4**
Aneurysmal formation	None	Partial disruption involving medial wall	Complete medial disruption with containment (intact EEL)	Complete disruption of arterial wall involving media and adventitia	—
Medial smooth muscle cell loss (depth and circumference)	None	Smooth muscle loss <25% of medial thickness	25%-50% of medial thickness	51%-75% of medial thickness	>75% of medial thickness
Calcifications	None	Focal, with <10% of region affected	Multifocal, with 10%-25% of region affected	Regionally with 26%-30% of region affected	Regionally diffuse, with >30% of region affected
Proteoglycan and collagen	None	<25% of area stains green-blue/yellow on Movat stain	25%-50% of area stains green-blue/yellow on Movat stain	51%-75% of area stains green-blue/yellow on Movat stain	>75% of area stains green-blue/yellow on Movat stain
Unresorbed fibrin, platelets, thrombus	None	Minimal, focal	Mild, multifocal	Moderate, regionally diffuse	Severe, marked diffuse or total luminal occlusion
Angiogenesis (location adventitial, medial, or neointimal)	None	Mild	Moderate	Severe	—

EEL, External elastic lamina.
*In addition to routine parameters evaluated in bare metal stents (see Table 3-1), the biologic mechanism of action of drug-eluting stents (i.e., a bioactive surface encompassing a carrier and the antiproliferative drug released over time) necessitates a detailed scrutiny of additional histologic features.

incomplete healing characterized by extensive fibrin and inflammatory cells, and local toxicity in the form of focal medial necrosis and intraintimal hemorrhage.[27] This preclinical finding appears to be associated with clinical outcomes and highlights the importance of a wide therapeutic window and the challenges of achieving an appropriate pharmacokinetic profile that maximizes neointimal suppression without promoting vascular toxicity. The QuaDS-QP stent (Quanam Medical, Santa Clara, California) was an early generation DES that eluted high-dose 7-hexanoyltaxol from multiple polyacrylate sleeves.[91] In patients treated for de novo lesions with this platform, a high rate of stent thrombosis and aneurysms was observed, thought to be a result of the toxic effect of the high-burst transfer of the paclitaxel analogue.[92]

Conversely, a DES platform that provided a precise and programmable delivery of paclitaxel (Conor Medsystems, Menlo Park, California)[93] was not noninferior compared with the paclitaxel-eluting Taxus stent in preventing restenosis in the Cobalt Chromium Stent with Antiproliferative for Restenosis (COSTAR) II trial, likely resulting from insufficient neointimal suppression with the particular pharmacokinetic elution profile selected (10 µg of paclitaxel over 30 days).[94]

NEWER GENERATION DRUG-ELUTING STENTS

Newer DES have been developed with the objective of improving overall healing but maintaining the clinical effect in reducing restenosis.[95-97] Incorporation of different metal alloys has allowed for reduced strut profiles to reduce vascular injury and foreign body reaction and enhance endothelialization.[28,29] More biocompatible nonabsorbable polymers have also been introduced.[98-100] In addition, bioabsorbable polymers and polymer-free systems are used in next-generation DES platforms.[32-34] Preclinical studies have shown that these changes have favorably affected the overall degree and time to resolution of peristrut inflammation, fibrin deposition, and healing compared with earlier generation DES platforms (Figure 3-7).[32,43,101]

DES platforms using everolimus and zotarolimus, sirolimus analogues, incorporate more biocompatible and thinner durable polymers that provide a similar total drug content and maintain a pharmacokinetics profile similar to the first-generation Cypher sirolimus-eluting stent.[102] The elution platform of the zotarolimus-eluting stent Endeavor (Medtronic, Santa Rosa, California) is a highly biocompatible phosphorylcholine coating. Preclinical data demonstrated that

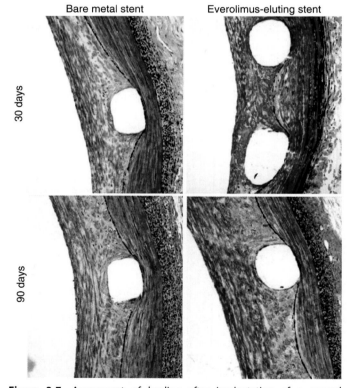

Bare metal stent   Everolimus-eluting stent

30 days

90 days

Figure 3-7 Assessment of healing after implantation of a second-generation DES. There is a lack of peristrut fibrin deposition at either time point in the bare metal stent *(left)* and resorption of fibrin between 30 and 90 days in the drug-eluting stent *(right).*

zotarolimus is released from this platform rapidly after stent implantation,[103] and subsequent clinical trials demonstrated less inhibition of neointimal proliferation compared with DES that elute sirolimus analogues.[104] In comparison, the zotarolimus-eluting Endeavor Resolute stent (Medtronic) uses a nonabsorbable highly compatible polymer (BioLinx) that results in sustained release (approximately 80% of the total dose by 60 days) comparable to other DES platforms. Clinical trials have demonstrated similar outcomes compared with everolimus-eluting stents.[105,106] These observations emphasize the importance of release kinetics, defined through preclinical testing, in determining biologic efficacy.

Bioresorbable Scaffolds and Bioabsorbable Stents

A bioresorbable scaffold further increases the complexity and volume of multidisciplinary research required to develop and validate a functional device (Figure 3-8). All the aspects to be addressed when developing a DES are still in place, now complicated by the fact that the entire scaffold is made of a material that is biochemically active over its entire life span within the arterial wall. The biochemical and mechanical properties of a bioresorbable scaffold change over time as a result of continuous biodegradation and resorption; these properties and their arterial responses may vary significantly among different materials and scaffold designs.[107] The ideal bioresorbable material must possess several characteristics, including adequate blood and tissue compatibility, durability to sustain the mechanical challenges of manufacturing (e.g., crimping), and ability to form an expandable scaffold to provide sufficient support to dilate plaque and resist acute recoil and chronic negative remodeling in addition to minimizing neointimal proliferation while the scaffold reabsorbs.[108] The structural material used by most bioresorbable scaffolds are polymers, in particular, different forms of polylactic acid. Bioresorbable metallic alloys have also been used; the most established body of evidence available is for magnesium.[109]

INITIAL BENCH TESTING

The tensile strengths and elongation breaking point of a scaffold made entirely from bioresorbable material are often much lower than those of traditional, bioinert stent metals, and so bioresorbable scaffolds must pass several durability tests. This is particularly challenging for polymers.[110] The scaffold must expand with adequate uniformity along its entire length and be devoid of regional deformation and underexpansion, both in isolation and against a simulated resistance of the arterial wall (often mimicked by a silicon tube). It must possess sufficient radial force and crush resistance, yet retain enough flexibility and plasticity not to break and fragment when being deployed against a lesion or suffer fatigue by thousands of motions.[108] The stresses resulting from cardiac contractions in the coronary territory differ from the stresses of the peripheral vessels, and the characteristics of the bioresorbable scaffold may need to be tuned to a specific vascular territory.[111] The durability of the scaffold is assessed through complex engineering tests that administer axial and perpendicular forces that stretch, flex, and crush the scaffolds akin to the stresses to which they will be exposed when implanted in the designated vascular territories. These tests are conducted in liquid baths at body temperature to simulate the moisture and temperature conditions in which the scaffold's inherent degradation occurs over time because the mechanical properties of the bioresorbable scaffold change as its molecular weight decreases through hydrolysis.

An ideal bioresorbable scaffold not only would acutely dilate the obstruction and sustain this result over time but also would allow for structural and functional remodeling of the treated segment.[112] Specifically, the compliance and vasoreactivity of the treated segment are expected to be restored eventually to those resembling a native artery without a stent.[113] For this reason, the intravascular use of a bioresorbable scaffold has been termed "vascular restoration therapy."[109] The optimal formula should result in a scaffold that retains its strength within the wall for long enough to withstand the forces of negative remodeling; when this mission to support the dilated vessel is fully accomplished, the scaffold should allow restoration of this arterial segment to a more natural shape, plasticity, and vasoreactivity.[108] Clinical experience indicates that the mechanical integrity of the scaffold should be retained for 6 to 9 months after implantation.[112] Clinical studies of magnesium bioresorbable stents demonstrated that any earlier loss of strength results in chronic recoil and negative remodeling.[114]

Difficulties in polymer production represent a major design challenge for bioresorbable scaffolds. Controlling the consistency of a complex polymeric material is harder than with metal. Different polymer batches even of theoretically identical chemical composition may possess subtle differences in purity and in the proportions of different components. These differences often translate into variability in the course of degradation, in terms of both the time frame of degradation and the array of by-products that are formed. This variability results in unpredictable changes in the mechanical properties of the resulting construct and in the biologic consequences of the scaffold degradation. In particular, the excessive release of oligomers resulting from overly rapid degradation can markedly aggravate the inflammatory and foreign body reaction that occurs after scaffold implantation within the artery. However, this variability in degradation also has potential design benefits. By adjusting the proportion of chains of different lengths or manipulating the relative proportion of different components of the multipolymer blend, the material can be individualized for specific performance needs and the desired time frame for bioabsorption.[110]

Another unique challenge resulting from the use of polymeric material instead of a metal is the way the scaffold deforms in response to regional external resistance, such as a hard eccentric lesion. With a biostable metallic stent, regional deformation has to be extreme to compromise other areas of the device, and application of higher inflation pressures (i.e., after dilation) can resolve such regional underexpansion because there is no concern that stent fracture will occur or that straightening one portion of the stent may unintentionally deform another portion. However, this is not the case for a bioresorbable scaffold, particularly a polymeric one; asymmetric loads are more likely to have severe consequences for a scaffold made from a less durable material than metal. Preclinical bench testing or use in animal models with a simulated hard eccentric lesion must simulate the consequences of atypical or uneven expansion.[115] The limits to which a scaffold can be pressurized and overexpanded beyond its nominal diameter are often narrower than those of conventional stents, and these must be defined for a particular scaffold before human application.

PRECLINICAL ANIMAL TESTING

When the scaffold's mechanical and biochemical properties are demonstrated to be consistent, satisfactory, and durable, preclinical animal testing can be considered. The methodologies used in animal testing of bioresorbable scaffolds resemble for the most part those used to

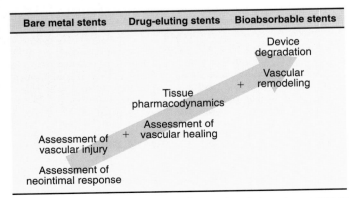

Figure 3-8 Evolution of endpoints and research techniques in response to the increasing complexity of stent technology.

validate DES. As for DES, the standard model for bioresorbable scaffold is the normal porcine artery, and the established histopathology techniques for DES are also the cornerstone for biocompatibility evaluation of bioresorbable scaffolds.[116] However, several aspects of this evaluation differ from DES as a result of the unique, dynamic nature of the bioresorbable scaffold. For example, with DES using durable polymers, the only component subject to pharmacokinetic evaluation is the drug, whereas the entire bioabsorbable scaffold is a chronically bioactive foreign body that acts as an indwelling long-term reservoir of bioactive substances and a source of metabolites released over time. The pharmacokinetics and pharmacodynamics of the scaffold material's biodegradation and bioabsorption are evaluated similarly to a depot form of a drug formulation. Scaffold degradation is studied by extracting treated arteries and performing histopathologic and biochemical analyses over sequential time points to assess the properties of the residual scaffold present in the arterial wall. Specifically, the molecular weight loss and scaffold mass loss over time are determined, and the levels and fate of intermediate and end metabolites are characterized to assess long-term safety. If the material is already well established in other biomedical applications (e.g., polylactic acid), some amount of this basic groundwork can be reduced, but the amount of predicate data that can be used depends on the particular scaffold and is generally limited because of the intraarterial application for the treatment of vascular disease.

Preclinical validation of bioresorbable scaffolds requires a long follow-up. The time point at which the maximum rate of mass loss occurs is scientifically and clinically relevant because it represents the inflection point when radial strength and structural continuity are lost, allowing the arterial segment to return to a more natural physiologic state[108]; this probably occurs before 12 months after implantation in the porcine model. However, a key aspect of bioresorbable scaffold validation is to define the time horizon when all scaffold residue is completely absorbed (full mass resorption) and when the scaffold is no longer metabolically active.[117] Preclinical studies characterizing this natural history of the bioresorbable scaffolds have required 3 to 4 years or more of follow-up.[109]

ENDOVASCULAR IMAGING VERSUS HISTOMORPHOMETRY

With metallic stents, endovascular imaging agrees well enough quantitatively with histomorphometry so as to serve as an acceptable surrogate of the latter.[118-120] However, with bioresorbable scaffolds, there is a marked discrepancy among quantitative measures of scaffold geometry and neointimal growth acquired through endovascular imaging and the corresponding morphometric parameters derived from histopathologic sections. This discrepancy has been reported to reach 83% to 100% in the case of strut thickness and strut void cross-sectional area.[121] In addition, there is a consistent exaggeration of lumen loss and stenosis by histomorphometry compared with endovascular imaging. A combination of factors is likely responsible for this disagreement. It is well documented in vessels without stenting that postmortem collapse of depressurized arterial segments results in significantly smaller dimensions on histomorphometry compared with in vivo. The arterial segments whose elasticity was restored by scaffold degradation may behave like an artery without a stent, and its collapse may not be fully compensated by pressurized fixation, resulting in marked alteration of select dimensions in histologic sections. Similarly, chemicals used in histopathologic processing (tissue fixation by formaldehyde, dehydration with ethanol, embedding and polymerization in methyl methacrylate, and subsequent deplasticization) may cause different dimensional changes depending on the composition and pH of the tissue and the temperature and concentration of the fixative.[122] The residual substances remaining in the spaces previously occupied by the scaffold struts are, in case of polylactic acid, highly water-containing acid mucopolysaccharides[109] and are likely susceptible to changes induced by this processing; this contributes to artifactual changes in histomorphometric parameters within the analyzed

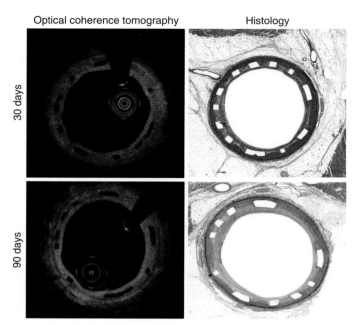

Optical coherence tomography   Histology

30 days

90 days

Figure 3-9   Bioabsorbable scaffold assessment in vivo by optical coherence tomography *(OCT) (left)* and corresponding histology sections *(right)*. OCT has become invaluable for bioabsorbable stent evaluation in vivo. The rectangular polymeric struts and bioabsorbable scaffolds allow light transmission, in contrast to the 100% light reflection from the metallic stents and resulting "blooming effect." Full strut thickness is visualized, rendering an unprecedented histology-like OCT image.

segment.[121] These issues have resulted in a paradigm shift in the preclinical evaluation of antirestenotic therapies; the application of histopathology for assessing bioresorbable scaffolds is confined to providing qualitative insights of biocompatibility, whereas endovascular imaging is indispensable in assessing the scaffold, neointima, and remodeling (Figure 3-9).

MEASURES OF EFFICACY FOR BIORESORBABLE SCAFFOLDS

In the naïve swine model, without interference from atherosclerosis or antiproliferative drug elution or both, bioresorbable polymer scaffolds are able to restore the ability of the treated segment to remodel outward and achieve a level transition between the caliber of the reference vessel and the scaffold-treated regions. This change over time in the ratio of the lumen area to reference vessel appears to be a phenomenon of vascular remodeling in response to the bioresorbable scaffold, which allows the treated segment and the adjacent proximal and distal host regions to establish a state of arterial homeostasis, a property augmented in the animal model, where arterial growth occurs.[123] A direct consequence of this property of bioresorbable scaffolds is that standard measures that rely on a consistent stent diameter over time, such as late loss, may be inaccurate for assessing restenosis and neointimal remodeling beyond the time point where bioresorbable stents lose mechanical strength. Metrics independent of acute gain, such as minimal luminal diameter and percentage diameter stenosis, may make better surrogates for restenosis.[124]

SPECIFIC BIORESORBABLE TECHNOLOGIES

Several bioresorbable scaffolds have undergone preclinical evaluation. Wiktor stents coated with five different types of biodegradable polymers all resulted in marked inflammation leading to neointimal hyperplasia or thrombus formation, or both, in porcine coronary arteries.[125] Subsequently, Lincoff and colleagues[126] demonstrated that in a porcine model a tantalum stent coated with high-molecular-weight (approximately 321 kDa) polylactic acid was well tolerated and effective, whereas a stent coated with low-molecular-weight (approximately 80 kDa) polylactic acid was associated with an intense inflammatory neointimal response. Feasibility of drug elution from the polylactic acid scaffold using dexamethasone was also demonstrated, although no suppression of neointimal hyperplasia was observed. In 1998, Yamawaki and coworkers[127] reported that in the porcine model the fully biodegradable polylactic acid stent with a tyrosine kinase inhibitor suppressed proliferative response caused by balloon injury. These pioneering experiments with high-molecular-weight polymer formulations culminated with the first human feasibility study of the Igaki-Tamai stent,[128] a coil stent made of polylactic acid monofilament. Several platforms now have substantial preclinical data and a growing body of clinical data.

ABSORB Bioresorbable Vascular Scaffold

The ABSORB Bioresorbable Vascular Scaffold (Abbott Laboratories, Abbott Park, Illinois) contains modified polylactic acid as the backbone material and in its clinical iteration elutes everolimus to inhibit neointimal proliferation. This device has accumulated the most substantial body of clinical evidence to date.[109] A landmark study correlated findings on intracoronary optical coherence tomography (OCT) with histology at 1 month and 2, 3, and 4 years after implantation of this device in a porcine coronary artery model.[129] The key finding was that struts that were still discernible by OCT at 2 years were compatible with largely bioresorbed struts as demonstrated by histologic and gel permeation chromatography analysis. At 3 and 4 years, both OCT and histology confirmed complete integration of the struts into the arterial wall. This study demonstrated that specific OCT findings of scaffold structures at different time points corresponded to specific histologic findings of the same structures. The study also demonstrated, through a preclinical animal experiment, that OCT is a reliable tool for monitoring the integration of bioabsorbable scaffold into the arterial wall. This study observed minimal inflammation on histopathology over very long-term follow-up. Chronic recoil was observed in the early clinical application of the first-generation ABSORB Bioresorbable Vascular Scaffold,[130] although this did not translate into excessive lumen loss and increased need for revascularization.[131] Nevertheless, a modified version was developed to improve the mechanical strength of the struts and reduce early and late recoil. First, this version has a new platform design with more uniform strut distribution and reduced maximum circular unsupported surface area, providing more uniform vessel wall support and drug transfer. Second, a modified manufacturing process ensures a slower hydrolysis (i.e., degradation) rate of the polymer, preserving mechanical integrity for a longer time period. Both of these modifications also provide increased radial strength and improved retention while the material and strut thickness remain unchanged.[109,132] These technologic changes resulted in favorable preclinical results, and a small clinical study demonstrated the restoration of pharmacologic vasomotion and no scaffold area loss at 12-month follow-up.[133]

Bioresorbable Magnesium Alloy Stent

The absorbable metallic stent (AMS-1; BIOTRONIK, Berlin, Germany) is a metallic biodegradable stent composed of 93% magnesium and 7% rare earth metals. In the porcine model, the AMS-1 has been shown to be rapidly endothelialized, and it is largely degraded into inorganic salts within 60 days with little associated inflammatory response.[134] Similar to observations with the first-generation ABSORB Bioresorbable Vascular Scaffold, in the first-in-man clinical trials of AMS-1, there was greater-than-expected chronic recoil not clearly predictable from preclinical testing. In the initial animal study, early recoil was noted at 10 days and 35 days, but at the longest follow-up of 56 days, positive remodeling was reported.[135] A subsequent study that examined this scaffold compared with BMS at 90 days after implantation did not identify negative remodeling as a serious issue.[134] The available preclinical information did not herald the excessive chronic recoil and subsequent significant lumen loss observed in human atherosclerotic vessels. A subsequent study published after the Clinical Performance Angiographic Results of Coronary Stenting with Absorbable Metal Stents (PROGRESS-AMS) clinical trial observed negative remodeling and late lumen loss at 90 days.[136] In retrospect, this first-generation device was probably programmed to degrade too rapidly to resist adequately the forces of negative remodeling occurring months after implantation. A redesign of the alloy and the scaffold extended the degradation time, mechanically strengthening the device for a more prolonged period, and eluted paclitaxel to suppress neointimal proliferation.[137] This second-generation device was tested in the BIOTRONIKS-Safety and Clinical Performance Of the First Drug-Eluting Generation Absorbable Metal Stent In Patients With de Novo Lesions in NatiVE Coronary Arteries (BIOSOLVE-I) study, which demonstrated reduced in-scaffolding diameter loss and on-scaffold neointimal hyperplasia compared with that observed in the PROGRESS-AMS trial.[138]

ReZolve Sirolimus-Eluting Bioresorbable Coronary Scaffold

The ReZolve Sirolimus-Eluting Bioresorbable Coronary Scaffold (REVA Medical, San Diego, California) consists of tyrosine-derived polycarbonate, which possesses several unique characteristics. The in vivo degradation rate of the polymer can be varied by changing the ratio of the esterized form to the nonesterized form of the monomer. The polymer can be iodinated and made radiopaque, in contrast to other bioresorbable polymeric scaffolds. The polymer can also serve as a stand-alone drug reservoir or act as a drug-eluting coating on a metallic surface. The scaffold is a balloon expandable design but also entails a slide-and-lock mechanism ratcheting the scaffold elements in an open position when the desired diameter is reached. As opposed to a conventional closed cell design that is prone to recoil when made from biodegradable polymer, this scaffold maintains its radial force through its structure, rather than the characteristic of the material itself. This design also permits a wide expansion range for a single diameter scaffold.[139]

The first generation of the ReZolve Sirolimus-Eluting Bioresorbable Coronary Scaffold has shown excellent biocompatibility in preclinical studies with more than 4 years of follow-up. In the porcine coronary model, the first-generation scaffold allowed restoration of the ability of the treated segment to remodel outward to achieve level lumen transition between the reference vessel and scaffold-treated regions, a process mediated by animal growth and scaffold degradation and consistently demonstrable over long-term follow-up.[123] The initial scaffold was redesigned after a first-in-man study with a non–drug-eluting device demonstrated a restenosis rate higher than desired. The polymer was refined to enhance its durability, and the slide-and-lock design, although retained in principle, was revised to reduce its thickness and minimize the segmented nature of the scaffold, while increasing the resistance to external forces. This second-generation design elutes sirolimus to reduce neointimal hyperplasia. After having cleared bench and animal studies, the ReZolve Sirolimus-Eluting Bioresorbable Coronary Scaffold at the present time is entering early clinical trials in the Safety Study of a Bioresorbable Coronary Stent (RESTORE) (clinicaltrials.gov identifier NCT01262703).[140]

Conclusion

The normal porcine model is the foundation of the preclinical assessment of BMS for the coronary arteries. The interdependence of vascular injury, inflammation, and neointimal hyperplasia and the consistent time course of these processes after implantation have enabled the standardization of stent assessment. This assessment includes qualitative scoring of injury and inflammation and semiquantitative, histomorphometric analyses of luminal area, diameter, neointimal thickness, and percent stenosis. DES validation is complicated by the addition of drug and polymer carrier, both of which are bioactive and whose effects change over time. Testing of the individual elements and the platform as a whole is required. The antirestenotic efficacy and the safety of DES critically depend on the pharmacokinetics of drug elution and the therapeutic window of the antiproliferative agent. Animal models of DES focus on the assessment of safety, using qualitative histologic scoring at various time points after implantation. Each class of DES displays a specific biologic signature on histology. Validation of bioresorbable scaffolds is even more complex because the entire scaffold is made of a material biochemically active over its entire life span within the arterial wall, and the mechanical characteristics of the scaffold are dynamic as it degrades over time. Endovascular imaging with OCT plays a more important role in the validation of bioresorbable platforms compared with BMS or DES. The challenges in validating the safety and efficacy of the bioresorbable scaffold and the development of porcine models displaying atherosclerosis herald a new chapter in the preclinical assessment of stents.

REFERENCES

1. Serruys PW, de Jaegere P, Kiemeneij F, et al. A comparison of balloon-expandable-stent implantation with balloon angioplasty in patients with coronary artery disease. Benestent Study Group. *N Engl J Med* 1994;331:489-495.
2. Tenaglia AN, Fortin DF, Califf RM, et al. Predicting the risk of abrupt vessel closure after angioplasty in an individual patient. *J Am Coll Cardiol* 1994;24:1004-1011.
3. Lincoff AM, Popma JJ, Ellis SG, et al. Abrupt vessel closure complicating coronary angioplasty: clinical, angiographic and therapeutic profile. *J Am Coll Cardiol* 1992;19:926-935.
4. Post MJ, Borst C, Kuntz RE. The relative importance of arterial remodeling compared with intimal hyperplasia in lumen renarrowing after balloon angioplasty: a study in the normal rabbit and the hypercholesterolemic Yucatan micropig. *Circulation* 1994;89:2816-2821.
5. Strauss BH, Chisholm RJ, Keeley FW, et al. Extracellular matrix remodeling after balloon angioplasty injury in a rabbit model of restenosis. *Circ Res* 1994;75:650-658.
6. Gertz SD, Gimple LW, Banai S, et al. Geometric remodeling is not the principal pathogenetic process in restenosis after balloon angioplasty: evidence from correlative angiographic-histomorphometric studies of atherosclerotic arteries in rabbits. *Circulation* 1994;90:3001-3008.
7. Dotter CT. Transluminally-placed coilspring endarterial tube grafts: long-term patency in canine popliteal artery. *Invest Radiol* 1969;4:329-332.
8. Dotter CT, Buschmann RW, McKinney MK, et al. Transluminal expandable nitinol coil stent grafting: preliminary report. *Radiology* 1983;147:259-260.
9. Cragg A, Lund G, Rysavy J, et al. Nonsurgical placement of arterial endoprostheses: a new technique using nitinol wire. *Radiology* 1983;147:261-263.
10. Sugita Y, Shimomitsu T, Oku T, et al. Nonsurgical implantation of a vascular ring prosthesis using thermal shape memory Ti/Ni alloy (Nitinol wire). *ASAIO Trans* 1986;32:30-34.
11. Maass D, Zollikofer CL, Largiader F, et al. Radiological follow-up of transluminally inserted vascular endoprostheses: an experimental study using expanding spirals. *Radiology* 1984;152:659-663.
12. Wright KC, Wallace S, Charnsangavej C, et al. Percutaneous endovascular stents: an experimental evaluation. *Radiology* 1985;156:69-72.
13. Palmaz JC, Sibbitt RR, Reuter SR, et al. Expandable intraluminal graft: a preliminary study. Work in progress. *Radiology* 1985;156:73-77.
14. Sigwart U, Puel J, Mirkovitch V, et al. Intravascular stents to prevent occlusion and restenosis after transluminal angioplasty. *N Engl J Med* 1987;316:701-706.
15. Roubin GS, Robinson KA, King 3rd SB, et al. Early and late results of intracoronary arterial stenting after coronary angioplasty in dogs. *Circulation* 1987;76:891-897.
16. Granada JF, Kaluza GL, Wilensky RL, et al. Porcine models of coronary atherosclerosis and vulnerable plaque for imaging and interventional research. *EuroIntervention* 2009;5:140-148.
17. Schook L, Beattie C, Beever J, et al. Swine in biomedical research: creating the building blocks of animal models. *Anim Biotechnol* 2005;16:183-190.
18. de Smet BJ, van der Zande J, van der Helm YJ, et al. The atherosclerotic Yucatan animal model to study the arterial response after balloon angioplasty: the natural history of remodeling. *Cardiovasc Res* 1998;39:224-232.
19. Suzuki Y, Yeung AC, Ikeno F. The representative porcine model for human cardiovascular disease. *J Biomed Biotechnol* 2011; 2011:195483.
20. Bollen PJA. *The Laboratory Swine*. Boca Raton: CRC Press; 1999.
21. Hughes GC, Post MJ, Simons M, et al. Translational physiology: porcine models of human coronary artery disease: implications for preclinical trials of therapeutic angiogenesis. *J Appl Physiol* 2003;94:1689-1701.
22. Crick SJ, Sheppard MN, Anderson RH, et al. A quantitative study of nerve distribution in the conduction system of the guinea pig heart. *J Anat* 1996;188(Pt 2):403-416.
23. Swindle MM, Horneffer PJ, Gardner TJ, et al. Anatomic and anesthetic considerations in experimental cardiopulmonary surgery in swine. *Lab Anim Sci* 1986;36:357-361.
24. Nakazawa G, Finn AV, Ladich E, et al. Drug-eluting stent safety: findings from preclinical studies. *Expert Rev Cardiovasc Ther* 2008;6:1379-1391.
25. Edelman ER, Rogers C. Pathobiologic responses to stenting. *Am J Cardiol* 1998;81:4E-6E.
26. Rogers C, Welt FG, Karnovsky MJ, et al. Monocyte recruitment and neointimal hyperplasia in rabbits: coupled inhibitory effects of heparin. *Arterioscler Thromb Vasc Biol* 1996;16: 1312-1318.
27. Farb A, Heller PF, Shroff S, et al. Pathological analysis of local delivery of paclitaxel via a polymer-coated stent. *Circulation* 2001;104:473-479.
28. Jabara R, Geva S, Ribeiro HB, et al. A third generation ultra-thin strut cobalt chromium stent: histopathological evaluation in porcine coronary arteries. *EuroIntervention* 2009;5:619-626.
29. Wilson GJ, Huibregtse BA, Stejskal EA, et al. Vascular response to a third generation everolimus-eluting stent. *EuroIntervention* 2010;6:512-519.
30. Suzuki T, Kopia G, Hayashi S, et al. Stent-based delivery of sirolimus reduces neointimal formation in a porcine coronary model. *Circulation* 2001;104:1188-1193.
31. Joner M, Nakazawa G, Finn AV, et al. Endothelial cell recovery between comparator polymer-based drug-eluting stents. *J Am Coll Cardiol* 2008;52:333-342.
32. Nakazawa G, Nakano M, Otsuka F, et al. Evaluation of polymer-based comparator drug-eluting stents using a rabbit model of iliac artery atherosclerosis. *Circ Cardiovasc Interv* 2011;4:38-46.
33. Koppara T, Joner M, Bayer G, et al. Histopathological comparison of biodegradable polymer and permanent polymer based sirolimus eluting stents in a porcine model of coronary stent implantation. *Thromb Haemost* 2012;107:161-171.
34. Abizaid A, Costa Jr JR. New drug-eluting stents: an overview on biodegradable and polymer-free next-generation stent systems. *Circ Cardiovasc Interv* 2010;3:384-393.
35. Gerrity RG, Naito HK, Richardson M, et al. Dietary induced atherogenesis in swine: morphology of the intima in prelesion stages. *Am J Pathol* 1979;95:775-792.
36. Grinstead WC, Rodgers GP, Mazur W, et al. Comparison of three porcine restenosis models: the relative importance of hypercholesterolemia, endothelial abrasion, and stenting. *Coron Artery Dis* 1994;5:425-434.
37. Gerrity RG, Natarajan R, Nadler JL, et al. Diabetes-induced accelerated atherosclerosis in swine. *Diabetes* 2001;50: 1654-1665.
38. Llano R, Winsor-Hines D, Patel DB, et al. Vascular responses to drug-eluting and bare-metal stents in diabetic/hypercholesterolemic and nonatherosclerotic porcine coronary arteries. *Circ Cardiovasc Interv* 2011;4:438-446.
39. Prescott MF, Hasler-Rapacz J, von Linden-Reed J, et al. Familial hypercholesterolemia associated with coronary atherosclerosis in swine bearing different alleles for apolipoprotein B. *Ann N Y Acad Sci* 1995;748:283-292; discussion 292-293.
40. Hasler-Rapacz J, Ellegren H, Fridolfsson AK, et al. Identification of a mutation in the low density lipoprotein receptor gene associated with recessive familial hypercholesterolemia in swine. *Am J Med Genet* 1998;76:379-386.
41. Prescott MF, McBride CH, Hasler-Rapacz J, et al. Development of complex atherosclerotic lesions in pigs with inherited hyper-LDL cholesterolemia bearing mutant alleles for apolipoprotein B. *Am J Pathol* 1991;139:139-147.
42. Tellez A, Krueger CG, Seifert P, et al. Coronary bare-metal stent implantation in homozygous LDL receptor deficient swine induces a neointimal formation pattern similar to humans. *Atherosclerosis* 2010;213:518-524.
43. Huibregtse BA, Tellez A, Seifert P, et al. Differential neointimal response to the implantation of coronary bare metal and everolimus eluting stents in a familial hypercholesterolemic swine. *J Am Coll Cardiol* 2010;56:B53.
44. Milewski K, Afari ME, Tellez A, et al. Evaluation of efficacy and dose response of different paclitaxel-coated balloon formulations in a novel swine model of iliofemoral in-stent restenosis. *J Am Coll Cardiol Interv* 2012;5:1081-1088.
45. Schwartz RS, Murphy JG, Edwards WD, et al. Restenosis after balloon angioplasty: a practical proliferative model in porcine coronary arteries. *Circulation* 1990;82:2190-2200.
46. Shimokawa H, Tomoike H, Nabeyama S, et al. Coronary artery spasm induced in miniature swine: angiographic evidence and relation to coronary atherosclerosis. *Am Heart J* 1985;110: 300-310.
47. Shimokawa H, Tomoike H, Nabeyama S, et al. Coronary artery spasm induced in atherosclerotic miniature swine. *Science* 1983;221:560-562.
48. van der Giessen WJ, Serruys PW, van Beusekom HM, et al. Coronary stenting with a new, radiopaque, balloon-expandable endoprosthesis in pigs. *Circulation* 1991;83:1788-1798.
49. Schwartz RS, Huber KC, Murphy JG, et al. Restenosis and the proportional neointimal response to coronary artery injury: results in a porcine model. *J Am Coll Cardiol* 1992;19: 267-274.
50. Karas SP, Gravanis MB, Santoian EC, et al. Coronary intimal proliferation after balloon injury and stenting in swine: an animal model of restenosis. *J Am Coll Cardiol* 1992;20: 467-474.
51. Garratt KN, Holmes Jr DR, Bell MR, et al. Restenosis after directional coronary atherectomy: differences between primary atheromatous and restenosis lesions and influence of subintimal tissue resection. *J Am Coll Cardiol* 1990;16: 1665-1671.
52. Kornowski R, Hong MK, Tio FO, et al. In-stent restenosis: contributions of inflammatory responses and arterial injury to neointimal hyperplasia. *J Am Coll Cardiol* 1998;31: 224-230.
53. Carter AJ, Laird JR, Farb A, et al. Morphologic characteristics of lesion formation and time course of smooth muscle cell proliferation in a porcine proliferative restenosis model. *J Am Coll Cardiol* 1994;24:1398-1405.
53a. Miller DD, Karim MA, Edwards WD, et al. Relationship of vascular thrombosis and inflammatory leukocyte infiltration to neointimal growth following porcine coronary artery stent placement. *Atherosclerosis* 1996;124:145-155.
54. van Beusekom HM, Serruys PW, van der Giessen WJ. Coronary stent coatings. *Coron Artery Dis* 1994;5:590-596.
55. US Food and Drug Administration. *Guidance for Industry: Coronary Drug-Eluting Stents—Nonclinical and Clinical Studies*. Rockville, MD: FDA; 2008.
56. Schwartz RS, Edelman ER, Carter A, et al. Drug-eluting stents in preclinical studies: recommended evaluation from a consensus group. *Circulation* 2002;106:1867-1873.
57. Gravanis MB, Roubin GS. Histopathologic phenomena at the site of percutaneous transluminal coronary angioplasty: the problem of restenosis. *Hum Pathol* 1989;20:477-485.
58. Schwartz RS, Chronos NA, Virmani R. Preclinical restenosis models and drug-eluting stents: still important, still much to learn. *J Am Coll Cardiol* 2004;44:1373-1385.
59. Schwartz RS, Edelman E, Virmani R, et al. Drug-eluting stents in preclinical studies: updated consensus recommendations for preclinical evaluation. *Circ Cardiovasc Interv* 2008;1: 143-153.
60. Brower V. Stents and biology combination for restenosis. *Nat Biotechnol* 1996;14:422.
61. Kirtane AJ, Gupta A, Iyengar S, et al. Safety and efficacy of drug-eluting and bare-metal stents: comprehensive meta-analysis of randomized trials and observational studies. *Circulation* 2009;119:3198-3206.
62. Nakazawa G, Vorpahl M, Finn AV, et al. One step forward and two steps back with drug-eluting-stents: from preventing restenosis to causing late thrombosis and nouveau atherosclerosis. *JACC Cardiovasc Imaging* 2009;2:625-628.
63. Finn AV, Nakazawa G, Joner M, et al. Vascular responses to drug eluting stents: importance of delayed healing. *Arterioscler Thromb Vasc Biol* 2007;27:1500-1510.
64. Azrin MA, Mitchell JF, Bow LM, et al. Effect of local delivery of heparin on platelet deposition during in-vivo balloon angioplasty using hydrogel-coated balloons. *Circulation* 1993;88: I-310.
65. Mitchel JF, Fram DB, Palme 2nd DF, et al. Enhanced intracoronary thrombolysis with urokinase using a novel, local drug delivery system: in vitro, in vivo, and clinical studies. *Circulation* 1995;91:785-793.
66. Fernandez-Ortiz AM, Meyer BJ, Mailhac A, et al. Intravascular local delivery: an iontophoretic approach. *Circulation* 1993; 88:308.
67. Wolinsky H, Thung SN. Use of a perforated balloon catheter to deliver concentrated heparin into the wall of the normal canine artery. *J Am Coll Cardiol* 1990;15:475-481.
68. Lovich MA, Edelman ER. Tissue average binding and equilibrium distribution: an example with heparin in arterial tissues. *Biophys J* 1996;70:1553-1559.
69. Fernández-Ortiz A, Meyer BJ, Mailhac A, et al. A new approach for local intravascular drug delivery: iontophoretic balloon. *Circulation* 1994;89:1518-1522.
70. Langer R. New methods of drug delivery. *Science* 1990;249: 1527-1533.
71. Agrawal CM, Haas KF, Leopold DA, et al. Evaluation of poly(L-lactic acid) as a material for intravascular polymeric stents. *Biomaterials* 1992;13:176-182.

72. Murphy JG, Schwartz RS, Edwards WD, et al. Percutaneous polymeric stents in porcine coronary arteries: initial experience with polyethylene terephthalate stents. *Circulation* 1992;86: 1596-1604.

73. Lincoff AM, can der Giessen WJ, Schwartz RS, et al. Biodegradable and biostable polymers may both cause vigorous inflammatory responses when implanted in the porcine coronary artery. *J Am Coll Cardiol* 1993;21:179A.

74. Zidar JP, Lincoff AM, Stack RS, Topol EJ, et al, eds. *Textbook of Interventional Cardiology*. 2nd ed. Philadelphia: Saunders; 1993.

75. Wilson GJ, Nakazawa G, Schwartz RS, et al. Comparison of inflammatory response after implantation of sirolimus- and paclitaxel-eluting stents in porcine coronary arteries. *Circulation* 2009;120:141-149.

76. Wilson GJ, Polovick JE, Huibregtse BA, et al. Overlapping paclitaxel-eluting stents: long-term effects in a porcine coronary artery model. *Cardiovasc Res* 2007;76:361-372.

77. Popma JJ, Califf RM, Topol EJ. Clinical trials of restenosis after coronary angioplasty. *Circulation* 1991;84:1426-1436.

78. Muller DW, Ellis SG, Topol EJ. Experimental models of coronary artery restenosis. *J Am Coll Cardiol* 1992;19:418-432.

79. Creel CJ, Lovich MA, Edelman ER. Arterial paclitaxel distribution and deposition. *Circ Res* 2000;86:879-884.

80. Hwang CW, Wu D, Edelman ER. Physiological transport forces govern drug distribution for stent-based delivery. *Circulation* 2001;104:600-605.

81. Hwang CW, Levin AD, Jonas M, et al. Thrombosis modulates arterial drug distribution for drug-eluting stents. *Circulation* 2005;111:1619-1626.

82. US Food and Drug Administration. *Guidance for Industry: Bioanalytical Method Validation*. Rockville, MD: FDA; 2001.

83. Volosov A, Napoli KL, Soldin SJ. Simultaneous simple and fast quantification of three major immunosuppressants by liquid chromatography—tandem mass-spectrometry. *Clin Biochem* 2001;34:285-290.

84. Streit F, Armstrong VW, Oellerich M. Rapid liquid chromatography-tandem mass spectrometry routine method for simultaneous determination of sirolimus, everolimus, tacrolimus, and cyclosporin A in whole blood. *Clin Chem* 2002;48: 955-958.

85. Zhang J, Reimer MT, Ji QC, et al. Accurate determination of an immunosuppressant in stented swine tissues with LC-MS/MS. *Anal Bioanal Chem* 2007;387:2745-2756.

86. Virmani R, Farb A, Kolodgie FD. Histopathologic alterations after endovascular radiation and antiproliferative stents: similarities and differences. *Herz* 2002;27:1-6.

87. Klugherz BD, Llanos G, Lieuallen W, et al. Twenty-eight-day efficacy and pharmacokinetics of the sirolimus-eluting stent. *Coron Artery Dis* 2003;13:183-188.

88. Axel DI, Kunert W, Goggelmann C, et al. Paclitaxel inhibits arterial smooth muscle cell proliferation and migration in vitro and in vivo using local drug delivery. *Circulation* 1997;96: 636-645.

89. Herdeg C, Oberhoff M, Baumbach A, et al. Local paclitaxel delivery for the prevention of restenosis: biological effects and efficacy in vivo. *J Am Coll Cardiol* 2000;35:1969-1976.

90. Parry TJ, Brosius R, Thyagarajan R, et al. Drug-eluting stents: sirolimus and paclitaxel differentially affect cultured cells and injured arteries. *Eur J Pharmacol* 2005;524:19-29.

91. Honda Y, Grube E, de La Fuente LM, et al. Novel drug-delivery stent: intravascular ultrasound observations from the first human experience with the QP2-eluting polymer stent system. *Circulation* 2001;104:380-383.

92. Liistro F, Stankovic G, Di Mario C, et al. First clinical experience with a paclitaxel derivate-eluting polymer stent system implantation for in-stent restenosis: immediate and long-term clinical and angiographic outcome. *Circulation* 2002;105:1883-1886.

93. Finkelstein A, McClean D, Kar S, et al. Local drug delivery via a coronary stent with programmable release pharmacokinetics. *Circulation* 2003;107:777-784.

94. Krucoff MW, Kereiakes DJ, Petersen JL, et al. A novel bioresorbable polymer paclitaxel-eluting stent for the treatment of single and multivessel coronary disease: primary results of the COSTAR (Cobalt Chromium Stent with Antiproliferative for Restenosis) II study. *J Am Coll Cardiol* 2008;51:1543-1552.

95. Stone GW, Ellis SG, Cox DA, et al. A polymer-based, paclitaxel-eluting stent in patients with coronary artery disease. *N Engl J Med* 2004;350:221-231.

96. Joner M, Finn AV, Farb A, et al. Pathology of drug-eluting stents in humans: delayed healing and late thrombotic risk. *J Am Coll Cardiol* 2006;48:193-202.

97. Moses JW, Leon MB, Popma JJ, et al. Sirolimus-eluting stents versus standard stents in patients with stenosis in a native coronary artery. *N Engl J Med* 2003;349:1315-1323.

98. Grube E, Buellesfeld L. BioMatrix Biolimus A9-eluting coronary stent: a next-generation drug-eluting stent for coronary artery disease. *Expert Rev Med Devices* 2006;3: 731-741.

99. Carter AJ, Brodeur A, Collingwood R, et al. Experimental efficacy of an everolimus eluting cobalt chromium stent. *Catheter Cardiovasc Interv* 2006;68:97-103.

100. Yan J, Bhat VD. Elixir Medical's bioresorbable drug eluting stent (BDES) programme: an overview. *EuroIntervention* 2009;5(Suppl F):F80-F82.

101. Nakazawa G, Finn AV, John MC, et al. The significance of preclinical evaluation of sirolimus-, paclitaxel-, and zotarolimus-eluting stents. *Am J Cardiol* 2007;100:36M-44M.

102. Kirchner GI, Meier-Wiedenbach I, Manns MP. Clinical pharmacokinetics of everolimus. *Clin Pharmacokinet* 2004;43: 83-95.

103. Carter A, Melder RJ, Udipl K, et al. *In vivo performance of a novel co-polymer system for extended release of zotarolimus in a next generation drug eluting stent.* Presented at Transcatheter Cardiovascular Therapeutics Annual Meeting, Washington, DC; 2006.

104. Stankovic G, Cosgrave J, Chieffo A, et al. Impact of sirolimus-eluting and paclitaxel-eluting stents on outcome in patients with diabetes mellitus and stenting in more than one coronary artery. *Am J Cardiol* 2006;98:362-366.

105. Silber S, Windecker S, Vranckx P, et al. Unrestricted randomised use of two new generation drug-eluting coronary stents: 2-year patient-related versus stent-related outcomes from the RESOLUTE All Comers trial. *Lancet* 2011;377: 1241-1247.

106. von Birgelen C, Basalus MW, Tandjung K, et al. A randomized controlled trial in second-generation zotarolimus-eluting Resolute stents versus everolimus-eluting Xience V stents in real-world patients: the TWENTE trial. *J Am Coll Cardiol* 2012; 59:1350-1361.

107. Zilberman M, Eberhart RC. Drug-eluting bioresorbable stents for various applications. *Annu Rev Biomed Eng* 2006;8: 153-180.

108. Oberhauser JP, Hossainy S, Rapoza RJ. Design principles and performance of bioresorbable polymeric coronary scaffolds. *EuroIntervention* 2009;5(Suppl F):F15-22.

109. Onuma Y, Serruys PW. Bioresorbable scaffold: the advent of a new era in percutaneous coronary and peripheral revascularization? *Circulation* 2011;123:779-797.

110. Vert M. Bioabsorbable polymers in medicine: an overview. *EuroIntervention* 2009;5(Suppl F):F9-F14.

111. Berglund J, Guo Y, Wilcox JN. Challenges related to development of bioabsorbable vascular stents. *EuroIntervention* 2009;5(Suppl F):F72-F79.

112. Ormiston JA, Serruys PW. Bioabsorbable coronary stents. *Circ Cardiovasc Interv* 2009;2:255-260.

113. Sarno G, Bruining N, Onuma Y, et al. Morphological and functional evaluation of the bioresorption of the bioresorbable everolimus-eluting vascular scaffold using IVUS, echogenicity and vasomotion testing at two year follow-up: a patient level insight into the ABSORB A clinical trial. *Int J Cardiovasc Imaging* 2012;28:51-58.

114. Erbel R, Di Mario C, Bartunek J, et al. Temporary scaffolding of coronary arteries with bioabsorbable magnesium stents: a prospective, non-randomised multicentre trial. *Lancet* 2007; 369:1869-1875.

115. Tellez A, Granada JF, Milewski KP, et al. Utility of a porcine in-vivo calcified high-grade arterial stenosis model in testing acute and chronic mechanical performance of metal and bioresorbable stents. *Am J Cardiol* 2009;104:185D.

116. Vorpahl M, Finn AV, Nakano M, et al. The bioabsorption process: tissue and cellular mechanisms and outcomes. *EuroIntervention* 2009;5(Suppl F):F28-F35.

117. Waksman R, Pakala R. Coating bioabsorption and chronic bare metal scaffolding versus fully bioabsorbable stent. *EuroIntervention* 2009;5(Suppl F):F36-F42.

118. Angiolillo DJ, Capranzano P, Goto S, et al. A randomized study assessing the impact of cilostazol on platelet function profiles in patients with diabetes mellitus and coronary artery disease on dual antiplatelet therapy: results of the OPTIMUS-2 study. *Eur Heart J* 2008;29:2202-2211.

119. Murata A, Wallace-Bradley D, Tellez A, et al. Accuracy of optical coherence tomography in the evaluation of neointimal coverage after stent implantation. *JACC Cardiovasc Imaging* 2010;3:76-84.

120. Templin C, Meyer M, Muller MF, et al. Coronary optical frequency domain imaging (OFDI) for in vivo evaluation of stent healing: comparison with light and electron microscopy. *Eur Heart J* 2010;31:1792-1801.

121. Gogas BD, Radu M, Onuma Y, et al. Evaluation with in vivo optical coherence tomography and histology of the vascular effects of the everolimus-eluting bioresorbable vascular scaffold at two years following implantation in a healthy porcine coronary artery model: implications of pilot results for future pre-clinical studies. *Int J Cardiovasc Imaging* 2012;28: 499-511.

122. Bahr GF, Bloom G, Friberg U. Volume changes of tissues in physiological fluids during fixation in osmium tetroxide or formaldehyde and during subsequent treatment. *Exp Cell Res* 1957;12:342-355.

123. Strandberg E, Zeltinger J, Schulz DG, et al. Late positive remodeling and late lumen gain contribute to vascular restoration by a non-drug eluting bioresorbable scaffold: a four-year intravascular ultrasound study in normal porcine coronary arteries. *Circ Cardiovasc Interv* 2012;5:39-46.

124. Bangalore S, Mauri L. Late loss in a disappearing frame of reference: is it still applicable to fully absorbable scaffolds? *EuroIntervention* 2009;5(Suppl F):F43-F48.

125. van der Giessen WJ, Lincoff AM, Schwartz RS, et al. Marked inflammatory sequelae to implantation of biodegradable and nonbiodegradable polymers in porcine coronary arteries. *Circulation* 1996;94:1690-1697.

126. Lincoff AM, Furst JG, Ellis SG, et al. Sustained local delivery of dexamethasone by a novel intravascular eluting stent to prevent restenosis in the porcine coronary injury model. *J Am Coll Cardiol* 1997;29:808-816.

127. Yamawaki T, Shimokawa H, Kozai T, et al. Intramural delivery of a specific tyrosine kinase inhibitor with biodegradable stent suppresses the restenotic changes of the coronary artery in pigs in vivo. *J Am Coll Cardiol* 1998;32:780-786.

128. Tamai H, Igaki K, Kyo E, et al. Initial and 6-month results of biodegradable poly-l-lactic acid coronary stents in humans. *Circulation* 2000;102:399-404.

129. Onuma Y, Serruys PW, Perkins LEL, et al. Intracoronary optical coherence tomography and histology at 1 month and 2, 3, and 4 years after implantation of everolimus-eluting bioresorbable vascular scaffolds in a porcine coronary artery model: an attempt to decipher the human optical coherence tomography images in the ABSORB trial. *Circulation* 2010;122: 2288-2300.

130. Tanimoto S, Bruining N, van Domburg RT, et al. Late stent recoil of the bioabsorbable everolimus-eluting coronary stent and its relationship with plaque morphology. *J Am Coll Cardiol* 2008;52:1616-1620.

131. Ormiston JA, Serruys PW, Regar E, et al. A bioabsorbable everolimus-eluting coronary stent system for patients with single de-novo coronary artery lesions (ABSORB): a prospective open-label trial. *Lancet* 2008;371:899-907.

132. Onuma Y, Piazza N, Ormiston JA, et al. Everolimus-eluting bioabsorbable stent—Abbot Vascular programme. *EuroIntervention* 2009;5(Suppl F):F98-F102.

133. Serruys PW, Onuma Y, Dudek D, et al. Evaluation of the second generation of a bioresorbable everolimus-eluting vascular scaffold for the treatment of de novo coronary artery stenosis: 12-month clinical and imaging outcomes. *J Am Coll Cardiol* 2011;58:1578-1588.

134. Waksman R, Pakala R, Kuchulakanti PK, et al. Safety and efficacy of bioabsorbable magnesium alloy stents in porcine coronary arteries. *Catheter Cardiovasc Interv* 2006;68:607-617; discussion 618-619.

135. Heublein B, Rohde R, Kaese V, et al. Biocorrosion of magnesium alloys: a new principle in cardiovascular implant technology? *Heart* 2003;89:651-656.

136. Maeng M, Jensen LO, Falk E, et al. Negative vascular remodelling after implantation of bioabsorbable magnesium alloy stents in porcine coronary arteries: a randomised comparison with bare-metal and sirolimus-eluting stents. *Heart* 2009;95: 241-246.

137. Waksman R. Current state of the absorbable metallic (magnesium) stent. *EuroIntervention* 2009;5(Suppl F):F94-F97.

138. Haude M, Erbel R, Verheye S, et al. Comparison of intermediate term late lumen loss after coronary implantation of bare or paclitaxel eluting absorbable metal scaffolds: results from Progress-AMS and Biosolve-1 trials. *J Am Coll Cardiol* 2012; 59:E203.

139. Zeltinger J, Schmid E, Brandom D, et al. Advances in the development of coronary stents. *Biomaterials Forum* 2004;26:8-9, 24.

140. Pollman MJ. Engineering a bioresorbable stent: REVA programme update. *EuroIntervention* 2009;5(Suppl F):F54-F57.

CHAPTER 4

Design, Analysis, and Interpretation of Comparative Effectiveness Studies and Randomized Clinical Trials of Coronary Stents

ROBERT W. YEH | NEIL J. WIMMER

KEY POINTS

- Randomized, controlled trials are the "gold standard" research design for establishing an unbiased treatment effect of a new technology or procedure and have been used extensively in the evaluation of coronary stents.

- Careful attention to study design and analysis, including selection of the appropriate patient population, comparator groups, randomization scheme, outcomes, blinding, and statistical analysis, is necessary for clinical trials to contribute to the understanding of stent safety and efficacy.

- Clinical trials may be impractical or lack feasibility to answer certain questions because of cost, lack of perceived equipoise, or inability to enroll large representative populations of patients.

- Observational approaches have been used to assess the comparative effectiveness of coronary stents, but such studies should be designed and evaluated with attention to bias and confounding.

- There are multiple approaches to control for confounding during the analysis of observational research, including the use of stratification, regression models, propensity scores, and instrumental variables. The purpose of these methods is to allow estimation of an unbiased treatment effect.

Introduction

Since the development of coronary angiography in 1958 by Sones and the subsequent introduction of coronary balloon angioplasty in 1977 by Gruentzig, cardiologists have attempted to demonstrate the effectiveness of techniques in interventional cardiology using sound clinical research methods. Innovators in the field and interested scientific investigators have taken multiple different approaches to evaluating the proliferation of evolving technology in clinical medicine. Over time, randomized clinical trials (RCTs) have become the center of this research, but other research methodologies have also been proven to be important. This chapter focuses on issues related to the design and interpretation of clinical trials and observational research studies in the investigation of coronary stents.

Palmaz initially introduced the concept of a stent mounted onto a balloon. In 1985, Palmaz and colleagues[1] described the results of a woven, stainless steel graft mounted on angioplasty balloon catheters and placed in the aortae and peripheral arteries of dogs by balloon expansion. Initial cases were performed on peripheral arteries. With refinement and miniaturization, stents began to be implanted in the coronary system. On March 28, 1986, Puel implanted the first coronary stent in a patient in Toulouse, France.[2] The first case series of coronary and peripheral artery stenting was published jointly from Toulouse, France, and Lausanne, Switzerland.[3] Shortly thereafter, the idea of coronary stenting was brought to the United States

when groups in Atlanta, Georgia, and San Antonio, Texas, published their initial cases in dogs.[4,5] By necessity, with the development of new technology, the initial published reports of coronary stenting were merely proof-of-concept studies in a small series of patients or animals.

Shortly after this initial proof of concept, investigators realized that to understand the true efficacy and limitations of this burgeoning technology, RCTs would need to be performed. Balloon angioplasty had been established as a treatment option in patients with coronary artery disease, but it was limited in many ways, most notably by the frequent occurrence of abrupt vessel closure. By 1991, two landmark RCTs of coronary stents had been designed and began enrolling patients. These trials were the European-based Benestent study and the North American–based Stent Restenosis (STRESS) study, both published in 1994.[6,7] Both studies randomly assigned patients with coronary artery disease either to balloon angioplasty alone or to the new treatment under study, coronary stenting with the Palmaz-Schatz stent. These initial studies incorporated many of the fundamental aspects of clinical trial design that would be repeated over the continued development of coronary stenting, including minimizing variation by strictly defining the eligible patient population and treatment protocols, randomization to treatment arms, and analysis by the principle of intention to treat (ITT).

Fundamentals of Clinical Trials Evaluating Coronary Stents

The objective of clinical trials is to establish the true effect of an intervention when it is used as intended. RCTs are the "gold standard" for doing so in clinical research. During a clinical trial, treatment effects are efficiently isolated by controlling for bias and confounding through minimizing variation between study arms. Key features of clinical trials that are used to meet this objective include randomization, adherence to ITT, blinding, and prospective evaluation.[8] Other fundamental issues in study design include clearly defining the research question, minimizing variation, selection of the appropriate control group, selection of the target population, selection of appropriate endpoints, planning for interim analyses, and planning for the final analysis and presentation of the results.

WHAT IS THE QUESTION?

The design of a clinical trial starts with a primary research question, for example, "Is stent A better than stent B?" However, this research question is too vague to be tested scientifically and must be honed down to a testable hypothesis. The formulation of this hypothesis often begins with understanding what the scientific claim is that an investigator would like to make at the end of a trial. The relevant design, data to be collected, and analytical approach may follow naturally from a clearly and precisely stated hypothesis. In interventional cardiology, in lieu of "Is stent A better than stent B?" a more precise question might be, "Is stent A more effective than stent B in preventing target lesion revascularization at 1 year in diabetic patients who present with stable angina and a greater than 70% de novo coronary lesion?"

MINIMIZING VARIATION

In any trial, there may be variation in trial conduct that occurs across physicians, study sites, and treatment arms. The larger the variation, the more difficult it is to isolate an effect of the treatment or device under study. Minimizing variation is a fundamental aspect of clinical trial design. Minimizing variation can be accomplished in numerous ways. One important method is the development of standardized clinical definitions and objective outcome measures (discussed later). In the study of coronary stents, this has often been supported by the use of angiographic core laboratories and blinded clinical event committees to provide uniform interpretation of data that are generated at diverse clinical centers.[9]

STRATIFIED RANDOMIZATION

Trials commonly employ stratified randomization by site or comorbid conditions in the study population to ensure that treatment groups are balanced with respect to confounding variables. In stratified randomization, treatment groups are balanced with respect to known important confounders. For instance, if diabetes is known to profoundly influence the development of restenosis at the site of stent implantation, two different randomization schedules can be used for patients with and without diabetes who enter a given clinical trial. However, stratification has important limitations. Although it can be effective in controlling confounding, subjects can be stratified only by known confounding variables. Attempts to stratify on many confounders can be hindered by the ability to enroll study subjects for each individual stratum and by the increased practical complexity for the enrolling sites.

RANDOMIZATION AND COMPARATORS

When feasible, RCTs are the preferred design for testing efficacy of various types of medical interventions. The key distinguishing feature of an RCT from other types of research that seek to establish the efficacy of an intervention is that after an initial assessment of patient eligibility, patients are randomly allocated to receive one of the possible alternative treatments under study. Random allocation in real RCTs can be complex and involve multiple factors or methodologies but conceptually can be understood as the flipping of a coin. After randomization, the groups (two or more) are followed in exactly the same way, and the only differences that are observed should be the result of the differences in their group assignment. The most important advantage of an RCT compared with other types of comparative effectiveness research is that proper randomization minimizes treatment selection bias by balancing both known and unknown factors that could otherwise be related to both the treatment selection and the outcome of interest. Randomized trials are the best way to understand what would have happened to a group of patients under study who are treated with a new device had that same group been treated differently. This idea, called the *counterfactual*, is central to the rationale of RCT design.

BLINDING

Blinding is a fundamental tool in clinical trial design and is a powerful method for preventing and reducing bias. Blinding refers to the practice of keeping study participants, investigators, endpoint assessors, or all three, unaware of the assigned intervention so that this knowledge would not affect their behavior (even if unintentionally or subtly).

When study participants are blinded, they may be less likely to have biased psychological or physical responses to the intervention. When investigators are blinded, they may be less likely to apply treatment algorithms differentially to patients being studied, known as *cointerventions*. When outcome assessors are blinded, they are less likely to have biases affect their outcome assessments. Investigators often label a study as "single-blind," referring to the blinding of one of these groups; "double-blind," referring to the blinding of two groups; and "triple-blind," referring to the blinding of all three groups. However, the terms are not specific; a "single-blind" study can be used to refer to blinding of the study subjects, the investigators, or the endpoint adjudicators. When a trial is conducted without blinding, it is often referred to as "open-label."

EQUIPOISE

In any RCT, there must be genuine uncertainty on behalf of the study investigators as to which treatment option, or study arm, is truly best for the patient being studied. This uncertainty provides the necessary equipoise, as described by Freedman,[10] to justify random allocation to treatment after due consent is given. There may be instances when a patient may be eligible to participate in a given RCT, but the treating physician believes that one of the trial options or courses of treatment is "best" for that given patient. In this case, the patient should not be entered into the RCT. Instead, the patient should be offered only treatment options that represent optimal treatment for the patient's particular condition.

The assumption of equipoise can often influence the generalizability of study results if there is a strong belief by clinicians that one treatment option is clearly preferred for certain patients, whether or not the data support this notion. In selectively removing patients that might benefit most from a given treatment, a study may not show benefit for that treatment in the remaining study population, potentially leading to the incorrect conclusion that the treatment was ineffective in general. The careful evaluation of the exclusion of patients on the basis of clinician preference owing to perceived lack of equipoise is an important and underappreciated consideration in the evaluation of therapies, including coronary stents.

SELECTION OF COMPARATORS

In the field of drug development, RCTs are often initially placebo-controlled when there are limited treatment options for a given condition. However, placebo-controlled trials would not be ethical when an established treatment exists for a given condition. In the history of the development of coronary stents, balloon angioplasty was already established as a routine practice at the time of early stent development. The first landmark RCTs in this field randomly allocated patients to either balloon angioplasty or coronary stent placement as described earlier. In the current era of RCTs that evaluate coronary stents, the devices or techniques under study must be tested against the current standard of care, which is often the preceding generation of stents. However, as stent technology has matured, some investigators have advocated the use of single-arm studies of the stent under investigation and comparing endpoints with relevant historical controls. An example of this approach was used in the trials of the Resolute zotarolimus-eluting stent (ZES). The Resolute ZES uses the same cobalt-chromium stent platform and antiproliferative agent as the previously developed Endeavor ZES, the only difference being that the Resolute ZES uses a hydrophilic biocompatible polymer that provides release of zotarolimus over a longer duration than the polymer used in the Endeavor ZES.[11] In the RESOLUTE US trial, investigators compared an active treatment arm of patients treated with the Resolute ZES with historical controls treated with the Endeavor ZES, allowing the trial to be conducted with fewer patients at a lower cost.[12] The limitation of this type of analysis is that the historical controls may not represent a population of patients treated under the same conditions as the patients currently under study, even if the inclusion criteria for the two studies are identical. More single-arm studies using historical controls for comparison are being planned and conducted to evaluate next-generation platforms of existing devices.

ENDPOINTS

The direct measure of clinical outcomes of interest is key in understanding the response of human subjects to new study devices.[13] The study endpoints that are selected for RCTs serve several purposes. Endpoints must have short-term or long-term pathophysiologic relevance to the performance of the device under study, or they must be clinically meaningful events. Endpoints also must be sufficiently well defined to be reproducibly assessed or adjudicated and subjected to statistical analysis. For a particular stent technology, most RCT programs begin with a focus on angiographic outcomes and mandate routine angiographic follow-up in a large proportion of study subjects.[14-21] As the technology matures, the focus of subsequent RCTs shifts to more clinically oriented endpoints (see the case study of TAXUS clinical trial program discussed later).

Angiographic Endpoints

Multiple angiographic endpoints have been developed and used to evaluate the efficacy of stent technology immediately after percutaneous coronary intervention (PCI) or at angiographic follow-up after the index procedure (Table 4-1). Acute gain is the change in minimum lesion diameter that occurs immediately after PCI. Angiographic success after PCI has traditionally been defined as the achievement of less than 30% residual diameter stenosis at the end of the procedure.[22] Several criteria have been used to describe angiographic restenosis after stent implantation. Binary angiographic restenosis is most often defined as a 50% or greater diameter stenosis at follow-up, although many other criteria have been used as well. Binary angiographic restenosis after stent placement may occur within the stent (i.e., in-stent restenosis), or within the 5-mm margins of the stent (i.e., "edge" restenosis or "in-segment"). In-stent or in-segment late lumen loss is defined as the difference in the minimum lesion diameter of the stent or segment at the end of the index procedure and the minimum lesion diameter at follow-up as measured in millimeters. Late lumen loss is a frequently used angiographic endpoint for coronary stent trials because of its monotonic correlation with the probability of restenosis.[23] Late lumen loss has been shown to be the most reliable angiographic variable for discriminating restenosis rates between new drug-eluting stent (DES) platforms across studies.[24] As binary restenosis rates have declined, the use of this surrogate endpoint has enabled smaller studies to be performed to demonstrate efficacy of newer stents.

Clinical Endpoints

Clinical endpoints commonly used in randomized trials evaluating coronary stents have included target lesion revascularization or target vessel revascularization, which may or may not be driven by clinical ischemia; target vessel myocardial infarction; stent thrombosis; and cardiac death (Tables 4-2 and 4-3). Pivotal clinical trials of coronary stents have used composite primary endpoints, such as target vessel or target lesion failure. Target vessel failure is commonly defined as death from cardiac causes, target vessel–related myocardial infarction, and repeat PCI or surgical revascularization of the target vessel; target lesion failure is commonly defined as death from cardiac causes, target vessel–related myocardial infarction, and target lesion revascularization. Clinical endpoints can also be considered "patient-oriented" or "device-oriented" (see Table 4-3). The primary endpoints used in the pivotal trials of the currently approved drug-eluting stents are shown in Table 4-4.

The Academic Research Consortium (ARC), an informal collaboration between academic research organizations, key regulatory agencies such as the U.S. Food and Drug Administration, and device manufacturers have generated a consensus set of standardized definitions for clinical endpoints of coronary stent trials.[25] These definitions can be used for the assessment of death, myocardial revascularization, repeat revascularization, stent thrombosis, and bleeding (see Tables 4-2 and 4-3).[26]

MONITORING TRIAL PROGRESS AND PERFORMING INTERIM ANALYSES

When RCTs are in progress, for reasons of safety of the patients treated in all of the study arms (both "active treatment" and "control"), data should be reviewed at prespecified intervals. These reviews are performed by an Independent Data Monitoring Committee (IDMC) (also referred to as Data Safety Monitoring Committee or Board) that is composed of clinical and statistical experts not involved in the planning, management, or conduct of the trial. Although an IDMC should be concerned with the relative efficacy of the treatment under study, issues of safety should be paramount. In extreme circumstances, serious safety issues may force early closure of a trial before completion of the prespecified follow-up time or subject recruitment. The IDMC arrives at this judgment from a combination of the trial data, external evidence related to new information generated since the trial was begun, and the collective experience of the IDMC members. In the planning stage of RCTs, specific plans for reporting to the IDMC should be made explicit. An interim report may include a formal statistical comparison of treatment efficacy. Because multiple testing can lead to inflation of the possible type I error (i.e., the null hypothesis is true but is rejected), this should be accounted for in the statistical analysis plan. The analysis plan for the study should also articulate termination procedures, or boundaries that when crossed by the interim data under review should prompt trial termination. In the evaluation of coronary stents, IDMCs are typically concerned with evidence of device malfunction and procedural complications such as coronary dissection and differences in stent-related endpoints including stent thrombosis. However, all serious adverse events that occur in a clinical trial are typically reviewed by the IDMC, whether or not they are believed to be related to the device under evaluation.

PATIENT POPULATIONS

Early RCTs of coronary stents focused on demonstrating efficacy compared with balloon angioplasty in ideal practice conditions. Patient populations in these trials were restricted in numerous ways. For example, in the Benestent study, patients were limited to having only stable angina from single-vessel disease and the target lesion was required to be less than 15 mm in length in a coronary vessel greater than 3 mm in diameter and to supply normally functioning myocardium. Patients with unstable symptoms, with ostial or bifurcation

TABLE 4-1	Common Angiographic Endpoints in Clinical Trials
Endpoint	**Definition**
Acute gain	Change in MLD (in mm) from before to immediately after PCI
Late loss	Loss after PCI that occurs during study follow-up period
Binary angiographic restenosis	Commonly defined as >50% diameter stenosis at follow-up
Applicable Segment	**Definition**
In-stent restenosis	When restenosis occurs within stent
Edge restenosis	When restenosis occurs within 5 mm of stent margins
In-segment (or in-lesion) restenosis	When restenosis occurs within segment between proximal and distal reference segments

PCI, Percutaneous coronary intervention; *MLD*, minimal luminal diameter.

TABLE 4-2	Academic Research Consortium Definitions of Clinical Endpoints in Coronary Stent Trials	
Classification of Death		
Cardiac death	Any death from proximate cardiac cause (e.g., myocardial infarction, low-output failure, fatal arrhythmia); unwitnessed death and death of unknown cause; and all procedure-related deaths, including deaths related to concomitant treatment, are classified as cardiac death	
Vascular death	Death caused by noncoronary vascular causes, such as cerebrovascular disease, pulmonary embolism, ruptured aortic aneurysm, dissecting aneurysm, or other vascular diseases	
Noncardiovascular death	Any death not covered by above definitions, such as death caused by infection, malignancy, sepsis, pulmonary causes, accident, suicide, or trauma	
Classification of Myocardial Infarction and Criteria for Diagnosis		
Classification	*Biomarker Criteria*	*Additional Criteria*
Periprocedural PCI	Troponin >3 times URL or CK-MB >3 times URL	Baseline value < URL
Periprocedural CABG	Troponin >5 times URL or CK-MB >5 times URL	Baseline value < URL and any of the following: new pathologic Q waves or LBBB, new native or graft vessel occlusion, imaging evidence of loss of viable myocardium
Spontaneous	Troponin > URL or CK-MB > URL	
Sudden death	Death before biomarkers obtained or before expected to be elevated	Symptoms suggestive of ischemia and any of the following: new ST segment elevation or LBBB, documented thrombus by angiography or autopsy
Reinfarction	Stable or decreasing values on 2 samples and 20% increase 3-6 hours after second sample	If biomarkers increasing or peak not reached, insufficient data to diagnose recurrent myocardial infarction
Classification of Repeat Revascularization		
TLR	TLR is defined as any repeat PCI of target lesion or bypass surgery of target vessel performed for restenosis or other complication of target lesion. All TLRs should be classified prospectively as clinically indicated or not clinically indicated by the investigator before repeat angiography. Target lesion is defined as the treated segment from 5 mm proximal to stent to 5 mm distal to stent	
TVR	TVR is defined as any repeat PCI or surgical bypass of any segment of target vessel. Target vessel is defined as the entire major coronary vessel proximal and distal to target lesion, which includes upstream and downstream branches and target lesion itself	
Clinically indicated revascularization	Revascularization is considered clinically indicated if angiography at follow-up shows percent diameter stenosis ≥50% (core laboratory QCA assessment) and if one of the following is present: (1) positive history of recurrent angina pectoris, presumably related to target vessel; (2) objective signs of ischemia at rest (ECG changes) or during exercise test (or equivalent), presumably related to target vessel; (3) abnormal results of any invasive functional diagnostic test (e.g., fractional flow reserve); (4) TLR or TVR with diameter stenosis ≥70% even in the absence of the above-mentioned ischemic signs or symptoms	
Classification of Stent Thrombosis		
Definite	Acute coronary syndrome with angiographic or autopsy evidence of thrombus or occlusion within or adjacent to stent	
Probable	Unexplained death within 30 days after stent implantation or acute myocardial infarction involving target vessel territory without angiographic confirmation	
Possible	Any unexplained death >30 days after procedure	
Timing of Stent Thrombosis		
Acute	Within 24 hours (excluding events within catheterization laboratory)	
Subacute	1-30 days	
Early	Within 30 days	
Late	30 days to 1 year	
Very late	>1 year	

CABG, Coronary artery bypass graft; CK-MB, creatine kinase myocardial band; ECG, electrocardiogram; LBBB, left bundle-branch block; PCI, percutaneous coronary intervention; QCA, quantitative coronary angiography; TLR, target lesion revascularization; TVR, target vessel revascularization; URL, upper reference limit, defined as 99th percentile of normal reference range.

Adapted from Cutlip DE, Windecker S, Mehran R, et al. Clinical end points in coronary stent trials: a case for standardized definitions. Circulation 2007;115:2344-2351.

lesions, with intracoronary thrombus, or with lesions in vessels supplied by bypass grafts were excluded.[6,7] As individual technologies have matured, the patient populations in clinical studies have expanded to evaluate safety and efficacy in specific and higher-risk clinical settings, such as in patients with acute myocardial infarction, diabetes, or previous coronary restenosis, or patients with more complex coronary anatomies, such as ostial lesions, bifurcation lesions, long lesions, or lesions in bypass grafts.

ANALYSIS OF RANDOMIZED CLINICAL TRIAL DATA

The type of statistical analysis used in RCTs depends on the characteristics of the data collected. Data may be binary, continuous, or time-to-event. Investigators also need to decide how to deal with missing or censored data. The primary role of statistics is to evaluate the possible role of chance or random variation in explaining observed differences between the groups being studied.[27] Statistical theory plays a key role in evaluating the results of RCTs. Statistical analysis for RCTs begins even before patient enrollment commences. Sample size calculations must be made to estimate the size of the trial needed to try to answer the scientific question being asked. The equation used to calculate sample size depends on the design of the trial. Regardless of the specific trial design, the sample size calculation requires the following components: the expected event rate of the primary outcome, the expected effect size of the intervention between the groups under study, the acceptable level of type I error, and the desired power of the study. Study power refers to the probability that the study will actually find a difference between the two groups being studied

TABLE 4-3	Composite Clinical Endpoints Used in Clinical Trials of Coronary Stents, According to Advanced Research Consortium Recommendations

Device-Oriented Composite (Hierarchical Order)

Cardiac death

Myocardial infarction (not clearly attributable to nontarget vessel)

TLR

Patient-Oriented Composite (Hierarchical Order)

All-cause mortality

Any MI (includes nontarget vessel territory)

Any repeat revascularization (includes all target and nontarget vessels)

TLR, Target lesion revascularization.
Adapted from Cutlip DE, Windecker S, Mehran R, et al. Clinical end points in coronary stent trials: a case for standardized definitions. Circulation 2007;115:2344-2351.

TABLE 4-4	Primary Endpoints in Pivotal Drug-Eluting Stent Trials	
Stent	**Trial**	**Primary Endpoint**
Sirolimus-eluting	SIRIUS[80]	Target vessel failure (defined as composite of death from cardiac causes, myocardial infarction, and repeat PCI or surgical revascularization of target vessel)
Paclitaxel-eluting	TAXUS IV[29]	Ischemia-driven TVR (defined as need for repeat PCI or surgical revascularization of target vessel)
Paclitaxel-eluting	TAXUS V[31]	Ischemia-driven TVR (defined as need for repeat PCI or surgical revascularization of target vessel)
Everolimus-eluting	SPIRIT IV[81]	Target lesion failure (defined as cardiac death, target vessel myocardial infarction, or ischemia-driven TLR)
Zotarolimus-eluting (Endeavor)	ENDEAVOR IV[82]	Target vessel failure (defined as cardiac death, myocardial infarction, or TVR)
Zotarolimus-eluting (Resolute)	RESOLUTE All-Comers[83]	Target lesion failure (defined as composite of death from cardiac causes, any myocardial infarction [not clearly attributable to nontarget vessel], or clinically indicated TLR)
Everolimus-eluting (Promus Element)	PLATINUM[60]	Target lesion failure (defined as composite of cardiac death [any death other than death confirmed to have noncardiac cause] related to target vessel, myocardial infarction related to target vessel, or ischemia-driven TLR)

PCI, Percutaneous coronary intervention; *TLR*, target lesion revascularization; *TVR*, target vessel revascularization.
Endeavor, Medtronic, Minneapolis, MN; Resolute, Medtronic, Minneapolis, MN; Promus Element, Boston Scientific, Natick, MA.

if one exists. The size of the clinical trial can be designed to target a specific number of enrolled patients or to target a specific number of outcome events.

Principle of Intention to Treat

The principle of intention to treat (ITT) is a fundamental concept in clinical trials, but it is frequently misunderstood. It essentially states to "analyze as randomized." When study participants have been randomly assigned, they are included in the analyses as part of the randomized regimen to which they were assigned regardless of adherence to the protocol, study completion, or anything else that occurs after randomization. An ITT approach can be considered an evaluation of the treatment "strategy" under study rather than an evaluation of treatment under ideal conditions. All patients randomly assigned should be accounted for in the analysis of RCTs as reviewed in detail in the Consolidation of the Standards of Reporting Trials (CONSORT) statement, which has been adopted by many leading journals (Figure 4-1).[28]

Per-Protocol Analyses

An alternative approach to an ITT analysis is to perform a per-protocol analysis, often defined as limiting the analysis to study participants who correctly completed the study protocol. Compared with a pharmacologic study that asks patients to take a study drug over a long period of time, per-protocol versus ITT issues are often less important in traditional coronary stent trials, where subjects undergo PCI shortly after randomization. However, subjects in coronary stent trials can still be randomly assigned and not complete the study protocol—for example, if a stent fails to be delivered or a different stent or stenting strategy is used than that to which the patient was randomly assigned. A per-protocol analysis may be subject to confounding because there may be systematic differences in the individuals who do not complete a study protocol in each group under study. A per-protocol analysis is not rooted in the same statistical foundation for inference as an ITT analysis.

Subgroup Analyses

Data in clinical trials should be evaluated to address the primary hypothesis of the study. Further subgroup analyses should be interpreted with care because of the multiple comparisons associated with testing large numbers of subgroups and the likelihood of type I, or false-positive, results. When possible, investigators should prespecify the secondary hypotheses they are interested in evaluating during the design phase of the trial and generate specific plans to address issues of multiple testing.

LIMITATIONS AND DISADVANTAGES OF RANDOMIZED CLINICAL TRIALS

The primary disadvantages of clinical trials are that they are complex, are expensive, and typically enroll a narrow spectrum of patients. Because of their immense complexity, clinical trials require large investments of time, effort, and money by a large number of investigators and research organizations compared with other potential methods for studying comparative effectiveness. Although clinical trials have become the "gold standard" design for demonstrating the effectiveness of a specific intervention, the limitations of time, effort, infrastructure, and cost often make them unrealistic for evaluating many important clinical questions. In addition, participants in clinical trials often represent a very compliant group of patients by virtue of the requirement to adhere to a strict protocol or may come from sites that are different in important ways from typical practice settings. These differences affect the generalizability of trial results—that is, whether or not the results observed are representative of results that might be seen in other patients or practice settings.

◈ Case Study: The TAXUS Paclitaxel-Eluting Stent Randomized Clinical Trial Program

As a case study evaluating the evolution of clinical trials in coronary stent development, we will highlight the series of RCTs that evaluated the safety and efficacy of the TAXUS paclitaxel-eluting stent (PES) (Boston Scientific, Natick, MA). The clinical safety and efficacy of the TAXUS PES was initially demonstrated in the TAXUS clinical trial program (Table 4-5).[17,18,29-31] TAXUS I and II evaluated TAXUS

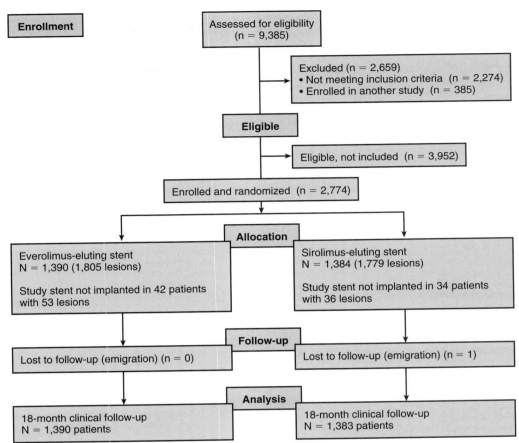

Figure 4-1   Example of a CONSORT diagram in a clinical trial from a randomized clinical trial comparing patients treated with everolimus-eluting and sirolimus-eluting stents. (From Jensen LO, Thayssen P, Hansen HS, et al. Randomized comparison of everolimus-eluting and sirolimus-eluting stents in patients treated with percutaneous coronary intervention: the Scandinavian Organization for Randomized Trials with Clinical Outcome IV [SORT OUT IV]. Circulation 2012;125:1246-1255.)

PES on the NIR stent platform in focal de novo lesions of native coronary arteries, whereas TAXUS V and VI investigated the TAXUS PES on the Express stent platform in more complex lesions with longer follow-up. Collectively, these trials demonstrated a marked decrease in binary restenosis in patients randomly assigned to PES compared with bare metal stents (BMS) and a significant reduction in the clinical endpoint of target lesion revascularization. In the pivotal TAXUS IV trial, 1314 patients with single, de novo lesions with visually estimated lengths of 10 to 28 mm in native coronary arteries with reference vessel diameters of 2.5 to 3.75 mm were randomly assigned to either a TAXUS sustained-release stent or Express BMS control. At 9 months, the primary endpoint of target vessel revascularization was reduced with the TAXUS PES from 12.0% to 4.7% (P < .001). Clinical and angiographic efficacy was present across a broad range of patient and lesion subtypes. Protocol-mandated angiographic follow-up was incorporated into all of the RCTs in the TAXUS program: TAXUS I, II, V, and VI mandated routine angiography in all enrolled subjects, whereas TAXUS IV specified routine angiographic follow-up in a subset of 732 patients out of the 1314 patients who were enrolled. Further RCTs evaluated TAXUS stents in more complex patient populations, including patients with ST segment elevation myocardial infarction,[32-35] left main coronary artery stenosis,[36] and saphenous vein graft stenoses (see Table 4-5).[37]

Because both the TAXUS PES and the Cypher sirolimus-eluting stent (SES) (Cypher stent, Cordis, Bridgewater, NJ) were approved for clinical use as the first generations of DES in the United States, more than 20 RCTs have been performed comparing the two stent platforms in an attempt to determine differences between their

performance in clinical use.[34,35,38-55] These RCTs have been performed in various patient populations using a variety of angiographic and clinical endpoints. The study cohorts for these comparisons have included unselected patients; patients limited to de novo lesions; diabetic patients; patients with lesions at "high risk" for restenosis, left main stenosis, long lesions, multivessel coronary disease, small vessels, bifurcation lesions, complex lesions, BMS restenosis, and prior SES restenosis; and patients presenting with ST segment elevation myocardial infarction. The primary endpoints of these trials have varied as well. Studies have evaluated late lumen loss, composite major adverse cardiovascular events, binary restenosis, target lesion revascularization, and intravascular ultrasound–assessed neointimal hyperplasia (Table 4-6).

More Recent Trends in Randomized Clinical Trials of Drug-Eluting Stents

ALL COMERS TRIALS

Although minimizing variation is a central theme in the design of clinical trials, there are instances when clinical trials should reflect "real world" practice. A more recent trend has been to design trials that enroll patients more representative of routine clinical practice instead of restricting enrollment to a highly specific population based on comorbid or lesion-specific factors. The RESOLUTE All Comers trial is an example of such a trial design.[56] This study had wide inclusion criteria, and patients were randomly assigned to coronary intervention with either zotarolimus-eluting stents or everolimus-eluting

TABLE 4-5	**Randomized Controlled Trials Comparing Paclitaxel-Eluting Stents with Bare Metal Stents**

Trial Name and Reference	Study Cohort	Number Randomized (Planned Angiographic Follow-up)	Latest Follow-up to Date	Principal Findings
TAXUS I[17]	Single de novo or restenotic lesions	61 (all)	5 years	6-month percent diameter stenosis was lower with PES compared with BMS (13.6% vs. 27.3%, $P < .001$), with improvements in IVUS findings with PES
TAXUS II[23]	Single de novo native coronary lesions	536 (all)	5 years	6-month net volume obstruction was lower with PES slow release vs. BMS (7.9% vs. 23.2%, $P < .001$) and PES moderate release compared with BMS. Reductions in TLR were maintained at 5 years with both PES formulations with no differences in death, myocardial infarction, or stent thrombosis
TAXUS IV[29]	Single de novo native coronary lesions	1314 (732)	5 years	PES was associated with lower rates of TLR compared with BMS at 9 months (4.7% vs. 12.0%, $P < .001$) and lower rates of angiographic restenosis. Reductions in TLR were maintained at 5 years with no differences in death, myocardial infarction, or stent thrombosis
TAXUS V[31]	Single lesions, including complex lesions	1156 (all)	5 years	PES reduced 9-month TVR compared with BMS (12.1% vs. 17.3%, $P = .02$), with reductions in angiographic restenosis overall and among patients with complex disease. At 5 years, reductions in clinical restenosis were maintained with similar rates of death, myocardial infarction, and stent thrombosis
TAXUS VI[30]	Single long complex lesions	448 (all)	5 years	9-month TVR rate was lower with PES moderate release compared with BMS (9.1% vs. 19.4%, $P = .0027$), with lower rates of angiographic restenosis. At 5 years, TVR rates were similar between both stents, although TLR was lower with PES moderate release
HORIZONS-AMI[32]	ST segment elevation myocardial infarction	3006 (1800)	3 years	PES was associated with lower rates of TLR compared with BMS at 1 year (4.5% vs. 7.5%, $P = .002$) and lower binary restenosis at 13 months (10.0% vs. 22.9%, $P < .001$). Reduction in TLR was maintained at 3 years, with no significant differences in death, myocardial infarction, or stent thrombosis observed
PASSION[33]	ST segment elevation myocardial infarction	619 (none)	2 years	PES was associated with non–statistically significantly lower rates of the primary endpoint of cardiac death, MI, and TLR (8.8% vs. 12.8%, $P = .09$) at 1 year, a finding that was maintained at 2 years
PASEO[34]	ST segment elevation myocardial infarction	270 including 90 SES (none)	4 years	PES was associated with a lower rate of TLR at 1 year compared with BMS (4.4% vs. 14.4%, $P = .023$), which was maintained at 4 years
SELECTION[84]	ST segment elevation myocardial infarction	80 (all)	7 months	Volume of neointimal hyperplasia by IVUS was lower with PES compared with BMS (4.6% vs. 20%, $P < .01$), with no differences in late malapposition seen between stent types
Erglis et al[85]	Left main stenosis	103 (all)	6 months	PES was associated with lower rates of binary angiographic restenosis at 6 months compared with BMS (6% vs. 22%, $P = .021$). IVUS measures were also improved with PES
SOS[37]	SVG	80 (all)	Median 1.5 years	Rate of binary angiographic restenosis was lower with PES compared with BMS (9% vs. 51%, $P < .001$). Similar rates of myocardial infarction and death were observed

BMS, Bare metal stent; IVUS, intravascular ultrasound; MI, myocardial infarction; PES, paclitaxel-eluting stent (slow-release); SES, sirolimus-eluting stent; SVG, saphenous vein grafts; TLR, target lesion revascularization; TVR, target vessel revascularization.

From Stone GW, Kirtane AJ. Bare metal and drug-eluting coronary stents. In: Topol E, Teirstein P, eds. Textbook of Interventional Cardiology, 6th ed. Philadelphia: Saunders; 2011.

TABLE 4-6	**Randomized Controlled Trials Comparing Sirolimus-Eluting Stents and Paclitaxel-Eluting Stents**

Trial Name and Reference	Study Cohort	Number Randomized (Planned Angiographic Follow-up)	Latest Follow-up to Date	Principal Findings
REALITY[38]	1-2 de novo coronary lesions	1386 (all)	1 year	Despite lower late loss with SES, rates of binary angiographic restenosis were similar with SES and PES (9.1% vs. 11.1%, $P = .31$), with similar rates of MACE at 1 year
Zhang et al[35]	De novo coronary lesions	673 including 224 Firebird stent (none)	1 year	At 1 year, rates of MACE were similar between SES and PES (8.4% vs. 11.2%)
SORT OUT II[39]	Unselected	2098 (none)	1.5 years	There were no significant differences between SES and PES in MACE (9.3% vs. 11.2%) or other endpoints, including death, myocardial infarction, or stent thrombosis
SIRTAX[40]	Unselected	1012 (approximately half)	5 years	SES was associated with a lower rate of MACE at 9 months compared with PES (6.2% vs. 10.8%, $P = .009$). However, at 5 years, the rates were similar, with an accrual of events in both stent groups

TABLE 4-6	Randomized Controlled Trials Comparing Sirolimus-Eluting Stents and Paclitaxel-Eluting Stents (Continued)			
Trial Name and Reference	Study Cohort	Number Randomized (Planned Angiographic Follow-up)	Latest Follow-up to Date	Principal Findings
TAXi[41]	Unselected	202 (none)	3 years	Rates of 6-month MACE were similar with SES and PES (6% vs. 4%, P = .8), with similar findings at 3 years
DES-DIABETES[42]	Diabetic patients	400 (all)	2 years	6-month in-segment restenosis was lower with SES compared with PES (3.4% vs. 18.2%, P < .001). At 2 years, rates of TLR remained lower with SES (3.5% vs. 11.0%, P = .004)
ISAR-DIABETES[43]	Diabetic patients	250 (all)	5 years (in pooled analyses)	In-segment late lumen loss was lower with SES compared with PES (0.43 mm vs. 0.67 mm, P= .002), with non–statistically significant rates of TLR at 9 months (6.4% vs. 12.0%, P = .13)
Kim et al[44]	Diabetic patients	169 (all)	6 months	Late lumen loss was similar with SES and PES (0.26 mm vs. 0.39 mm, P = .36); rates of TLR were similar at 6 months
DiabeDES[45]	Diabetic patients	153 (all)	8 months	In-stent late lumen loss was lower with SES compared with PES (0.23 mm vs. 0.52 mm, P = .025). Rates of TLR and MACE were similar with both types of stents
ISAR LEFT MAIN[46]	Left main stenosis	607 (all)	2 years	Similar rates of angiographic restenosis were observed with SES and PES (19.4% vs. 16.0%, P = .30), with no differences observed in death, myocardial infarction, or TLR
LONG DES II[47]	Long lesions	500 (all)	9 months	In-segment binary restenosis was lower with SES compared with PES (3.3% vs. 14.6%, P < .001), with a lower rate of 9-month TLR
Han et al[48]	Multivessel CAD	416 (all)	19.5 months	Rates of MACE were similar with SES and PES over follow-up period (6.4% vs. 8.8%), with no differences in minimum lumen diameter
ISAR-SMART 3[49]	Small vessels	360 (all)	5 years (in pooled analyses)	Late lumen loss at 6-8 months was greater with PES compared with SES (0.56 mm vs. 0.25 mm, P < .001), with greater TLR (14.7% vs. 6.6%, P = .008)
Pan et al[50]	Bifurcation lesions	205 (all)	2 years	SES was associated with lower rates of binary angiographic restenosis, less late lumen loss, and lower rate of TLR at 2 years compared with PES (4% vs. 13%, P < .021)
Petronio et al[51]	Complex lesions	100 (all)	9 months	By IVUS, area of neointimal hyperplasia was significantly lower with SES than with PES (7.4% vs. 15.4%, P < .001) at 9 months
Cervinka et al[52]	Complex CAD	70 (all)	6 months	IVUS-assessed neointimal hyperplasia volume was lower with SES compared with PES (4.1 mm³ vs. 17.4 mm³, P = .001)
ISAR-DESIRE[53]	BMS restenosis	300 including 100 balloon angioplasty patients (all)	5 years (in pooled analyses)	Angiographic restenosis was lower with both SES (14.3%) and PES (21.7%) compared with balloon angioplasty at 6 months (44.6%). TVR was lower with SES compared with PES (8% vs. 19%, P = .02)
ISAR-DESIRE 2[54]	SES restenosis	450 (all)	1 year	There were no differences in late lumen loss (0.40 vs. 0.38, P = .85) or other angiographic or clinical endpoints with SES or PES for treatment of SES restenosis
PROSIT[55]	ST segment elevation myocardial infarction	308 (all)	1 year	In-segment restenosis was lower with SES compared with PES (5.9% vs. 14.8%, P = .03), with similar rates of TLR and MACE
PASEO[34]	ST segment elevation myocardial infarction	270 including 90 BMS (none)	4 years	Similar reductions in TLR were seen with SES and PES (relative to BMS); this was maintained throughout follow-up period

BMS, Bare metal stent; CAD, coronary artery disease; MACE, major adverse coronary event; PES, paclitaxel-eluting stent; SES, sirolimus-eluting stent; TLR, target lesion revascularization; TVR, target vessel revascularization.
From Stone GW, Kirtane AJ. Bare metal and drug-eluting coronary stents. In: Topol E, Teirstein P, eds. Textbook of Interventional Cardiology, 6th ed. Philadelphia: Saunders; 2011.

stents; patients were also stratified into simple or complex lesion groups. Both stent platforms appeared to be safe and effective in this study, but there were significantly more frequent adverse events in the patients with complex lesions compared with patients with simple lesions. As the need to increase the generalizability of clinical trials and reduce trial costs becomes more paramount, pragmatic clinical trial designs with broad enrollment criteria and less protocolized treatment algorithms are likely to grow in number.

SINGLE-ARM TRIALS WITH HISTORICAL CONTROLS

Another trend in the study of new coronary stent platforms harks back to the initial development of coronary stents. As manufacturers develop products with small design changes, there has been a desire to simplify the trials needed for their clinical approval by regulatory agencies. The technology of coronary stents is relatively mature, and the requirement for testing each new technologic advance against an active comparison group has been seen by some investigators and Sponsors as an onerous burden. Single-arm trials are best used when the natural history of the disease is well understood and there are minimal or nonexistent placebo effects. With regard to DES, abundant data are available that were derived using techniques and equipment that are still currently in use. The comparison of small technologic improvements with an existing DES platform would be an appropriate setting for a single-arm trial that compares patients receiving active treatment with historical controls comprising patients who received previous iterations of the DES under study. As described earlier, the Resolute ZES (Medtronic, Minneapolis, MN) is similar to the previously approved Endeavor ZES (Medtronic, Minneapolis, MN) except for release kinetics of the antiproliferative agent that is used. The RESOLUTE US clinical trial compared the Resolute ZES with the Endeavor ZES using patient-level, historical control data from previously published ENDEAVOR studies and by adjusting for patient-level covariates between the groups using propensity scores.[12,57] For selected subgroups in which there were insufficient historical controls to employ this methodology (i.e., the 2.25-mm diameter and 38-mm length Resolute ZES), the primary endpoint was tested against a numerically based performance goal.

Equivalence and Noninferiority Trials

Noninferiority trials have become more important in the study of coronary stents as technology of BMS and DES has matured. The objective of a noninferiority trial differs from the objective of a traditional superiority trial, which is used to test whether an intervention is superior to a control treatment. A noninferiority design is appropriate when it would be desirable to show that the intervention is "at least as good as" or "no worse than" the active control. Generally, noninferiority trials should be evaluated in the context of several general principles (Box 4-1).[59] These pertain to the noninferiority margin that is selected, the appropriateness of and outcomes observed in the control group, the findings of the ITT and per-protocol analyses, the quality of trial conduct, and the ability to detect the endpoints that are used in the trial.

EXAMPLE OF A NONINFERIORITY TRIAL OF CORONARY STENTS: PLATINUM TRIAL

There are several examples of noninferiority studies in the coronary stent literature. The PLATINUM trial was a noninferiority design that randomly assigned 1530 patients to either the cobalt-chromium everolimus-eluting stent or the platinum-chromium everolimus-eluting stent; the primary endpoint was target lesion failure.[60] The investigators performed both an ITT analysis and a per-protocol analysis. The noninferiority margin was chosen as an absolute 3.5% difference in the primary endpoint between groups, and one-sided testing was performed. The rate of target lesion failure at 12 months in the per-protocol population occurred in 2.9% of patients assigned to the cobalt-chromium stent and 3.4% of patients assigned to the platinum-chromium stent (mean difference, 0.5%). The one-sided 95% upper confidence limit of the mean difference was 2.1%, which is less than the prespecified noninferiority margin of 3.5%. The primary endpoint of noninferiority was met ($P_{noninferiority}$ = .001).

CONTROL ARMS IN NONINFERIORITY STUDIES

The control group in a noninferiority trial should be selected carefully. The active control ideally has clinical efficacy that is of substantial magnitude that has been demonstrated repeatedly in the clinical setting of interest (i.e., assurance that the active control would be superior to placebo if a placebo was employed is a key feature in the design of these studies).

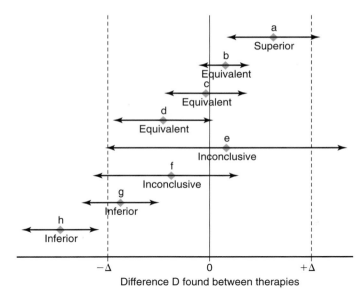

Figure 4-2 How comparisons are made in noninferiority trials. (From Christensen E. Methodology of superiority vs. equivalence trials and noninferiority trials. J Hepatol 2007;46:947-954.)

NONINFERIORITY MARGIN

A noninferiority margin (M) is selected, and if treatment differences between the intervention and active control can be shown to fall within this margin, noninferiority can be claimed.[58] Specifically, a one-sided confidence interval for the difference between study arms is calculated, and the 95% limit of this confidence interval must be within the bounds of the noninferiority margin. For example, if the primary endpoint is binary, a confidence interval for the difference in the response rates to the two treatments can be constructed. If the lower limit of the confidence interval is greater than −M, important differences can be ruled out with reasonable confidence, and noninferiority can be claimed (Figure 4-2). Noninferiority studies are difficult to design because selection of the noninferiority margin is a complex issue. Generally, the noninferiority margin should be viewed as the "maximum treatment difference between the two arms of the study that would be considered acceptable." Interpretation of this value can change depending on the audience for the study, so investigators performing trials with this design should be prepared to face scrutiny over the clinical validity of the noninferiority margin that is chosen.

INTENTION TO TREAT AND PER-PROTOCOL ANALYSES IN NONINFERIORITY TRIALS

Analyzing the findings of a noninferiority trial is different from analysis of a traditional superiority trial. In a superiority trial, an ITT analysis is most often used because it may minimize the observed differences between study arms and is considered the most conservative approach. However, in the setting of a noninferiority trial, a bias toward finding no difference between the treatment groups would be a bias toward a "positive" result (i.e., declaring noninferiority), and an ITT analysis is not the conservative approach. Investigators typically perform both ITT and per-protocol analyses in noninferiority trials (see "Example of a Noninferiority Trial of Coronary stent: PLATINUM Trial," earlier).

Observational Studies to Determine Comparative Effectiveness

Although RCTs represent the "gold standard" for determining the effectiveness of a particular treatment, not all clinical questions are

TABLE 4-7	Types of Observational Study Designs	
Descriptive Observational Studies	**Analytical Observational Studies**	
Case reports	Cohort studies	
Case series	Case-control studies	
Analyses of secular trends	Hybrid studies	
	Nested case-control studies	
	Case-crossover studies	
	Case-cohort studies	

TABLE 4-8	Prototypical 2 × 2 Table	
	Diseased	Nondiseased
Exposed	A	B
Nonexposed	C	D

amenable to study with an RCT, often owing to the cost or complexity that an appropriately designed RCT would require. Table 4-7 lists several types of observational study designs.

ANALYTICAL STRATEGIES FOR NONRANDOMIZED COMPARATIVE EFFECTIVENESS STUDIES

The starting point in the analytical process for nonrandomized comparative effectiveness studies in interventional cardiology is the estimation of the crude effect of the exposure of interest (e.g., stent type) on the outcome of interest (e.g., restenosis or major adverse cardiovascular events). In addition to deriving estimates of effects that can be adjusted for confounding, inferential statistics are needed to evaluate the role of chance as an explanation for the observed association. The strategies for determining crude estimates are given in the following sections.

Cohort Studies

Data from cohort studies can be based on counts (e.g., cumulative incidence) or population time (e.g., incidence rates). The data layout for a cohort using count data is the prototypical 2 × 2 table as shown in Table 4-8, where the "exposure" may be one stent type versus another, and the "disease" may be the development of the outcome of interest (e.g., restenosis). Cumulative incidence is defined as the proportion of people who become diseased in a specified time period and is a measure of risk that ranges from 0 to 1; it can also be thought of as the probability of developing the disease over a specific time period (i.e., the average risk for the population). Use of cumulative incidence to determine the measure of effect assumes that everyone in the population would have survived without development of the disease to the end of the study period (i.e., no competing risks). The relative risk (or risk ratio) is the basic measure of association in cohort studies and reflects the relative increase in risk of developing the disease in the "exposed" (e.g., receiving a particular stent) compared with the "unexposed" (e.g., not receiving the particular stent). The relative risk is calculated by taking the ratio of the cumulative incidence in the exposed group to the cumulative incidence in the unexposed group. Using data arranged in the 2 × 2 table, the risk ratio is derived from the following formula:

$$\text{Risk ratio} = (a/[a+b])/(c/[c+d])$$

Case-Control Studies

When determining crude associations from case-control studies, one cannot directly estimate the rate of disease because it is fixed based on the sampling scheme of cases and controls. The same analytical strategy used in cohort studies cannot be used in case-control studies. Instead, the measure of effect used in case-control studies is the odds

ratio, which is similar to the relative risk when the outcome of interest is rare. The odds ratio is calculated as follows:

$$\text{Odds ratio} = (a/[1-a])/(c/[1-c]) = (a/b)/(c/d) = ad/bc$$

A case-control design is particularly useful when studying rare outcomes such as stent thrombosis. Cayla and associates[61] used a case-control study of 123 patients with definite stent thrombosis and 246 matched controls and found that three genetic variants were independently associated with early stent thrombosis.

ANALYTICAL CONTROL FOR CONFOUNDING

Observational studies provide particular challenges to overcome, most notably, confounding by variables that are unevenly distributed between treatment comparison groups. Analytical techniques to adjust for confounding include stratified analyses using Mantel-Haenszel methods and multivariable adjustment using statistical methods such as logistic regression. More recently, the use of propensity score analyses and instrumental variable analyses have been used in this field as well. The choice of analytical strategy to handle confounding in comparative effectiveness research depends on numerous factors, including study design, the measure of effect of interest, the number of potential confounders, and the sample size. No matter what the analytical approach, investigators should have an idea of potential confounders and their hypothesized effect on the study estimate before performing any statistical adjustments. The following sections briefly discuss the potential methods used to adjust for confounding and give selected examples where they have been used in the interventional cardiology literature.

Stratified Analyses

Stratified analyses accomplish two goals. First, by stratifying an analysis on variables known or expected to be confounders, separate analyses within each stratum are unconfounded by the stratification variable. Second, stratification can help investigators understand and evaluate effect modification (or interactions). Effect modification exists when the effect of an exposure on the outcome under study is modified, depending on a third variable.[62] The steps involved in performing stratified analyses are straightforward. First, the crude estimates of effect (i.e., odds ratio or relative risk) are calculated. Second, the data are stratified, and the stratum-specific effect estimates are calculated. Third, the effect estimates are compared, often qualitatively, across the strata. Fourth, a summary effect estimate is calculated, depending on whether the effect estimates are uniform across strata. If the effect estimates are uniform, a summary effect estimate is calculated using the Mantel-Haenszel formula for relative risk or odds ratios.

Compared with regression analyses, stratification is not often used in the study of coronary stents; however, there are instances when the simplicity of the technique makes it attractive. In a study to elucidate the impact of low-dose versus high-dose aspirin on the incidence of stent thrombosis after DES implantation, Lotfi and colleagues[63] stratified patients by the type of stent used (to account for differences between the DES as a possible confounder) and combined effect measures with the Mantel-Haenszel formula across strata to generate a uniform measure of effect of the impact of low-dose compared with high-dose aspirin.

Stratification is intuitively simple and easy to perform, but there can be significant limitations to its application. For example, there may be an insufficient number of individuals in each stratum to make appropriate statistical inferences. When stratifying on more than one factor, the number of strata quickly becomes excessive, and interpretation becomes difficult.

Regression Analyses

Regression analyses are extensions of stratified analyses that allow for the simultaneous adjustment for multiple confounders. Logistic regression is used for binary outcomes, and Cox regression models are used when dealing with person-time or survival data. A full explanation of the mathematics behind regression models is beyond the scope of this chapter. In general, the logistic regression model evaluating the relationship between an exposure x_1 and potential confounding variables x_2 to x_n, and the outcome y is:

$$(y)/(1-y) = e^{\beta_0 + \beta_1 x_1 + \beta_2 x_2 + \ldots + \beta_n x_n}$$

The interpretation for the model is simple. The odds ratio describing the relationship between the exposure and the outcome of interest while holding all other variables in the model constant can be represented by e^{β_1}. Similar models can be generated for survival data as well using Cox regression.

Both logistic regression and Cox models can be used to determine predictors of adverse events with different types of stents. In a single-center study evaluating outcomes with sirolimus-eluting stents compared with BMS, Munir and colleagues[64] generated logistic regression models to evaluate predictors of 30-day major adverse cardiovascular events and Cox regression models to determine independent predictors of long-term outcomes. The authors found that stent type was not associated with major cardiovascular events at 30 days (odds ratio, 0.95; 95% confidence interval, 0.51-1.77), but target vessel failure at 3 years was significantly greater with BMS treatment (hazard ratio, 1.37; 95% confidence interval, 1.20-1.56).

Regression models are limited by several factors. First, the models rely on assumptions related to the mathematical relationships in which clinical variables are modeled. Second, models account only for confounders that have been measured and included in the model. If the investigator does not consider a given confounder, no amount of statistical or methodologic sophistication would provide an unbiased estimate of the relationship between the exposure and treatment of interest. Third, the stability of the model depends on the number of events—when there are too few events in traditional regression models, the model can be unstable. A typical rule for stability requires a ratio of predictors to outcomes of greater than 10:1.[65]

Propensity Scores

Another method for dealing with potential confounding involves the use of propensity scores that may provide better adjustment for confounding than traditional multivariable modeling.[66] The propensity score method involves two steps, the first of which is calculating the propensity score itself. Operationally, propensity scores are derived from logistic regression models that predict the probability that patients will receive the treatment of interest by using a set of variables that may be related to the treatment selection. Most commonly, patients who did and did not receive the treatment are matched with respect to their propensity scores and are compared according to the outcome of interest. Alternatively, a second regression model can be generated predicting the outcome of interest that includes the exposure of interest in addition to each patient's propensity score as a continuous covariate. This second model (or matched groups) can be used to approximate an unconfounded estimate of the exposure on the outcome. Stratified analyses based on propensity score groups or weighted regression analyses based on the inverse of the propensity score have also been employed. Douglas and coworkers[67] used this approach in an analysis of data from more than 262,000 elderly patients in the National Cardiovascular Data Registry (NCDR). In this study, clinical outcomes of patients receiving DES versus BMS were compared with estimated cumulative incidence rates with inverse probability weighted estimators. The investigators found that patients receiving DES had significantly better clinical outcomes than their BMS counterparts, without an associated increase in bleeding or stroke, throughout the study follow-up time of 30 months and across all subgroups studied.

Propensity score analysis has several potential advantages. First, it can be simpler to model the probability of treatment exposure than it can in some circumstances to model the outcome. Second, because the propensity score models the likelihood of receiving a particular treatment, investigators are not usually limited by a small number of outcome events. In the setting of too few events, traditional regression

models can be unstable. However, when building propensity score models, there are usually a large number of subjects who received both treatments under study, so stable models can be generated with large numbers of predictor variables. Propensity score matching works well when there is significant overlap in the propensity score distributions in both groups of individuals when stratified on the exposure variable. If there is not significant overlap between the propensity scores of subjects who are exposed and subjects who are not exposed to the treatment of interest, matching becomes difficult, and a large proportion of the study population may be excluded from the final analysis.

Propensity scores have been used extensively in the comparison of coronary stents, most notably in the comparison of DES with BMS. Mauri and colleagues[68] compared 2-year outcomes of patients with acute myocardial infarction undergoing PCI in Massachusetts with either DES or BMS. The authors performed 1:1 propensity score matching among the more than 7000 patients included in the study and found that 2-year repeat revascularization and mortality rates were lower for patients receiving DES. The safety of DES in patients with myocardial infarction was later confirmed in RCTs.[32,69,70]

INSTRUMENTAL VARIABLE ANALYSES

Instrumental variables methodology is a class of methods that have been used extensively in economics for many years, and the methods are gaining popularity in the health sciences.[71,72] An instrumental variable, or instrument, is a variable that is associated with a predictor of interest but is not associated with the outcome of interest except through its relationship with the predictor (Figure 4-3). When an instrument is identified, investigators estimate how much variation in the treatment variable is induced by changes in the instrument. The best example of an instrumental variable is the treatment arm of an RCT. The randomization arm is a perfect or near-perfect (when there is noncompliance or crossover) predictor of the treatment but is not associated with outcomes except through its relationship with the treatment.

The most difficult part of research with instruments is identifying appropriate instruments outside of the randomized trial setting. The identification of appropriate instrumental variables is difficult for two reasons. First, there must not be a direct relationship between the instrument and the outcome. If such a backdoor relationship exists, the estimate of the treatment effect is biased. Second, many proposed instruments do not induce much variation in the treatment variable and provide little statistical power. If the instrument is weak, the natural variation in the treatment would be masked by random error in the system, and true effects between the outcome of interest and the treatment of interest would not be uncovered during the study. Examples follow.

CASE STUDY OF METHODS TO CONTROL FOR CONFOUNDING: IS THERE A MORTALITY BENEFIT WITH DRUG-ELUTING STENTS COMPARED WITH BARE METAL STENTS?

We focus on two studies to illustrate how an identical research question can be approached in multiple ways. Yeh and colleagues[73] and

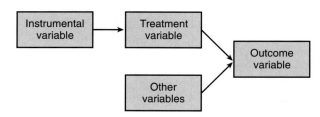

Figure 4-3 Relationship of instrumental variable to the treatment and outcome variables being studied.

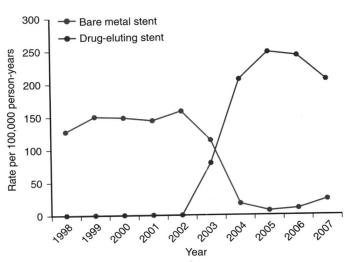

Figure 4-4 Example of instrumental variable analysis. The eras before and after the change in rates represent an appropriate instrumental variable for the study of mortality when comparing DES with BMS. (From Yeh RW, Chandra M, McCulloch CE, et al. Accounting for the mortality benefit of drug-eluting stents in percutaneous coronary intervention: a comparison of methods in a retrospective cohort study. BMC Med 2011;9:78.)

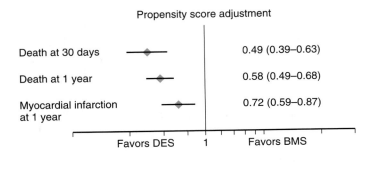

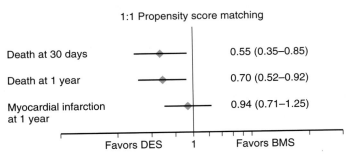

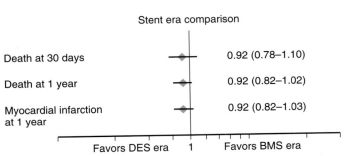

Figure 4-5 Mortality differences in an observational cohort study of more than 35,000 patients treated with bare metal stents *(BMS)* or drug-eluting stents *(DES)* according to different methods for controlling for confounding. Although the use of propensity score adjustment and propensity score matching demonstrated a mortality benefit with DES, this was not seen with instrument variable analysis that used stent era as the instrument. Unobserved factors that influence stent selection in observational studies may account for the observed mortality benefit of DES that was not seen in randomized clinical trials. (From Yeh RW, Chandra M, McCulloch CE, et al. Accounting for the mortality benefit of drug-eluting stents in percutaneous coronary intervention: a comparison of methods in a retrospective cohort study. BMC Med 2011;9:78.)

Venkitachalam and associates[74] examined the question of whether DES provide a mortality benefit compared with BMS in routine practice. In "real world" clinical practice, there are large differences in baseline characteristics between patients who receive DES and BMS. This phenomenon suggests the presence of strong treatment selection bias that may be incompletely characterized by traditional regression analyses or propensity score–based methods because of numerous confounders that are difficult to capture. Yeh and colleagues[73] compared rates of all-cause mortality at 30 days and 1 year for patients undergoing PCI with DES or BMS from 1998 to 2007 in a retrospective cohort study of patients within Kaiser Permanente Northern California. The comparison between DES and BMS was made using propensity score adjustment (i.e., modeling the propensity of receiving DES compared with BMS), propensity score matching, and an instrumental variable approach. Because patients treated before 2003 were uniformly treated with BMS, whereas patients treated after 2003 were predominantly treated with DES, procedure era (before or after the introduction of DES in 2003) was used as the instrument (Figure 4-4). After propensity score adjustment, DES were associated with significantly lower death rates at 30 days and 1 year (odds ratio, 0.49; 95% confidence interval, 0.39-0.63, and OR, 0.58; 95% confidence interval, 0.49-0.68). Mortality was also significantly decreased with DES after propensity score matching. In contrast, when using the instrument variable of stent era, there was no significant difference in mortality between DES and BMS, similar to findings observed in clinical trials (Figure 4-5).

Venkitachalam and associates[74] used a similar set of methods to address the question of a mortality difference between patients treated with DES or BMS. These authors evaluated 9266 patients who underwent nonemergent PCI at 55 centers across the United States from 2004 to 2007. They evaluated whether there was a mortality difference at 1 year between patients who received DES or BMS in unadjusted analyses, multivariable-adjusted analyses with traditional regression models, propensity matched analyses, and an instrumental variable analysis using procedure era as the instrument—in this case taking advantage of the decline in DES use in later years. The results were concordant with the results of Yeh and colleagues; in the regression and the propensity matched analyses, there was a significant mortality benefit seen in patients receiving DES compared with patients receiving BMS. In the instrumental variable analysis, however, there was

no significant difference in 1-year mortality (predicted absolute difference of 2.0%; 95% CI, −1.8%-5.7%) (Figure 4-6). No significant difference in target vessel revascularization was observed between DES and BMS in this study, most likely because of the weak association between the instrumental variable and stent type.[75]

Both of these studies demonstrate that even with rigorous risk adjustment and the availability of detailed clinical descriptors, sophisticated analytical techniques for dealing with observational data may still be limited in providing unbiased estimates of treatment effects, likely owing to unmeasured confounders. Instrumental variables eliminate the need for these concerns to a large degree, but the major limitation to their use is the difficulty in identifying appropriate instruments that significantly influence the exposure but do not have a backdoor pathway that may influence the outcome directly.

COMPARISON OF RISK-ADJUSTED CLINICAL OUTCOMES BY STENT TYPE

Variable	Death (95% CI)	P Value	TLR (95% CI)	P Value
Multivariable regression*				
HR	0.50 (0.37 to 0.69)	<0.001	0.49 (0.37 to 0.63)	<0.001
Risk difference, %	−2.4 (−3.8 to −1.0)	0.001	−3.3 (−4.9 to −1.8)	<0.001
Propensity-matched regression*				
HR	0.51 (0.36 to 0.71)	<0.001	0.50 (0.38 to 0.67)	<0.001
Risk difference, %	−1.8 (−3.3 to −0.3)	0.02	−3.0 (−4.5 to −1.4)	<0.001
Instrumental variable analysis*				
Risk difference, %	2.0 (−1.8 to 5.7)	0.30	−4.2 (−8.9 to 0.4)	0.07

Figure 4-6 Different methods for controlling for confounding can result in substantially different conclusions. In an observational study of more than 9000 patients undergoing nonemergent PCI, DES provided a mortality benefit compared with BMS according to multivariable and propensity-matched regression but not by instrumental variable analysis. *Negative values indicate lower rates of the outcome with DES versus BMS use. (*CI,* Confidence interval; *HR,* hazard ratio; *TLR,* target lesion revascularization.) (From Venkitachalam L, Lei Y, Magnuson EA, et al. Survival benefit with drug-eluting stents in observational studies: fact or artifact? Circ Cardiovasc Qual Outcomes 2011;4:587-594.)

Other Types of Studies

SYSTEMATIC REVIEWS

Systematic research reviews, also known as quantitative literature reviews, are formal summaries of the existing literature on a given scientific question. In contrast to simple narrative research reviews, these studies use a logical framework, formal literature search criteria, and some form of objective and systematic evaluation of the literature on a given topic. Systematic reviews often are used to identify areas of consensus in the literature and to highlight the nature and cause of disagreements. They are used to identify areas where further research questions exist and can frame research results so that they can be translated into clinical practice. These types of reviews often form the basis for summative or "evidence-based" guidelines.

META-ANALYSES

Meta-analyses represent a subset of systematic reviews that use statistical techniques to analyze data from a large number of studies evaluating a similar research question comparing two treatments or treatment strategies. They are often performed as a way to integrate the findings of disparate studies or to evaluate subpopulations that are difficult to study in a single trial. Combining trial data allows for the increase in the precision of summary estimates. These studies can also resolve issues relating to conflicting results from individual trials. Kirtane and associates[76] performed a meta-analysis of 22 randomized clinical trials and 34 observational studies to compare the effectiveness and safety of DES versus BMS. The authors found similar rates of death or myocardial infarction between stent types in RCTs but reduced rates of death and myocardial infarction with DES in observational studies, possibly owing to residual confounding. Finally, combining studies through the use of meta-regression allows investigators to estimate relationships between the effects of study-level variables.

NETWORK META-ANALYSES

A network meta-analysis is a study in which multiple (three or more) treatments are compared using both direct comparisons of interventions within randomized controlled trials and indirect comparisons across trials based on a common comparator (Figs. 4-7 and 4-8). These studies have become popular in the study of coronary stents, likely because there are various stent platforms but few head-to-head comparisons of DES. Several network meta-analyses have been published in this field.[77,78] Because of the indirect comparisons between studies

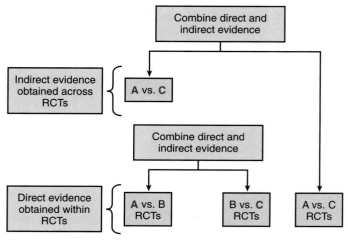

Figure 4-7 Schematic of a network meta-analysis. This type of analysis combines direct evidence obtained within randomized clinical trials *(RCTs)* (*A* vs. *B*, *B* vs. *C*, and *A* vs. *C*) and indirect evidence obtained across RCTs through a common comparator (*A* vs. *B* and *B* vs. *C*). (From Li T, Puhan MA, Vedula SS, et al. Network meta-analysis: highly attractive but more methodological research is needed. BMC Med 2011;9:79.)

in network meta-analyses, investigators must be careful to design these analyses rigorously and pay careful attention to study inclusion and exclusion criteria in regard to the quality of the evidence up for comparison.[79] Without clear understanding of what is being evaluated in each study and how each study is conducted, biased comparisons can easily lead to erroneous results.

Conclusion

The development of the field of interventional cardiology and, in particular, coronary stents has been shaped by the continued desire to answer new scientific questions using clinical research techniques. Randomized, controlled trials are the "gold standard" research design for establishing an unbiased treatment effect of a new technology or procedure and have been used extensively in the evaluation of coronary stents. Key aspects of RCT design include the selection of an appropriate patient population, comparator groups, randomization scheme, outcomes, blinding, and statistical analysis approach.

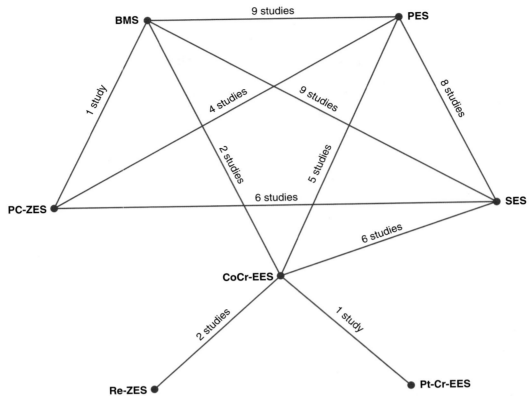

Figure 4-8 Evidence network for stents included in a meta-analysis comparing several types of drug-eluting stents and bare metal stents *(BMS)* with each other. This figure demonstrates the complexity of network meta-analyses and the associated indirect comparisons across the web of studies that are performed when using this study design. *Co-Cr-EES,* Cobalt chromium everolimus-eluting stent; *PC-ZES,* phosphorylcholine polymer-based zotarolimus eluting stent; *PES,* paclitaxel-eluting stent; *Pt-Cr-EES,* platinum chromium everolimus-eluting stent; *Re-ZES,* Resolute zotarolimus-eluting stent; *SES,* sirolimus-eluting stent. (From Palmerini T, Biondi-Zoccai G, Della Riva D, et al. Stent thrombosis with drug-eluting and bare-metal stents: evidence from a comprehensive network meta-analysis. Lancet 2012;379:1393-1402.)

Randomized trials may be impractical or lack feasibility to answer certain questions because of cost, lack of perceived equipoise, or inability to enroll large representative populations of patients. As the DES field matures, randomized clinical trials to evaluate small incremental technologic changes in newer generation DES is increasingly burdensome, and single-arm studies have been used to compare patients receiving active treatment with historical control patients who received previous iterations of the DES under evaluation. Observational research designs have been used to assess the comparative effectiveness of coronary stents but should be designed and interpreted with particular attention to bias and confounding. Moving forward, rigorous study design and thoughtful study interpretation are keys to pushing the field in new, data-driven directions for the betterment of patients.

REFERENCES

1. Palmaz JC, Sibbitt RR, Reuter SR, et al. Expandable intraluminal graft: a preliminary study. Work in progress. *Radiology* 1985;156:73-77.
2. Puel J, Joffre F, Rousseau H, et al. [Self-expanding coronary endoprosthesis in the prevention of restenosis following transluminal angioplasty: preliminary clinical study] [in French]. *Arch Mal Coeur Vaiss* 1987;80:1311-1312.
3. Sigwart U, Puel J, Mirkovitch V, et al. Intravascular stents to prevent occlusion and restenosis after transluminal angioplasty. *N Engl J Med* 1987;316:701-706.
4. Roubin GS, Robinson KA, King 3rd SB, et al. Early and late results of intracoronary arterial stenting after coronary angioplasty in dogs. *Circulation* 1987;76:891-897.
5. Schatz RA, Palmaz JC, Tio FO, et al. Balloon-expandable intracoronary stents in the adult dog. *Circulation* 1987;76:450-457.
6. Serruys PW, de Jaegere P, Kiemeneij F, et al. A comparison of balloon-expandable-stent implantation with balloon angioplasty in patients with coronary artery disease. Benestent study group. *N Engl J Med* 1994;331:489-495.
7. Fischman DL, Leon MB, Baim DS, et al. A randomized comparison of coronary-stent placement and balloon angioplasty in the treatment of coronary artery disease. Stent restenosis study investigators. *N Engl J Med* 1994;331:496-501.
8. Machin D. *Textbook of Clinical Trials.* Hoboken, NJ: Wiley; 2004.
9. Moer R, van Weert AW, Myreng Y, et al. Variability of quantitative coronary angiography: an evaluation of on-site versus core laboratory analysis. *Int J Cardiovasc Imaging* 2003;19:457-464.
10. Freedman B. Equipoise and the ethics of clinical research. *N Engl J Med* 1987;317:141-145.
11. Udipi K, Chen M, Cheng P, et al. Development of a novel biocompatible polymer system for extended drug release in a next-generation drug-eluting stent. *J Biomed Mater Res A* 2008;85:1064-1071.
12. Yeung AC, Leon MB, Jain A, et al. Clinical evaluation of the Resolute zotarolimus-eluting coronary stent system in the treatment of de novo lesions in native coronary arteries: the Resolute US Clinical Trial. *J Am Coll Cardiol* 2011;57:1778-1783.
13. Kereiakes DJ, Kuntz RE, Mauri L, et al. Surrogates, substudies, and real clinical end points in trials of drug-eluting stents. *J Am Coll Cardiol* 2005;45:1206-1212.
14. Morice MC, Serruys PW, Sousa JE, et al. A randomized comparison of a sirolimus-eluting stent with a standard stent for coronary revascularization. *N Engl J Med* 2002;346:1773-1780.
15. Schampaert E, Cohen EA, Schluter M, et al. The Canadian Study of the Sirolimus-Eluting Stent in the treatment of patients with long de novo lesions in small native coronary arteries (C-SIRIUS). *J Am Coll Cardiol* 2004;43:1110-1115.
16. Schofer J, Schluter M, Gershlick AH, et al. Sirolimus-eluting stents for treatment of patients with long atherosclerotic lesions in small coronary arteries: double-blind, randomised controlled trial (E-SIRIUS). *Lancet* 2003;362:1093-1099.
17. Grube E, Silber S, Hauptmann KE, et al. TAXUS I: six- and twelve-month results from a randomized, double-blind trial on a slow-release paclitaxel-eluting stent for de novo coronary lesions. *Circulation* 2003;107:38-42.
18. Colombo A, Drzewiecki J, Banning A, et al. Randomized study to assess the effectiveness of slow- and moderate-release polymer-based paclitaxel-eluting stents for coronary artery lesions. *Circulation* 2003;108:788-794.
19. Kandzari DE, Leon MB, Popma JJ, et al. Comparison of zotarolimus-eluting and sirolimus-eluting stents in patients with native coronary artery disease: a randomized controlled trial. *J Am Coll Cardiol* 2006;48:2440-2447.
20. Meredith IT, Worthley S, Whitbourn R, et al. Clinical and angiographic results with the next-generation Resolute stent system: a prospective, multicenter, first-in-human trial. *JACC Cardiovasc Interv* 2009;2:977-985.
21. Serruys PW, Ong AT, Piek JJ, et al. A randomized comparison of a durable polymer everolimus-eluting stent with a bare metal coronary stent: the SPIRIT FIRST trial. *EuroIntervention* 2005;1:58-65.

22. Levine GN, Bates ER, Blankenship JC, et al. 2011 ACCF/AHA/SCAI guideline for percutaneous coronary intervention: a report of the American College of Cardiology Foundation/American Heart Association Task Force on Practice Guidelines and the Society for Cardiovascular Angiography and Interventions. *Circulation* 2011;124:e574-e651.

23. Mauri L, Orav EJ, Kuntz RE. Late loss in lumen diameter and binary restenosis for drug-eluting stent comparison. *Circulation* 2005;111:3435-3442.

24. Mauri L, Orav EJ, Candia SC, et al. Robustness of late lumen loss in discriminating drug-eluting stents across variable observational and randomized trials. *Circulation* 2005;112:2833-2839.

25. Cutlip DE, Windecker S, Mehran R, et al. Clinical end points in coronary stent trials: a case for standardized definitions. *Circulation* 2007;115:2344-2351.

26. Mehran R, Rao SV, Bhatt DL, et al. Standardized bleeding definitions for cardiovascular clinical trials: a consensus report from the bleeding academic research consortium. *Circulation* 2011;123:2736-2747.

27. Rosner B. *Fundamentals of Biostatistics*. Boston: Brooks/Cole, Cengage Learning; 2011.

28. Begg C, Cho M, Eastwood S, et al. Improving the quality of reporting of randomized controlled trials. The CONSORT statement. *JAMA* 1996;276:637-639.

29. Stone GW, Ellis SG, Cox DA, et al. A polymer-based, paclitaxel-eluting stent in patients with coronary artery disease. *N Engl J Med* 2004;350:221-231.

30. Dawkins KD, Grube E, Guagliumi G, et al. Clinical efficacy of polymer-based paclitaxel-eluting stents in the treatment of complex, long coronary artery lesions from a multicenter, randomized trial: support for the use of drug-eluting stents in contemporary clinical practice. *Circulation* 2005;112:3306-3313.

31. Stone GW, Ellis SG, Cannon L, et al. Comparison of a polymer-based paclitaxel-eluting stent with a bare metal stent in patients with complex coronary artery disease: a randomized controlled trial. *JAMA* 2005;294:1215-1223.

32. Stone GW, Lansky AJ, Pocock SJ, et al. Paclitaxel-eluting stents versus bare-metal stents in acute myocardial infarction. *N Engl J Med* 2009;360:1946-1959.

33. Laarman GJ, Suttorp MJ, Dirksen MT, et al. Paclitaxel-eluting versus uncoated stents in primary percutaneous coronary intervention. *N Engl J Med* 2006;355:1105-1113.

34. Di Lorenzo E, De Luca G, Sauro R, et al. The PASEO (Paclitaxel or Sirolimus-Eluting Stent versus Bare Metal Stent in Primary Angioplasty) randomized trial. *JACC Cardiovasc Interv* 2009;2:515-523.

35. Zhang Q, Zhang RY, Zhang JS, et al. One-year clinical outcomes of Chinese sirolimus-eluting stent in the treatment of unselected patients with coronary artery disease. *Chin Med J (Engl)* 2006;119:165-168.

36. Erglis A, Narbute I, Kumsars I, et al. A randomized comparison of paclitaxel-eluting stents versus bare-metal stents for treatment of unprotected left main coronary artery stenosis. *J Am Coll Cardiol* 2007;50:491-497.

37. Brilakis ES, Lichtenwalter C, de Lemos JA, et al. A randomized controlled trial of a paclitaxel-eluting stent versus a similar bare-metal stent in saphenous vein graft lesions the SOS (Stenting Of Saphenous Vein Grafts) trial. *J Am Coll Cardiol* 2009;53:919-928.

38. Morice MC, Colombo A, Meier B, et al. Sirolimus- vs paclitaxel-eluting stents in de novo coronary artery lesions; the REALITY trial: a randomized controlled trial. *JAMA* 2006;295:895-904.

39. Galloe AM, Thuesen L, Kelbaek H, et al. Comparison of paclitaxel- and sirolimus-eluting stents in everyday clinical practice: the Sort Out II randomized trial. *JAMA* 2008;299:409-416.

40. Windecker S, Remondino A, Eberli FR, et al. Sirolimus-eluting and paclitaxel-eluting stents for coronary revascularization. *N Engl J Med* 2005;353:653-662.

41. Goy JJ, Stauffer JC, Siegenthaler M, et al. A prospective randomized comparison between paclitaxel and sirolimus stents in the real world of interventional cardiology: the TAXi trial. *J Am Coll Cardiol* 2005;45:308-311.

42. Lee SW, Park SW, Kim YH, et al. A randomized comparison of sirolimus- versus paclitaxel-eluting stent implantation in patients with diabetes mellitus. *J Am Coll Cardiol* 2008;52:727-733.

43. Dibra A, Kastrati A, Mehilli J, et al. Paclitaxel-eluting or sirolimus-eluting stents to prevent restenosis in diabetic patients. *N Engl J Med* 2005;353:663-670.

44. Kim MH, Hong SJ, Cha KS, et al. Effect of paclitaxel-eluting versus sirolimus-eluting stents on coronary restenosis in Korean diabetic patients. *J Intervent Cardiol* 2008;21:225-231.

45. Maeng M, Jensen LO, Galloe AM, et al. Comparison of the sirolimus-eluting versus paclitaxel-eluting coronary stent in patients with diabetes mellitus: the Diabetes and Drug-Eluting Stent (DIABEDES) randomized angiography trial. *Am J Cardiol* 2009;103:345-349.

46. Mehilli J, Kastrati A, Byrne RA, et al. Paclitaxel- versus sirolimus-eluting stents for unprotected left main coronary artery disease. *J Am Coll Cardiol* 2009;53:1760-1768.

47. Kim YH, Park SW, Lee SW, et al. Sirolimus-eluting stent versus paclitaxel-eluting stent for patients with long coronary artery disease. *Circulation* 2006;114:2148-2153.

48. Han YL, Wang XZ, Jing QM, et al. [Comparison of rapamycin and paclitaxel eluting stent in patients with multi-vessel coronary disease] [in Chinese]. *Zhonghua Xin Xue Guan Bing Za Zhi* 2006;34:123-126.

49. Mehilli J, Dibra A, Kastrati A, et al. Randomized trial of paclitaxel- and sirolimus-eluting stents in small coronary vessels. *Eur Heart J* 2006;27:260-266.

50. Pan M, Suarez de Lezo J, Medina A, et al. Drug-eluting stents for the treatment of bifurcation lesions: a randomized comparison between paclitaxel and sirolimus stents. *Am Heart J* 2007;153:15.e11-15.e17.

51. Petronio AS, De Carlo M, Branchitta G, et al. Randomized comparison of sirolimus and paclitaxel drug-eluting stents for long lesions in the left anterior descending artery: an intravascular ultrasound study. *J Am Coll Cardiol* 2007;49:539-546.

52. Cervinka P, Costa MA, Angiolillo DJ, et al. Head-to-head comparison between sirolimus-eluting and paclitaxel-eluting stents in patients with complex coronary artery disease: an intravascular ultrasound study. *Cathet Cardiovasc Interv* 2006;67:846-851.

53. Kastrati A, Mehilli J, von Beckerath N, et al. Sirolimus-eluting stent or paclitaxel-eluting stent vs balloon angioplasty for prevention of recurrences in patients with coronary in-stent restenosis: a randomized controlled trial. *JAMA* 2005;293:165-171.

54. Mehilli J, Byrne RA, Tiroch K, et al. Randomized trial of paclitaxel- versus sirolimus-eluting stents for treatment of coronary restenosis in sirolimus-eluting stents: the ISAR-DESIRE 2 (Intracoronary Stenting and angiographic Results: Drug Eluting Stents for In-Stent Restenosis 2) study. *J Am Coll Cardiol* 2010;55:2710-2716.

55. Lee JH, Kim HS, Lee SW, et al. Prospective randomized comparison of sirolimus- versus paclitaxel-eluting stents for the treatment of acute ST-elevation myocardial infarction: PROSIT trial. *Cathet Cardiovasc Interv* 2008;72:25-32.

56. Stefanini GG, Serruys PW, Silber S, et al. The impact of patient and lesion complexity on clinical and angiographic outcomes after revascularization with zotarolimus- and everolimus-eluting stents: a substudy of the Resolute All Comers trial (a randomized comparison of a zotarolimus-eluting stent with an everolimus-eluting stent for percutaneous coronary intervention). *J Am Coll Cardiol* 2011;57:2221-2232.

57. Mauri L, Leon MB, Yeung AC, et al. Rationale and design of the clinical evaluation of the Resolute zotarolimus-eluting coronary stent system in the treatment of de novo lesions in native coronary arteries (the Resolute US Clinical Trial). *Am Heart J* 2011;161:807-814.

58. Rothmann MD, Wiens BL, Chan ISF. *Design and Analysis of Non-inferiority Trials*. Boca Raton, FL: Chapman & Hall/CRC; 2011.

59. Evans SR. Clinical trial structures. *J Exp Stroke Transl Med* 2010;3:8-18.

60. Stone GW, Teirstein PS, Meredith IT, et al. A prospective, randomized evaluation of a novel everolimus-eluting coronary stent: the PLATINUM (a prospective, randomized, multicenter trial to assess an everolimus-eluting coronary stent system [Promus Element] for the treatment of up to two de novo coronary artery lesions) trial. *J Am Coll Cardiol* 2011;57:1700-1708.

61. Cayla G, Hulot JS, O'Connor SA, et al. Clinical, angiographic, and genetic factors associated with early coronary stent thrombosis. *JAMA* 2011;306:1765-1774.

62. Rothman KJ. Causes. *Am J Epidemiol* 1976;104:587-592.

63. Lotfi A, Cui J, Wartak S, et al. Influence of low-dose aspirin (81 mg) on the incidence of definite stent thrombosis in patients receiving bare-metal and drug-eluting stents. *Clin Cardiol* 2011;34:567-571.

64. Munir M, Aliota J, Ahmed A, et al. Sirolimus-eluting stents versus bare-metal stents in routine clinical use: a nonrandomized comparison. *Tex Heart Inst J* 2011;38:508-515.

65. Katz MH. Multivariable analysis: a primer for readers of medical research. *Ann Intern Med* 2003;138:644-650.

66. Rubin DB. On principles for modeling propensity scores in medical research. *Pharmacoepidemiol Drug Saf* 2004;13:855-857.

67. Douglas PS, Brennan JM, Anstrom KJ, et al. Clinical effectiveness of coronary stents in elderly persons: results from 262,700 Medicare patients in the American College of Cardiology-National Cardiovascular Data Registry. *J Am Coll Cardiol* 2009;53:1629-1641.

68. Mauri L, Silbaugh TS, Garg P, et al. Drug-eluting or bare-metal stents for acute myocardial infarction. *N Engl J Med* 2008;359:1330-1342.

69. Vink MA, Dirksen MT, Suttorp MJ, et al. 5-year follow-up after primary percutaneous coronary intervention with a paclitaxel-eluting stent versus a bare-metal stent in acute ST-segment elevation myocardial infarction: a follow-up study of the PASSION (Paclitaxel-eluting versus Conventional Stent in Myocardial Infarction with ST-Segment Elevation) trial. *JACC Cardiovasc Interv* 2011;4:24-29.

70. Spaulding C, Teiger E, Commeau P, et al. Four-year follow-up of typhoon (trial to assess the use of the Cypher sirolimus-eluting coronary stent in acute myocardial infarction treated with balloon angioplasty). *JACC Cardiovasc Interv* 2011;4:14-23.

71. Newhouse JP, McClellan M. Econometrics in outcomes research: the use of instrumental variables. *Annu Rev Public Health* 1998;19:17-34.

72. Greenland S. An introduction to instrumental variables for epidemiologists. *Int J Epidemiol* 2000;29:722-729.

73. Yeh RW, Chandra M, McCulloch CE, et al. Accounting for the mortality benefit of drug-eluting stents in percutaneous coronary intervention: a comparison of methods in a retrospective cohort study. *BMC Med* 2011;9:78.

74. Venkitachalam L, Lei Y, Magnuson EA, et al. Survival benefit with drug-eluting stents in observational studies: fact or artifact? *Circ Cardiovasc Qual Outcomes* 2011;4:587-594.

75. Yeh RW, Mauri L. Choosing methods to minimize confounding in observational studies: do the ends justify the means? *Circ Cardiovasc Qual Outcomes* 2011;4:581-583.

76. Kirtane AJ, Gupta A, Iyengar S, et al. Safety and efficacy of drug-eluting and bare metal stents: comprehensive meta-analysis of randomized trials and observational studies. *Circulation* 2009;119:3198-3206.

77. Palmerini T, Biondi-Zoccai G, Della Riva D, et al. Stent thrombosis with drug-eluting and bare-metal stents: evidence from a comprehensive network meta-analysis. *Lancet* 2012;379:1393-1402.

78. Bangalore S, Kumar S, Fusaro M, et al. Short- and long-term outcomes with drug-eluting and bare-metal coronary stents: a mixed-treatment comparison analysis of 117 762 patient-years of follow-up from randomized trials. *Circulation* 2012;125:2873-2891.

79. Li T, Puhan MA, Vedula SS, et al. Network meta-analysis: highly attractive but more methodological research is needed. *BMC Med* 2011;9:79.

80. Moses JW, Leon MB, Popma JJ, et al. Sirolimus-eluting stents versus standard stents in patients with stenosis in a native coronary artery. *N Engl J Med* 2003;349:1315-1323.

81. Stone GW, Rizvi A, Newman W, et al. Everolimus-eluting versus paclitaxel-eluting stents in coronary artery disease. *N Engl J Med* 2010;362:1663-1674.

82. Leon MB, Mauri L, Popma JJ, et al. A randomized comparison of the Endeavor zotarolimus-eluting stent versus the Taxus paclitaxel-eluting stent in de novo native coronary lesions: 12-month outcomes from the ENDEAVOR IV trial. *J Am Coll Cardiol* 2010;55:543-554.

83. Serruys PW, Silber S, Garg S, et al. Comparison of zotarolimus-eluting and everolimus-eluting coronary stents. *N Engl J Med* 2010;363:136-146.

84. Chechi T, Vittori G, Biondi Zoccai GG, et al. Single-center randomized evaluation of paclitaxel-eluting versus conventional stent in acute myocardial infarction (SELECTION). *J Interv Cardiol* 2007;20:282-291.

85. Erglis A, Narbute I, Kumsars I, et al. A randomized comparison of paclitaxel-eluting stents versus bare-metal stents for treatment of unprotected left main coronary artery stenosis. *J Am Coll Cardiol* 2007;50:491-497.

CHAPTER 5

Pathology of Drug-Eluting Stents in Humans

FUMIYUKI OTSUKA | MASATAKA NAKANO | FRANK D. KOLODGIE | RENU VIRMANI | ALOKE V. FINN

KEY POINTS

- Pathologic studies have identified incomplete endothelialization or neointimal coverage of drug-eluting stent struts as the primary substrate responsible for late and very late stent thrombosis.

- Vessel healing at culprit sites in patients with acute myocardial infarction treated with first-generation drug-eluting stents (sirolimus-eluting stents and paclitaxel-eluting stents) is substantially delayed compared with nonculprit sites and culprit sites in patients receiving drug-eluting stents for stable angina, emphasizing the importance of underlying plaque morphology in arterial healing and the risk of late and very late stent thrombosis after drug-eluting stent implantation.

- Arterial healing at bifurcation lesions treated with drug-eluting stents is impaired, with greater delays in healing at the flow divider (high shear) compared with the lateral wall sites (low shear), which may be caused by a combination of drug effect and differences in flow conditions.

- Grade V stent fracture (multiple strut fractures with acquired transection with gap in the stent body) is associated with adverse pathologic findings, including late and very late stent thrombosis and restenosis. Longer stent length, use of a sirolimus-eluting stent, and longer duration of implant are independent predictors of stent fracture.

- Localized hypersensitivity reaction is exclusive to sirolimus-eluting stents as an underlying mechanism of late and very late stent thrombosis, whereas malapposition secondary to excessive peristrut fibrin deposition is associated with paclitaxel-eluting stent implants.

- Persistently uncovered struts are identified in both sirolimus-eluting stents and paclitaxel-eluting stents with implant durations beyond 12 months, particularly in stents placed for off-label indications.

- In-stent neoatherosclerosis occurs in both bare metal stents and drug-eluting stents; however, the development of neoatherosclerosis is more rapid and frequent with drug-eluting stents and may be another important contributing factor to very late stent thrombosis.

- Future pathologic studies should address the long-term safety of newer generations of drug-eluting stents, including second-generation zotarolimus-eluting stents and everolimus-eluting stents, biodegradable polymer-coated and polymer-free drug-eluting stents, and completely bioresorbable scaffolds, in terms of improvements in reendothelialization, decreased inflammation and fibrin deposition, and a lower incidence of neoatherosclerosis, all of which may contribute to a reduced risk of late and very late stent thrombosis and improved patient outcomes.

Introduction

Percutaneous coronary interventions (PCIs) involving stenting are the most widely performed procedures for the treatment of symptomatic coronary disease.[1] Drug-eluting stents (DES) have dramatically reduced restenosis rates and have become the standard of care for the treatment of atherosclerotic coronary artery disease.[2-4] However, concern exists about the long-term safety of DES technology because observational studies have shown an increase in very late stent thrombosis associated with first-generation DES (sirolimus-eluting stents

[SES] and paclitaxel-eluting stents [PES]), and pathologic studies have suggested delayed reendothelialization as an important substrate for this phenomenon.[5-7] More recently, the development of atherosclerotic changes within the neointima (neoatherosclerosis) has been identified as another important mechanism of very late stent thrombosis.[8] DES have been implanted in millions of patients worldwide; understanding histopathologic findings seen after deployment of such devices in patients in the global practice of medicine is of paramount importance. This chapter reviews the pathologic mechanisms of late and very late stent thrombosis after first-generation DES implantation, the differential vascular response between SES and PES, and characteristics of neoatherosclerosis after first-generation DES compared with bare metal stents (BMS) in human coronary arteries.

Endothelial Coverage as a Morphometric Predictor for Late and Very Late Stent Thrombosis

To determine the pathologic correlates of late and very late stent thrombosis after DES implantation, we investigated 62 coronary lesions from 46 human autopsy cases with first-generation DES implanted for greater than 30 days[7] (Box 5-1). We identified stent thrombosis in 28 lesions (23 patients) and compared those lesions with 34 lesions (23 patients) of similar duration without stent thrombosis (duration of implant, 254 ± 235 days for lesions with late and very late stent thrombosis vs. 244 ± 289 days for lesions without thrombosis, P = not significant). In cases with late and very late stent thrombosis, 13 occlusive and 15 nonocclusive thrombi were detected. In these lesions with thrombus formation, there were 16 SES (14 lesions) and 22 PES (14 lesions), whereas lesions without thrombi included 23 SES (18 lesions) and 17 PES (16 lesions).

We found that neointimal thickness was less in thrombosed DES lesions (median 0.074 interquartile range [0.033, 0.129] mm vs. 0.11 [0.071, 0.19] mm, P = .05), and the percentage of endothelialization was significantly less in thrombosed DES lesions compared with patent DES lesions (40.5 ± 29.8% vs. 80.0 ± 25.2%, P < .0001). Total stent length was longer in thrombosed stents (25.9 ± 11.5 mm vs. 20.3 ± 9.6 mm, P = .04), and an average stent length without neointimal coverage was significantly greater in thrombosed compared with nonthrombosed lesions (20.1 ± 11.5 mm vs. 9.9 ± 10.1 mm, P = .0004). The mean number of uncovered struts per section was also significantly greater in DES lesions with thrombosis versus DES lesions without thrombosis (5.0 ± 2.7 vs. 2.0 ± 2.7, P < .0001), and the ratio of uncovered struts to total struts per section was greater in thrombosed versus nonthrombosed lesions (0.50 ± 0.23 vs. 0.19 ± 0.25, P < .0001).

The average distance between individual stent struts was significantly shorter in DES lesions with thrombus formation compared with patent DES lesions (0.52 ± 0.24 mm vs. 0.70 ± 0.25 mm, P = .004). There was also a good correlation between the mean number of uncovered struts per section and the average distance between stent struts ($r = -0.41$, P = .001), with most uncovered stent struts showing less interstrut distance than covered stent struts. On further examination, we found heterogeneity of coverage of stent struts, both within individual cross-sections and between sections from the same stent. Within the same DES, although some struts show healing as demonstrated by neointimal growth, others remain bare and serve as a nidus for thrombus formation (Figure 5-1). Within a DES, the middle section of the stent (vs. the proximal and distal ends) was the most common location of stent struts lacking neointimal coverage, and this was also the most common site of thrombus formation.

Multivariable logistic generalized estimating equations modeling demonstrated that endothelialization was the best predictor of late and very late stent thrombosis. The morphometric parameter that best correlated with endothelialization was the ratio of uncovered to total stent struts per section. In a stent with greater than 30% uncovered struts, the odds ratio (OR) for thrombosis was 9.0 (95% confidence interval [CI], 3.5-22.0) compared with a stent with complete coverage.

The mechanisms by which the first-generation DES induces non-uniform incomplete healing are not fully understood; however, lesion characteristics, drug properties, total drug dose, drug release profile and distribution, and polymer biocompatibility together all play an important role in inducing neointimal suppression. Although sirolimus and paclitaxel reduce neointimal formation by impeding smooth muscle cell proliferation and migration, these drugs also impair the normal healing process of the injured arterial wall.[9-11] Underlying plaque morphology may also affect the rate of healing when stent struts penetrate deeply into a necrotic core and are not in contact with cellular areas.[12] Eccentric plaques may prevent uniform strut deployment, increasing local toxicity owing to higher concentrations of drug and polymer. Sections with evidence of thrombosis showed significantly lower interstrut distances, and this correlated with lower neointimal growth. Local concentration of drug is ultimately highly dependent on spacing of stent struts, and the variance in distance between struts amplifies differences in concentrations leading to biologic effects.[13] Heterogeneity in loaded dose of drug varies from strut to strut with greater retention of lipophilic drugs in different regions of plaque affecting arterial drug concentration and resulting in non-uniform healing.[14] Coating defects can explain some of these differences.[15] The relationship between local drug concentration and cellular repair is clarified further by data from overlapping versus nonoverlapping SES and PES, which illustrate less coverage of stent struts in overlapping segments compared with nonoverlapping stent struts in the rabbit iliac model.[16]

The underlying pathology in cases of late and very late stent thrombosis indicates incomplete stent strut coverage as the most important morphometric predictor of late and very late stent thrombosis and is the most powerful surrogate of endothelialization. Both plaque-related and device-related issues play a role in promoting uneven healing.

🔹 Delayed Arterial Healing in First-Generation Drug-Eluting Stents Implanted for Acute Myocardial Infarction

Given that acute myocardial infarction is one of the only clinical presentations in which PCI has been shown to decrease the risk of death compared with medical therapy alone, the long-term outcomes after DES for acute myocardial infarction are of substantial clinical importance.[17,18] Using our autopsy database of patients dying after DES implantation with duration of implant greater than 30 days, we compared the vascular pathologic responses to DES implantation in patients receiving first-generation DES for acute myocardial infarction (n = 17) with the vascular pathologic responses of patients receiving first-generation DES for stable angina (n = 18).[19] Histologic sections were evaluated for the identification of culprit and nonculprit sites. Culprit sites in the setting of acute myocardial infarction were defined as the stented segments with underlying presence of a necrotic core and a thin cap with ruptured fibrous cap, whereas culprit sites in the setting of stable angina were identified as the sections with the largest underlying necrotic core and overlying thick fibrous cap (>100 μm). We compared culprit sites in patients with acute myocardial infarction with culprit sites in patients with stable angina and with nonculprit sites within each stent.

CULPRIT STENT THROMBOSIS SITES IN PATIENTS TREATED WITH DRUG-ELUTING STENTS FOR ACUTE MYOCARDIAL INFARCTION COMPARED WITH STABLE ANGINA

The incidence of late and very late stent thrombosis was significantly higher in patients with acute myocardial infarction (7 of 17, 41%) compared with patients with stable angina (2 of 18, 11%; $P = .04$). Very late stent thrombosis (>1 year) was observed in two patients with acute myocardial infarction (12%) and in no patients with stable angina. Morphometric analysis showed that culprit acute myocardial infarction sites versus stable plaque had significantly less neointimal thickness (0.04 [0.02, 0.09] mm vs. 0.11 [0.07, 0.21] mm, $P = .008$), greater fibrin deposition (63 ± 28% vs. 36 ± 27%, $P = .008$) and inflammation (35 [27, 49]% vs. 17 [7, 25]%, $P = .003$), and higher prevalence of uncovered struts (49 [16, 96]% vs. 9 [0, 39]%, $P = .01$). Images of culprit sites from patients with acute myocardial infarction and patients with stable angina are presented in Figure 5-2.

CULPRIT SITES COMPARED WITH NONCULPRIT SITES

In patients with acute myocardial infarction, neointimal thickness was significantly less at culprit sites compared with nonculprit sites (0.04 [0.02, 0.09] mm vs. 0.07 [0.04, 0.20] mm, $P = .008$), whereas this difference was not observed in patients with stable angina (0.11 [0.07, 0.21] mm vs. 0.11 [0.08, 0.19] mm, $P = .56$). Similarly, the percentage of struts with fibrin (63 ± 28% vs. 52 ± 27%, $P = .04$), struts with inflammation (35 [27, 49]% vs. 30 [13, 38]%, $P = .04$), and uncovered struts (49 [16, 96]% vs. 19 [3, 34]%, $P = .02$) was significantly greater at the culprit sites compared with nonculprit sites in patients with acute myocardial infarction, whereas there were no significant differences in these parameters in patients with stable angina.

FIBROUS CAP THICKNESS AND STENT STRUT COVERAGE

In this cohort, fibrous cap thickness and the presence of uncovered struts were significantly and negatively correlated (i.e., the thinner the fibrous cap, the more the presence of uncovered struts) ($R = -0.60$, $P = .0006$). There was also a significant but weaker negative correlation between duration of stent implants and the presence of uncovered struts ($R = -0.39$, $P = .01$). Similarly, fibrous cap thickness and neointimal thickness had a significant positive correlation ($R = 0.68$, $P = .0001$), whereas a weaker correlation was observed between neointimal thickness and duration of implant ($R = 0.38$, $P = .03$).

These findings, among others,[7] demonstrate the heterogeneity of healing that may occur within the same stent. Plaque rupture is the most frequent cause of acute myocardial infarction,[20] and this underlying plaque morphology is the most reasonable explanation for the delayed healing at culprit sites from patients with acute myocardial infarction as opposed to nonculprit sites and culprit sites from stable

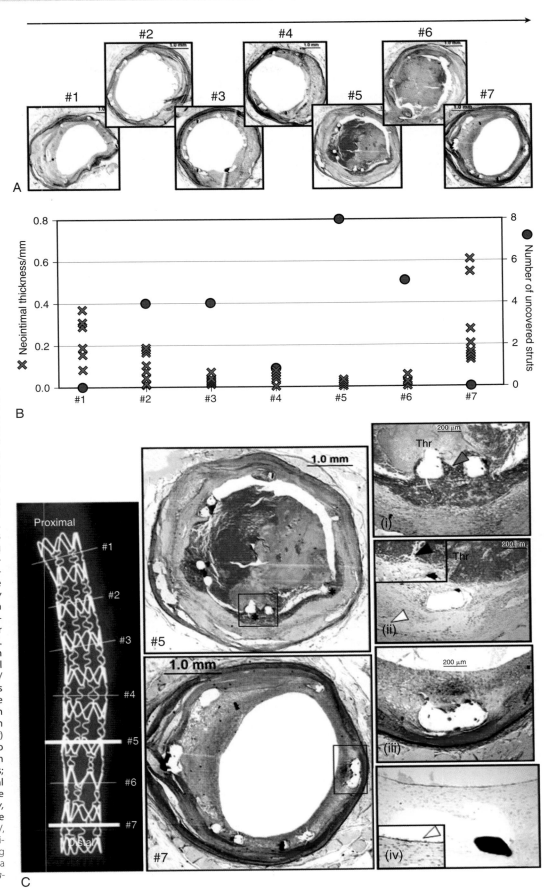

Figure 5-1 Heterogeneity of neointimal healing after DES placement. A 34-year-old woman underwent placement of one SES (22 mm × 3 mm) stent in the proximal left circumflex artery for acute myocardial infarction 2 years before her death. The patient was admitted to the emergency department with ST segment elevation myocardial infarction and subsequently died. Consecutive sections of the SES were cut 3 mm apart and stained with Movat Pentachrome **(A)**, and neointimal thickness (above each strut) and the number of uncovered stent struts were measured **(B)**. There is greater neointimal growth above each strut *(x)* and fewer uncovered stent struts *(red circle)* within the proximal and distal stented portions, with absence of luminal thrombus formation. At the site of thrombus formation (sections #5 and #6), neointimal thickness is minimal, and the number of uncovered stent struts is maximal. Movat Pentachrome–stained sections #5 and #7 **(C)** show detailed histology. There is a platelet-rich thrombus surrounding stent struts lacking neointima *(*)* in section #5. High-power images *(i* and *ii)* show uncovered stent struts with extensive underlying fibrin deposition *(gray arrowhead)*, luminal platelet-rich thrombus *(Thr)*, and lack of endothelialization *(ii, black arrowhead)* after immunostaining for CD31/CD34. However, positive staining (brown area) is observed within medial microvessels containing CD31/CD34-positive endothelial cells *(white arrowhead)*. In contrast, there is a well-healed neointima with complete strut coverage in section #7. High-power images *(iii* and *iv)* show stent struts embedded into neointima composed of smooth muscle cells and proteoglycans; there is an absence of luminal thrombus, and endothelial cells are abundant above stent struts *(iv, white arrowhead)* with positive staining (brown area). (From Finn AV, Joner M, Nakazawa G, et al. Pathological correlates of late drug-eluting stent thrombosis: strut coverage as a marker of endothelialization. *Circulation.* 2007;115:2435-2441.)

AMI LESIONS (WITH PLAQUE RUPTURE)

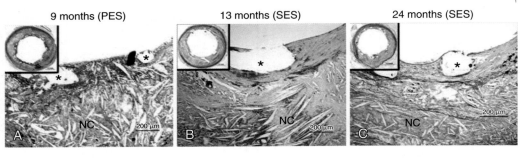

9 months (PES)   13 months (SES)   24 months (SES)

STABLE LESIONS (WITH FIBROATHEROMA AND THICK CAP)

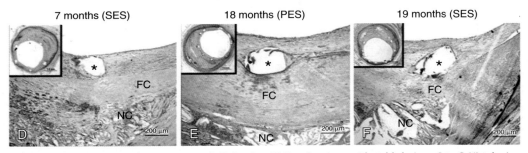

7 months (SES)   18 months (PES)   19 months (SES)

Figure 5-2 Histologic sections from patients with acute myocardial infarction *(AMI)* and patients with stable lesions. **A to C,** Histologic sections from patients with acute myocardial infarction: a 64-year-old woman who died of congestive heart failure 9 months after paclitaxel-eluting stent *(PES)* implantation **(A)**, a 49-year-old man who died from a noncardiac cause 13 months after sirolimus-eluting stent *(SES)* implantation **(B)**, and a 34-year-old woman who died as a result of late stent thrombosis 24 months after SES implantation **(C)**. Struts with a necrotic core *(NC)* were observed with fibrin deposition and absence of endothelial coverage **(A)**. Stents in **B** and **C** showed minimal coverage of struts above the NC at 13 months' and 24 months' duration. **D to F,** Histologic sections from patients with stable lesions: a 61-year-old man who died from a noncardiac cause 7 months after SES implantation **(D)**, a 53-year-old man who died suddenly 18 months after PES implantation **(E)**, and a 68-year-old man who died from a noncardiac cause 19 months after SES implantation **(F)**. All patients had underlying fibroatheroma with a thick fibrous cap *(FC)*. High-magnification images show underlying NC and thick FC with varying degrees of neointimal formation above the stent struts. Asterisks indicate stent strut. (From Nakazawa G, Finn AV, Joner M, et al. Delayed arterial healing and increased late stent thrombosis at culprit sites after drug-eluting stent placement for acute myocardial infarction patients: an autopsy study. *Circulation.* 2008;118:1138-1145.)

patients. Because sirolimus and paclitaxel are highly lipophilic,[14] it is likely that these agents have high affinity for lipid-rich plaques (i.e., necrotic core) and dwell there for longer periods because of greater strut penetration compared with when struts are exposed to adjacent inflamed regions of the plaque. In addition, the lipid-rich necrotic cores are avascular and have fewer smooth muscle cells within the fibrous cap. These areas are less likely to be covered by migrating and proliferating cells from adjacent regions. Higher drug concentrations in these areas may also heavily influence healing by retarding smooth muscle cell proliferation and endothelial regrowth. In addition, thrombus burden may play a role by increasing uptake of drug.[21]

Long-term, 3- to 5-year follow-up data from randomized clinical trials in patients with ST segment elevation acute myocardial infarction treated with either BMS or DES have demonstrated that the incidence of all-cause mortality, stent thrombosis, and myocardial infarction did not differ between BMS and DES.[22-28] Spaulding and associates[27] reported 4-year follow-up results from TYPHOON (Trial to Assess the Use of the CYPHer Sirolimus-Eluting Coronary Stent in Acute Myocardial Infarction Treated with BallOON Angioplasty), in which no significant differences in freedom from cardiac death (SES 97.6% vs. BMS 95.9%, $P = .37$), from repeat myocardial infarction (SES 94.8% vs. BMS 95.6%, $P = .85$), and from definite or probable stent thrombosis (SES 4.4% vs. BMS 4.8%, $P = .83$) were identified between the groups, although complete data were available in only 70% of patients (n = 501). All-cause mortality was also similar between the groups (SES 5.8% vs. BMS 7.0%, $P = .61$), whereas freedom from target lesion revascularization (TLR) was significantly better in the SES group compared with the BMS group (92.4% vs. 85.1%, $P = .002$). Vink and colleagues[28] reported a 5-year follow-up study of the PASSION (Paclitaxel-Eluting Vs. Conventional Stent

in Myocardial Infarction with ST-Segment Elevation) trial (n = 619 patients), in which the occurrence of the composite of cardiac death, recurrent myocardial infarction, or TLR was comparable between PES and BMS (18.6% vs. 21.8%; hazard ratio, 0.82; 95% CI, 0.58-1.18; $P = .28$), and the rate of TLR was similar between PES and BMS (7.7% vs. 10.5%, $P = .21$). The incidence of definite or probable stent thrombosis, which includes acute, subacute, late, and very late stent thrombosis, was not different between PES and BMS (4.2% vs. 3.4%, $P = .68$); however, the PES group had a higher incidence of very late definite or probable stent thrombosis compared with the BMS group (3.5% vs. 1.1%, $P = .06$), and the incidence of very late definite stent thrombosis was significantly higher in PES compared with BMS (3.3% vs. 0.7%, $P = .04$).

In a large prospective single-center registry of patients undergoing primary PCI over more than a decade, which included consecutive patients receiving DES (SES, PES, or second-generation DES; n = 368) or BMS (n = 1095) for ST segment elevation myocardial infarction, the rate of definite/probable stent thrombosis was similar between DES and BMS at 1 year (4.0% vs. 5.1%) but increased more with DES after the first year (DES, 1.9%/year; BMS, 0.6%/year).[29] Landmark analysis (>1 year) revealed that DES had a significantly higher incidence of very late stent thrombosis ($P < .001$) and reinfarction ($P = .003$), and DES was the only independent determinant of very late stent thrombosis (hazard ratio, 3.79; 95% CI, 1.64-8.79; $P = .002$). These findings are similar to findings of previous long-term registries, in which very late stent thrombosis after primary PCI was noted only with DES.[30,31] Randomized trials generally recruit patients with fewer comorbidities who are more likely to comply with study protocols, whereas registries include "all-comers," who may have multiple comorbidities, are noncompliant, or cannot afford close follow-up and long-term medical treatment. However, unmeasured confounders may affect the findings of nonrandomized registries that compare outcomes among patients treated with DES or BMS. Our data offer a pathophysiologic underpinning for the possibility that the benefits of opening an infarct-related artery with DES might be outweighed by long-term risks of death and myocardial infarction associated with DES-driven late and very late stent thrombosis.

Vessel healing at culprit sites in patients with acute myocardial infarction treated with first-generation DES is substantially delayed compared with nonculprit sites and culprit sites in patients receiving DES for stable angina, emphasizing the importance of underlying plaque morphology in arterial healing and the risk of late and very late stent thrombosis after DES implantation.

Pathologic Findings in Bifurcation Stenting

Atherosclerotic lesions tend to form at specific regions of the coronary vasculature where flow is disturbed, in particular, in areas of low shear.[32-34] Because dramatic hemodynamic alterations occur at branch points within the arterial tree, coronary bifurcations are extraordinarily susceptible to atherosclerosis. Our human pathologic data in coronary bifurcation lesions without stents demonstrated that low shear areas (i.e., the lateral wall) had significantly greater intimal thickness and necrotic core size compared with high shear areas (i.e., the flow divider).[35] The use of DES at bifurcation lesions has reduced restenosis rates compared with BMS; however, long-term outcomes are tempered by an increased risk of stent thrombosis,[36] which raises the possibility that delayed healing seen after DES implantation might be exacerbated at bifurcation sites. Given the difference in

atherosclerotic plaque burden between low and high shear regions, neointimal growth after stent implantation also may be different between these lesions.

To investigate this hypothesis, we evaluated the pathologic arterial response to bifurcation stenting with DES and BMS.[35] From our stent registry, 40 stented bifurcation lesions (DES = 19 and BMS = 21) from 40 patients were reviewed. Duration of implant was similar between the DES and BMS groups (330 [188, 680] days vs. 150 [54, 540] days, $P = .14$). To assess the impact of flow disturbance on arterial healing in stented lesions, the differences between high shear (flow divider) and low shear (lateral wall) regions were compared. Neointimal thickness was significantly less at the high shear (flow divider) site compared with the low shear (lateral wall) site in DES (0.07 [0.03, 0.15] mm vs. 0.17 [0.09, 0.23] mm, $P = .001$), whereas this difference did not reach statistical significance for BMS (0.26 [0.16, 0.73] mm vs. 0.44 [0.17, 0.67] mm, $P = .25$). Similarly, the percentage of uncovered struts was significantly greater at high shear sites compared with low shear sites in DES (40 [16, 76]% vs. 0 [0, 15]%, $P = .001$), whereas there was no significant difference in BMS (0 [0, 21]% vs. 0 [0, 0]%, $P = .09$). Fibrin deposition was also frequently higher at sites of high shear blood flow compared with low shear and was observed only in DES (60 [21, 67]% vs. 17 [0, 55]%, $P = .01$). A numerically greater incidence of late and very late stent thrombosis was documented in the DES group compared with the BMS group at bifurcation sites (main vessel, 75% vs. 36%, $P = .06$; side branch, 42% vs. 14%, $P = .19$), although this difference did not reach statistical significance, possibly because of a limited sample size. Most of the thrombi originated at the flow divider sites where uncovered struts were frequently observed (Figure 5-3). Consistent with these findings, greater neointimal formation has been shown to occur in the lateral compared with

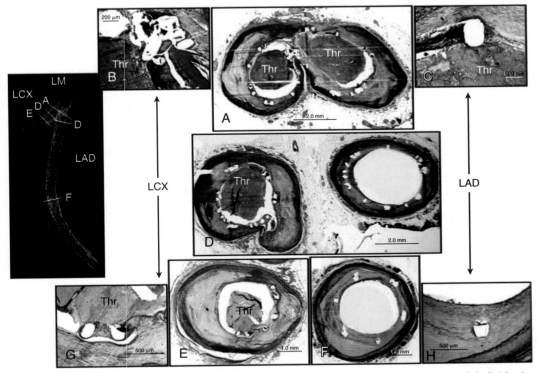

Figure 5-3 Late DES thrombosis in a bifurcation lesion. A 55-year-old man with a history of smoking, hypertension, and dyslipidemia received two PES in the distal left main artery (ostium of left anterior descending coronary artery [LAD] and left circumflex [LCX]) with overlapping Taxus stents placed in the LAD. **A,** The patient died suddenly 2 years after stent implantation. Radiograph shows a mildly calcified coronary artery. Both stents are occluded with platelet-rich thrombus *(Thr)* at the ostium of the LAD and LCX. **B** and **C,** High-magnification images showed adherent thrombus in the region of the uncovered struts at the flow divider. **D, E,** and **G,** Uncovered struts and adherent thrombus were also observed in all sections of the LCX stent. **D, F,** and **H,** The middle to distal portion of the LAD stent showed an absence of thrombus and healed luminal surface with mild neointimal thickening. (From Nakazawa G, Yazdani SK, Finn AV, et al. Pathological findings at bifurcation lesions: the impact of flow distribution on atherosclerosis and arterial healing after stent implantation. *J Am Coll Cardiol.* 2010;55:1679-1687.)

the flow divider region after stent implantation in a porcine iliofemoral bifurcation model.[37] Significant differences between the lateral and flow divider regions did not occur with BMS, possibly because of more rapid healing and more uniform neointimal formation after BMS compared with DES implantation. A combination of drug effect and blood flow disturbance is likely to accelerate the delayed healing in a bifurcation lesion.

In summary, arterial healing at bifurcation lesions with first-generation DES is impaired with greater delay at the flow divider (high shear) compared with the lateral wall sites (low shear), which may be caused by a combination of drug effect and differences in flow conditions.

Impact of Stent Fracture on Adverse Pathologic Findings

Stent fracture has emerged as a complication after DES implantation and is recognized as a contributor to in-stent restenosis[38-40] and stent thrombosis.[41,42] Stent fracture has been observed in 1% to 2% of patients at 8- to 10-month follow-up angiography,[38,43] although the sensitivity of angiography to detect stent fracture is limited. Stent fracture can be classified as follows (Table 5-1): grade I, single strut fracture; grade II, two or more strut fractures without deformation; grade III, two or more strut fractures with deformation; grade IV, multiple strut fractures with acquired transection but without gap; and grade V, multiple strut fractures with acquired transection with gap in the stent body.

The incidence of stent fracture at autopsy using high-contrast film-based radiography was assessed in 177 consecutive lesions (SES = 77 and PES = 101, 1 lesion with both SES and PES), and the impact of stent fracture on the pathologic findings and clinical outcomes was evaluated.[44] Stent fracture was documented in 51 lesions (29%; grade I = 9, grade II = 14, grade III = 11, grade IV = 6, and grade V = 9). There was no significant difference in age, gender, and cause of death between patients with fracture and patients without fracture. Lesions with stent fracture had longer duration of implant compared with lesions without fracture (172 [31-630] days vs. 44 [7-270] days, P = .004), whereas no statistical difference in duration of implant was identified between each grade of stent fracture (grade I, 31 [5, 616] days; grade II, 105 [27, 1095] days; grade III, 376 [72, 570] days; grade IV, 331 [31, 833] days; and grade V, 172 [44, 450] days; P = .70). Lesions with stent fracture showed a higher rate of SES usage (63% vs. 36%, P = .001), longer stent length (30.0 [22.0-40.0] mm vs. 20.0 [14.0-27.3] mm, P < .0001), and a higher rate of overlapping stents (45% vs. 22%, P = .003) compared with lesions without stent fracture. A forward stepwise logistic regression analysis demonstrated that longer stent length (OR, 1.07; 95% CI, 1.036-1.100; P < .0001), use of SES (OR, 3.40; 95% CI, 1.57-7.33; P = .002), and longer duration of implant (OR, 1.002; 95% CI, 1.001-1.003; P = .002) were independent determinants of stent fracture.

Histologic evaluation showed that neointimal thickness was similar between lesions with stent fracture and lesions without fracture (0.11 [0.06, 0.19] mm vs. 0.11 [0.03, 0.19] mm; P = .62). There was no significant difference in fibrin deposition (fibrin score, fracture (+) 1.0 [0.1, 1.5] vs. fracture (−) 1.4 [0.4, 2.0]) and inflammation (inflammatory score, fracture (+) 1.0 [0.5, 1.6] vs. fracture (−) 1.4 [0.4, 2.0]),

including a similar degree of giant cell and eosinophil infiltration. There were no differences in these parameters among various fracture grades (i.e., grades I through V). Six adverse events (five thrombosis and one restenosis) were associated with grade V fracture (67%), whereas there were no fracture site–related adverse pathologic findings in stents with grade I to IV fracture except for one stented lesion with grade IV fracture, which had a long overlapping stent (grade I-IV vs. grade V, P < .0001). A representative case of grade V fracture of DES is shown in Figure 5-4.

The lack of stent integrity, leading to distortion or acquired underexpansion, may play an important role in the occurrence of adverse events after stent fracture, although the mechanism of adverse events in this setting is not fully understood. Clinical studies have reported that the main risk factors for stent fracture are longer stent length, right coronary artery or saphenous vein graft lesion location, lesion with high motion, overlapping stent, and SES use.[38,40,45] In pathology studies, the flexible N-shaped, undulating longitudinal inter–sinusoidal-ring linker segment of the SES, which are smaller in width than the sinusoidal-ring portion, is the most frequent location of fractures. The relationship between longer implant duration and higher incidence of stent fracture suggests that stent fracture may result from continuous stress over time to the implant, which leads to greater metal fatigue and eventual fracture. However, stent fracture was seen even in the patients who died shortly after stent implantation; in these cases, fracture was probably procedure related (e.g., high pressure or oversized balloon, overlapping stent).

In summary, the incidence of DES fracture was 29% of stented lesions at autopsy, which is much higher than clinically reported. A high rate of adverse pathologic findings is observed in lesions with grade V fracture, whereas grade I through IV fracture does not appear to have a significant impact on the clinical outcome. Longer stent length, SES usage, and longer duration of stent implant are independent predictors of stent fracture.

Coronary Responses and Differential Mechanisms of Late and Very Late Stent Thrombosis Attributed to Sirolimus-Eluting Stents and Paclitaxel-Eluting Stents

Previous clinical trials have reported differences in angiographic late lumen loss in patients receiving SES or PES.[46] It is unclear whether the long-term histologic responses to each stent type are different and how this relates to the time course of arterial healing and mechanisms of late and very late stent thrombosis. The vascular healing response and the mechanisms of late and very late stent thrombosis in patients with first-generation DES were evaluated in 174 patients (230 DES lesions) from an autopsy registry; histomorphometry was performed on coronary stents from 127 patients (171 lesions) who died 30 days or more after receiving stent implants.[47] Analysis of individual lesions with duration of implant less than 30 days (SES = 25 and PES = 34) revealed that the incidence of early stent thrombosis was similar for lesions with SES and PES (44% vs. 38%, P = .79). Histologically, no differences in the extent of inflammation and fibrin deposition were noted between SES and PES implants with less than 30 days' duration.

The lesions with duration of implant 30 days or greater included 77 SES and 94 PES lesions; of these, 40 SES (52%) and 53 PES (56%) lesions were treated for off-label indications, which included stents deployed for acute myocardial infarction or bifurcation lesions, left main artery, bypass graft, restenosis, chronic total occlusion, or lesion lengths greater than 30 mm.[48] There was no significant difference in the incidence of late and very late stent thrombosis between SES and PES (21% vs. 27%, P = .47). Neointimal thickness was significantly greater in PES compared with SES (0.13 [0.03, 0.20] mm vs. 0.10 [0.04, 0.15] mm, P = .04). Similarly, PES had greater maximum neointimal thickness than SES (0.23 [0.13, 0.37] mm vs. 0.17 [0.06, 0.28] mm, P = .04). The heterogeneity in neointimal thickness

TABLE 5-1	Classification of Stent Fracture
Grade I	Fracture of single strut
Grade II	Fracture of two or more struts without stent deformation
Grade III	Fracture of two or more struts with stent deformation
Grade IV	Fracture of multiple struts with acquired stent transection but without gap in stent body
Grade V	Fracture of multiple struts with acquired stent transection and gap in stent body

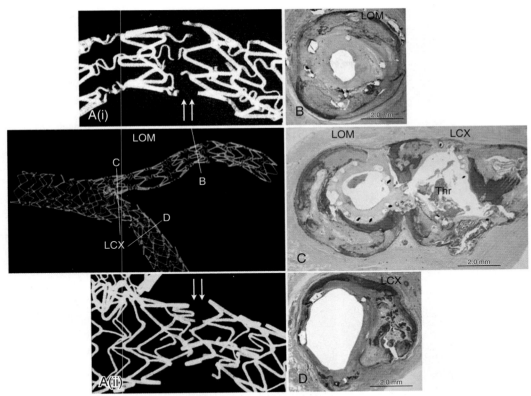

Figure 5-4 Grade V stent fracture: SES and PES. A 68-year-old woman died suddenly as a result of stent thrombosis in the left circumflex artery *(LCX)* 172 days after stent implantation. **A,** Radiograph shows the stented LCX and left obtuse marginal artery *(LOM)*. A grade V SES fracture *(double arrows)* is present, highlighted in the magnified image *(i)*, and another grade V fracture *(double arrows)* is present at the bifurcation site in the PES *(ii)*. **B,** SES in the LOM with grade V fracture was associated with restenosis. **C,** The PES fracture in the LCX was located in the area close to the bifurcation site, where the thrombus *(Thr)* was located. **D,** The stented LCX segment distal to the fracture was widely patent. (From Nakazawa G, Finn AV, Vorpahl M, et al. Incidence and predictors of drug-eluting stent fracture in human coronary artery a pathologic analysis. *J Am Coll Cardiol.* 2009;54:1924-1931.)

between sections was also significantly greater for PES versus SES (0.14 [0.08, 0.31] mm vs. 0.10 [0.03, 0.22] mm, $P = .02$). The percentage of uncovered struts was similar between PES and SES (20% vs. 21%, $P = .72$). There was a progressive and significant increase in neointimal thickness beyond 9 and 18 months' duration in lesions with PES without evidence of late and very late stent thrombosis ($P = .009$); although similar trends were observed for SES, findings were of borderline significance ($P = .08$).

Accumulated fibrin as assessed by fibrin score was significantly greater in PES compared with SES (1.8 [1.0, 2.5] vs. 0.8 [0.0, 2.0], $P = .001$). In contrast, SES implants were associated with a significantly greater inflammatory score compared with PES (1.3 [0.5, 2.0] vs. 1.0 [0.5, 1.5], $P = .007$). The contributing cells resulting in greater inflammation observed with SES were predominantly eosinophils and giant cells. The incidence of malapposition was comparable between SES and PES (14% vs. 19%, $P = .40$), although the mechanism of this phenomenon was different (see later). A further analysis revealed near-complete healing in stents placed for on-label indications with implant durations of greater than 12 months, whereas most DES with off-label usage remained unhealed beyond this similar time point.

Underlying pathologic causes of late and very late stent thrombosis were determined as penetration of necrotic core, bifurcation stenting, long or overlapping stents, stent underexpansion, isolated uncovered struts, localized hypersensitivity reaction, and malapposition from excessive fibrin deposition. The underlying cause of late and very late stent thrombosis was significantly different between SES and PES. For SES, there were localized hypersensitivity reactions, consisting of eosinophils, lymphocytes, and giant cells, throughout the stented segment (Figure 5-5, A), whereas late and very late stent thrombosis in PES was attributed to malapposition secondary to excessive fibrin

deposition on the abluminal surface (Figure 5-5, B). Localized hypersensitivity was documented in five cases involving seven lesions treated by SES that developed late and very late stent thrombosis, whereas no PES lesion showed this reaction. Most patients with hypersensitivity reaction after SES implantation died in the very late phase (>1 year; mean duration of implant, 649 days). Malapposition was observed in five lesions (71%) with a mean section of struts from the vessel wall of 944 µm. In most SES with severe inflammation, positive remodeling of the vessel occurred resulting in a malapposition. In contrast, malapposition secondary to excessive strut fibrin as the primary contributor to late and very late stent thrombosis was observed only in PES (seven lesions from six patients) with mean implant duration of 611 days. The mean distance separating the struts from the vessel wall was 404 µm. The luminal surface generally lacked endothelial cell coverage and evidence of granulation tissue consisting of macrophages or smooth muscle cell or proteoglycan matrix (see Figure 5-5, B).

As previously described, mechanisms of late and very late stent thrombosis are likely multifactorial.[6] Although there is a certain commonality in the mechanism of late and very late stent thrombosis for both SES and PES in that all cases demonstrated poor endothelialization, our findings indicate the final stimulus for thrombus development may differ according to DES type. The disparities in vascular responses are likely attributable to differences in the loading drug, polymer coating, and unique elution profile of each device. The hypersensitivity reaction observed with SES is likely attributable to the polymer rather than drug,[49] which is completely eluted by 3 months. Preclinical DES implants in porcine coronary arteries showed escalating amounts of inflammation over time,[50] which is consistent with our findings showing that most hypersensitivity cases

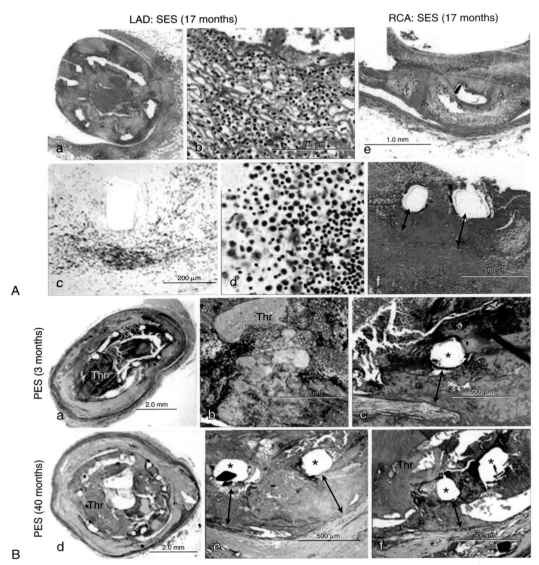

Figure 5-5 Representative images of late and very late stent thrombosis in sirolimus-eluting stents *(SES)* and paclitaxel-eluting stents *(PES)*. **A,** Histologic sections from SES. A 40-year-old woman died suddenly 4 days after surgical removal of melanoma (wide excision); she had received two SES, one in the left anterior descending artery *(LAD)* and one in the right coronary artery *(RCA)*, 17 months before her death. Antiplatelet therapy (aspirin and clopidogrel) was discontinued 5 days before the melanoma surgery. Histologic sections of the SES in the LAD showed total thrombotic occlusion and diffuse inflammation *(a)*. Numerous inflammatory cells were observed within the neointimal area *(b)*. The inflammatory reaction predominantly consists of T lymphocytes (CD45Ro) *(c)* and eosinophils (Luna stain) *(d)*. The same reaction was observed in the SES in the RCA *(e)*, and severe inflammation resulted in malapposition of the stent struts *(double arrows) (f)*. **B,** Histologic sections from a PES showing malapposition. A 69-year-old man who received a PES in a saphenous vein graft died suddenly 3 months after stent placement. Histologic sections showed thrombotic occlusion *(Thr)* in the PES *(a and b)*; malapposition is present secondary to severe fibrin deposition *(c)*. A 48-year-old man with PES implantation in the proximal LAD died suddenly 40 months after stent placement. Histologic sections showed thrombotic occlusion of the PES *(d)*. Most struts are malapposed with fibrin deposition underneath the stent struts *(e and f)*. Asterisks indicate stent strut, and double arrows indicate malapposition of the stent struts. (From Nakazawa G, Finn AV, Vorpahl M, et al. Coronary responses and differential mechanisms of late stent thrombosis attributed to first-generation sirolimus- and paclitaxel-eluting stents. *J Am Coll Cardiol.* 2011;57:390-398.)

were documented in devices more than 1 year old. Greater fibrin accumulation around struts in human PES cases is consistent with preclinical findings that showed a dose-dependent increase in fibrin deposition and medial necrosis after deployment of PES in rabbit iliac arteries[51] and similar findings of a dose escalation study in a porcine model.[52] We believe that paclitaxel itself is responsible for excessive fibrin deposition.

The heterogeneity of arterial healing with PES may result from an uneven distribution of drug and polymer because histologic sections of PES demonstrating the thinnest neointima are typically accompanied by persistent fibrin. Scanning electron microscopy studies demonstrating webbing and delamination of polymer, which is a frequent finding in PES, provide further support for variations in available paclitaxel within a single stent.[15]

First-generation DES exhibit divergent mechanisms of late and very late stent thrombosis in which hypersensitivity likely plays a significant role in SES, whereas for PES, the etiology appears to be associated with excessive fibrin deposition on the abluminal surface with malapposition. Another important finding was near-complete healing in DES placed for greater than 12 months with confirmed on-label usage, whereas off-label indications of both stents resulted in incomplete healing in DES beyond 12 months. This observation may have implications for the appropriate duration of dual antiplatelet therapy after first-generation DES placement.

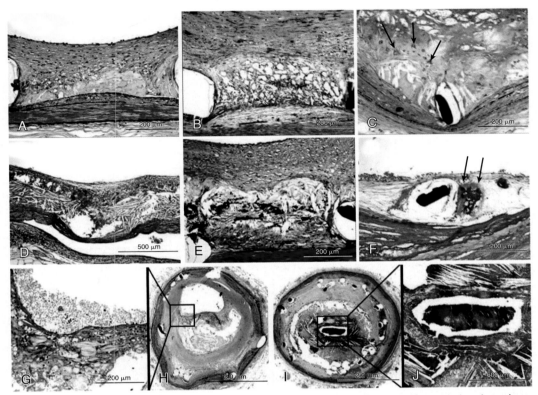

Figure 5-6 Representative images of the various stages of newly formed atherosclerotic changes within the neointima (neoatherosclerosis) after stent implantation. **A,** Foamy macrophage clusters in the peristrut region of SES implanted for 13 months before the patient's death. **B,** Fibroatheroma with foamy macrophage-rich lesions and early necrotic core formation in SES of 13 months' duration. **C,** Fibroatheroma with peristrut early necrotic core, cholesterol clefts, surface foamy macrophages, and early calcification (arrow) in SES of 13 months' duration. **D,** Peristrut late necrotic core in the neointima characterized by a large aggregate of cholesterol cleft in SES of 17 months' duration. **E,** Fibroatheroma with calcification in the necrotic core in SES of 10 months' duration. **F,** Peristrut calcification (arrow) with fibrin in SES of 7 months' duration. Low-power **(H)** and high-power **(G)** magnifications of a severely narrowed BMS implanted 61 months with a thin-cap fibroatheroma. Macrophage infiltration and a discontinuous thin fibrous cap are apparent **(G). I,** Low-magnification image shows plaque rupture with an acute thrombus that has totally occluded the lumen in a BMS implanted 61 months before the patient's death. **J,** High-magnification image of the same BMS in **I** shows a discontinuous thin cap with occlusive luminal thrombus. (From Nakazawa G, Otsuka F, Nakano M, et al. The pathology of neoatherosclerosis in human coronary implants bare-metal and drug-eluting stents. *J Am Coll Cardiol.* 2011;57:1314-1322.)

Late Increases in Neointima after Drug-Eluting Stent Implantation

Progressive neointimal growth, although slow to develop, is likely related to persistent fibrin and inflammation. In both DES platforms, biologic signs of a drug effect such as fibrin remain beyond the reported durations of drug release. Fibrin degradation products, in particular, fibrin fragment E, are a known initiator of smooth muscle cell migration and proliferation,[53,54] a phase that generally occurs early after BMS placement. In addition to fibrin, persistent inflammation is another plausible explanation for the late increases in neointimal formation associated with DES. Nonerodible polymers used in first-generation DES are associated with chronic inflammation and, in particular for SES, eosinophils,[6,16,49,55] lymphocytes, and giant cells, especially in the presence of hypersensitivity vasculitis. However, hypersensitivity cases do not show an increase in neointimal thickness. Clinical studies have shown that target vessel revascularization rates increase with time,[56-58] and gradual growth of neointima may partly account for this phenomenon.

Comparative Pathology of Neoatherosclerosis after Bare Metal Stent or Drug-Eluting Stent Implantation

Atherosclerosis is characterized by the accumulation of lipid-laden foamy macrophages in native coronary arteries that develops over decades, whereas newly formed atherosclerotic changes within the neointima (neoatherosclerosis) after BMS and DES implantation occur much faster. The incidence, character, and temporal development of neoatherosclerosis occurring within BMS and DES at autopsy were examined in a cohort of 299 consecutive cases (142 BMS, 157 DES [81 SES and 76 PES] cases) with 406 lesions with duration of implant greater than 30 days (197 BMS, 209 DES [103 SES and 106 PES] lesions).[8] Stent-related deaths from thrombosis were significantly more frequent with DES compared with BMS (20% vs. 4%, $P < .001$), whereas restenosis as a cause of death was more frequent with BMS compared with DES (28% vs. 7%, $P < .001$). The median duration of implant was shorter in lesions treated with DES versus BMS (DES 361 [172, 540] days vs. BMS 721 [271, 1801] days, $P < .001$). Of DES, 85% (177 lesions) were implanted for 2 years or less with no lesions extending beyond 6 years, whereas 45% (88 lesions) of BMS were implanted for 2 years or less, and 17% (33 lesions) had durations of more than 6 years. Stent lengths were significantly longer in DES compared with BMS (22.0 [15.5, 30.0] mm vs. 16.0 [12.0, 24.0] mm, $P < .001$), and the underlying plaque morphology was also different with unstable lesions (i.e., ruptured plaques and thin-cap fibroatheromas) more commonly found in DES compared with BMS ($P = 0.008$).

Representative images of various stages of neoatherosclerosis after stent implantation are shown in Figure 5-6. The earliest duration of implant with foamy macrophage accumulation was 70 days for PES, 120 days for SES, and 900 days for BMS.[8] Necrotic core formation was identified at 270 days for PES, 360 days for SES, and 900 days for

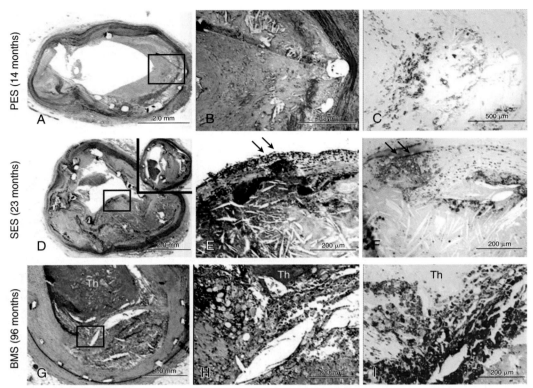

Figure 5-7   Representative cases showing atherosclerotic change after bare metal stent *(BMS)*, sirolimus-eluting stent *(SES)*, and paclitaxel-eluting stent *(PES)* implantation. **A-C,** Histologic sections from a 65-year-old woman who died of traumatic brain injury and had a PES implanted in the left circumflex artery 14 months before her death. **A,** Low-power image shows a patent lumen with moderate neointimal growth. **B,** Foamy macrophage infiltration and necrotic core formation with cholesterol clefts are seen at high magnification. **C,** Same section as **B** shows CD68-positive macrophages in the neointima. **D-F,** Histologic sections from a 59-year-old man with SES implanted for 23 months before he died of stent thrombosis. **D,** Thrombus was more apparent in the distal section taken 3 mm apart. **E,** Note thin-cap fibroatheroma with fibrous cap disruption *(arrows)* from the boxed area in **D. F,** CD68-positive macrophages in the fibrous cap and in the underlying necrotic core. **G-I,** Histologic section from a 47-year-old man who had BMS implanted 8 years before his death. *Th,* Thrombus. **G,** There is occlusive thrombus (Th) in the lumen and ruptured plaque *(boxed area).* **H,** Thrombus and ruptured plaque are shown at higher magnification, with large numbers of macrophages within the lumen and at the ruptured cap. **I,** Large number of CD68-positive macrophages at the site of rupture. (From Nakazawa G, Otsuka F, Nakano M, et al. The pathology of neoatherosclerosis in human coronary implants bare-metal and drug-eluting stents. *J Am Coll Cardiol.* 2011;57:1314-1322.)

BMS. Figure 5-7, *A-C,* shows representative images of fibroatheroma with necrotic core from a PES implant of 14 months' duration. More advanced lesions (i.e., lesions with the unstable features of thin-cap fibroatheromas and in-stent plaque rupture) (see Figure 5-6, *G-J,* and Figure 5-7, *D-I*) were identified in both BMS (n = 7, 4%) and DES (n = 3, 1%). In these cases, most BMS were of greater than 5 years' duration (average implant duration 6.1 ± 1.5 years), whereas for DES, unstable neoatherosclerotic lesions were identified with devices implanted 2 years or less (1.1 years, 1.4 years, and 1.9 years).

The overall incidence of neoatherosclerosis was significantly greater in DES compared with BMS (31% vs. 16%, P < .001) despite longer duration of implant for BMS. For implants of 2 years' or less duration, DES had a greater incidence of any neoatherosclerosis (DES 29% vs. BMS 0%, P < .001), represented by a greater incidence of foamy macrophage clusters (DES 14% vs. BMS 0%, P < .001) and fibroatheromas (DES 13% vs. BMS 0%, P < .001). For durations between 2 and 6 years, the DES group still expressed a higher incidence of neoatherosclerosis (DES 41% vs. BMS 22%, P = .053). The incidence of any neoatherosclerosis was greater in SES than PES for implant durations of 2 years or less (SES 37% vs. PES 21%, P = .021), although there were no differences among the DES implanted for 2 to 6 years (SES 44% vs. PES 38%, P = .719). Figure 5-8 shows the cumulative incidence of any neoatherosclerosis over time after implantation of BMS versus SES and PES; neoatherosclerosis was observed more frequently and at earlier time points in first-generation

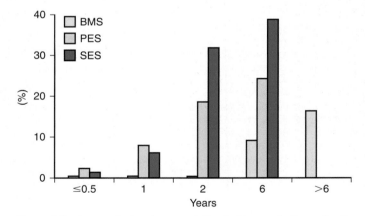

Figure 5-8   Bar graph showing cumulative incidence of atherosclerotic change with time after implantation of bare metal stents *(BMS)* versus sirolimus-eluting stents *(SES)* and paclitaxel-eluting stents *(PES).* Both SES and PES show earlier onset of neoatherosclerosis and a higher incidence of lesion formation compared with BMS. No DES were available beyond 6 years. (From Nakazawa G, Otsuka F, Nakano M, et al. The pathology of neoatherosclerosis in human coronary implants: bare-metal and drug-eluting stents. *J Am Coll Cardiol.* 2011;57:1314-1322.)

DES compared with BMS. Younger age (OR, 0.963; 95% CI, 0.942-0.983; $P < .001$), longer implant duration (OR, 1.028; 95% CI, 1.017-1.041; $P < .001$), SES usage (OR, 6.534; 95% CI, 3.387-12.591; $P < .001$), PES usage (OR, 3.200; 95% CI, 1.584-6.469; $P = .001$), and underlying unstable plaque (OR, 2.387; 95% CI, 1.326-4.302; $P = .004$) were identified as independent determinants of the development of neoatherosclerosis.

Although the underlying processes responsible for the development of neoatherosclerosis after stent implantation are likely multifactorial, the inability to maintain a fully functional endothelialized luminal surface within the stented segment likely plays a central role. The endothelium normally provides an efficient barrier against the excessive uptake of circulating lipid, whereas the endothelial cells within the stented segment in DES show poorly formed cell junctions, reduced expression of antithrombotic molecules, and decreased nitric oxide production.[59,60] Local inflammation induced by drugs or polymers may also be associated with immature reendothelialization through their deleterious effect on the endothelium. An inefficient barrier of the endothelium within the stented segment is characterized by increased permeability with poor cell-to-cell contact and increased inflammation, which allow a greater amount of lipoproteins to enter the subendothelial space where matrix proteins such as proteoglycans promote their retention.[61] Retained lipoproteins in the subendothelial space further undergo oxidative modifications, which lead to production of chemoattractant and inflammatory mediators such as monocyte chemoattractant protein-1 and vascular cell adhesion molecule-1, which are involved in the recruitment and attachment of monocytes.[62] Also, stent-induced flow disturbances contribute to complex spatiotemporal shear stress, which, through mechanotransduction, leads to changes in endothelial phenotype characterized by increased expression of transmembrane proteins that further allow inflammatory cell attachment and migration to subendothelial spaces.[63,64] In addition to lipid uptake, macrophage and smooth muscle cell death may dictate the development of neoatherosclerosis. The death of resident macrophages that particularly localize near stent struts may contribute to the pool of free cholesterol and cholesterol esters, forming a necrotic core.[65] Natural and drug-induced smooth muscle cell death may also yield free cholesterol and cholesterol esters, which may further attract macrophages.[66] Along similar lines, experimental evidence suggests that neoatherosclerosis is associated with delayed arterial healing compounded by lethal injury to smooth muscle cells and endothelial cells. Implantation of a ^{32}P β-emitting stent with activities ranging from 6 to 48 μCi resulted in focal evidence of neoatherosclerosis within normal arteries of New Zealand White rabbits at 6-month and 12-month follow-up.[67] Because atherosclerosis does not develop in normal rabbit arteries in the absence of hypercholesterolemia, this finding supports the contention that neoatherogenesis is the result of processes occurring around the stent itself.

In summary, in-stent neoatherosclerosis occurs in both BMS and DES; however, it is observed more frequently and at an earlier time point with DES implants compared with BMS. Neoatherosclerosis in DES show unstable characteristics by 2 years after implant, whereas similar features in BMS occur at relatively later time points (average implant duration of 6 years). The development of neoatherosclerosis may be another important contributing factor for very late stent thrombosis.

Conclusion

Stent thrombosis is an infrequent but catastrophic complication after stent implantation. First-generation DES have dramatically reduced restenosis; however, increases in late and very late stent thrombosis have raised concern about the long-term safety of this technology. Pathologic studies identified incomplete neointimal coverage of stent struts as the most important predictor of late and very late stent thrombosis after first-generation DES implantation and showed that delayed arterial healing is associated with penetration of necrotic core, long or overlapping stents, and bifurcation stenting especially in the flow divider (high shear) region. Grade V stent fracture is also associated with adverse pathologic findings including late and very late stent thrombosis and restenosis. Localized hypersensitivity reaction is exclusive to SES as an underlying mechanism of late and very late stent thrombosis, whereas malapposition secondary to excessive peristrut fibrin deposition is associated with PES implants. In addition, persistently uncovered struts are identified in both SES and PES with implant durations greater than 12 months, particularly in stents placed for off-label indications. Neoatherosclerosis has been recognized as another important contributing factor for very late stent thrombosis and is observed in both BMS and DES; however, DES are associated with rapid and more frequent development of neoatherosclerosis compared with BMS, which is potentially attributable to more incompetent regenerated endothelium in DES compared with BMS. Future pathologic studies should address the long-term safety of newer generations of DES, including second-generation zotarolimus-eluting stents and everolimus-eluting stents, biodegradable polymer-coated and polymer-free DES, and completely bioerodible scaffolds, in terms of improvements in reendothelialization, decreased inflammation and fibrin deposition, and a lower incidence of neoatherosclerosis, all of which may contribute to a reduced risk of late and very late stent thrombosis and better patient outcomes.

REFERENCES

1. Serruys PW, Kutryk MJ, Ong AT. Coronary-artery stents. *N Engl J Med* 2006;354:483-495.
2. Morice MC, Serruys PW, Sousa JE, et al. A randomized comparison of a sirolimus-eluting stent with a standard stent for coronary revascularization. *N Engl J Med* 2002;346:1773-1780.
3. Ryan J, Linde-Zwirble W, Engelhart L, et al. Temporal changes in coronary revascularization procedures, outcomes, and costs in the bare-metal stent and drug-eluting stent eras: results from the US Medicare program. *Circulation* 2009;119:952-961.
4. Stone GW, Ellis SG, Cox DA, et al. A polymer-based, paclitaxel-eluting stent in patients with coronary artery disease. *N Engl J Med* 2004;350:221-231.
5. Lagerqvist B, Carlsson J, Frobert O, et al. Stent thrombosis in Sweden: a report from the Swedish Coronary Angiography and Angioplasty Registry. *Circ Cardiovasc Interv* 2009;2:401-408.
6. Joner M, Finn AV, Farb A, et al. Pathology of drug-eluting stents in humans: delayed healing and late thrombotic risk. *J Am Coll Cardiol* 2006;48:193-202.
7. Finn AV, Joner M, Nakazawa G, et al. Pathological correlates of late drug-eluting stent thrombosis: strut coverage as a marker of endothelialization. *Circulation* 2007;115:2435-2441.
8. Nakazawa G, Otsuka F, Nakano M, et al. The pathology of neoatherosclerosis in human coronary implants bare-metal and drug-eluting stents. *J Am Coll Cardiol* 2011;57:1314-1322.
9. Marx SO, Jayaraman T, Go LO, et al. Rapamycin-FKBP inhibits cell cycle regulators of proliferation in vascular smooth muscle cells. *Circ Res* 1995;76:412-417.
10. Poon M, Marx SO, Gallo R, et al. Rapamycin inhibits vascular smooth muscle cell migration. *J Clin Invest* 1996;98:2277-2283.
11. Wiskirchen J, Schober W, Schart N, et al. The effects of paclitaxel on the three phases of restenosis: smooth muscle cell proliferation, migration, and matrix formation: an in vitro study. *Invest Radiol* 2004;39:565-571.
12. Farb A, Burke AP, Kolodgie FD, et al. Pathological mechanisms of fatal late coronary stent thrombosis in humans. *Circulation* 2003;108:1701-1706.
13. Hwang CW, Wu D, Edelman ER. Physiological transport forces govern drug distribution for stent-based delivery. *Circulation* 2001;104:600-605.
14. Levin AD, Vukmirovic N, Hwang CW, et al. Specific binding to intracellular proteins determines arterial transport properties for rapamycin and paclitaxel. *Proc Natl Acad Sci USA* 2004;101:9463-9467.
15. Basalus MW, Ankone MJ, van Houwelingen GK, et al. Coating irregularities of durable polymer-based drug-eluting stents as assessed by scanning electron microscopy. *EuroIntervention* 2009;5:157-165.
16. Finn AV, Kolodgie FD, Harnek J, et al. Differential response of delayed healing and persistent inflammation at sites of overlapping sirolimus- or paclitaxel-eluting stents. *Circulation* 2005;112:270-278.
17. Bavry AA, Kumbhani DJ, Quiroz R, et al. Invasive therapy along with glycoprotein IIb/IIIa inhibitors and intracoronary stents improves survival in non-ST-segment elevation acute coronary syndromes: a meta-analysis and review of the literature. *Am J Cardiol* 2004;93:830-835.
18. Keeley EC, Boura JA, Grines CL. Primary angioplasty vs. intravenous thrombolytic therapy for acute myocardial infarction: a quantitative review of 23 randomised trials. *Lancet* 2003;361:13-20.
19. Nakazawa G, Finn AV, Joner M, et al. Delayed arterial healing and increased late stent thrombosis at culprit sites after drug-eluting stent placement for acute myocardial infarction patients: an autopsy study. *Circulation* 2008;118:1138-1145.
20. Virmani R, Kolodgie FD, Burke AP, et al. Lessons from sudden coronary death: a comprehensive morphological classification scheme for atherosclerotic lesions. *Arterioscler Thromb Vasc Biol* 2000;20:1262-1275.
21. Hwang CW, Levin AD, Jonas M, et al. Thrombosis modulates arterial drug distribution for drug-eluting stents. *Circulation* 2005;111:1619-1626.

22. Di Lorenzo E, Sauro R, Varricchio A, et al. Long-term outcome of drug-eluting stents compared with bare metal stents in ST-segment elevation myocardial infarction: results of the paclitaxel- or sirolimus-eluting stent vs. bare metal stent in Primary Angioplasty (PASEO) Randomized Trial. *Circulation* 2009;120: 964-972.

23. Tebaldi M, Arcozzi C, Campo G, et al. The 5-year clinical outcomes after a randomized comparison of sirolimus-eluting vs. bare-metal stent implantation in patients with ST-segment elevation myocardial infarction. *J Am Coll Cardiol* 2009;54: 1900-1901.

24. Kaltoft A, Kelbaek H, Thuesen L, et al. Long-term outcome after drug-eluting vs. bare-metal stent implantation in patients with ST-segment elevation myocardial infarction: 3-year follow-up of the randomized DEDICATION (Drug Elution and Distal Protection in Acute Myocardial Infarction) Trial. *J Am Coll Cardiol* 2010;56:641-645.

25. Violini R, Musto C, De Felice F, et al. Maintenance of long-term clinical benefit with sirolimus-eluting stents in patients with ST-segment elevation myocardial infarction 3-year results of the SESAMI (Sirolimus-Eluting Stent vs. Bare-Metal Stent in Acute Myocardial Infarction) trial. *J Am Coll Cardiol* 2010; 55:810-814.

26. Atary JZ, van der Hoeven BL, Liem SS, et al. Three-year outcome of sirolimus-eluting vs. bare-metal stents for the treatment of ST-segment elevation myocardial infarction (from the MISSION! Intervention Study). *Am J Cardiol* 2010; 106:4-12.

27. Spaulding C, Teiger E, Commeau P, et al. Four-year follow-up of TYPHOON (Trial to Assess the Use of the CYPHer Sirolimus-Eluting Coronary Stent in Acute Myocardial Infarction Treated With BallOON Angioplasty). *JACC Cardiovasc Interv* 2011; 4:14-23.

28. Vink MA, Dirksen MT, Suttorp MJ, et al. 5-Year follow-up after primary percutaneous coronary intervention with a paclitaxel-eluting stent vs. a bare-metal stent in acute ST-segment elevation myocardial infarction: a follow-up study of the PASSION (Paclitaxel-Eluting Vs. Conventional Stent in Myocardial Infarction With ST-Segment Elevation) trial. *JACC Cardiovasc Interv* 2011;4:24-29.

29. Brodie B, Pokharel Y, Fleishman N, et al. Very late stent thrombosis after primary percutaneous coronary intervention with bare-metal and drug-eluting stents for ST-segment elevation myocardial infarction: a 15-year single-center experience. *JACC Cardiovasc Interv* 2011;4:30-38.

30. Kukreja N, Onuma Y, Garcia-Garcia H, et al. Primary percutaneous coronary intervention for acute myocardial infarction: long-term outcome after bare metal and drug-eluting stent implantation. *Circ Cardiovasc Interv* 2008;1:103-110.

31. Leibundgut G, Nietlispach F, Pittl U, et al. Stent thrombosis up to 3 years after stenting for ST-segment elevation myocardial infarction vs. for stable angina—comparison of the effects of drug-eluting vs. bare-metal stents. *Am Heart J* 2009;158: 271-276.

32. Ku DN, Giddens DP, Zarins CK, et al. Pulsatile flow and atherosclerosis in the human carotid bifurcation: positive correlation between plaque location and low oscillating shear stress. *Arteriosclerosis (Dallas, Tex)* 1985;5:293-302.

33. Friedman MH, Bargeron CB, Deters OJ, et al. Correlation between wall shear and intimal thickness at a coronary artery branch. *Atherosclerosis* 1987;68:27-33.

34. Prosi M, Perktold K, Ding Z, et al. Influence of curvature dynamics on pulsatile coronary artery flow in a realistic bifurcation model. *J Biomech* 2004;37:1767-1775.

35. Nakazawa G, Yazdani SK, Finn AV, et al. Pathological findings at bifurcation lesions: the impact of flow distribution on atherosclerosis and arterial healing after stent implantation. *J Am Coll Cardiol* 2010;55:1679-1687.

36. Iakovou I, Schmidt T, Bonizzoni E, et al. Incidence, predictors, and outcome of thrombosis after successful implantation of drug-eluting stents. *JAMA* 2005;293:2126-2130.

37. Richter Y, Groothuis A, Seifert P, et al. Dynamic flow alterations dictate leukocyte adhesion and response to endovascular interventions. *J Clin Invest* 2004;113:1607-1614.

38. Aoki J, Nakazawa G, Tanabe K, et al. Incidence and clinical impact of coronary stent fracture after sirolimus-eluting stent implantation. *Catheter Cardiovasc Interv* 2007;69:380-386.

39. Lee MS, Jurewitz D, Aragon J, et al. Stent fracture associated with drug-eluting stents: clinical characteristics and implications. *Catheter Cardiovasc Interv* 2007;69:387-394.

40. Shaikh F, Maddikunta R, Djelmami-Hani M, et al. Stent fracture, an incidental finding or a significant marker of clinical in-stent restenosis? *Catheter Cardiovasc Interv* 2008; 71:614-618.

41. Leong DP, Dundon BK, Puri R, et al. Very late stent fracture associated with a sirolimus-eluting stent. *Heart Lung Circ* 2008;17:426-428.

42. Shite J, Matsumoto D, Yokoyama M. Sirolimus-eluting stent fracture with thrombus, visualization by optical coherence tomography. *Eur Heart J* 2006;27:1389.

43. Lee SH, Park JS, Shin DG, et al. Frequency of stent fracture as a cause of coronary restenosis after sirolimus-eluting stent implantation. *Am J Cardiol* 2007;100:627-630.

44. Nakazawa G, Finn AV, Vorpahl M, et al. Incidence and predictors of drug-eluting stent fracture in human coronary artery a pathologic analysis. *J Am Coll Cardiol* 2009;54:1924-1931.

45. Yang TH, Kim DI, Park SG, et al. Clinical characteristics of stent fracture after sirolimus-eluting stent implantation. *Int J Cardiol* 2009;131:212-216.

46. Windecker S, Remondino A, Eberli FR, et al. Sirolimus-eluting and paclitaxel-eluting stents for coronary revascularization. *N Engl J Med* 2005;353:653-662.

47. Nakazawa G, Finn AV, Vorpahl M, et al. Coronary responses and differential mechanisms of late stent thrombosis attributed to first-generation sirolimus- and paclitaxel-eluting stents. *J Am Coll Cardiol* 2011;57:390-398.

48. Marroquin OC, Selzer F, Mulukutla SR, et al. A comparison of bare-metal and drug-eluting stents for off-label indications. *N Engl J Med* 2008;358:342-352.

49. Virmani R, Guagliumi G, Farb A, et al. Localized hypersensitivity and late coronary thrombosis secondary to a sirolimus-eluting stent: should we be cautious? *Circulation* 2004;109: 701-705.

50. Nakazawa G, Finn AV, Ladich E, et al. Drug-eluting stent safety: findings from preclinical studies. *Expert Rev Cardiovasc Ther* 2008;6:1379-1391.

51. Farb A, Heller PF, Shroff S, et al. Pathological analysis of local delivery of paclitaxel via a polymer-coated stent. *Circulation* 2001;104:473-479.

52. Heldman AW, Cheng L, Jenkins GM, et al. Paclitaxel stent coating inhibits neointimal hyperplasia at 4 weeks in a porcine model of coronary restenosis. *Circulation* 2001;103:2289-2295.

53. Ishida T, Tanaka K. Effects of fibrin and fibrinogen-degradation products on the growth of rabbit aortic smooth muscle cells in culture. *Atherosclerosis* 1982;44:161-174.

54. Naito M, Stirk CM, Smith EB, et al. Smooth muscle cell outgrowth stimulated by fibrin degradation products: the potential role of fibrin fragment E in restenosis and atherogenesis. *Thromb Res* 2000;98:165-174.

55. Wilson GJ, Nakazawa G, Schwartz RS, et al. Comparison of inflammatory response after implantation of sirolimus- and paclitaxel-eluting stents in porcine coronary arteries. *Circulation* 2009;120:141-149.

56. Morice MC, Serruys PW, Barragan P, et al. Long-term clinical outcomes with sirolimus-eluting coronary stents: five-year results of the RAVEL trial. *J Am Coll Cardiol* 2007;50:1299-1304.

57. Nakagawa Y, Kimura T, Morimoto T, et al. Incidence and risk factors of late target lesion revascularization after sirolimus-eluting stent implantation (3-year follow-up of the j-Cypher Registry). *Am J Cardiol* 2010;106:329-336.

58. Ellis SG, Stone GW, Cox DA, et al. Long-term safety and efficacy with paclitaxel-eluting stents: 5-year final results of the TAXUS IV clinical trial (TAXUS IV-SR: Treatment of De Novo Coronary Disease Using a Single Paclitaxel-Eluting Stent). *JACC Cardiovasc Interv* 2009;2:1248-1259.

59. Joner M, Nakazawa G, Finn AV, et al. Endothelial cell recovery between comparator polymer-based drug-eluting stents. *J Am Coll Cardiol* 2008;52:333-342.

60. Nakazawa G, Nakano M, Otsuka F, et al. Evaluation of polymer-based comparator drug-eluting stents using a rabbit model of iliac artery atherosclerosis. *Circ Cardiovasc Interv* 2011;4:38-46.

61. Skalen K, Gustafsson M, Rydberg EK, et al. Subendothelial retention of atherogenic lipoproteins in early atherosclerosis. *Nature* 2002;417:750-754.

62. Simionescu M. Implications of early structural-functional changes in the endothelium for vascular disease. *Arterioscler Thromb Vasc Biol* 2007;27:266-274.

63. Jimenez JM, Davies PF. Hemodynamically driven stent strut design. *Ann Biomed Eng* 2009;37:1483-1494.

64. Davies PF. Hemodynamic shear stress and the endothelium in cardiovascular pathophysiology. *Nat Clin Pract Cardiovasc Med* 2009;6:16-26.

65. Tabas I. Consequences and therapeutic implications of macrophage apoptosis in atherosclerosis: the importance of lesion stage and phagocytic efficiency. *Arterioscler Thromb Vasc Biol* 2005; 25:2255-2264.

66. Tulenko TN, Chen M, Mason PE, et al. Physical effects of cholesterol on arterial smooth muscle membranes: evidence of immiscible cholesterol domains and alterations in bilayer width during atherogenesis. *J Lipid Res* 1998;39:947-956.

67. Farb A, Shroff S, John M, et al. Late arterial responses (6 and 12 months) after (32)P beta-emitting stent placement: sustained intimal suppression with incomplete healing. *Circulation* 2001; 103:1912-1919.

CHAPTER 6

Bioresorbable Coronary Scaffolds

JOHN A. ORMISTON | MARK W.I. WEBSTER | YOSHINOBU ONUMA |
PATRICK W. SERRUYS

KEY POINTS

- To limit restenosis, a stent or scaffold needs to prevent the negative constrictive remodeling after percutaneous coronary intervention (PCI) for about 3 months during healing. After this, a permanent stent is unnecessary and may be detrimental.

- Controlled delivery of an antiproliferative drug is needed to limit neointimal hyperplasia, which also contributes to late luminal loss and restenosis.

- Potential advantages of a resorbable scaffold include reduction of late events related to foreign material–induced inflammation, return of vasomotion in response to physiologic need, remodeling to accommodate plaque or atheroma, improved vessel imaging with CT and MRI, facilitation of repeat PCI or surgery, and patient and cardiologist preference.

- Although the first iterations of scaffolds constructed from magnesium resorbed too quickly to prevent restenosis, results with subsequent iterations are improving because they resorb more slowly and release an antiproliferative drug.

- The Absorb bioresorbable vascular scaffold (BVS) consists of a polylactide, everolimus-eluting scaffold that metabolizes to carbon dioxide and water. It is the most studied BVS to date, with up to 5 years of follow-up data in simple coronary anatomy, in which clinical results appear similar to those of metallic drug-eluting stents.

- Other polymeric scaffolds in clinical trials are the REVA sirolimus-eluting device, Elixir novolimus-eluting device, and ART device, which is being tested without an antiproliferative drug.

A bioresorbable coronary stent or bioresorbable vascular scaffold (BVS) is an attractive alternative to permanent metallic stents for percutaneous coronary intervention (PCI) because scaffolding of the coronary artery is only needed during the early healing process, perhaps 3 to 6 months. Lifelong support is not necessary for a transient problem. Compared with balloon angioplasty, stents or scaffolds improve immediate outcomes after PCI by holding back intimal tissue flaps to optimize vessel caliber and reduce the likelihood of acute vessel occlusion. They reduce subsequent restenosis by preventing negative remodeling or vessel shrinkage.[1-3] Controlled release of anti-proliferative agents from the stent coating reduces the intimal hyperplastic healing response to the vessel injury that is induced by PCI.[4,5]

Since immediate outcomes after PCI have improved, the focus in interventional cardiology has turned to outcomes over the longer term. This chapter considers the promise of improvement in such outcomes with bioresorbable scaffolds and reviews the different bioresorbable scaffolds that have been evaluated clinically.

Potential Advantages of Bioresorbable Scaffolds

Potential advantages of having the scaffold disappear from the treated site include the following: (1) a possible reduction in late thrombotic events; (2) improved lesion imaging with computed tomography (CT) or magnetic resonance imaging (MRI); (3) facilitation of repeat percutaneous revascularization or the subsequent placement of a

surgical graft anastomosis to the treated site; (4) restoration of coronary vasomotion; (5) freedom from side branch obstruction by stent struts; (6) freedom from strut fracture–induced restenosis; and (7) the fact that many patients and their cardiologists prefer an effective temporary implant rather than a permanent prosthesis.[6-8]

Another potentially significant advantage of a bioresorbable scaffold is that it may preserve the ability of the vessel to undergo positive outward remodeling. Traditional metallic stents prevent exposure of the vessel wall to the pulsatile flow and shear stress that may be necessary for such optimal vascular health.[9] When bioresorbable scaffolds have partially resorbed and no longer cage the vessel, the vessel may still remodel positively, which may allow the vessel to accommodate intimal hyperplasia or neoatheroma without significant luminal narrowing.[10-12] Beyond intervention for atherosclerotic coronary disease, bioresorbable scaffolds have a potential role in pediatric interventional procedures because they allow for vessel growth and do not require eventual surgical removal. They may also have a role in peripheral intervention.

Late thrombosis after the implantation of a drug-eluting stent (DES) has been a major concern with first-generation DES, as randomized trials and registry data suggest an unremitting incidence of approximately 0.6%/year.[13-17] Use of DES worldwide declined after the initial systematic identification of this phenomenon. The long-term thrombotic risk of current-generation DES appears lower than with first-generation DES; a recent meta-analysis has even suggested that the rates of stent thrombosis associated with an everolimus-eluting fluoropolymer-coated stent are lower than of a bare metal stent (BMS) or other types of DES.[18] Similarly, in the Swedish Coronary Angiography and Angioplasty Registry (SCAAR), the rates of stent thrombosis, restenosis, and death were all lower with newer-generation DES than with BMS or older-generation DES during the first 18 months after implantation.[19]

Although stent thrombosis may no longer be as significant a concern during the first 1 or 2 years after implantation of newer DES, bioresorbable scaffolds may improve other later events associated with DES and BMS. A 15- to 20-year clinical and angiographic follow-up study after BMS implantation has found that beyond 4 years, there is progressive luminal narrowing and an annual rate of target lesion revascularization (TLR) of approximately 2%.[20] A 5-year follow-up in the SIRolimus-eluting versus pacliTAXel-eluting stents for coronary revascularization (SIRTAX) trial, a late randomized comparison of sirolimus with paclitaxel stents demonstrated a continuous increase in angiographic late lumen loss; beyond 1 year, the major adverse cardiac event (MACE) rate was 2% to 3%/year.[21] In the large Japanese Cypher registry of almost 13,000 patients, the ongoing annual rates of stent thrombosis and TLR were 0.26% and 2.2%, respectively, without attenuation over time.[22] Although the incidence of restenosis is lower with newer compared with older DES,[19] late MACEs, including TLR, occur after the implantation of other permanent DES designs.[23,24]

Multiple factors may contribute to MACE that occur late after metallic stent implantation. Ongoing inflammation has been observed in arteries stented with DES[25,26] or BMS[20] and may contribute to neoatheroma development, late catch-up, and stent thrombosis.[27] Malapposition of stent struts is associated with late stent thrombosis. In addition, late fracture of permanent metallic stent struts may contribute to stent thrombosis and restenosis.[7] A fully resorbed scaffold will not incite an ongoing inflammatory response[28] and, once the stent is absorbed, there is no risk of strut fracture or adverse events from malapposition.

There was no evidence of inflammation at 3 or 4 years after implantation of the fully bioresorbable poly-ʟ-lactic acid Absorb BVS everolimus-eluting scaffold (Abbott Vascular, Santa Clara, Calif) in normal porcine coronary arteries,[28] suggesting a vascular substrate at very low risk for adverse events. This is in contrast with both DES and BMS.[20,27] Although a BVS is resorbing, the vessel is no longer caged by a rigid stent, so it can undergo positive outward remodeling, which can accommodate the formation of intimal hyperplasia or neoatheroma and thereby limit the severity of luminal stenosis.[10,12]

Very late follow-up (17 years) after balloon angioplasty without stenting shows that although there is some stenosis progression at the dilated site, late repeat intervention is rare.[29] The late outcomes after balloon angioplasty may provide some insight into outcomes after the temporary scaffolding provided by fully resorbable platforms.

It has been further argued that bioresorbable scaffolds may stabilize plaque. An optical coherence tomography (OCT) study of neointimal formation 6 and 12 months after implantation of the Absorb BVS scaffold has demonstrated a neointimal layer that resembles a thick fibrous cap. This property may potentially stabilize vulnerable plaques,[30] although further evaluation is needed to confirm this hypothesis.

🔷 Bioresorbable Scaffold Technologies

Challenges in making an effective bioresorbable scaffold include ensuring that the scaffold absorbs while providing sufficient duration of vessel support to overcome early vessel negative remodeling after PCI. Polymers such as poly-ʟ-lactic acid have less tensile strength than metal alloys, and polymeric stent struts may be more likely to fracture when stretched beyond their working range.[31]

IGAKI-TAMAI BIOABSORBABLE SCAFFOLD

The Igaki-Tamai stent (Kyoto Medical Planning, Kyoto, Japan) was the first resorbable scaffold implanted in humans. It is constructed from poly-ʟ-lactic acid,[32] which is absorbed through the hydrolysis of bonds between repeating lactide units. This produces lactic acid that subsequently enters the Krebs cycle and is metabolized to carbon dioxide and water. Small particles, less than 2 μm in diameter, are phagocytosed by macrophages. Poly-ʟ-lactic acid is approved for use for many medical implants, ranging from absorbable sutures to orthopedic plates and screws.

The Igaki-Tamai bioabsorbable scaffold design consists of sinusoidal hoops that are largely out of phase, with adjacent hoops linked by three connectors (Figure 6-1). The struts are 170 μm thick and provide 24% vessel coverage, both of which are greater than those of contemporary metallic stents, although this strut thickness is similar to that of other bioresorbable scaffolds.[8] The scaffold resorbs by bulk erosion. The delivery system consists of a balloon-mounted, self-expanding sheathed system in which expansion is hastened by dilation with warmed contrast medium. Because poly-ʟ-lactic acid is radiolucent, gold markers at each end provide radiopacity for scaffold identification under fluoroscopy. The scaffold does not release an antiproliferative agent. At 10-year follow-up of the first prospective, nonrandomized clinical trial of 50 patients,[33] stent thrombosis occurred in two patients, one acutely and the other related to a sirolimus-eluting DES implanted in a new lesion adjacent to the Igaki-Tamai scaffold. The study confirmed the safety of poly-ʟ-lactic acid in human coronary arteries. Interestingly, in the small number of patients who were restudied with angiography, luminal enlargement was observed between 9-month and 3-year follow-up.[33] Beyond this study, there have been no further human coronary implants of the Igaki-Tamai bioabsorbable scaffold.

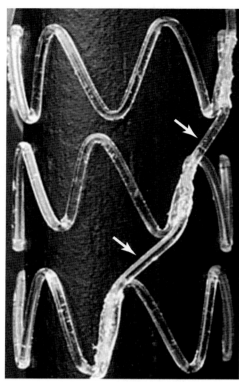

Figure 6-1 The Igaki-Tamai scaffold. The design of this scaffold consists of sinusoidal hoops that are largely out of phase, with adjacent hoops linked by three connectors *(arrows)*. There are gold radiopaque markers at each end (not shown).

BIOABSORBABLE MAGNESIUM STENT

Magnesium possesses several properties that make it an attractive material for a resorbable scaffold but also has features that create challenges. Advantages of magnesium over polymeric scaffolds include greater radial strength, resulting in less immediate stent recoil after deployment, and the capability of post-dilation without strut rupture. An example of the 3.0-mm scaffold that has been post-dilated to 5.3 mm without damage to stent struts is shown in Figure 6-2. In contrast, some 3.0-mm polymeric designs can only be dilated slightly greater than nominal diameter (e.g., 3.8 mm) before significant strut disruption occurs. Because magnesium is radiolucent, accurate post-dilation and additional stent placement without gaps or long overlap may be a challenge. To overcome this limitation, tantalum composite radiopaque markers have been added to the design of the third-generation absorbable metallic stent (AMS; see Figure 6-2).

One limitation of magnesium stents is the challenge of prolonging resorption sufficiently to resist the negative remodeling forces that occur after PCI and that are a major contributor to restenosis after balloon angioplasty. Resorption of magnesium stents is by surface erosion, so struts become thinner with time. The first generation (see Figure 6-2) of the balloon expandable bioabsorbable magnesium alloy stents, AMS-1 (Biotronik, Berlin), was studied in the Clinical Performance Angiographic Results of Coronary Stenting with Absorbable Metal Stents (PROGRESS-AMS) First-In-Human trial.[34] The stent resorbed so rapidly that it lost its radial support within weeks.[35] In this study, the restenosis rate at 4 months was almost 50%; the rate of target vessel revascularization at 1 year was 45% because it was unable to resist negative vessel remodeling and did not release an antiproliferative agent to suppress the neointimal hyperplastic response to balloon injury.[34] However, the study demonstrated that the AMS-1 was safe, with a high procedural success, and the stent

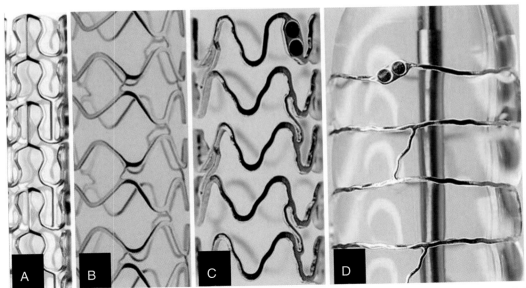

Figure 6-2   Absorbable magnesium stents. **A,** First-generation, uncoated absorbable magnesium stent (AMS-1) before expansion. **B,** The next generation stent, AMS-3, elutes paclitaxel. Its design consists of out of phase sinusoidal hoops linked by three connectors per hoop. **C,** The AMS-4 stent has in-phase sinusoidal hoops, with two S-shaped connectors linking each hoop. The connectors link midway between the peaks and valleys. This scaffold releases sirolimus from a resorbable coating and has tantalum composite radiopaque markers at each end. **D,** A 3-mm AMS-4 stent post-dilated to 5.4 mm without strut fracture, in contrast to the phenomenon observed with most polymeric scaffolds.

degraded without distal embolism. In addition, it was shown that the stented vessel was still vasoreactive in response to the administration of nitrate, an endothelium-independent vasodilator.[36]

Longer degradation times were achieved with the next generation stent, AMS-3, by modifying the alloy with the addition of zirconium, yttrium, and other rare earth elements. The strut thickness of the AMS-3 is thinner than that of the AMS-1 (120 vs. 165 μm, respectively), and the AMS-3 has a fast-degrading, thin (1-μm) PLGA (poly[lactic-co-glycolic acid]) coating for the controlled elution of the antiproliferative agent, paclitaxel, over 3 months. The design of this stent consists of out of phase sinusoidal hoops linked by three straight connectors angled from the stent long axis that are somewhat offset from the hoop peaks (see Figure 6-2). This stent was evaluated in the Biotroniks Safety and Clinical Performance Of the First Drug-Eluting Generation Absorbable Metal Stent In Patients With de Novo Lesions in Native Coronary Arteries (BIOSOLVE)-1 prospective, multicenter first-in-human trial.[36a] This trial enrolled patients with single de novo lesions with a reference diameter of 3.0 to 3.5 mm and lesion length of less than 12 mm; devices that were 3.0 and 3.5 mm in diameter and 16 mm in length were implanted. Of the 46 patients enrolled, 22 were enrolled in cohort 1 and underwent 6-month and optional 12-month imaging, whereas cohort 2 enrolled 24 patients with optional 6-month and mandatory 12-month invasive imaging. Device success was 100%. There were no deaths or episodes of scaffold thrombosis and, at 6 months, 2 patients (4.3%) had repeat revascularization. In cohort 1, in-stent late lumen loss at 6 months (n = 20) was 0.64 ± 0.50 mm, which is less than that observed with the BMS but more than with contemporary DES. Although the details regarding the mechanism of the late loss have yet to be elucidated, it may be more likely to result from negative remodeling associated with premature scaffold absorption rather than from neointimal hyperplasia.

The AMS-4 sirolimus-eluting magnesium scaffold has in-phase sinusoidal hoops (see Figure 6-2), with two connectors per hoop linking midway between peaks and valleys and with radiopaque markers at each end. To date, it has not yet entered clinical trials.

ABSORB EVEROLIMUS-ELUTING BIORESORBABLE VASCULAR SCAFFOLD

The Absorb BVS (Abbott Vascular, Santa Clara, CA) has a bioresorbable polymer backbone of poly-L-lactic acid with a polymer coating of poly-D,L-lactide that contains and controls the release of everolimus (Novartis, Basel, Switzerland).[37] The device design has undergone several iterations over three generations (Figure 6-3). Two adjacent platinum markers at each end allow for radiographic identification. The design of the first-generation Absorb BVS scaffold consists of circumferential out of phase sinusoidal hoops with a strut thickness (including the drug coating layer) of 156 μm, linked directly or by straight bridges (see Figure 6-3). The strut thickness is similar to that of the Cypher sirolimus-eluting stent (Cordis, Miami Lakes, Fla) and the crossing profile of 1.4 mm is slightly larger than that of contemporary metallic stents, which are generally around 1.1 mm.

Cohort A Design and Outcomes

The acute performance of the Absorb BVS is similar to or slightly inferior to that of the Xience cobalt chromium stents (Abbott Vascular, Santa Clara, Calif).[38] Immediate recoil was similar to that of a cobalt chromium stent,[39] and radial strength was of the same order as that of the original Multi-Link stent.[37] In Cohort A of the Absorb trial, a 3.0-mm-diameter Absorb BVS scaffold of 12 or 18 mm in length was implanted in 30 patients with simple, de novo, native coronary artery stenoses. The device was safe, with only one ischemia-driven major adverse cardiac event (a non–Q-wave myocardial infarction) at 5-year follow-up. This occurred at the site of metallic stent deployment at 46 days in a scaffold that had likely been damaged at the time of implantation. At 6 months, although there was no change in the area within the external elastic lamina, consistent with an absence of vessel remodeling, there was shrinkage of the scaffold itself, with an area reduction of 11% to 12%. This, in addition to the development of some intimal hyperplasia, resulted in a 16.8% reduction in luminal area and an angiographic late lumen loss of 0.44 mm.[38] The endolumen often appeared corrugated as a result of the scaffold

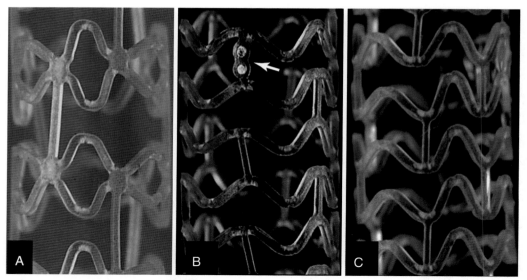

Figure 6-3   Absorb bioresorbable vascular scaffold—three generations of design. Each generation is constructed from poly-L-lactic acid and coated with a faster resorbing poly-D,L-lactide coating releasing everolimus. **A,** The first-generation Absorb bioresorbable vascular scaffold consists of pairs of out of phase sinusoidal hoops directly linked at each peak and valley. Each of these pairs is linked by three straight connectors. This design was used in Cohort A of the ABSORB trial. **B,** The second-generation Absorb scaffold, tested in Cohort B of the ABSORB trial, has in-phase sinusoidal hoops linked at peaks and valleys by three straight connectors. All three Absorb scaffold designs have platinum radiopaque markers at each end *(arrow)*. **C,** In the third-generation stent (the commercialized Absorb design), there have been small changes in the shape of the bends in the hoops, changes in strut thickness and width, and processing changes to facilitate post-dilation to a larger diameter without damage. Strut thickness is increased from 150 to 155 μm and strut width increased from 163 to 188 μm, respectively, for the 2.5- and 3.0-mm third-generation Absorb devices; the 3.5-mm third-generation device has a strut thickness of 155 μm and strut width of 213 μm. The 3.0-mm third-generation scaffold can be post-dilated safely to 3.5 mm and the 3.5-mm device to 4.0 mm.

shrinkage. The angiographic late loss of 0.44 mm was historically similar to that of some metallic DES but greater than sirolimus-eluting or sirolimus analogue–eluting stents.[38]

Although the scaffold shrinkage at 6 months is consistent with potentially insufficient mechanical support, the area obstruction within the scaffold was only 5% by intravascular ultrasound, consistent with an appropriate suppression of any excessive healing response by the antiproliferative drug that was eluted, and is similar to that observed with the everolimus-eluting Xience stent at 6 months in the Spirit First Trial.[38,40,41] Interestingly, between 6 months and 2 years, imaging by intravascular ultrasound (IVUS) and OCT demonstrated enlargement of the lumen, without change in scaffold size.[6] There was a significant decrease in plaque volume, partly resulting from scaffold absorption; this observation was not confirmed in the Absorb Cohort B trial.[12] There was no change in the angiographic late lumen loss. Echogenicity, virtual histology, OCT, and preclinical studies have shown that by 2 years, the scaffold used in the Absorb Cohort A trial is incorporated into the vessel wall and bioresorbed.[6,28] In addition, in the small number of patients tested, vasoactivity was present at 2 years within the scaffolded segment, with vasoconstriction induced by methylergonovine maleate and vasodilation induced by nitroglycerin.[6] This observation raises the possibility of a return of a physiologic response to vasoactive stimuli such as exercise and the potential for the artery to dilate in response to local ischemia, consistent with a normally functioning, healthy vessel.

Cohort B Design and Outcomes

A second-generation scaffold was designed to overcome the shortcomings of the Cohort A design (i.e., scaffold shrinkage and angiographic late loss), presumed to be caused by the premature loss of scaffold integrity (see Figure 6-3). This design was used in Cohort B of the Absorb trial. It is constructed from the same polymeric material as the prior generation but with different processing, which results in a slower rate of hydrolysis, increasing the duration of radial support

and delaying full resorption.[42] Although the strut thickness is unchanged, the design provides for more uniform vessel support and drug application. In addition, it can be stored at room temperature rather than needing refrigeration. The security of the scaffold on the delivery balloon has also been increased.

The Absorb Cohort B trial evaluated this second-generation scaffold in 101 patients with simple coronary lesions. The first 45 patients (Cohort B1) had invasive follow-up at 6 months and 2 years, and the subsequent 56 patients (Cohort B2) underwent invasive follow-up at 1 and 3 years. At 2 years, the hierarchical MACE rate was 6.8%; the angiographic late loss was 0.16 mm at 6 months and increased to 0.27 mm at 24 months.[12] In contrast with that observed in Cohort A, there was no evidence of endoluminal corrugation or scaffold area loss at 6 months; in contradistinction, scaffold enlargement was detected by IVUS and OCT between 6 months and 2 years. This enlargement reflects the programmed disappearance of the mechanical integrity of the scaffold, which was also demonstrated by the return of vasomotion in Cohort B2 at 1 year.[43] Although signs of bioresorption at 2 years were observed with IVUS and OCT, this was slower than in Cohort A.[42] There were significant increases in total plaque area and plaque area behind the struts on IVUS, together with an increase in neointimal growth, between 6 and 24 months.[12] Because the neointimal tissue growth was in part accommodated by vessel expansive remodeling, there was, depending on imaging modality, no or limited late luminal compromise between 6 and 24 months.[12] At 2 years, 99% of struts were covered, and only one scaffold showed malapposition. In summary, compared with the first-generation scaffold, the second-generation scaffold appeared to abolish scaffold area reduction at 6 months and provided an angiographic late lumen loss comparable to metallic, everolimus-eluting stents. At 24-month follow-up, intravascular imaging suggested persistence of the proliferating healing process with increasing neointima but with enlargement of the scaffold area, which could potentially herald further late lumen enlargement at 3 and 4 years.[12]

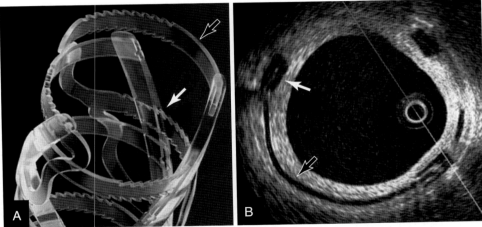

Figure 6-4 The REVA bioresorbable scaffold. **A,** The REVA bioresorbable scaffold has a unique slide and lock mechanism *(white arrow)* that permits scaffold lumen enlargement without the strain that is concentrated at the hinge points with standard polymeric scaffolds. After expansion of the ReZolve scaffold, the lock mechanism maintains acute gain and provides radial strength. **B,** Optical coherence tomography image. The strut (thickness, 120 μm) is shown by the *black arrow;* the *white arrow* indicates the ratchet (strut thickness, 250 μm).

Side Branches

Although a favorable outcome after resorbable scaffold placement across side branches has been predicted because the struts are resorbed, few data are available, and the reality may be more complex. In a patient from Cohort A, the struts overhanging the branch at 6 months appeared thickened and covered with tissue. At 2 years, there was partial clearing of struts from the ostium, but struts distal in relation to the side branch ostium formed a ridge or rim extending proximally from the carina.[44]

Future Studies

The ABSORB Extend Trial (clinicaltrials.gov identifier, NCT01023789) is a continued access, nonrandomized registry using the second-generation device in up to 1000 patients in 100 centers and permitting treatment of longer lesions with longer scaffolds and allowing scaffold overlap. The ABSORB II trial (clinicaltrials.gov identifier, NCT01425281) will enroll approximately 500 patients with simple de novo lesions to be randomized to receive a second-generation Absorb everolimus-eluting scaffold or a Xience Prime stent eluting everolimus from a cobalt chromium platform. The coprimary endpoints are vasomotion at 2 years and minimum luminal diameter at 2 years. The ABSORB III trial (clinicaltrials.gov identifier, NCT01751906) is a planned randomized, clinical trial that will evaluate whether the Absorb everolimus-eluting scaffold is noninferior with regard to clinical outcomes (in specific, target lesion failure) compared with the Xience V/Prime stent, for the purposes of U.S. Food and Drug Administration (FDA) approval in the United States. The third-generation Absorb scaffold, sometimes called the TEM design, was commercially released in 2012 (see Figure 6-3). Compared with the Cohort B design, there have been small changes in the shape of the bends in the hoops and changes in strut thickness and width, along with processing changes to facilitate post-dilation to a larger diameter without damage.

REVA BIOABSORBABLE STENT

The first-generation, non–drug-eluting REVA device (Reva Medical, San Diego, Calif) was tested in the RESORB prospective, nonrandomized, single-arm safety study, which enrolled 27 patients. An interim analysis found unfavorable results between 4 and 6 months after implantation, with a higher than anticipated target lesion revascularization rate driven mainly by reduced stent diameter caused by focal scaffold failure.[8] The ReZolve device is the result of design modifications and polymer processing changes to overcome this issue, as well as the addition of sirolimus that elutes from the abluminal

surface (Figure 6-4). It is constructed from an absorbable, tyrosine-derived polycarbonate polymer that metabolizes to amino acids, ethanol, and carbon dioxide. Iodination of the desaminotyrosine ring makes the device radiopaque.[45] During deployment of a standard deformable polymeric scaffold, significant strain is concentrated at the hinge points, with a potential important loss of mechanical strength. In contrast, the ReZolve scaffold is balloon expandable, with a redesigned slide and lock (i.e., ratchet) mechanism that allows stent expansion without material deformation (see Figure 6-4).

After expansion, the lock mechanism maintains acute gain and provides radial strength. This device has sliding struts that are 120 μm thick, except at the sites of the backbone mechanism, where the thickness is 250 μm. The 3- × 18-mm device is suitable for vessels between 2.9 and 3.3 mm, and scaffold integrity is maintained with post-dilation up to 3.8 mm, where the last ratchet tooth holds. The scaffold is sheathed for delivery, has a crossing profile of 1.88 mm, and is compatible with a 7-Fr guide. The next-generation ReZolve2, which has approximately 30% more radial strength than the first-generation device, is not sheathed, has a crossing profile of 1.52 mm, and is compatible with a 6-Fr guide. The ReZolve scaffold retains radial strength for 3 to 4 months. In long-term porcine studies, the first-generation scaffold underwent positive outward remodeling, which began at 6 months, peaked at 2 years, and remained at that level at 55 months.[11] The absorption time can be modified by modification of the polymer. Most resorption (by bulk erosion) occurs within 4 years. The Safety Study of a Bioresorbable Coronary Stent (RESTORE) trial (clinical trials.gov identifier, NCT01262703) is a prospective, multicenter study of the ReZolve device in 26 patients. The primary endpoint is freedom from symptomatic TLR at 6 months, and there are invasive imaging endpoints at 12 months.

ELIXIR BIORESORBABLE SCAFFOLD

The Elixir Medical (Sunnyvale, Calif) scaffold has 150-μm-thick struts constructed from a poly-L-lactic acid-derived polymer that ultimately metabolizes to carbon dioxide and water. The body of the scaffold has sinusoidal in-phase hoops with three straight bridges per hoop linking adjacent peaks and troughs (Figure 6-5). The end design differs with a pair of out of phase hoops linked by straight connectors between peaks and troughs. There are two adjacent platinum radiopaque markers at each end. A 3-μm-thick, poly-D,L-lactide coating resorbs more quickly and contains and controls the release of a sirolimus analogue, either myolimus (Novartis, Basel, Switzerland) or novolimus (Elixir Medical, Sunnyvale, Calif), which is an active

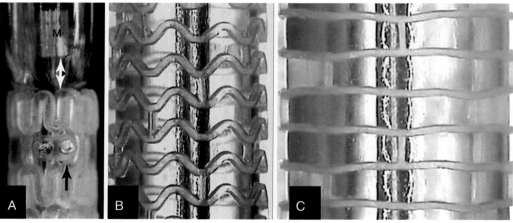

Figure 6-5   The Elixir Medical DESolve bioresorbable scaffold. The scaffold is constructed from a poly-L-lactic acid–based polymer and elutes novolimus or myolimus from a coating <3 μm thick that resorbs more quickly. **A,** Balloon-mounted scaffold. *Black arrow,* Radiopaque markers; *white arrowheads,* gap between the balloon marker *(M)* and scaffold. **B,** The design of the scaffold consists of in-phase sinusoidal hoops linked by three straight connectors. **C,** A scaffold that has been post-dilated to 4.75 mm without strut fracture.

metabolite of sirolimus. The scaffold is balloon expandable; the 3-mm diameter device has a crossing profile of 1.47 mm. Radial strength is preserved for approximately 3 months, which appears to be of sufficient duration to resist early negative remodeling forces. Immediate recoil is slightly greater than the Elixir metallic DES. After deployment, there is small self-expansion of the scaffold. There is evidence that the 3-mm scaffold can, in some cases, be post-dilated up to 4.75 mm without strut rupture (see Figure 6-5), but more data are needed from a sizable sample of patients to confirm this observation; the degree of scaffold radial strength after such expansion is unknown. Bioresorption is by bulk erosion and is expected to be complete by 1.5 to 2 years. Currently, there are no data about the time to appearance of vasomotion.

The DESolve First-in-Man (FIM) study is a prospective, multi-center, single-arm study enrolling a total of 16 patients with a single de novo lesion eligible for treatment with a single 3.0- × 14-mm scaffold that elutes myolimus at a rate of 3 mg/mm. At 6 months, the angiographic and volumetric results were favorable: angiographic, in-scaffold, late lumen loss was 0.19 mm, and the percent neointimal volume by IVUS was 7%, with no evidence of scaffold shrinkage or late malapposition. This amount of angiographic in-scaffold late lumen loss is similar to that of contemporary permanent DES.[46] There was no significant increase in scaffold size at 6 months. In-segment target lesion revascularization occurred in 1 patient, and there were no episodes of stent thrombosis.[47] The Elixir Medical Clinical Evaluation of the Novolimus-Eluting Coronary Stent System: A Randomized Study with a Single Arm Registry (EXCELLA II) trial will further evaluate the safety and efficacy of this platform in a total of 120 patients with the resorbable scaffold coated with 5 μg of novolimus per millimeter of stent.

ARTERIAL REMODELING TECHNOLOGIES

The ART scaffold design (ART18Z, Arterial Remodeling Technologies [ART], Paris) consists of pairs of out of phase zigzag hoops directly linked at crowns. The adjacent pairs are linked by two straight bridges (Figure 6-6). The struts are 170 μm thick, and the scaffold is compatible with a 6-Fr guide. The 3-mm-diameter device can be overexpanded by 25% without cracking. Stent and vessel coverage is less than 25%. The scaffold does not have an antiproliferative drug coating. The scaffold is constructed from semicrystalline poly-D,L-lactide, rather than highly crystalline poly-L-lactide, so that it resorbs relatively quickly, with an approximate 75% reduction in molecular weight by 90 days and full resorption expected within 18 to 24 months. The scaffold surrenders its primary scaffolding function

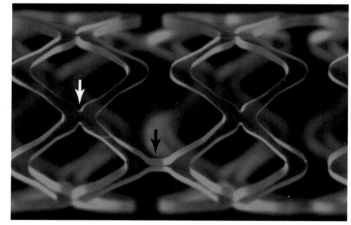

Figure 6-6   The Arterial Remodeling Technologies (ART) bioresorbable scaffold. The design of this scaffold consists of pairs of out of phase zigzag hoops constructed from poly-L-lactic acid directly linked at crowns *(white arrow).* Adjacent pairs of hoops are linked by two straight bridges *(black arrow).* The struts are 170 μm thick, and the device is compatible with a 6-Fr guide. The 3.0-mm device can be expanded by 25% (to 3.75 mm) without cracking or crazing. There is 25% stent and vessel coverage, and the 3-mm scaffold increases in diameter to 3.2 mm after deployment.

by 3 months, which is thought to be long enough for the healing process to stabilize the artery after the trauma of PCI and to avoid recoil and constrictive remodeling. Positive remodeling can occur after 3 months. In preclinical studies, inflammation appeared stable and similar to that of other polylactic acid bioresorbable scaffolds in the first 9 months and decreased thereafter. It was hypothesized that an antiproliferative drug coating is not necessary because the intimal hyperplastic response to PCI trauma peaks at about 6 months and then regresses.[48-50] In addition, because the scaffold is no longer caging the vessel, positive remodeling can accommodate the intimal hyperplasia and limit restenosis.

Consistent with this observation, late lumen loss becomes negative at 9 months in the porcine coronary artery model, with an increased scaffold area. Moreover, the lack of an antiproliferative coating may permit the more rapid return of normal endothelial function and maintain an efficient endothelial barrier, limiting plaque progression.[27] Theoretically, neoatheroma development may be less of a problem with the ART device compared with DES or BMS because of the combination of a competent endothelium and the absence of a foreign body reaction. First-in-human trials have not yet been completed.

Summary

An ideal stent or scaffold should enhance acute outcomes after PCI by sealing intimal flaps and optimizing lumen size. It should reduce restenosis by preventing negative remodeling and limiting neointimal proliferation by delivery of an antiproliferative drug. Beyond 6 months, a permanent implant has no apparent useful function and may be detrimental by contributing to late adverse clinical events. The concept of a stent that performs its function and then disappears has appeal.[51] A number of different materials ranging from magnesium to a variety of polymers have been used to construct scaffolds of different designs. Some of these are being tested in clinical trials. The Absorb BVS everolimus-eluting scaffold has the largest body of data available and is commercially available in some countries. Further data are needed, in particular for the treatment of more complex disease. Clinical results with the magnesium resorbable stents have shown promise. Outcomes in the small trial with the Elixir resorbable drug-eluting scaffold are impressive but much more clinical data are needed. Clinical results from trials with the REVA and ART devices are awaited. There will likely be many more players in this field as the advantages of bioresorbable scaffolds are recognized. If proven safe and efficacious, bioresorbable scaffolds may represent a paradigm shift in the interventional treatment of obstructive coronary artery disease.

REFERENCES

1. Lafont A, Guzman L, Whitlow P, et al. Restenosis after experimental angioplasty. Intimal, medial and adventitial changes associated with constrictive remodeling. Circ Res 1995;76:996-1002.
2. Mintz G, Popma J, Pichard A, et al. Arterial remodeling after coronary angioplasty: a serial intravascular ultrasound study. Circulation 1996;94:35-43.
3. Kimura T, Kaburagi S, Tamura T, et al. Remodeling responses of human coronary arteries undergoing coronary angioplasty and atherectomy. Circulation 1997;96:475-483.
4. Morice M, Serruys PW, Sousa J, et al. A randomized comparison of a sirolimus-eluting stent with a standard stent for coronary revascularization. N Engl J Med 2002;346:1773-1780.
5. Colombo A, Drzewiecki J, Banning A, et al. Randomized study to assess the effectiveness of slow- and moderate-release polymer-based paclitaxel-eluting stents for coronary artery disease. Circulation 2003;108:788-794.
6. Serruys PW, Ormiston J, Onuma Y, et al. Absorb Trial first-in-man evaluation of a bioabsorbable everolimus-eluting coronary stent system: two-year outcomes and results from multiple imaging modalities. Lancet 2009;373:897-910.
7. Nakazawa G, Finn A, Vorpahl M, et al. Incidence and predictors of drug-eluting stent fracture in human coronary artery. J Am Coll Cardiol 2009;54:1924-1931.
8. Ormiston J, Serruys PW. Bioresorbable coronary stents. Circ Cardiovasc Interv 2009;2:255-260.
9. Malek A, Alper S, Izumo S. Hemodynamic shear stress and its role in atherosclerosis. JAMA 1992;282:2035-2042.
10. Glagov S, Weisenberg E, Zarins C, et al. Compensatory enlargement of human atherosclerotic coronary arteries. N Engl J Med 1987;316:1372-1375.
11. Strandberg E, Zeltinger J, Schultz D, et al. Late positive remodeling and late lumen gain contribute to vascular restoration by a non–drug-eluting bioresorbable scaffold: a four-year intravascular ultrasound study in normal porcine coronary arteries. Circ Cardiovasc Interv 2012;5:39-46.
12. Ormiston J, Serruys PW, Onuma Y, et al. First serial assessment at 6 months and 2 years of the second generation of Absorb everolimus-eluting bioresorbable vascular scaffold: a multi-imaging modality study. Circ Cardiovasc Interv 2012;5:620-632.
13. Camenzind E, Steg P, Wijns W. A cause for concern. Circulation 2007;115:1440-1455.
14. Nordmann A, Briel M, Bucher H. Mortality in randomized controlled trials comparing drug-eluting vs. bare metal stents in coronary artery disease: a meta-analysis. Eur Heart J 2006;27:2784-2814.
15. Pfisterer M, Brunner-La Rocca H, Buser P, et al. Late clinical events after clopidogrel discontinuation may limit the benefit of drug-eluting stents: an observational study of drug-eluting versus bare-metal stents. J Am Coll Cardiol 2006;48:2584-2591.
16. Largerqvist B, Carlsson J, Frobert O, et al. Stent thrombosis in Sweden : a report from the Swedish Coronary Angiography and Angioplasty Registry. Circ Cardiovasc Interv 2009;2:401-408.
17. Daemen J, Wenaweser P, Tsuchida K, et al. Early and late coronary stent thrombosis of sirolimus-eluting and paclitaxel-eluting stents in routine clinical practice: data from a large two-institutional cohort study. Lancet 2007;369:667-678.
18. Palmerini T, Biondi-Zoccai G, Della Riva D, et al. Stent thrombosis with drug-eluting and bare-metal stents: evidence from a comprehensive network meta-analysis. Lancet 2012;379:1393-1402.
19. Sarno G, Largerqvist B, Frobert O, et al. Lower risk of stent thrombosis and restenosis with unrestricted access of "new generation" drug-eluting stents: a report from the nationwide Swedish Coronary Angiography and Angioplasty Registry. Eur Heart J 2012;33:606-613.
20. Yamaji K, Kimura T, Morimoto T, et al. Very long-term (15-20 years) clinical and angiographic outcome after coronary bare metal stent implantation. Circ Cardiovasc Interv 2010;3:468-475.
21. Raber L, Wohlwend L, Wigger M, et al. Five-year clinical and angiographic outcomes of a randomized comparison of sirolimus-eluting and paclitaxel-eluting stents: results of the sirolimus-eluting versus paclitaxel-eluting stents for coronary revascularization LATE trial. Circulation 2011;123:2819-2828.
22. Kimura T, Morimoto T, Nakagawa Y, et al. Very late stent thrombosis and late target lesion revascularization after sirolimus-eluting stent implantation: five-year outcome of the j-Cypher Registry. Circulation 2012;125:584-591.
23. Stone G, Rizvi A, Sudhir K, et al. Randomized comparison of everolimus- and paclitaxel-eluting stents. 2-year follow-up from the SPIRIT (Clinical evaluation of the XIENCE V Everolimus-eluting stent system) IV trial. J Am Coll Cardiol 2011;58:19-25.
24. Jensen L, Thayssen P, Hansen H, et al. Randomized comparison of everolimus-eluting and sirolimus-eluting stents in patients treated with percutaneous coronary intervention: the Scandinavian Organization for Randomized Trials with Clinical Outcome (SORT OUT IV). Circulation 2012;125:1246-1255.
25. Virmani R, Guagliumi G, Farb A, et al. Localized hypersensitivity and late coronary thrombosis secondary to a sirolimus-eluting stent: should we be cautious? Circulation 2004;109:701-705.
26. Cook S, Ladich E, Nakazawa G, et al. Correlation of intravascular ultrasound findings with histological analysis of thrombus aspriates in patients with very late drug-eluting stent thrombosis. Circulation 2009;120:391-399.
27. Nakazawa G, Otsuka F, Nakano M, et al. The pathology of neoatherosclerosis in human coronary implants. Bare-metal and drug-eluting stents. J Am Coll Cardiol 2011;57:1314-1322.
28. Onuma Y, Serruys PW, Perkins L, et al. Intracoronary optical coherence tomography and histology at 1 month and 2,3, and 4 years after implantation of everolimus-eluting bioresorabable scaffolds in a porcine coronary artery model: an attempt to decipher the human optical coherence tomography images in the Absorb trial. Circulation 2010;122:2288-2300.
29. Hatrick R, Ormiston J, Ruygrok P, et al. Very late changes in the dilated lesion following coronary balloon angioplasty: a 17-year serial quantitative angiographic study. EuroIntervention 2009;5:121-124.
30. Brugaletta S, Radu M, Garcia-Garcia H, et al. Circumferential evaluation of the neointima by optical coherence tomography after ABSORB bioresorbable vascular scaffold implantation: can the scaffold cap the plaque? Atherosclerosis 2012;221:106-112.
31. Ormiston J, De Vroey F, Serruys PW, et al. Bioresorbable polymeric vascular scaffolds: a cautionary tale. Circ Cardiovasc Interv 2011;4:535-538.
32. Tamai H, Igaki K, Kyo E, et al. Initial and 6-month results of biodegradable poly-L-lactic acid coronary stents in humans. Circulation 2000;102:399-404.
33. Nishio S, Kosuga K, Igaki K, et al. Long-term (>10 years) clinical outcomes of the first-in-human biodegradable poly-L-lactic acid coronary stents: Igaki-Tamai stents. Circulation 2012;125:2343-2353
34. Erbel R, Di Mario C, Bartunek J, et al. Temporary scaffolding of coronary arteries with bioabsorbable magnesium stents: a prospective, non-randomized multicentre trial. Lancet 2007;369:1869-1875.
35. Waksman R. Current state of the absorbable metallic (magnesium) stent. EuroIntervention 2009;5(Suppl F):F94-F97.
36. Ghimire G, Spiro J, Kharbanda R, et al. Initial evidence for the return of coronary vasoreactivity following the absorption of bioresorbable magnesium alloy coronary stents. EuroIntervention 2009;4:481-484.
36a. Haude M, Erbel R, Erne P, et al, Safety and performance of the drug-eluting absorbable metal scaffold (DREAMS) in patients with de-novo coronary lesions: 12 month results of the prospective, multicentre, first-in-man BIOSOLVE-I trial. Lancet. 2013 Jan 14. doi: 10.1016/S0140-6736(12)61765-6. [Epub ahead of print.]
37. Ormiston J, Webster M, Armstrong G. First-in-human implantation of a fully bioabsorbable drug-eluting stent: the BVS poly-L-lactic acid everolimus-eluting coronary stent. Catheter Cardiovasc Interv 2007;69:128-131.
38. Ormiston J, Serruys PW, Regar E, et al. A bioabsorbable everolimus-eluting coronary stent system with single de-novo coronary artery lesions (ABSORB): a prospective open-label trial. Lancet 2008;371:899-907.
39. Tanimoto S, Serruys P, Thuesen L, et al. Comparison of in vivo acute stent recoil between the bioabsorbable everolimus-eluting coronary stent and the everolimus-eluting cobalt chromium coronary stent: insights from the ABSORB and SPIRIT trials. Catheter Cardiovasc Interv 2007;70:515-523.
40. Serruys PW, Ong A, Piek J, et al. One-year results of a durable polymer everolimus-eluting stent in de novo coronary narrowings (the Spirit First Trial). EuroIntervention 2005;1:266-272.
41. Grube E, Sonoda S, Ikeno F, et al. Six- and twelve-month results from first human experience using everolimus-eluting stents with bioabsorbable polymer. Circulation 2004;109:2168-2171.
42. Brugaletta S, Gomez-Lara J, Serruys PW, et al. Serial in vivo intravascular ultrasound-based echogenicity changes of everolimus-eluting bioresorbable vascular scaffold during the first 12 months. JACC Cardiovasc Interv 2011;4:1281-1289.
43. Serruys PW, Onuma Y, Dudek D, et al. Evaluation of the second generation of a bioresorbable everolimus-eluting vascular scaffold. J Am Coll Cardiol 2011;58:1578-1588.
44. Okamura T, Onuma Y, Garcia-Garcia H, et al. 3-Dimensional optical coherence tomographic assessment of jailed side-branches by bioresorbable scaffolds: a proposed classification. JACC Cardiovasc Interv 2010;3:836-844.
45. Pollman M. Engineering a bioresorbable stent: REVA programme update. EuroIntervention 2009;5(Suppl F):F54-F57.
46. Stone G, Midei M, Newman W, et al. Comparison of an everolimus-eluting stent and a paclitaxel-eluting stent in patients with coronary artery disease: a randomized trial. JAMA 2008;299:1903-1913.
47. Verheye S. EuroPCR, presented May 16, 2012, Paris, France.
48. Virmani R, Kolodgie F, Farb A, et al. Drug eluting stents: are human and animal studies comparable? Heart 2003;89:133-138.
49. Ormiston J, Stewart F, Roche A, et al. Late regression of the dilated site after coronary angioplasty. A five-year quantitative angiographic study. Circulation 1997;96:468-474.
50. Kimura T, Yokoi H, Nakagawa Y, et al. Three-year follow-up after implantation of metallic coronary-artery stents. N Engl J Med 1996;334:561-566.
51. Waksman R. Biodegradable stents: they do their job and disappear. J Invasive Cardiol 2006;18:70-74.

Clinical Use

CHAPTER 7

Efficacy and Safety of Bare Metal and Drug-Eluting Stents

KARTHIK GUJJA | AMAR NARULA | GREGG W. STONE | AJAY J. KIRTANE

KEY POINTS

- The coronary stent, acting as a scaffold within the treated coronary artery, was devised to stabilize the results of balloon angioplasty. Stent implantation results in a larger initial lumen (or acute gain in luminal diameter) and seals dissections resulting from stand-alone angioplasty, preventing acute and subacute abrupt closure.

- Despite the success of early stents in stabilizing and improving on the early and late results of stand-alone balloon angioplasty, widespread adoption of stent technology was initially hindered by high rates of subacute stent thrombosis and rates of in-stent restenosis that approached 20% to 40% within the first year after implantation.

- Drug-eluting stents, which maintain the mechanical advantages of bare metal stents while delivering pharmacologic therapy locally to the arterial wall to prevent restenosis, effectively inhibit neointimal hyperplasia after stent implantation, decreasing the rates of repeat revascularization procedures to less than 10%.

- Despite the clearly demonstrated efficacy of first-generation drug-eluting stents observed in initial and subsequent randomized trials of these devices, early observational data derived from studies examining more unselected use revealed possible concerns regarding stent safety.

- Data are emerging that demonstrate improvements in safety outcomes with second-generation compared with first-generation drug-eluting stents. These findings, in conjunction with superior or similar efficacy of second-generation drug-eluting stents, suggest that the comparison between second-generation drug-eluting stents and bare metal stents may be even more favorable than prior studies comparing first-generation drug-eluting stents with bare metal stents.

Introduction

More than 2 decades ago, the advent of the bare metal stent (BMS) revolutionized the role of percutaneous coronary intervention (PCI) for the treatment of coronary artery disease. Despite the initial efforts of Gruentzig and others in establishing balloon angioplasty as a viable, minimally invasive treatment for coronary artery disease, the results of stand-alone balloon angioplasty before the introduction of the coronary stent were often unpredictable. Although many patients were successfully treated, balloon-mediated dissections leading to acute and subacute abrupt closure in other patients rendered the procedure a risky proposition. Arterial recoil and chronic constrictive remodeling in many cases led to late luminal compromise and clinical restenosis, which in some cases could be occlusive. These subacute and late complications of balloon angioplasty limited the overall scope of the procedure. It was not until the more widespread use of coronary stents that PCI became an accessible procedure for operators with a wide range of training experiences and procedural volumes. PCI has now become the default strategy for coronary revascularization for many patients with symptomatic coronary artery disease. This chapter describes the key clinical studies that have led to the acceptance of coronary stenting as the standard of care for PCI; it also provides an overview to aid the clinician in gaining an appreciation not only for the appropriate historical perspective on stent-related studies, but also for the strengths and limitations of the current clinical evidence base.

Bare Metal Stents

The coronary stent, acting as a scaffold within the treated coronary artery, was devised to stabilize the results of balloon angioplasty. Stent implantation created a larger initial lumen (or acute gain in luminal diameter) and sealed dissections resulting from stand-alone angioplasty, preventing acute and subacute abrupt closure. Because of the persistence of a scaffold within the artery that resisted radial forces of elastic recoil and vascular remodeling, stents had the potential to increase the durability of the angioplasty procedure. In 1986, Puel and Sigwart implanted the first stents in human patients.[1] Although this self-expanding stent had high rates of thrombotic occlusion,[2] patients without thrombosis had low rates of angiographic restenosis, suggesting that stenting could improve late patency of PCI in addition to stabilizing acute angioplasty results. A second stent under investigation at that time, the balloon-expandable Gianturco-Roubin coil stent, was efficacious in reversing acute or threatened vessel closure after angioplasty,[3] which led to the first U.S. Food and Drug Administration (FDA) approval for a coronary stent in June 1993.

However, because of limitations of these early devices, neither of these two stents heralded the "stent revolution" of the 1990s, which ultimately was attributed to the introduction of the Palmaz-Schatz stent, a slotted tube stent with a central 1-mm articulating bridge connecting two rigid 7-mm slotted segments. The Palmaz-Schatz stent was investigated in two landmark clinical trials randomly assigning patients to elective stenting with this device or balloon angioplasty. In the STRESS and BENESENT-1 trials, the use of the Palmaz-Schatz stent was associated with a 20% to 30% reduction in clinical and angiographic restenosis compared with conventional balloon angioplasty,[4,5] a finding that ultimately led to approval of this stent by the FDA in 1994. In these trials, the use of the Palmaz-Schatz stent resulted in markedly improved initial angiographic results, with a larger minimal luminal diameter (acute gain) and fewer residual dissections after the procedure, reducing the rate of subacute vessel closure. However, angiographic late lumen loss was greater with the BMS compared with stand-alone angioplasty, leading to the observation that late restenotic events occurring after coronary stent implantation were influenced by the tradeoff of acute luminal gain versus late luminal loss. This observation led to the "bigger is better" concept in stent deployment, as coined by Kuntz and colleagues[6]; that is, the late results after coronary stenting depended on the adequacy of acute luminal gain at the time of initial stent implantation.

Despite the success of early stents in stabilizing and improving on the early and late results of stand-alone balloon angioplasty, widespread adoption of stent technology was initially hindered by high rates of subacute stent thrombosis. To try to overcome stent thrombosis, patients were treated in the peri-stent and post-stent periods with adjunctive pharmacotherapies consisting of combinations of aspirin, dextran, dipyridamole, heparin, and warfarin. These therapies were not without bleeding risk, particularly given the large arterial sheaths required to deliver early stents. As stent thrombosis rates and bleeding complications remained daunting, additional progress in the stent procedure itself, as well as adjunctive pharmacotherapy, was required. Nakamura and colleagues[7] were able to lower rates of sub-acute stent thrombosis with more aggressive use of intravascular ultra-sound (IVUS), routine high-pressure dilation (>14 atm), and use of aspirin and a second antiplatelet agent (ticlopidine, a thienopyridine) rather than prolonged warfarin therapy. These modifications reduced the incidence of stent thrombosis to a more acceptable range of approximately 1% to 2% and resulted in a lower incidence of vascular and bleeding complications.[8] The confirmation of these initial find-ings in randomized clinical trials comparing dual antiplatelet therapy with warfarin anticoagulation facilitated the more widespread adop-tion of coronary stenting as the therapy of choice for patients under-going PCI by the late 1990s.[9-12]

Notwithstanding initial concerns regarding potentially diminished efficacy of coronary stents with more generalized use of these devices,[13] abundant randomized and nonrandomized data exist comparing stent-ing with balloon angioplasty across a range of patient and lesion subsets, almost universally demonstrating an advantage to coronary stenting over conventional balloon angioplasty.[14-16] In addition, long-term follow-up (up to 15 years) of BMS has demonstrated that most restenosis occurs within the first year after stent implantation. From 1 to 5 years after coronary stent implantation, there are few observed late clinical or angiographic recurrences,[17,18] with slight and progres-sive decrements in luminal size thereafter extending beyond 10 years.[19] It is unknown whether more aggressive medical therapy may modify the progression of disease in originally stented segments. The mechanisms of this late progression of disease are not well understood, but the development of new atherosclerosis within the stented segment has been hypothesized to result in late disease progression and ultimately restenosis.[19]

Drug-Eluting Stents

In-stent restenosis has limited the use of BMS as the default adjunc-tive therapy to balloon angioplasty for patients undergoing coronary revascularization by PCI. BMS have been demonstrated to reduce the rate of abrupt closure and even late arterial recoil. However, the neointimal hyperplastic response to BMS with resulting late luminal loss and subsequent clinical restenosis has been termed the "Achilles heel" of PCI with BMS. Despite attempts to maximize acute gain through an upfront "bigger-is-better" stent optimization strategy, rates of clinical restenosis after BMS implantation approached 20% to 40%, with even higher rates observed among patients with greatest risk, such as diabetic patients, and certain lesion subsets, such as long lesions and small reference vessel diameters.

Drug-eluting stents (DES), which maintain the mechanical advan-tages of BMS while delivering pharmacologic therapy locally to the arterial wall to prevent restenosis, effectively inhibit neointimal hyperplasia after stent implantation. As a result, DES are currently implanted in most of the greater than 2 million patients undergoing PCI each year. By combining a BMS platform with a drug carrier that controls the release of one or more pharmacologic agents to prevent restenosis (Figure 7-1), DES were designed specifically to prevent the neointimal hyperplasia resulting after conventional BMS placement and have been highly successful in this regard.[20-22]

First-Generation Drug-Eluting Stents

SIROLIMUS-ELUTING STENT

The first DES to attain approval for human use was the Cypher sirolimus-eluting stent (SES) (Cordis Corporation, Miami Lakes, FL). Initial first-in-man studies and subsequent clinical trials led to its approval in Europe in 2002 and the United States in 2003. This stent

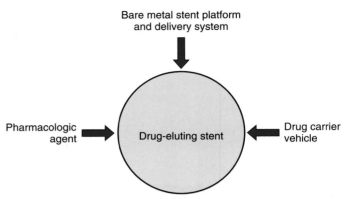

Figure 7-1   Components of drug-eluting stents.

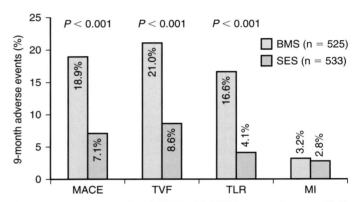

Figure 7-2   Primary results of SIRIUS trial. *BMS*, Bare metal stents; *MACE*, major adverse cardiac events; *MI*, myocardial infarction; *SES*, sirolimus-eluting stent; *TLR*, revascularization of target lesion; *TVF*, target vessel failure.

elutes sirolimus from the thick-strutted Bx-Velocity stainless steel stent via a biostable polymer. The landmark Randomized Study with the Sirolimus-Eluting Velocity Balloon-Expandable Stent in the Treatment of Patients with De Novo Native Coronary Artery Lesions (RAVEL) trial was the first randomized trial conducted with a DES.[20] In this study, 238 patients with de novo coronary lesions (lesion length ≤18 mm in coronary arteries 2.5 to 3.5 mm in diameter) were randomly assigned to either the Cypher SES or the uncoated Bx-Velocity BMS. The SES essentially eliminated late loss at 6 months compared with the BMS (mean of −0.01 mm vs. 0.80 mm, P < .001), with a corresponding reduction in the rate of angiographic restenosis (0% vs. 26%, P < .001). After the success of RAVEL, the Sirolimus-Eluting Balloon Expandable Stent in the Treatment of Patients with De Novo Native Coronary Artery Lesions (SIRIUS) trial—the pivotal U.S. randomized trial that led to FDA approval of SES—was conducted.[21] This was a randomized trial comprising 1058 patients that compared the Cypher SES with the uncoated Bx-Velocity in patients with vessel diameters of 2.5 to 3.5 mm and lesion lengths of 15 to 30 mm. The primary endpoint, the rate of target vessel failure (TVF), a composite of cardiac death, myocardial infarction, or target vessel revascularization (TVR), was improved at 9 months in SES-treated patients (8.6% vs. 21.0%, P < .001) (Figure 7-2). Additionally, SES resulted in a 60% to 80% relative reduction in composite adverse events in all examined subgroups in the trial, including diabetic patients, and the magnitude of this reduction did not depend on vessel size or lesion length. Among the 703 patients in whom 8-month routine angiographic follow-up was performed, mean in-stent late loss was markedly lower with SES (0.17 mm vs. 1.00 mm; P < .001).

On the basis of these results, in April 2003 the Cypher SES became the first DES approved by the FDA. To date, this stent has been one of the most studied devices in modern history, with numerous randomized trials and observational studies assessing its efficacy and safety. Collectively, these data demonstrate extremely low levels of in-stent late loss (averaging approximately 0.15 mm across studies), with an approximate 70% to 80% reduction in angiographic restenosis and clinical revascularization of the target lesion (TLR) compared with BMS. Longer-term follow-up with this device has extended to 5 years and beyond and has confirmed these findings. In these analyses, treatment with SES has resulted in sustained reductions in clinical restenosis endpoints with similar rates of death, myocardial infarction, and stent thrombosis in both SES and BMS arms.[23]

PACLITAXEL-ELUTING STENT

The other first-generation DES that came to market soon after approval of the SES was the Taxus paclitaxel-eluting stent (PES) (Boston Scientific Corporation, Natick, MA), evaluated in the TAXUS clinical program.[22,24-27] TAXUS I and II evaluated the performance of the Taxus PES on the Nir stent platform in focal de novo disease, whereas TAXUS IV, V, and VI investigated the Taxus Express stent in more complex lesions. Most clinical studies except for TAXUS VI and one arm of TAXUS II evaluated the slow-release formulation of the PES; all formulations have eluted paclitaxel from a polyolefin-derivative biostable polymer. Collectively, these trials have demonstrated significant reductions in the rate of binary restenosis with PES compared with BMS, with an approximately 60% to 75% reduction in the need for TLR, an effect that has been consistent across a range of patient and lesion subtypes. The study that ultimately led to device approval in the United States was the TAXUS IV trial, which enrolled 1314 patients with single de novo lesions with visually estimated lengths of 10 to 28 mm in native coronary arteries with a reference vessel diameter of 2.5 to 3.75 mm.[22] Patients were assigned to either a Taxus slow-release stent or Express BMS control. The primary endpoint of TVR assessed at 9 months was reduced with the Taxus PES from 12.0% to 4.7% ($P < .001$) (Figure 7-3). Follow-up angiography at 9 months demonstrated marked reductions in mean in-stent late loss (0.39 mm vs. 0.92 mm, $P < .001$) and in the rate of binary in-segment restenosis (7.9% vs. 26.6%, $P < .001$).

Since approval by the FDA in March 2004, the Taxus slow-release PES has been studied in numerous randomized trials and observational analyses, across a range of patient indications and lesion subsets. The studies have demonstrated consistent reductions in measures of neointimal hyperplasia and resultant reductions in clinical restenosis endpoints compared with BMS. Longer-term follow-up (≥5 years) with this device has confirmed these findings.[22] In these

analyses, treatment with PES has resulted in sustained reductions in clinical restenosis endpoints, with similar rates of death, myocardial infarction, and stent thrombosis with PES and BMS. In addition, a series of comparisons between the first two approved devices (Cypher SES and Taxus PES) were made to determine whether superiority could be established for a particular DES. The totality of evidence appears to indicate similar performance of SES and PES in routine de novo coronary artery lesions, despite a lower amount of neointimal hyperplasia with SES as assessed by intravascular ultrasound and angiography.[28-31] Given the greater degree of late loss suppression with the SES, it has been hypothesized that this stent would hold an advantage over the PES in patients and lesions with the highest risk for restenosis. However, in the absence of a large-scale, adequately powered randomized trial, these potential benefits remain unproven.

The commercially available PES has undergone several iterations. The initially approved Taxus Express slow-release stent was subsequently replaced by the Taxus Liberté stent, which uses the same drug and polymer formulation as the Taxus Express slow-release stent but uses an improved and more flexible stent platform. This stent was approved after several nonrandomized single-arm studies in which outcomes in patients treated with the Taxus Liberté were compared with outcomes in the treatment arms from prior TAXUS trials with the Express PES.[32] More recently, the Liberté PES has been replaced by the Taxus Element stent, which also uses the same drug and polymer formulation as the original Taxus Express slow-release stent but with an iterated stent platform using a platinum chromium alloy. The Taxus Element stent (or ION stent) is the current commercially available version of the PES in the United States. This stent was studied in the Prospective Evaluation in a Randomized Trial of the Safety and Efficacy of the Use of the TAXUS Element Paclitaxel-Eluting Coronary Stent System (PERSEUS) trial, which evaluated 1262 patients with de novo "workhorse" atherosclerotic coronary lesions allocated in a 3:1 randomization to the Taxus Element versus the Taxus Express.[33] The Taxus Element was shown to be noninferior to Taxus Express with respect to the primary endpoint of 12-month target lesion failure (TLF) (5.6% vs. 6.1%) and the secondary endpoint of percentage diameter stenosis at 9-month angiographic follow-up (3.1% vs. 3.1%). No differences in clinical outcomes were observed between the two randomized groups in this trial. The Taxus Element stent has also been evaluated in smaller vessels in a prospective single-arm trial comparing 224 patients treated with this stent with 125 lesion-matched historical Express BMS control subjects from the TAXUS V trial.[34] In this analysis, the Taxus Element was superior to the Express BMS with respect to late lumen loss (0.38 mm vs. 0.80 mm, $P < .001$) and TLF (7.3% vs. 19.5%, $P < .001$).

Second-Generation Drug-Eluting Stents

Despite the demonstrated efficacy of first-generation SES and PES as observed in initial and subsequent randomized trials of these devices, early observational data derived from studies examining more unselected use of first-generation DES revealed possible concerns regarding DES safety.[35] Specifically, late reactions to first-generation DES polymers and delayed endothelialization and adverse vessel responses were described,[36,37] potentially resulting in the most devastating complication of stent placement—late stent thrombosis.

To mitigate some of the abnormal vessel responses associated with first-generation DES, several new devices have been introduced, with specific modifications implemented on first-generation technology. These so-called second-generation DES have incorporated more deliverable, thinner strut stents with polymers that have been specifically designed for biologic compatibility. The drug used to combat neointimal hyperplasia in most of these newer devices is one of several sirolimus analogues. These devices include everolimus-eluting stents (EES; Xience V/Promus and everolimus-eluting platinum chromium stent [Promus Element]), zotarolimus-eluting stents (ZES; Endeavor and Resolute), and Biolimus A9-eluting stents (BES; Biomatrix). Because these devices were largely introduced after approval of SES

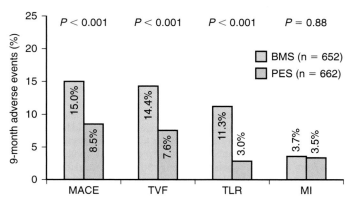

Figure 7-3   Primary results of TAXUS IV trial. *BMS*, Bare metal stents; *MACE*, major adverse cardiac events; *MI*, myocardial infarction; *PES*, paclitaxel-eluting stent; *TLR*, revascularization of target lesion; *TVF*, target vessel failure.

and PES, there are limited comparative data between second-generation DES and BMS. Most of these data consist of comparisons between second-generation DES and earlier first-generation DES.

EVEROLIMUS-ELUTING STENTS

Xience V/Promus

The Xience V EES (Abbott Vascular, Santa Clara, CA) is a thin-strutted cobalt-chromium stent that elutes everolimus from a stable, biocompatible fluoropolymer. In the Clinical Evaluation of the XIENCE V Everolimus-Eluting Coronary Stent System in the Treatment of Patients With De Novo Coronary Artery Lesions (SPIRIT) First trial, it was first shown to markedly reduce the extent of angiographic late loss at 6 months and 12 months compared with the otherwise identical cobalt-chromium Vision BMS.[38] Subsequently, the EES has been studied in multiple randomized trials comparing this device with PES, SES, ZES, and BMS (Table 7-1).[39-50]

The large SPIRIT IV trial,[50] enrolling 3687 patients with stable coronary artery disease undergoing PCI of up to three lesions, was a pivotal FDA-approval study of the EES that randomly assigned patients to EES or PES (Taxus Express platform). Although this study had broader inclusion criteria than first-generation DES approval studies, patients with unstable acute coronary syndromes, myocardial infarction, thrombus, chronic occlusions, vein graft lesions, and true bifurcation lesions were excluded. The primary endpoint of TLF, a composite of cardiac death, target vessel myocardial infarction, or ischemia-driven TLR, was significantly lower at 1 year with EES compared with PES (3.9% vs. 6.6%, $P = .0008$). Rates of stent thrombosis (0.3% vs. 1.1%, $P = .003$), myocardial infarction (1.9% vs. 3.1%, $P = .02$), and TLR (2.3% vs. 4.5%, $P = .0008$) were also lower with EES compared with PES. Longer-term follow-up (up to 3 years) of SPIRIT IV[45] has demonstrated sustained reductions in TLF, myocardial infarction, and stent thrombosis with EES over PES but narrowing of the initially observed differences in TLR (6.2% vs. 7.8%, $P = .06$). However, at 3 years, further clinical differences between EES and PES have emerged: both all-cause mortality (3.2% vs. 5.1%, $P = .02$), and death or myocardial infarction (5.9% vs. 9.1%, $P = .001$) were reduced with EES compared with PES. These data from SPIRIT IV parallel results from the unrestricted all-comer Everolimus-Eluting Stents and Paclitaxel-Eluting Stents for Coronary Revascularization in Daily Practice (COMPARE) trial, in which 1800 patients were randomly assigned to EES vs. PES (Taxus Liberté platform). The primary endpoint of major adverse cardiovascular events (MACE) at 1 year (death, myocardial infarction, or TVR) was lower with EES compared with PES (6.2% vs. 9.1%, $P = .02$), driven by reductions in stent thrombosis (0.7% vs. 2.6%, $P = .002$), myocardial infarction (2.8% vs. 5.4%, $P = .007$), and TLR (1.7% vs. 4.8%, $P = .0002$). Between 1 and 3 years in this high-risk study cohort (in whom only approximately 15% of patients were maintained on dual antiplatelet therapy), less stent thrombosis, myocardial infarction, and TLR occurred with EES compared with PES.[40]

In contrast to that observed between EES and PES, randomized trials have demonstrated fewer clinically apparent differences between EES and SES. In the Scandinavian Organization for Randomized Trials with Clinical Outcome (SORT OUT) IV trial,[47] 2774 unselected patients in Denmark were randomly assigned to either EES or SES and followed through the Danish Civil Registration System. Similar 9-month outcomes were observed between patients treated with EES and SES, although definite stent thrombosis occurred in fewer patients treated with EES compared with SES at both 9 months and 18 months (18 months, 0.2% vs. 0.9%). In the BAsel Stent Kosten Effektivitäts Trial PROspective Validation Examination (BASKET-PROVE) multicenter, randomized trial, 2314 patients with lesions with reference vessel diameters greater than 3.0 mm were randomly assigned to receive EES, SES, or the cobalt-chromium Vision BMS.[51] EES, SES, and BMS were associated with similar rates of cardiac death or nonfatal myocardial infarction at 2 years, and the rate of TVR was similar comparing EES and SES. However, the rate of TVR was significantly

lower with both EES and SES compared with BMS (3.1% for EES, 3.7% for SES, 8.9% for BMS). Therefore the drug-eluting stents were beneficial, even in larger arteries with low rates of restenosis after bare metal stenting. Most trials comparing EES with SES have demonstrated largely similar angiographic outcomes,[49,52,53] except for the Everolimus-Eluting Stent Versus Sirolimus-Eluting Stent Implantation for De Novo Coronary Artery Disease in Patients with Diabetes Mellitus (ESSENCE-DIABETES) trial,[48] a trial confined to diabetic patients, in which EES were associated with lower rates of angiographic late loss and binary restenosis at 8 months compared with SES. With the exception of the results of this trial, the current randomized trial dataset does not address whether there exist clinically apparent efficacy differences between EES and SES in the highest risk subgroups of patients and lesions.

One performance advantage of EES that has emerged relative to other stents is the low rate of stent thrombosis, particularly very late stent thrombosis, that has been observed. First demonstrated in SPIRIT IV and COMPARE, these findings have also been validated in several other studies, including a meta-analysis of 13 randomized trials involving EES and a total of 17,101 patients that demonstrated lower rates of stent thrombosis with EES compared with non-EES DES.[54] These data, combined with that of further observational studies,[55] appear to support the use of the second-generation EES over previously existing first-generation DES with respect to safety in addition to efficacy. Whether EES can achieve lower or noninferior overall rates of stent thrombosis compared with BMS is an area of active interest, piqued by studies such as the randomized EXAMINATION trial of 1504 patients with ST segment elevation myocardial infarction,[56] in which the rate of definite or probable stent thrombosis at 1 year was significantly lower in patients treated with EES compared with patients treated with BMS (0.9% vs. 2.6%, $P = .01$).

Promus Element

Another iteration of the EES has involved the use of everolimus eluted by the same stable fluoropolymer as that of the original EES but using a platinum chromium stent platform (Promus Element, Boston Scientific Corporation, Natick, MA). This stent was evaluated in the randomized Prospective, Randomized, Multicenter Trial to Assess an Everolimus-Eluting Coronary Stent System [PROMUS Element] for the Treatment of Up to Two de Novo Coronary Artery Lesions (PLATINUM) trial,[57] which randomly assigned 1530 patients undergoing PCI of one or two de novo native lesions to treatment with either the standard EES or the Promus Element stent. The rates of efficacy and safety outcomes were very similar with both stents in this trial, which ultimately led to FDA approval of this EES platform.

In a broad cross-section of patients undergoing PCI, EES have shown significant improvements in safety and efficacy outcomes compared with PES and more modest improvements (more related to safety rather than efficacy) compared with SES. The finding of lower rates of stent thrombosis with EES compared with predecessor DES systems is notable and suggests that if these findings can be validated further in larger, adequately powered clinical trials, this stent may have set a new standard for DES safety.

ZOTAROLIMUS-ELUTING STENTS

Endeavor

Although studied contemporaneously with first-generation SES and PES, the zotarolimus-eluting Endeavor stent (ZES-Endeavor, Medtronic CardioVascular, Santa Rosa, CA) was originally conceived as a "second-generation" DES, rapidly eluting zotarolimus over 30 days from a flexible cobalt alloy stent with a biocompatible phosphorylcholine polymer. The Endeavor I First-In-Man study[58] demonstrated that the ZES-Endeavor provided a low rate of TLR despite a mean in-stent late lumen loss of 0.61 mm at 12 months. The ZES-Endeavor was subsequently compared with its base BMS (the Driver stent) in the Randomized Controlled Trial to Evaluate the Safety and Efficacy

TABLE 7-1	Randomized Controlled Trials of Everolimus-Eluting Stents				
Trial	Study Cohort	EES vs.	Number Randomized (Planned Angiographic Follow-up)	Latest Follow-up to Date	Principal Findings
SPIRIT First[38,94]	Noncomplex CAD	BMS	60 (all)	5 years	EES vs. BMS resulted in markedly reduced late loss and neointimal volume obstruction
SPIRIT II[42]	Noncomplex CAD; up to 2 lesions	PES(E)	300 (all)	5 years	EES vs. PES(E) resulted in lower 6-month angiographic in-stent late loss (0.11 ± 0.27 mm vs. 0.36 ± 0.39 mm, $P < .0001$)
SPIRIT III[43,95]	Noncomplex CAD; up to 2 lesions	PES(E)	1002 (564)	5 years	EES vs. PES(E) resulted in lower 8-month angiographic in-segment late loss (0.14 ± 0.41 mm vs. 0.28 ± 0.48 mm, $P = .004$), noninferior 9-month rates of TVF (7.2% vs. 9.0%, $P = .31$), and reduced rates of MACE at 1 year (5.9% vs. 9.9%, $P = .02$) and 5 years (13.7% vs. 20.2%, $P = .007$)
SPIRIT IV[45,50]	Noncomplex CAD; up to 3 lesions	PES(E)	3687 (none)	3 years	EES vs. PES(E) resulted in lower 1-year rates of TLF (3.9% vs. 6.6%, $P = .0008$) and ischemia-driven TLR (2.3% vs. 4.5%, $P = .0008$), with similar rates of cardiac death or target vessel MI (2.2% vs. 3.2%, $P = .09$). EES also resulted in lower rates of MI and stent thrombosis. At 3 years, these results were maintained, although the difference in TLR was no longer significant (6.2% vs. 7.8%, $P = .06$). The 3-year mortality and death or MI was reduced with EES compared with PES (see text)
COMPARE[40,96]	All-comers	PES(L)	1800 (none)	3 years	EES vs. PES(L) resulted in lower 1-year rates of the primary composite endpoint death, MI, or TVR (6.2% vs. 9.1%, $P = .02$). EES also resulted in lower rates of MI, stent thrombosis, and TLR (see text). Between 1 and 3 years, EES resulted in less stent thrombosis, MI, and TLR
SPIRIT V Diabetes[39]	Diabetes	PES(L)	324 (all)	1 year	EES vs. PES(L) resulted in lower 9-month rates of angiographic in-stent late loss (0.19 ± 0.37 mm vs. 0.39 ± 0.49 mm, $P = .0001$)
BASKET-PROVE[51]	Large coronary arteries (≥3.0-mm stents)	SES, BMS	2314 (none)	2 years	EES and SES resulted in lower rates of TVR compared with BMS (3.1% and 3.7% vs. 8.9%). There were no differences between the three stent types in the rates of death, MI, or stent thrombosis at 2 years
EXECUTIVE[41]	MVD, otherwise noncomplex CAD	PES(L)	200 (all)	9 months	EES vs. PES(L) resulted in lower 9-month angiographic in-stent late loss (0.11 ± 0.27 mm vs. 0.36 ± 0.39 mm, $P = .008$)
ISAR-TEST-4[46,52]	Simple and complex CAD	SES	1304 (all)	3 years	EES vs. SES resulted in nonsignificant different rates of in-segment late loss at 24 months (0.29 ± 0.51 mm vs. 0.31 ± 0.58 mm, $P = .59$). At 3 years, rates of clinical outcomes were similar between EES and SES (for TLR, 12.8% vs. 15.5%, $P = .15$)
SORT OUT IV[47]	Unselected patients	SES	2774 (none)	18 months	EES vs. SES resulted in similar rates of composite endpoint of death, MI, stent thrombosis, or clinically driven TVR at 9 and 18 months (7.2% vs. 7.6%, $P = .64$). Definite stent thrombosis at 18 months was lower with EES (0.2% vs. 0.9%, $P = .03$)
EXAMINATION[56]	STEMI	BMS	1504 (none)	1 year	EES vs. BMS resulted in similar rates of composite death, MI, or revascularization but lower rates of TLR (2.2% vs. 5.1%, $P = .003$). Definite and probable stent thrombosis at 1 year was lower in EES patients (0.9% vs. 2.6%, $P = .01$)
EXCELLENT[49]	Noncomplex CAD	SES	1443 (all)	9 months	EES vs. SES resulted in similar in-segment late loss at 9 months (0.10 mm vs. 0.05 mm, P for noninferiority = .02). Low rates of MACE were seen in both groups
LONG-DES-III[53]	Long (≥25 mm) native coronary lesions	SES	450 (all)	9 months	EES vs. SES resulted in higher in-segment late loss (0.17 mm vs. 0.09 mm, $P = .046$) but similar in-stent late loss and in-stent binary restenosis as well as other clinical endpoints at 9 months
ESSENCE-DIABETES[48]	Diabetes	SES	300 (all)	1 year	EES vs. SES resulted in lower 8-month angiographic in-segment late loss (mean, 0.23 mm vs. 0.37 mm, $P = .02$) and lower binary restenosis (0.9% vs. 6.5%, $P = .04$). There were no differences in clinical outcomes between the two stents

Continued on following page

TABLE 7-1	Randomized Controlled Trials of Everolimus-Eluting Stents (Continued)				
Trial	Study Cohort	EES vs.	Number Randomized (Planned Angiographic Follow-up)	Latest Follow-up to Date	Principal Findings
RESOLUTE All-Comers[44,74]	Unselected patients	ZES(R)	2292 (460)	2 years	EES vs. ZES(R) resulted in comparable 1-year rates of TLF (8.3% vs. 8.2%, P = .92) and TLR (3.4% vs. 3.9%, P = .50), although less definite stent thrombosis (0.3% vs. 1.2%, P = .01) and definite and probable stent thrombosis (0.7% vs. 1.6%, P = .05) were noted at 1 year. At 2 years, similar rates of clinical endpoints were observed, with a trend toward less definite and probable stent thrombosis (1.0% vs. 1.9%, P = .077)
TWENTE[75]	Unselected patients	ZES(R)	1391 (none)	1 year	EES vs. ZES(R) resulted in similar rates of TVR (8.1% vs. 8.2%, P = .94) and other clinical endpoints, including stent thrombosis at 1 year
PLATINUM[57]	1 or 2 de novo native lesions	Pt-Cr EES	1530 (none)	1 year	EES vs. Pt-Cr EES resulted in similar rates of TLF (2.9% vs. 3.4%, P = .60) and other clinical endpoints at 1 year

BMS, Bare metal stents; CAD, coronary artery disease; EES, everolimus-eluting stents (Xience V/Promus); MACE, major adverse cardiac events (cardiac death, myocardial infarction, or target lesion revascularization); MI, myocardial infarction; MVD, multivessel disease; PES(E), paclitaxel-eluting stents (Taxus Express platform); PES(L), paclitaxel-eluting stents (Taxus Liberté platform); Pt-Cr EES, platinum chromium everolimus-eluting stents; SES, sirolimus-eluting stents; TLF, target lesion failure (cardiac death, target vessel myocardial infarction, or TLR); TLR, target lesion revascularization; TVF, target vessel failure (cardiac death, myocardial infarction, or TVR); TVR, target vessel revascularization; ZES(R), zotarolimus-eluting stents (Resolute platform).

of the Medtronic AVE ABT-578 Eluting Driver Coronary Stent in De Novo Native Coronary Artery Lesions (ENDEAVOR II),[59,60] conducted in 1197 patients with noncomplex lesions. In this trial, the ZES-Endeavor was associated with lower rates of TVF and TLR at 9 months compared with BMS; these results were sustained at follow-up to 5 years. In this trial, 9-month angiographic in-stent late loss (0.61 mm) was greater than previously seen with either SES or PES, but nonetheless in-segment binary restenosis compared with BMS was reduced from 35.0% to 13.2% (P < .0001).

Based on these data, head-to-head DES studies in the ENDEAVOR clinical trial program were launched with a 436-patient study, the Randomized Controlled Trial of the Medtronic Endeavor Drug [ABT-578] Eluting Coronary Stent System Versus the Cypher Sirolimus-Eluting Coronary Stent System in De Novo Native Coronary Artery Lesions (ENDEAVOR III), designed to demonstrate angiographic noninferiority of the ZES-Endeavor to the Cypher SES. In this trial, the ZES-Endeavor failed to meet its primary endpoint, and the amount of late loss and rate of restenosis were significantly greater with the ZES-Endeavor than SES.[61] Despite these findings, the overall rates of clinical restenosis endpoints were not substantially different. In the larger, clinical endpoint-oriented Randomized Comparison of Zotarolimus- and Paclitaxel-Eluting Stents in Patients with Coronary Artery Disease (ENDEAVOR IV) (N = 1548), patients with noncomplex coronary lesions were randomly assigned to treatment with the ZES-Endeavor versus PES. Despite greater late loss and angiographic restenosis with the ZES-Endeavor compared with PES, the ZES-Endeavor had noninferior 9-month rates of TVF and comparable 12-month rates of TLR.[62] TLR rates were lowest and comparable among patients assigned to receive clinical follow-up alone (rather than routine angiographic follow-up) (Figure 7-4), emphasizing the clinical trial phenomenon referred to as the oculostenotic reflex, which can increase differential revascularization rates based on nonclinically significant differences in late loss in the setting of mandated surveillance angiography. The ENDEAVOR IV findings ultimately led to device approval of the ZES-Endeavor in the United States. At 5-year follow-up, rates of TLR were similar for the Endeavor-ZES compared with PES (7.7% vs. 8.6%, P = .70).[63] The ZES-Endeavor appeared to demonstrate a superior late safety profile with a lower rate of very late stent thrombosis (0.4% vs. 1.8%, P = .012) and lower overall incidence of cardiac death or myocardial infarction (6.4% vs. 9.1%, P = .048) compared with PES.

Several trials have compared the ZES-Endeavor with other DES in unrestricted patient populations. In the SORT OUT III trial,[64] 2333

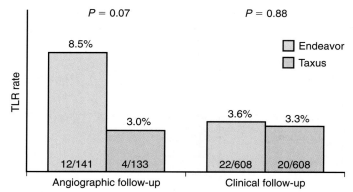

Figure 7-4 Rates of revascularization of the target lesion *(TLR)* in the ENDEAVOR IV trial according to performance of angiographic follow-up. The differences in repeat revascularization rates among patients with or without mandated follow-up angiography is likely a function of the oculostenotic reflex, in that differences in late loss between stents, although not clinically significant, influenced treatment decisions.

patients (nearly 50% of whom presented with acute coronary syndromes) were randomly assigned to the ZES-Endeavor or SES. In this trial, treatment with the ZES-Endeavor was associated with higher rates of 9-month MACE (cardiac death, myocardial infarction, or TVR; 6% vs. 3%, P = .0002) and higher rates of myocardial infarction, stent thrombosis, and TLR. These differences, with the exception of stent thrombosis, persisted at 18 months. The Intracoronary Stenting and Angiographic Results: Test Efficacy of Three Limus-Eluting Stents (ISAR-TEST-2) trial was a three-way 1:1:1 randomized trial in 1007 patients of an investigational combination sirolimus/probucol–eluting stent versus ZES-Endeavor versus SES.[65,66] Compared with SES, the ZES-Endeavor resulted in higher rates of late loss, angiographic restenosis (the primary endpoint), and TLR at 6 to 8 months, with similar rates of death, myocardial infarction, and stent thrombosis. A larger study, the Comparison of the Efficacy and Safety of Zotarolimus-Eluting Stent with Sirolimus-Eluting and Paclitaxel-Eluting Stents for Coronary Lesions (ZEST) trial, randomly assigned 2645 patients with simple and complex coronary artery disease to ZES-Endeavor, SES, or PES.[67,68] In this trial, SES demonstrated the lowest degree of late loss and binary restenosis, and the ZES-Endeavor was intermediate between SES and PES with respect to rates of MACE, TVR, and TLR.

There were no significant differences in the 2-year rates of death, myocardial infarction, or stent thrombosis among the three stents.

Overall, both the approval trials within the ENDEAVOR clinical program and investigator-initiated clinical trials demonstrate less neointimal suppression with the ZES-Endeavor than either SES or PES, resulting in inferiority of this stent with respect to angiographic endpoints (e.g., late loss and binary restenosis). However, the ZES-Endeavor is superior in efficacy to BMS and likely comparable to other stent platforms in reducing clinical restenosis in less complex lesions, particularly in the absence of routine angiographic follow-up. The very low rates of late adverse safety events with the ZES-Endeavor, including very late stent thrombosis and cardiac death or myocardial infarction,[69] are important findings, particularly in light of the potential ongoing thrombotic risks of SES and PES.[70] The Patient Related OuTcomes with Endeavor versus Cypher stenting Trial (PROTECT) randomly assigned 8709 all-comer patients to the ZES-Endeavor or SES, with a primary endpoint of definite and probable stent thrombosis at 3 years.[71] No evidence of superiority of ZES-Endeavor compared with SES in definite or probable stent thrombosis rates was noted at 3 years (hazard ratio 0.81, 95% CI 0.58-1.14, P = 0.22).[71a]

Resolute

The zotarolimus-eluting Resolute stent (ZES-Resolute, Medtronic CardioVascular, Santa Rosa, CA) is similar to the ZES-Endeavor stent in that zotarolimus is eluted from a thin-strut cobalt alloy stent platform. However, to extend the elution of zotarolimus over a longer time (180 days), the ZES-Resolute uses the BioLinx tripolymer coating, consisting of a hydrophilic endoluminal component and a hydrophobic component adjacent to the stent surface. In the single-arm RESOLUTE first-in-human trial,[72] in-stent late lumen loss at 9 months was 0.22 mm, and the in-segment binary restenosis rate was 2.1%, both less than seen in other studies of ZES-Endeavor or BMS. Low rates of MACE, TLR, and Academic Research Consortium–defined definite or probable stent thrombosis were also observed. The 2-year data from this study have shown TLR, TVR, and TVF rates of 1.4%, 1.4%, and 7.9% with no late stent thrombosis events.[73]

The large RESOLUTE All-Comers trial randomly assigned 2292 patients to ZES-Resolute or EES.[44] This trial enrolled a more unselected patient population compared with prior pivotal DES trials. The rate of the primary endpoint of TLF at 1 year was similar with the ZES-Resolute and EES (8.2% vs. 8.3%, P for noninferiority < .001). With respect to other clinical endpoints, the rates of death, cardiac death, myocardial infarction, and TLR were similar with both stents, but both definite and definite or probable stent thrombosis occurred less frequently with EES at 1 year. In-segment late loss among the 460 patients undergoing angiographic follow-up at 13 months (after ascertainment of the primary clinical endpoints) was slightly greater with the ZES-Resolute compared with EES (0.15 mm vs. 0.06 mm; P = .04), but there were no differences in rates of binary restenosis. Similar rates of clinical endpoints including TLF, TVF, myocardial infarction, TLR, and TVR were observed at 2 years, with a trend toward less stent thrombosis with EES (1.0% vs. 1.9%, P = .077), predominantly driven by events within the first year.[74] Three patients in each group (0.3%) had very late stent thrombosis (i.e., occurring >1 year after stent placement). In the investigator-initiated Real-World Endeavor Resolute Versus XIENCE V Drug-Eluting SteNt Study: Head-to-head Comparison of Clinical Outcome after Implantation of Second Generation Drug-eluting Stents in a Real World Scenario (TWENTE) trial,[75] 1391 unselected patients were randomly assigned to ZES-Resolute or EES. The indication for stent implantation was off-label in greater than 75% of patients enrolled. At 1 year, the primary endpoint of TVF was similar with both stents (8.1% vs. 8.2%, P = .94), with no observed differences in other clinical endpoints, including definite or probable stent thrombosis (0.9% for ZES-Resolute vs. 1.2% for EES).

The ZES (Resolute platform) is the first stent to demonstrate comparable overall safety and efficacy to the EES, notwithstanding slight differences in angiographic and clinical outcomes between these stent platforms. Larger studies and longer term follow-up are required to assess whether device-specific performance characteristics influence outcomes in actual clinical practice.

BIOLIMUS A9-ELUTING STENTS

BioMatrix is a BES that releases drug using a biodegradable poly-L-lactic acid polymer that is gone from the stent by 6 to 9 months after implantation. The Nobori DES is a similar BES that releases biolimus using the same polymer system but with a different stent platform. The Nobori DES (Terumo Corporation, Tokyo, Japan) has demonstrated favorable results compared with PES and SES in three modestly sized randomized trials.[76-78] The BioMatrix BES (Biosensors International, Morges, Switzerland) was first tested in the randomized STent Eluting A9 BioLimus Trial in Humans (STEALTH) trial; 120 patients with single de novo coronary lesions received either a BES or a bare metal S stent.[79] Treatment with BES resulted in lower in-stent late loss at 6 months (0.26 mm vs. 0.74 mm, P < .001).

The Biolimus-Eluting Stent with Biodegradable Polymer versus Sirolimus-Eluting Stent with Durable Polymer for Coronary Revascularization (LEADERS) trial is the largest randomized study examining the safety and efficacy of BES. This trial randomly assigned 1707 all-comer patients (55% of whom had acute coronary syndromes) to BES or SES (Figure 7-5).[80] Similar rates of all clinical endpoints were observed at 9 months with BES or SES, including the primary study endpoint, which was the composite of cardiac death, myocardial infarction, or TVR (9.2% vs. 10.5%, P = .39). Among the 427 patients

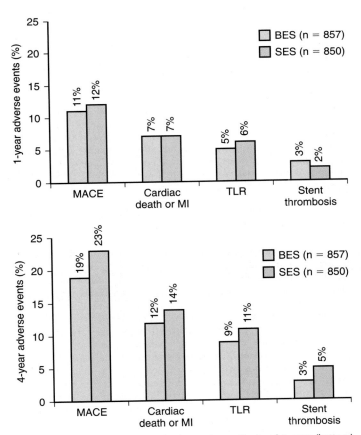

Figure 7-5 Principal clinical endpoints at 1 year (top) and 4 years (bottom) from the randomized all-comers LEADERS trial. Cardiac death, myocardial infarction (MI), and clinically indicated target vessel revascularization (TVR) are included in major adverse cardiac events (MACE). Stent thrombosis refers to Academic Research Consortium definite or probable events. BES, Biolimus-eluting stent; SES, sirolimus-eluting stent.

allocated to angiographic follow-up at 9 months, in-stent late loss and binary restenosis were similar. At 4-year follow-up, the rate of the composite primary endpoint of cardiac death, myocardial infarction, or clinically indicated TVR was lower with BES compared with SES (19% vs. 23%, P = .039), with gradual separation of respective event curves over time.[81] Although overall definite or probable stent thrombosis rates were not significantly different (3% for BES vs. 5% for SES, P = .20), the rate of very late definite or probable stent thrombosis was significantly lower with BES (6 events [1%] vs. 20 events [2%], P = .005). Similar results were observed when assessing the endpoint of definite stent thrombosis.

Collectively, these data demonstrate that BES has similar efficacy to first-generation devices, with a favorable safety profile that appears to emerge beyond 1 year. However, a much larger and adequately powered study is required to determine whether BES or other devices with bioabsorbable polymers offer true and sustained clinical advantages to the best-in-class second-generation DES with durable polymers.

Comparisons of Drug-Eluting Stents versus Bare Metal Stents and Concerns Regarding Safety of Drug-Eluting Stents

The evidence base for initial DES approvals by the FDA has consisted largely of randomized controlled trials enrolling patients with mostly stable coronary artery disease and relatively noncomplex, de novo coronary artery lesions. Data from these early randomized clinical trials have suggested that overall rates of death and myocardial infarction are similar among patients treated with DES and BMS,[82,83] perhaps because of the offsetting risks and benefits of DES (i.e., a reduction in restenosis events with increase in late stent thrombosis events).[84] However, because of their potent efficacy, DES are used off-label in higher risk patients and with more complex lesions in 60% to 70% of cases.[85] This has led to concern about the safety and appropriateness of the routine use of DES in the real-world setting. Most comparative randomized studies have included primary outcomes of interest that focused on stent efficacy rather than absolute safety. Evidence of the safety of DES has come from two sources—randomized controlled trials, which are usually small to modest in size and typically underpowered to assess individual safety endpoints such as death, myocardial infarction, and stent thrombosis, and large-scale observational registries, which assess the "real world" use of DES in clinical practice and allow more generalizability.

Concomitant with the large amount of clinical trial data comparing SES, PES, and BMS, numerous analyses amalgamate trial data across clinical studies to increase overall sample size. In particular, these studies have attempted to address one of the prominent limitations of individual DES studies—the limited power to detect differences in low-frequency safety endpoints. By aggregating data across trials, these DES meta-analyses have also served as means of summarizing the large number of clinical studies in the published and nonpublished domains. The largest and most comprehensive meta-analysis of first-generation DES versus BMS studies included 9470 patients from 22 randomized trials and 182,901 patients from 34 observational studies. In this analysis, the use of DES in randomized trials was associated with comparable rates of mortality and myocardial infarction, with significant reductions in TVR (55%) compared with BMS (Figure 7-6).[82] There were no detectable differences in death or myocardial infarction with DES compared with BMS when the analysis was restricted to either off-label or on-label studies (Figure 7-7). In the observational studies included in this analysis, treatment with DES was associated with significant reductions in overall death, myocardial infarction, and TVR, although significant heterogeneity among studies was detected. The differences observed among the findings of randomized trials and observational studies included in this analysis highlight the difficulty in assessing nonrandomized active treatment comparisons through an observational study design. In another

meta-analysis, Stettler and colleagues[86] incorporated comparative data from SES versus BMS trials, PES versus BMS trials, and SES versus PES trials in a statistical "network" of trials to discern treatment effects across all included trials. In this analysis of 38 trials, including data from 18,023 patients, TLR was lower with SES and PES compared with BMS, with similar mortality among patients treated with SES, PES, and BMS. A reduction in the hazard of myocardial infarction was observed with SES compared with both BMS (hazard ratio, 0.81; 95% confidence interval, 0.66-0.97; P = .030) and PES (hazard ratio, 0.83; 95% confidence interval 0.71-1.00; P = .045).

In addition to these and other meta-analyses, numerous observational comparative analyses have focused on the examination of low-frequency safety endpoints with first-generation DES compared with BMS. More than 50 nonrandomized comparisons between DES and BMS have been published or presented to date. Aside from the initial publication of data from the Swedish Angiography and Angioplasty Registry (SCAAR) registry,[87] which was subsequently revised with the addition of longer-term follow-up,[88] most of these studies have demonstrated favorable safety for DES compared with BMS. In the largest such analysis, the use of DES was associated with lower rates of death (13.5% vs. 16.5%, P < .001) and myocardial infarction (7.5% vs. 8.9%, P < .001) with minimal differences in bleeding in 262,700 Medicare beneficiaries in the United States.[89]

Despite the reassuring findings from numerous observational registries suggesting that DES may reduce mortality compared with BMS, data from these nonrandomized comparisons of DES versus BMS should be considered exploratory at best and potentially misleading. This conclusion is based on several notable observations: (1) nonrandomized treatment comparisons are subject to significant confounding that cannot be adequately accounted for using conventional statistical methodology; (2) mortality reductions have never been observed in randomized trials comparing first-generation DES with BMS[31]; and (3) in propensity matched observational analyses comparing DES with BMS, most of the benefit of DES compared with BMS was evident within the first 30 days after implantation, a difference that does not appear to have an adequate pathophysiologic explanation.[90] These limitations notwithstanding, the abundance of randomized trial and registry study data with first-generation DES is reassuring because it demonstrates efficacy of DES in reducing clinical restenosis with no major safety concerns compared with BMS. As described in the previous section on second-generation DES, data are now emerging demonstrating improvements in safety outcomes with ZES-Endeavor, EES, and BES compared with first-generation DES. These findings, in conjunction with superior or similar efficacy of second-generation DES, suggest that the comparison between second-generation DES and BMS may be even more favorable than prior studies comparing first-generation DES with BMS. However, this remains unproven at the present time because direct comparisons between second-generation DES and BMS are lacking.

The most concerning adverse outcome associated with the use of DES is the risk of stent thrombosis, specifically thrombotic events that occur late (>30 to 360 days) or very late (>1 year) after stent implantation. Stent thrombosis is significant despite its low incidence because of substantial morbidity, with rates of death approximately 30% and rates of myocardial infarction greater than 60%.[91] When concerns regarding late stent thrombotic events were initially raised,[35] the early trials comparing DES with BMS were reexamined. One meta-analysis of 14 randomized controlled trials, including the pivotal approval trials of SES, found no differences in rates of stent thrombosis in the first 12 months or overall, but in years 1 to 5, the overall risk of stent thrombosis was 0.6% among SES-treated patients and 0.05% among BMS-treated patients (P = .02).[92] Similarly, in an analysis of nine of the original randomized controlled trials comparing SES or PES with BMS, the overall rates of stent thrombosis at 4 years were similar.[83] However, between years 1 and 4, both DES were associated with significantly higher rates of stent thrombosis (SES 0.6% vs. BMS 0%, P = .025, and PES 0.7% vs. BMS 0.2%, P = .028) compared with their BMS counterparts.

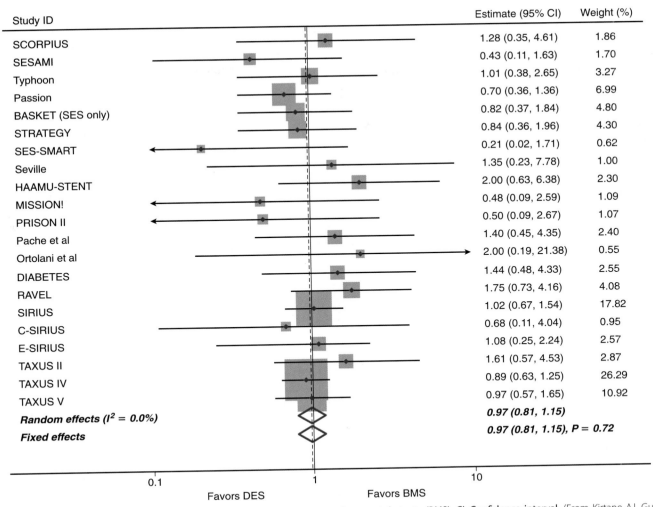

Figure 7-6   Mortality in randomized trials of drug-eluting stents *(DES)* versus bare metal stents *(BMS)*. *CI,* Confidence interval. (From Kirtane AJ, Gupta A, Iyengar S, et al. Safety and efficacy of drug-eluting and bare-metal stents: comprehensive meta-analysis of randomized trials and observational studies. *Circulation.* 2009;119:3198-206.)

Because very late stent thrombosis is an extremely rare event, differences in the risk of stent thrombosis associated with the various DES are difficult to ascertain with statistical confidence. To date, all randomized DES trials are underpowered to detect a difference in stent thrombosis between treatment arms. Assuming a baseline stent thrombosis rate of 2% with a particular stent, an individual clinical trial would have to enroll about 8000 patients to adequately detect a doubling of the risk of stent thrombosis. Given this difficulty, Garg and associates[93] developed a decision analytic model comparing DES with BMS strategies for a contemporary PCI population in which they examined the potential net benefit of DES given varying rates of very late stent thrombosis. The analysis concluded that when assuming identical rates of very late stent thrombosis between DES and BMS, DES were superior to BMS. However, the risk-benefit calculation was very sensitive to small, incremental changes in the rate of very late stent thrombosis. Over a 4-year follow-up period, the threshold excess risk for very late stent thrombosis above which BMS would become the preferred strategy was only 0.14% per year. This model quantitatively demonstrates the clinical significance of late stent thrombotic events; although thrombotic events are rare, they typically have severe clinical sequelae, counteracting the benefits of DES in reducing typically less severe clinical restenosis events.

Conclusion: Balancing Safety and Efficacy

In evaluating the clinical benefit of DES, the potent antirestenotic benefits of these devices must be weighed against their potential adverse effects and a prolonged and in some cases ongoing risk period during which the patient may experience stent thrombosis. The clinical benefits of DES over BMS are driven primarily, but not solely, by a reduction in TLR. This reduction in TLR comes with either a null or a positive effect in reducing mortality in most randomized trials and observational studies. This benefit also must be examined in the context of a slightly increased risk of late stent thrombosis with DES, particularly with first-generation DES, which if numerically frequent enough become associated with increases in hard clinical endpoints such as myocardial infarction and death. In this regard, the data demonstrating improved long-term safety outcomes with second-generation DES (including ZES, EES, and BES) are reassuring. As further adoption and development of second-generation and third-generation DES technology occurs, the landscape of the evidence regarding safety and efficacy of DES will continue to evolve. With many different DES options now available, the continued interest in head-to-head trials of DES in unselected patient populations will continue to define optimally the most efficacious and safest choices for coronary stenting.

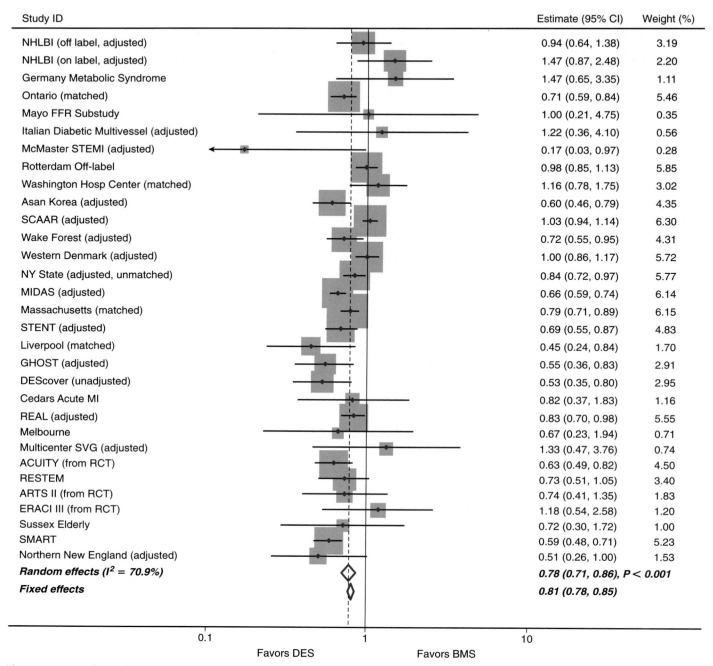

Study ID		Estimate (95% CI)	Weight (%)
NHLBI (off label, adjusted)		0.94 (0.64, 1.38)	3.19
NHLBI (on label, adjusted)		1.47 (0.87, 2.48)	2.20
Germany Metabolic Syndrome		1.47 (0.65, 3.35)	1.11
Ontario (matched)		0.71 (0.59, 0.84)	5.46
Mayo FFR Substudy		1.00 (0.21, 4.75)	0.35
Italian Diabetic Multivessel (adjusted)		1.22 (0.36, 4.10)	0.56
McMaster STEMI (adjusted)		0.17 (0.03, 0.97)	0.28
Rotterdam Off-label		0.98 (0.85, 1.13)	5.85
Washington Hosp Center (matched)		1.16 (0.78, 1.75)	3.02
Asan Korea (adjusted)		0.60 (0.46, 0.79)	4.35
SCAAR (adjusted)		1.03 (0.94, 1.14)	6.30
Wake Forest (adjusted)		0.72 (0.55, 0.95)	4.31
Western Denmark (adjusted)		1.00 (0.86, 1.17)	5.72
NY State (adjusted, unmatched)		0.84 (0.72, 0.97)	5.77
MIDAS (adjusted)		0.66 (0.59, 0.74)	6.14
Massachusetts (matched)		0.79 (0.71, 0.89)	6.15
STENT (adjusted)		0.69 (0.55, 0.87)	4.83
Liverpool (matched)		0.45 (0.24, 0.84)	1.70
GHOST (adjusted)		0.55 (0.36, 0.83)	2.91
DEScover (unadjusted)		0.53 (0.35, 0.80)	2.95
Cedars Acute MI		0.82 (0.37, 1.83)	1.16
REAL (adjusted)		0.83 (0.70, 0.98)	5.55
Melbourne		0.67 (0.23, 1.94)	0.71
Multicenter SVG (adjusted)		1.33 (0.47, 3.76)	0.74
ACUITY (from RCT)		0.63 (0.49, 0.82)	4.50
RESTEM		0.73 (0.51, 1.05)	3.40
ARTS II (from RCT)		0.74 (0.41, 1.35)	1.83
ERACI III (from RCT)		1.18 (0.54, 2.58)	1.20
Sussex Elderly		0.72 (0.30, 1.72)	1.00
SMART		0.59 (0.48, 0.71)	5.23
Northern New England (adjusted)		0.51 (0.26, 1.00)	1.53
Random effects (I^2 = 70.9%)		*0.78 (0.71, 0.86), P < 0.001*	
Fixed effects		*0.81 (0.78, 0.85)*	

0.1   1   10

Favors DES   Favors BMS

Figure 7-7 Mortality in observational studies of drug-eluting stents *(DES)* versus bare metal stents *(BMS)*. *CI,* Confidence interval. (From Kirtane AJ, Gupta A, Iyengar S, et al. Safety and efficacy of drug-eluting and bare-metal stents: comprehensive meta-analysis of randomized trials and observational studies. *Circulation.* 2009;119:3198-206.)

REFERENCES

1. Sigwart U, Puel J, Mirkovitch V, et al. Intravascular stents to prevent occlusion and restenosis after transluminal angioplasty. *N Engl J Med* 1987;316:701-706.
2. Serruys PW, Strauss BH, Beatt KJ, et al. Angiographic follow-up after placement of a self-expanding coronary-artery stent. *N Engl J Med* 1991;324:13-17.
3. George BS, Voorhees 3rd WD, Roubin GS, et al. Multicenter investigation of coronary stenting to treat acute or threatened closure after percutaneous transluminal coronary angioplasty: clinical and angiographic outcomes. *J Am Coll Cardiol* 1993; 22:135-143.

4. Fischman DL, Leon MB, Baim DS, et al. A randomized comparison of coronary-stent placement and balloon angioplasty in the treatment of coronary artery disease. Stent Restenosis Study Investigators. *N Engl J Med* 1994;331:496-501.
5. Serruys PW, de Jaegere P, Kiemeneij F, et al. A comparison of balloon-expandable-stent implantation with balloon angioplasty in patients with coronary artery disease. Benestent Study Group. *N Engl J Med* 1994;331:489-495.
6. Kuntz RE, Gibson CM, Nobuyoshi M, et al. Generalized model of restenosis after conventional balloon angioplasty, stenting and directional atherectomy. *J Am Coll Cardiol* 1993;21:15-25.

7. Nakamura S, Colombo A, Gaglione A, et al. Intracoronary ultrasound observations during stent implantation. *Circulation* 1994;89:2026-2034.
8. Colombo A, Hall P, Nakamura S, et al. Intracoronary stenting without anticoagulation accomplished with intravascular ultrasound guidance. *Circulation* 1995;91:1676-1688.
9. Bertrand ME, Legrand V, Boland J, et al. Randomized multicenter comparison of conventional anticoagulation versus antiplatelet therapy in unplanned and elective coronary stenting. The Full Anticoagulation versus Aspirin and Ticlopidine (FANTASTIC) study. *Circulation* 1998;98:1597-1603.

10. Leon MB, Baim DS, Popma JJ, et al. A clinical trial comparing three antithrombotic-drug regimens after coronary-artery stenting. Stent Anticoagulation Restenosis Study Investigators. *N Engl J Med* 1998;339:1665-1671.
11. Schomig A, Neumann FJ, Kastrati A, et al. A randomized comparison of antiplatelet and anticoagulant therapy after the placement of coronary-artery stents. *N Engl J Med* 1996;334:1084-1089.
12. Urban P, Macaya C, Rupprecht HJ, et al. Randomized evaluation of anticoagulation versus antiplatelet therapy after coronary stent implantation in high-risk patients: the multicenter aspirin and ticlopidine trial after intracoronary stenting (MATTIS). *Circulation* 1998;98:2126-2132.
13. Antoniucci D, Valenti R, Santoro GM, et al. Restenosis after coronary stenting in current clinical practice. *Am Heart J* 1998; 135:510-518.
14. Agostoni P, Biondi-Zoccai GG, Gasparini GL, et al. Is bare-metal stenting superior to balloon angioplasty for small vessel coronary artery disease? Evidence from a meta-analysis of randomized trials. *Eur Heart J* 2005;26:881-889.
15. Nordmann AJ, Hengstler P, Leimenstoll BM, et al. Clinical outcomes of stents versus balloon angioplasty in non-acute coronary artery disease: a meta-analysis of randomized controlled trials. *Eur Heart J* 2004;25:69-80.
16. Al Suwaidi J, Berger PB, Holmes Jr DR. Coronary artery stents. *JAMA* 2000;284:1828-1836.
17. Cutlip DE, Chhabra AG, Baim DS, et al. Beyond restenosis: five-year clinical outcomes from second-generation coronary stent trials. *Circulation* 2004;110:1226-1230.
18. Kimura T, Abe K, Shizuta S, et al. Long-term clinical and angiographic follow-up after coronary stent placement in native coronary arteries. *Circulation* 2002;105:2986-2991.
19. Yamaji K, Kimura T, Morimoto T, et al. Very long-term (15 to 20 years) clinical and angiographic outcome after coronary bare metal stent implantation. Clinical perspective. *Circ Cardiovasc Interv* 2010;3:468-475.
20. Morice MC, Serruys PW, Sousa JE, et al. A randomized comparison of a sirolimus-eluting stent with a standard stent for coronary revascularization. *N Engl J Med* 2002;346:1773-1780.
21. Moses JW, Leon MB, Popma JJ, et al. Sirolimus-eluting stents versus standard stents in patients with stenosis in a native coronary artery. *N Engl J Med* 2003;349:1315-1323.
22. Stone GW, Ellis SG, Cox DA, et al. A polymer-based, paclitaxel-eluting stent in patients with coronary artery disease. *N Engl J Med* 2004;350:221-231.
23. Caixeta A, Leon MB, Lansky AJ, et al. 5-year clinical outcomes after sirolimus-eluting stent implantation: insights from a patient-level pooled analysis of 4 randomized trials comparing sirolimus-eluting stents with bare-metal stents. *J Am Coll Cardiol* 2009;54:894-902.
24. Grube E, Silber S, Hauptmann KE, et al. TAXUS I: six- and twelve-month results from a randomized, double-blind trial on a slow-release paclitaxel-eluting stent for de novo coronary lesions. *Circulation* 2003;107:38-42.
25. Colombo A, Drzewiecki J, Banning A, et al. Randomized study to assess the effectiveness of slow- and moderate-release polymer-based paclitaxel-eluting stents for coronary artery lesions. *Circulation* 2003;108:788-794.
26. Stone GW, Ellis SG, Cannon L, et al. Comparison of a polymer-based paclitaxel-eluting stent with a bare metal stent in patients with complex coronary artery disease: a randomized controlled trial. *JAMA* 2005;294:1215-1223.
27. Dawkins KD, Grube E, Guagliumi G, et al. Clinical efficacy of polymer-based paclitaxel-eluting stents in the treatment of complex, long coronary artery lesions from a multicenter, randomized trial: support for the use of drug-eluting stents in contemporary clinical practice. *Circulation* 2005;112:3306-3313.
28. Morice M-C, Colombo A, Meier B, et al. Sirolimus- vs paclitaxel-eluting stents in de novo coronary artery lesions: the REALITY trial: a randomized controlled trial. *JAMA* 2006; 295:895-904.
29. Lee SW, Park SW, Kim YH, et al. A randomized comparison of sirolimus-versus paclitaxel-eluting stent implantation in patients with diabetes mellitus. *J Am Coll Cardiol* 2008;52:727-733.
30. Galloe AM, Thuesen L, Kelbaek H, et al. Comparison of paclitaxel- and sirolimus-eluting stents in everyday clinical practice: the SORT OUT II randomized trial. *JAMA* 2008;299: 409-416.
31. Petronio AS, De Carlo M, Branchitta G, et al. Randomized comparison of sirolimus and paclitaxel drug-eluting stents for long lesions in the left anterior descending artery: an intravascular ultrasound study. *J Am Coll Cardiol* 2007;49:539-546.
32. Turco MA, Ormiston JA, Popma JJ, et al. Polymer-based, paclitaxel-eluting TAXUS Liberte stent in de novo lesions: the pivotal TAXUS ATLAS trial. *J Am Coll Cardiol* 2007;49: 1676-1683.
33. Kereiakes DJ, Cannon LA, Feldman RL, et al. Clinical and angiographic outcomes after treatment of de novo coronary stenoses with a novel platinum chromium thin-strut stent: primary results of the PERSEUS (Prospective Evaluation in a Randomized Trial of the Safety and Efficacy of the Use of the TAXUS Element Paclitaxel-Eluting Coronary Stent System) trial. *J Am Coll Cardiol* 2010;56:264-271.
34. Cannon LA, Kereiakes DJ, Mann T, et al. A prospective evaluation of the safety and efficacy of TAXUS Element paclitaxel-eluting coronary stent implantation for the treatment of de novo coronary artery lesions in small vessels: the PERSEUS Small Vessel trial. *EuroIntervention* 2011;6:920-927.
35. Daemen J, Wenaweser P, Tsuchida K, et al. Early and late coronary stent thrombosis of sirolimus-eluting and paclitaxel-eluting stents in routine clinical practice: data from a large two-institutional cohort study. *Lancet* 2007;369:667-678.
36. Cook S, Wenaweser P, Togni M, et al. Incomplete stent apposition and very late stent thrombosis after drug-eluting stent implantation. *Circulation* 2007;115:2426-2434.
37. Cook S, Ladich E, Nakazawa G, et al. Correlation of intravascular ultrasound findings with histopathological analysis of thrombus aspirates in patients with very late drug-eluting stent thrombosis. *Circulation* 2009;120:391-399.
38. Serruys PW, Ong AT, Piek JJ, et al. A randomized comparison of a durable polymer Everolimus-eluting stent with a bare metal coronary stent: The SPIRIT first trial. *EuroIntervention* 2005;1: 58-65.
39. Grube E. *SPIRIT V diabetic RCT: 9 month angiographic and 1 year clinical follow-up. Presented at Transcatheter Cardiovascular Therapeutics*. Washington, DC, 2010.
40. Smits PC. *COMPARE trial: 3-year follow-up. Presented at Transcatheter Cardiovascular Therapeutics*. San Francisco, CA, 2011.
41. Ribichini F. *EXECUTIVE: a prospective randomized trial of everolimus-eluting stents compared to paclitaxel-eluting stents in patients with multivessel coronary artery disease. Presented at Transcatheter Cardiovascular Therapeutics*. Washington, DC, 2010.
42. Serruys PW, Ruygrok P, Neuzner J, et al. A randomised comparison of an everolimus-eluting coronary stent with a paclitaxel-eluting coronary stent: the SPIRIT II trial. *EuroIntervention* 2006;2:286-294.
43. Stone GW, Midei M, Newman W, et al. Comparison of an everolimus-eluting stent and a paclitaxel-eluting stent in patients with coronary artery disease: a randomized trial. *JAMA* 2008;299:1903-1913.
44. Serruys PW, Silber S, Garg S, et al. Comparison of zotarolimus-eluting and everolimus-eluting coronary stents. *N Engl J Med* 2010;363:136-146.
45. Stone GW. *A large scale randomized comparison of everolimus-eluting and paclitaxel-eluting stents: three-year outcomes from the SPIRIT IV trial. Presented at Transcatheter Cardiovascular Therapeutics*. San Francisco, CA, 2011.
46. Byrne RA, Kastrati A, Kufner S, et al. Randomized, non-inferiority trial of three limus agent-eluting stents with different polymer coatings: the Intracoronary Stenting and Angiographic Results: Test Efficacy of 3 Limus-Eluting Stents (ISAR-TEST-4) trial. *Eur Heart J* 2009;30:2441-2449.
47. Jensen LO, Thayssen P, Hansen HS, et al. Randomized comparison of everolimus-eluting and sirolimus-eluting stents in patients treated with percutaneous coronary intervention (the SORT OUT IV trial). *Circulation* 2012;125:1246-1255.
48. Kim WJ, Lee SW, Park SW, et al. Randomized comparison of everolimus-eluting stent versus sirolimus-eluting stent implantation for de novo coronary artery disease in patients with diabetes mellitus (ESSENCE-DIABETES): results from the ESSENCE-DIABETES trial. *Circulation* 2011;124:886-892.
49. Park KW, Chae IH, Lim DS, et al. Everolimus-eluting versus sirolimus-eluting stents in patients undergoing percutaneous coronary intervention: the EXCELLENT (Efficacy of Xience/Promus Versus Cypher to Reduce Late Loss After Stenting) randomized trial. *J Am Coll Cardiol* 2011;58:1844-1854.
50. Stone GW, Rizvi A, Newman W, et al. Everolimus-eluting versus paclitaxel-eluting stents in coronary artery disease. *N Engl J Med* 2010;362:1663-1674.
51. Kaiser C, Galatius S, Erne P, et al. Drug-eluting versus bare-metal stents in large coronary arteries. *N Engl J Med* 2010;363: 2310-2319.
52. Byrne RA, Kastrati A, Massberg S, et al. Biodegradable polymer versus permanent polymer drug-eluting stents and everolimus-versus sirolimus-eluting stents in patients with coronary artery disease: 3-year outcomes from a randomized clinical trial. *J Am Coll Cardiol* 2011;58:1325-1331.
53. Park DW, Kim YH, Song HG, et al. Comparison of everolimus- and sirolimus-eluting stents in patients with long coronary artery lesions: a randomized LONG-DES-III (Percutaneous Treatment of LONG Native Coronary Lesions With Drug-Eluting Stent-III) Trial. *JACC Cardiovasc Interv* 2011;4:1096-1103.
54. Baber U, Mehran R, Sharma SK, et al. Impact of the everolimus-eluting stent on stent thrombosis: a meta-analysis of 13 randomized trials. *J Am Coll Cardiol* 2011;58:1569-1577.
55. Räber L, Magro M, Stefanini GG, et al. Very late coronary stent thrombosis of a newer generation everolimus-eluting stent compared with early generation drug-eluting stents: a prospective cohort study. *Circulation* 2012;125:1110-1121.
56. Sabate M, Cequier A, Iniguez A, et al. Rationale and design of the EXAMINATION trial: a randomised comparison between everolimus-eluting stents and cobalt-chromium bare-metal stents in ST-elevation myocardial infarction. *EuroIntervention* 2011;7:977-984.
57. Stone GW, Teirstein PS, Meredith IT, et al. A prospective, randomized evaluation of a novel everolimus-eluting coronary stent: the PLATINUM (a Prospective, Randomized, Multicenter Trial to Assess an Everolimus-Eluting Coronary Stent System [PROMUS Element] for the Treatment of Up to Two de Novo Coronary Artery Lesions) trial. *J Am Coll Cardiol* 2011;57: 1700-1708.
58. Meredith IT, Ormiston J, Whitbourn R, et al. First-in-human study of the Endeavor ABT-578-eluting phosphorylcholine-encapsulated stent system in de novo native coronary artery lesions: Endeavor I Trial. *EuroIntervention* 2005;1:157-164.
59. Eisenstein EL, Wijns W, Fajadet J, et al. Long-term clinical and economic analysis of the Endeavor drug-eluting stent versus the Driver bare-metal stent: 4-year results from the ENDEAVOR II trial (Randomized Controlled Trial to Evaluate the Safety and Efficacy of the Medtronic AVE ABT-578 Eluting Driver Coronary Stent in De Novo Native Coronary Artery Lesions). *JACC Cardiovasc Interv* 2009;2:1178-1187.
60. Fajadet J, Wijns W, Laarman GJ, et al. Randomized, double-blind, multicenter study of the Endeavor zotarolimus-eluting phosphorylcholine-encapsulated stent for treatment of native coronary artery lesions: clinical and angiographic results of the ENDEAVOR II Trial. *Minerva Cardioangiol* 2007;55:1-18.
61. Kandzari DE, Leon MB, Popma JJ, et al. Comparison of zotarolimus-eluting and sirolimus-eluting stents in patients with native coronary artery disease: a randomized controlled trial. *J Am Coll Cardiol* 2006;48:2440-2447.
62. Leon MB, Mauri L, Popma JJ, et al. A randomized comparison of the ENDEAVOR zotarolimus-eluting stent versus the TAXUS paclitaxel-eluting stent in de novo native coronary lesions: 12-month outcomes from the ENDEAVOR IV trial. *J Am Coll Cardiol* 2010;55:543-554.
63. Kandzari D. *The "final" five-year follow-up from the ENDEAVOR IV trial: comparing a zotarolimus-eluting stent with a paclitaxel-eluting stent. Presented at Transcatheter Cardiovascular Therapeutics*. San Francisco, CA, 2011.
64. Rasmussen K, Maeng M, Kaltoft A, et al. Efficacy and safety of zotarolimus-eluting and sirolimus-eluting coronary stents in routine clinical care (SORT OUT III): a randomised controlled superiority trial. *Lancet* 2010;375:1090-1099.
65. Byrne RA, Kastrati A, Tiroch K, et al. 2-year clinical and angiographic outcomes from a randomized trial of polymer-free dual drug-eluting stents versus polymer-based Cypher and Endeavor [corrected] drug-eluting stents. *J Am Coll Cardiol* 2010;55: 2536-2543.
66. Byrne RA, Mehilli J, Iijima R, et al. A polymer-free dual drug-eluting stent in patients with coronary artery disease: a randomized trial vs. polymer-based drug-eluting stents. *Eur Heart J* 2009;30:923-931.
67. Park SJ. *The ZEST trial: 2-year final outcomes. Presented at Transcatheter Cardiovascular Therapeutics*. Washington, DC, 2010.
68. Park DW, Kim YH, Yun SC, et al. Comparison of zotarolimus-eluting stents with sirolimus- and paclitaxel-eluting stents for coronary revascularization: the ZEST (comparison of the efficacy and safety of zotarolimus-eluting stent with sirolimus-eluting and paclitaxel-eluting stent for coronary lesions) randomized trial. *J Am Coll Cardiol* 2010;56:1187-1195.
69. Mauri L, Massaro JM, Jiang S, et al. Long-term clinical outcomes with zotarolimus-eluting versus bare-metal coronary stents. *JACC Cardiovasc Interv* 2010;3:1240-1249.
70. Wenaweser P, Daemen J, Zwahlen M, et al. Incidence and correlates of drug-eluting stent thrombosis in routine clinical practice: 4-year results from a large 2-institutional cohort study. *J Am Coll Cardiol* 2008;52:1134-1140.
71. Camenzind E, Wijns W, Mauri L, et al. Rationale and design of the Patient Related OuTcomes with Endeavor versus Cypher stenting Trial (PROTECT): randomized controlled trial comparing the incidence of stent thrombosis and clinical events after sirolimus or zotarolimus drug-eluting stent implantation. *Am Heart J* 2009;158:902.e5-909.e5.
71a. Camenzind E, Wijns W, Mauri L. Stent thrombosis and major clinical events at 3 years after zotarolimus-eluting or sirolimus-eluting coronary stent implantation: a randomised, multicentre, open-label, controlled trial. *Lancet* 2012;380(9851):1396-1405.
72. Meredith IT, Worthley S, Whitbourn R, et al. Clinical and angiographic results with the next-generation resolute stent system: a prospective, multicenter, first-in-human trial. *JACC Cardiovasc Interv* 2009;2:977-985.
73. Meredith IT, Worthley SG, Whitbourn R, et al. Long-term clinical outcomes with the next-generation Resolute Stent System: a report of the two-year follow-up from the RESOLUTE clinical trial. *EuroIntervention* 2010;5:692-697.
74. Silber S, Windecker S, Vranckx P, et al. Unrestricted randomised use of two new generation drug-eluting coronary stents: 2-year patient-related versus stent-related outcomes from the RESOLUTE All Comers trial. *Lancet* 2011;377:1241-1247.
75. von Birgelen C, Basalus MWZ, Tandjung K, et al. A randomized controlled trial in second-generation zotarolimus-eluting resolute stents versus everolimus-eluting Xience V stents in real-world patients: the TWENTE trial. *J Am Coll Cardiol* 2012;59: 1350-1361.
76. Chevalier B, Silber S, Park SJ, et al. Randomized comparison of the Nobori Biolimus A9-eluting coronary stent with the Taxus Liberte paclitaxel-eluting coronary stent in patients with stenosis in native coronary arteries: the NOBORI 1 trial—phase 2. *Circ Cardiovasc Interv* 2009;2:188-195.
77. Ostojic M, Sagic D, Beleslin B, et al. First clinical comparison of Nobori-Biolimus A9 eluting stents with Cypher-Sirolimus eluting stents: Nobori Core nine months angiographic and one year clinical outcomes. *EuroIntervention* 2008;3:574-579.
78. Kadota K, Muramatsu T, Iwabuchi M, et al. Randomized comparison of the Nobori Biolimus A9-eluting stent with the sirolimus-eluting stent in patients with stenosis in native coronary arteries. *Catheter Cardiovasc Interv* 2012;80:789-796.
79. Grube E, Hauptmann KE, Buellesfeld L, et al. Six-month results of a randomized study to evaluate safety and efficacy of a Biolimus A9 eluting stent with a biodegradable polymer coating. *EuroIntervention* 2005;1:53-57.

80. Windecker S, Serruys PW, Wandel S, et al. Biolimus-eluting stent with biodegradable polymer versus sirolimus-eluting stent with durable polymer for coronary revascularisation (LEADERS): a randomised non-inferiority trial. *Lancet* 2008; 372:1163-1173.

81. Stefanini GG, Kalesan B, Serruys PW, et al. Long-term clinical outcomes of biodegradable polymer biolimus-eluting stents versus durable polymer sirolimus-eluting stents in patients with coronary artery disease (LEADERS): 4 year follow-up of a randomised non-inferiority trial. *Lancet* 2011;378:1940-1948.

82. Kirtane AJ, Gupta A, Iyengar S, et al. Safety and efficacy of drug-eluting and bare metal stents: comprehensive meta-analysis of randomized trials and observational studies. *Circulation* 2009;119:3198-3206.

83. Stone GW, Moses JW, Ellis SG, et al. Safety and efficacy of sirolimus- and paclitaxel-eluting coronary stents. *N Engl J Med* 2007;356:998-1008.

84. Stone GW, Ellis SG, Colombo A, et al. Offsetting impact of thrombosis and restenosis on the occurrence of death and myocardial infarction after paclitaxel-eluting and bare metal stent implantation. *Circulation* 2007;115:2842-2847.

85. Win HK, Caldera AE, Maresh K, et al. Clinical outcomes and stent thrombosis following off-label use of drug-eluting stents. *JAMA* 2007;297:2001-2009.

86. Stettler C, Wandel S, Allemann S, et al. Outcomes associated with drug-eluting and bare-metal stents: a collaborative network meta-analysis. *Lancet* 2007;370:937-948.

87. Lagerqvist B, James SK, Stenestrand U, et al. Long-term outcomes with drug-eluting stents versus bare-metal stents in Sweden. *N Engl J Med* 2007;356:1009-1019.

88. James SK, Stenestrand U, Lindback J, et al. Long-term safety and efficacy of drug-eluting versus bare-metal stents in Sweden. *N Engl J Med* 2009;360:1933-1945.

89. Douglas PS, Brennan JM, Anstrom KJ, et al. Clinical effectiveness of coronary stents in elderly persons: results from 262,700 Medicare patients in the American College of Cardiology-National Cardiovascular Data Registry. *J Am Coll Cardiol* 2009;53:1629-1641.

90. Mauri L, Silbaugh TS, Garg P, et al. Drug-eluting or bare-metal stents for acute myocardial infarction. *N Engl J Med* 2008;359:1330-1342.

91. Cutlip DE, Baim DS, Ho KK, et al. Stent thrombosis in the modern era: a pooled analysis of multicenter coronary stent clinical trials. *Circulation* 2001;103:1967-1971.

92. Kastrati A, Mehilli J, Pache J, et al. Analysis of 14 trials comparing sirolimus-eluting stents with bare-metal stents. *N Engl J Med* 2007;356:1030-1039.

93. Garg P, Cohen DJ, Gaziano T, et al. Balancing the risks of restenosis and stent thrombosis in bare-metal versus drug-eluting stents: results of a decision analytic model. *J Am Coll Cardiol* 2008;51:1844-1853.

94. Wiemer M, Serruys PW, Miquel-Hebert K, et al. Five-year long-term clinical follow-up of the XIENCE V everolimus eluting coronary stent system in the treatment of patients with de novo coronary artery lesions: the SPIRIT FIRST trial. *Catheter Cardiovasc Interv* 2010;75:997-1003.

95. Stone GW. *Comparison of everolimus-eluting and paclitaxel-eluting stents: first report of the five-year clinical outcomes from the SPIRIT III Trial. Presented at Transcatheter Cardiovascular Therapeutics.* San Francisco, CA, 2011.

96. Kedhi E. *COMPARE-AMI: two-year outcomes from a prospective randomized trial of everolimus-eluting stents compared to paclitaxel-eluting stents in patients with STEMI. Presented at Transcatheter Cardiovascular Therapeutics.* Washington, DC, 2010.

CHAPTER 8

Clinical Presentation, Evaluation, and Treatment of Restenosis

GEORGIOS J. VLACHOJANNIS | JENNIFER YU | ROXANA MEHRAN

KEY POINTS

- In-stent restenosis after percutaneous coronary intervention leads to repeat coronary revascularization, increased medical costs, and substantial increases in patient morbidity.

- In-stent restenosis is mainly caused by neointimal hyperplasia, which occurs in response to local arterial injury sustained during percutaneous coronary intervention leading to complex inflammatory and reparative processes.

- The efficacy of a coronary stent generally is highly dependent on its composition, including the stent platform and, in the case of drug-eluting stents, the active drug and the polymer in which it has been packaged (drug carrier).

- Interactions between the arterial tissue and the implanted stent are influenced by patient characteristics (e.g., risk profile, genetics, clinical presentation), type of stent, biologic factors (e.g., drug resistance, hypersensitivity), mechanical factors (e.g., stent underexpansion, nonuniform drug distribution, stent fracture), and technical factors (e.g., geographic miss, stent gap), forging the risk of restenosis.

- The temporal presentation, pattern, and response to treatment may differ between bare metal stent and drug-eluting stent restenosis.

- Drug-eluting stents are superior to bare metal stents because they reduce the risk of restenosis across all coronary lesions and patient subsets.

- The rates of restenosis differ among various drug-eluting stent platforms, in particular between first-generation and newer generation drug-eluting stents.

- Various clinical, angiographic, and procedural predictors of restenosis have been defined.

- Most cases of in-stent restenosis manifest with recurrent symptoms, including unstable angina and acute myocardial infarction.

- Coronary angiography is the "gold standard" for assessment of coronary restenosis severity.

- Computed tomography coronary angiography is a valuable imaging modality for assessing coronary artery disease, but its diagnostic value in the assessment of in-stent restenosis is limited in heavily calcified arteries, intermediate or small arteries or stents, thick stent struts, and regions of stent overlap.

- For bare metal stent restenosis, the treatment of choice is a drug-eluting stent.

- The optimal therapeutic approach for drug-eluting stent restenosis is unclear.

- Next-generation drug-eluting stents show promise in continuing to decrease the occurrence of restenosis after percutaneous coronary intervention through the use of novel antiproliferative drugs, improved stent platforms with better biocompatible or biodegradable polymers, or nonpolymeric drug-eluting stent surfaces or depots.

Introduction

The introduction of bare metal stents (BMS) improved outcomes of percutaneous coronary interventions (PCIs) by reducing the incidence of arterial recoil and acute vessel closure compared with the previous treatment option, balloon angioplasty. However, BMS implantation gave rise to the iatrogenic problem of in-stent neointimal hyperplasia, resulting in a restenosis rate of 20% to 30%.[1,2] First-generation drug-eluting stents (DES), including sirolimus-eluting stents (SES) and paclitaxel-eluting stents (PES), drastically reduced rates of restenosis and target lesion revascularization (TLR) compared with BMS.[3,4] Despite further advancements in stent design with newer generation DES, such as everolimus-eluting stents (EES) and zotarolimus-eluting stents (ZES), a small but significant number of patients continue to experience restenosis. Many preclinical and clinical studies have been conducted to determine the frequency, timing, causes, predictors, and optimal treatment of in-stent restenosis (ISR). In this chapter, we provide an overview of the underlying mechanisms, clinical presentation, methods of evaluation, and medical interventions for ISR.

Definition

Restenosis, or ISR, is a frequent complication after PCI. Arterial barotrauma occurring during the procedure leads to reactive neointimal tissue proliferation within the stented arterial segment and subsequent reduction of the vessel luminal diameter. *Binary angiographic restenosis* generally refers to a luminal narrowing of 50% or greater as measured by follow-up angiography.[5] Box 8-1 presents an angiographic classification of restenosis. *Late loss* or late lumen loss is the difference in millimeters between the diameter of a stented segment immediately after PCI and the diameter measured by a follow-up angiogram, which is usually done 6 to 9 months later (Box 8-2). The most widely accepted definition of clinical restenosis at the present time is the one proposed by the Academic Research Consortium. This definition requires either a luminal narrowing of at least 50% of the vessel diameter with associated evidence of functional significance by symptoms of ischemia or abnormal fractional flow reserve or luminal narrowing of at least 70% or greater in the absence of ischemic symptoms.[6]

Pathophysiology

ISR is mainly caused by neointimal hyperplasia, which occurs in response to local arterial injury sustained during PCI, leading to complex inflammatory and reparative processes (Figure 8-1).[7,8] Neointimal formation involves the activation, proliferation, and migration of vascular smooth muscle cells and increased production of extracellular matrix components. Tissue accumulation within the stent peaks at 3 to 12 months, depending on stent type.[9,10] Recoil and arterial vessel remodeling, phenomena that were seen after balloon angioplasty,[11] have been virtually abolished by stent implantation.[1,2]

The restenosis process depends on multiple, complex biologic events, each one regulated by interrelated molecular and cellular mechanisms.[12] In the early phase (days to weeks after the index procedure), arterial injury results in apoptosis of medial vascular smooth muscle cells, thrombus deposition, and leukocyte trafficking to the stent site. Together, these initial responses provide the foundation for the inflammatory aggregation and reparative processes.[13-16] The late phase (weeks to months after the index procedure) is characterized by phenotypic modification of medial vascular smooth muscle cells, which leads to their migration to and proliferation within the intima. Extracellular matrix secretion within the intima contributes to the increasing volume of neointimal tissue.[17] These steps are controlled by interactions between multiple pathways involving growth factors, cytokines, secondary messengers, and microRNAs as well as additional epigenetic and genetic modifications that are involved in transcription, translation, and posttranslational events.[12,18-21]

Stent thrombosis and ISR are distinct entities. Target lesion revascularization (TLR) occurring within 30 days after stent implantation is likely due to procedural complications or subacute stent thrombosis because clinically significant neointimal hyperplasia takes longer to develop. However, it is possible that processes of restenosis and thrombosis may occur concomitantly because both might include the features of neointimal hyperplasia and focal stent thrombosis. Angiographic characteristics (e.g., length of stent, previous ISR), features on intravascular ultrasound (IVUS) or optical coherence tomography (OCT), and intraprocedural findings provide valuable information that can help differentiate ISR from stent thrombosis.

Factors Contributing to Restenosis

Interactions between the arterial tissue and the implanted stent are influenced by the biologic characteristics and genetic background of the individual, the type of clinical presentation, the type of implanted stent, and the PCI technique used. The efficacy of a coronary stent is highly dependent on its composition, including the stent platform and, in the case of DES, the active drug and the polymer in which it has been packaged (drug carrier). The temporal presentation, morphology, and response to treatment differ to some extent between BMS and DES restenosis. In addition to stent characteristics, various mechanical and technical variables are encountered during PCI that contribute to the risk of ISR after stent implantation (Box 8-3).

BIOLOGIC FACTORS

Drug Resistance

Resistance to the antiproliferative agent eluted by the DES may play a role in DES failure. Sirolimus (also known as rapamycin) and its derivatives (rapalogues [e.g., everolimus, zotarolimus]) inhibit the mammalian target of rapamycin (mTOR) pathway, which is vital for cell metabolism and growth.[22] The ultimate effect is cytostatic, suppressing smooth muscle cell migration and proliferation.[19] In contrast, paclitaxel (taxol) is cytotoxic and acts by binding specifically to the β-tubulin subunit of microtubules, interfering with the turnover of key cytoskeletal proteins and causing cell cycle arrest in mitosis.[19] Primary and acquired resistance to these drugs has been described, and increasing data show that cells may acquire resistance with or without mutagenesis.[23,24] Whether sirolimus analogues such as everolimus and zotarolimus are also associated with drug resistance and whether they affect the rates of ISR remain unknown.

Hypersensitivity

The stent platform for most BMS and first-generation DES is 316L stainless steel. This material contains nickel and molybdenum, which are potentially allergenic and may increase the risk of ISR.[25] Newer generation BMS and DES that use cobalt-chromium or platinum-chromium, which have a lower nickel content than 316L stainless steel, appear to reduce hypersensitivity.[25]

The drug or the drug-carrying polymer in DES also can cause hypersensitivity reactions. In one study, the U.S. Food and Drug Administration (FDA) surveyed 5783 patients after PCI with first-generation DES. A hypersensitivity reaction was reported in 261 patients; DES appeared to be the cause of hypersensitivity reactions in 17 patients, 4 of whom died 4 to 18 months after PCI.[26] The underlying pathology was stent thrombosis, either alone or in combination with late restenosis. This report raised alarm about a possible causative role of the suboptimal biocompatibility of the durable DES polymers that reside on the stent surface after drug elution. Newer generation DES using polymers with better biocompatibility, biodegradable polymers, nonpolymeric stent surfaces, and improved metal alloys have been designed to overcome problems with hypersensitivity.

MECHANICAL FACTORS

Stent Underexpansion

Stent underexpansion, a consequence of insufficient stent expansion during PCI, is a potentially preventable risk factor for ISR.[27] Stent underexpansion can be difficult to detect by angiography, particularly in the setting of calcified lesion. Definitive diagnosis of underexpansion can be made by IVUS or OCT, which can show that the underexpanded site has a considerably smaller stent cross-sectional area than the reference lumen area.[28] An in-stent minimal lumen area of at least 90% of the average reference lumen area is consistent with excellent stent expansion.[29]

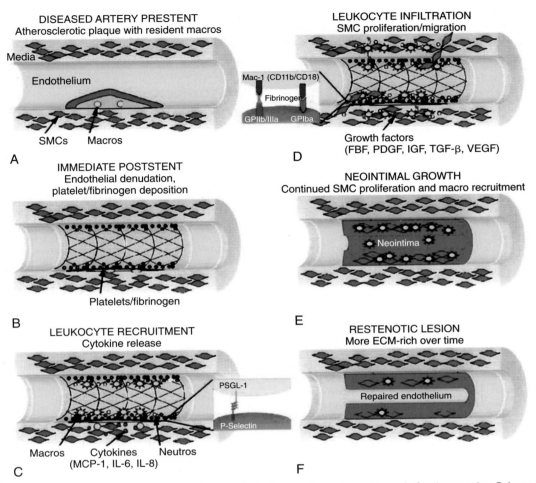

Figure 8-1 Integrated cascade underlying the mechanism of restenosis. **A,** Mature atherosclerotic plaque before intervention. **B,** Immediate result of stent placement with endothelial denudation and platelet/fibrinogen deposition. **C** and **D,** Leukocyte recruitment, infiltration, and smooth muscle cell proliferation and migration in the days after injury. **E,** Neointimal thickening in the weeks after injury, with continued smooth muscle cell proliferation and monocyte recruitment. **F,** Long-term (weeks to months) change from a predominantly cellular to a less cellular and more extracellular matrix–rich plaque. *ECM,* extracellular matrix; *FBF,* fibroblast growth factor; *GP,* glycoprotein; *IGF,* insulin-like growth factor; *IL,* interleukin; *MCP-1,* monocyte chemoattractant protein-1; *PDGF,* platelet-derived growth factor; *PSGL-1,* P-selectin glycoprotein ligand-1; *SMC,* smooth muscle cell; *TGF,* transforming growth factor; *VEGF,* vascular endothelial growth factor. (From Costa MA, Simon. Molecular basis of restenosis and drug-eluting stents. *Circulation.* 2005;111:2257-2273.)

BOX 8-3 POSSIBLE MECHANISMS OF RESTENOSIS AFTER STENT PLACEMENT

Biologic

Drug resistance*
Hypersensitivity

Mechanical

Stent underexpansion
Nonuniform stent strut distribution
Stent fracture
Nonuniform drug deposition*
Polymer peeling*

Technical

Barotrauma outside stented segment
Stent gap
Residual uncovered atherosclerotic plaques

*Applies exclusively to drug-eluting stents.

Stent underexpansion should not be confused with stent malapposition, in which stent struts are not apposed to the vessel wall, seen on IVUS or OCT as a space between the stent struts and the vessel wall. Typically, acute stent malapposition follows the implantation of undersized stents or occurs in vessels with substantial tortuosity, ectasia, or fluctuations in the arterial lumen diameter within the area of target lesion. Malapposition is potentially associated with stent thrombosis.[30]

Nonuniform Drug Distribution

The uniformity of drug elution might be hindered by local blood flow, polymer damage, and strut overlap.[31,32] Periprocedural difficulties in stent placement may damage and shred the polymeric material, which might lead to compromised local drug elution. Treatment of complex bifurcation lesions, especially with two-stent techniques and multiple balloon dilations, may also result in nonuniform drug distribution and susceptibility to restenosis.

Stent Fracture

Stent fracture refers to the complete or partial separation of stent struts after PCI.[33] On IVUS, partial stent fracture appears as an absence of stent struts over at least one third of the circumference of the stent; complete stent fracture appears as complete separation of the stent into two or more pieces separated by image slices with no visible stent struts.[33] Stent fracture results in reduced local radial strength of the stent and drug elution in the case of DES, contributing to the risk of ISR.[34] The need for revascularization in cases of stent fracture is estimated to be 15% to 60%.[35-37]

Reported rates of stent fracture after PCI with BMS and DES range from 1% to 8%.[35-38] However, autopsy data suggest an occurrence of 29%.[39] Various anatomic and procedural characteristics have been identified as risk factors for stent fracture, including PCI of ostial lesions, segments with severe tortuosity or angulation, right coronary artery lesions, use of overlapping stents, long stents, and use of the Cypher SES (Cordis Corporation, East Bridgewater, New Jersey) owing to its rigid closed-cell structure.[35-38] Although there are isolated reports of stent fracture with newer generation DES, the precise incidence is unknown.[40]

TECHNICAL FACTORS

Geographic Miss and Barotrauma Outside Stented Segment

The term "geographic miss" in the context of PCI describes the failure to cover completely the injured or diseased arterial segment with a stent. As reported by an early randomized trial of SES, the area at the margin of the deployed stent, which is injured by balloon angioplasty but not covered by the stent, is the most likely site for restenosis.[4] The same study indicated that restenosis arose mainly at the proximal stent margin after SES placement. The Stent Deployment Techniques on Clinical Outcomes of Patients Treated With the Cypher Stent (STLLR) trial, which studied outcomes in 1557 patients treated with SES, found that residual uncovered atherosclerotic plaques after PCI were associated with increased target vessel revascularization (TVR) and myocardial infarction at 1 year.[41] Occurrence of this phenomenon declined in later studies because of advances in procedural techniques, particularly the use of shorter balloons for predilation and post-dilation and single-stent use for covering the entire area of balloon injury.[42,43] The use of direct stenting where appropriate may minimize proximal and distal edge trauma and subsequent restenosis.[44]

Stent Gap

Similar to stent fracture, gaps between two stented segments result in discontinuous stent coverage, typically of areas that have undergone balloon barotrauma from either predilation or post-dilation. In the case of PCI with DES, drug elution is interrupted at the gap site, which may lead to insufficient concentrations of antiproliferative drug at the vessel wall, predisposing that region to restenosis. Given the safety and efficacy of overlapping contiguous stents, short stent gaps should be avoided.[45,46]

🏷 Incidence

Stent design is a key determinant of restenosis risk.[47,48] Stent type (e.g., coil, tube, slotted), stent length, percentage of metal coverage, number of struts, strut thickness, strut cross-section (square or round), surface finish, symmetry, and stent material all have been shown to affect subsequent restenosis rates.[49] The introduction of DES marked a milestone in interventional cardiology that has led to a significant reduction in ISR rates. The incidence of restenosis after PCI with DES, as reported in randomized trials, is shown in Table 8-1. However, despite progress in stent design and procedural techniques, ISR has not been eliminated, and certain anatomic and clinical scenarios continue to be problematic.

BARE METAL STENTS

An early comparison of balloon angioplasty with BMS PCI treatment of native coronary artery disease showed a reduction in restenosis at 6 months from 42.1% to 31.6%.[2] A larger study of greater than 3370 patients who underwent PCI with BMS placement for de novo coronary lesions found that nearly one third of patients had restenosis at 6 months after the index procedure; stent type was an independent determinant of restenosis risk.[50]

DRUG-ELUTING STENTS

First-Generation Drug-Eluting Stents

First-generation DES displayed advantages compared with BMS in reducing the extent of neointimal proliferation and, consequently, the incidence of clinical restenosis and the need for revascularization.[51]

Sirolimus-Eluting Stent

The Cypher SES was the first FDA-approved DES. The pivotal SES versus Standard Stents in Patients with Stenosis in a Native Coronary Artery (SIRIUS) trial showed a significant reduction of binary ISR at 8 months, from 35.4% in the BMS arm to 3.2% in the Cypher arm.[4] A randomized trial of all-comers undergoing elective PCI showed an 8-month binary restenosis rate of 25.5% in the BMS group versus 8.3% in the SES group[52]; the rate of TLR was 18.8% with BMS and 7.2% with SES.

Paclitaxel-Eluting Stent

The TAXUS IV trial, which was pivotal in the approval of the Taxus Express PES (Boston Scientific, Natick, Massachusetts), reported a binary restenosis rate at 9 months of 7.9% and 26.6% in the PES and BMS groups[53]; TLR was reduced to 3.0% with PES from 11.3% with BMS.

Second-Generation Drug-Eluting Stents

Second-generation DES differ from first-generation DES with regard to all three stent components: (1) the polymer carrier, which affects drug kinetics and biocompatibility; (2) the stent platform, including strut thickness and material; and (3) the antiproliferative drug itself. These changes have improved the safety and efficacy of stent implantation.[54]

Zotarolimus-Eluting Stent

The second-generation Endeavor ZES (Medtronic, Minneapolis, Minnesota) showed superiority compared with BMS in the ENDEAVOR II study with significantly reduced in-stent late luminal loss, binary restenosis at 9 months (9.4% with ZES vs. 33.5% with BMS), and reduced TLR (4.6% vs. 11.8%).[55] Compared with PES and SES, the ZES had numerically higher rates of binary restenosis at 8 months (15.3% in ZES and 10.4% in PES, $P = .284$; 11.7% in ZES and 4.3% in SES, $P = .04$) and TLR (at 12 months, 4.5% in ZES and 3.2% in PES, $P = .228$; at 9 months, 6.3% in ZES and 3.5% in SES, $P = .34$) in the ENDEAVOR III and IV trials.[56,57] However, the absolute difference in TLR between ZES and SES and PES decreased over time to 0.5% at 3 years (6.5% in ZES vs. 6.1% in PES, $P = .662$)[58] and 1.6% at 5 years (8.1% in ZES vs. 6.5% in SES, $P = .68$).[59]

Everolimus-Eluting Stent

The EES (Xience V; Abbott Vascular, Santa Clara, California, and Promus; Boston Scientific, Natwick, Massachusetts) have consistently demonstrated safety and efficacy. The Clinical Evaluation of the XIENCE V Everolimus Eluting Coronary Stent System IV (SPIRIT IV) study demonstrated in 3690 patients undergoing PCI of a previously untreated native coronary artery lesion the superiority of EES compared with PES with reduced rates of TLR (2.5% vs. 4.6%) at 12 months.[60] The Second-generation Everolimus-eluting and Paclitaxel-eluting Stents in Real-life Practice (COMPARE) study, which recruited 1800 patients, was the first all-comers trial comparing EES and PES (using the second-generation Taxus Liberté stent [Boston Scientific, Natwick, Massachussetts]). The patient population was more complex than the population studied in SPIRIT IV. A quarter

TABLE 8-1	Incidence of Restenosis after Drug-Eluting Stent Implantation in Randomized Clinical Trials							
	No. DES Treated Patients	Clinical Setting	Follow-up Angiography Rate (%)	Follow-up Period (months)	Binary In-Stent Restenosis (%)	In-Segment Restenosis (%)	Longest Clinical Follow-up (months)	TLR at Longest Clinical Follow-up (%)
SES								
RAVEL[197,198]	120	Elective simple lesions	89	6	0	0	60	10.3
SIRIUS[4,199]	533	U.S. pivotal approval trial	66	8	3.2	8.9	60	9.4
E-SIRIUS[43]	175	Elective long lesions, small vessels, overlapped stents	92	8	3.9	5.9	—	—
C-SIRIUS[42]	50	Canadian approval trial	88	8	0	2.3	—	—
SES SMART[200,201]	129	Small vessel	95	8	4.9	9.8	24	7.9
DIABETES[202,203]	80	Diabetic patients	93	9	3.9	7.8	48	8.1
PES								
TAXUS II SR[204,205]	131	Simple lesions	98	6	2.3	5.5	60	10.3
TAXUS II MR[204,205]	135	Simple lesions	96	6	4.7	8.6	60	4.5
TAXUS IV[53,206]	662	Pivotal approval trial	44	9	5.5	7.9	60	9.1
TAXUS V[207,208]	577	Complex lesions	86	9	13.7	18.9	60	17.0
TAXUS V ISR[163,166]	195	Treatment for bare metal ISR	88	9	7.0	14.5	24	10.1
TAXUS VI[209,210]	219	Long complex lesions	96	9	9.1	12.4	60	14.6
ZES								
ENDEAVOR II[55,211]	598	Elective simple lesions	88.5	8	9.4	13.2	60	7.5
SES versus PES								
REALITY[212]								
SES	648	Unselected	93	8	7.0	9.6	—	—
PES	669		91	8	8.3	11.1	—	—
SIRTAX[213,214]								
SES	503	Unselected	53	8	3.2	6.6	60	14.9
PES	569		54	8	7.5	11.7		17.9
ISAR-DIABETIC[215]								
SES	180	Diabetic patients	86	6-8	8.0	11.4	—	—
PES	180		88	6-8	14.9	19.0	—	—
ISAR-SMART 3[216]								
SES	100	Small vessels, nondiabetic	91	6-8	11.0	14.3	—	—
PES	100		92	6-8	18.5	21.7	—	—
ISAR-DESIRE[171]								
SES	125	ISR	82	6-8	4.9	6.9	—	—
PES	125		82	6-8	13.6	16.5	—	—
ZES versus SES								
ENDEAVOR III[56,59]								
ZES	323	Elective	87	8	9.2	11.7	60	8.1
SES	113		83	8	2.1	4.3		6.5
ZES versus PES								
ENDEAVOR IV[58]								
ZES	770	Elective	19	8	13.3	15.3	36	6.5
PES	772		18	8	6.7	10.4		6.0
EES versus PES								
SPIRIT II[217,218]								
EES	223	Elective	92	6	1.3	3.4	48	5.9
PES	77		92	6	3.5	5.8		12.7
EES versus PES								
SPIRIT III[219,220]								
EES	669	Elective	51	8	2.3	4.7	36	5.4
PES	332		50	8	5.7	8.9		8.9
BES versus SES								
LEADERS[221,222]								
BES	857	Stable angina or acute coronary syndrome	20	9	17.5	16.4	48	10
SES	850		20	9	19.6	18.5		13

BES, Biolimus-eluting stents; DES, drug-eluting stents; EES, everolimus-eluting stents; ISR, in-stent restenosis; PES, paclitaxel-eluting stents; SES, sirolimus-eluting stents; TLR, target lesion revascularization; ZES, zotarolimus-eluting stents.

DES, Drug-eluting stent; *ISR,* in-stent restenosis.

of COMPARE subjects had ST segment elevation myocardial infarction, and a relatively high percentage of patients had calcified lesions, bifurcations, multivessel disease, and diabetes. The rate of TLR at 12 months was lower for EES than for PES (2.0% vs. 5.3%).[61] In a meta-analysis of 13 randomized clinical trials (N = 17,101), Baber and colleagues[62] reported that compared with other available DES, EES significantly reduced stent thrombosis, TVR, and myocardial infarction without any statistically significant difference between the groups in regard to cardiac mortality.

PREDICTORS OF RESTENOSIS

A plethora of studies have examined the clinical, angiographic, and procedural predictors of restenosis. Early studies were hampered by a high frequency of restenosis that weakened the predictive values of single variables. In addition, there was a high heterogeneity of study populations between trials, making comparisons of outcomes difficult. Although the main pathophysiologic processes of restenosis are similar between BMS and DES, variances therein are reflected in minor alterations of the restenosis predictors for each of the two stent types. Despite differences in study design and stent types, there is a general consensus regarding the main determinants of restenosis. These factors can be classified as related to patient, lesion, or procedure (Box 8-4).

PATIENT-RELATED FACTORS

Advanced age is associated with increased comorbidities known to increase the risk of restenosis. However, age has also been independently associated with increased restenosis rates.[63] The incidence of restenosis among women has been reported to be greater than among men.[64,65] Women generally experience coronary disease at a later age compared with men and have a higher prevalence of comorbid diseases; women also generally have a smaller coronary artery diameter. Some studies have shown that, after correcting for differences in age and comorbidities, there was no independent association between incidence of restenosis and female gender.[66,67]

Diabetes mellitus is an important predictor of ISR after BMS implantation, but data from DES studies have shown conflicting results.[68-76] Diabetes increases the risk of restenosis by approximately 30% to 50% after BMS implantation.[77-80] A study of patients undergoing PCI with BMS of lesion lengths up to 28 mm and a minimum reference diameter of 2.5 mm reported a 50% increase in the rate

of ISR in patients with diabetes compared with patients without diabetes.[53] Similarly, a post hoc analysis of the Prevention of Restenosis with Tranilast and Its Outcomes (PRESTO) trial found that diabetes increased the risk of BMS restenosis by approximately 45%.[80] In contrast, in patients with diabetes in the TAXUS IV trial, PES decreased the risk of restenosis by greater than 80% compared with BMS.[53] Similarly, a meta-analysis showed that the incidence of ISR in diabetic patients was approximately 8% after DES implantation compared with 41% after BMS implantation.[81] A large PCI registry that included data from 35,478 DES implantations reported that the adjusted risk of restenosis was higher in patients with diabetes compared with patients without diabetes and that there were important differences between different DES types.[82]

Patients with end-stage renal failure on hemodialysis have been reported to have a high risk of restenosis. Several small studies have reported restenosis rates of 50%, and renal failure has been described as an independent predictor.[71,83,84]

LESION-RELATED FACTORS

Small vessel size and long lesion length are strong predictors of restenosis after PCI and implantation of BMS or DES.[76,85-88] The substudy of the PRESTO trial analyzed 1312 patients who underwent angiographic follow-up and demonstrated that lesion lengths greater than 20 mm, ostial lesions, American College of Cardiology/American Heart Association (ACC/AHA) type C lesions, and PCI for prior ISR all were associated with higher incidence of BMS restenosis.[80] A meta-analysis including 2926 patients who underwent PCI with BMS confirmed that longer lesion length and smaller vessel diameter predict restenosis.[89] In another study, BMS ISR was associated with ostial lesions, bifurcations, and left anterior descending artery lesions.[86] In a study of 238 consecutive patients with complex coronary artery disease treated with SES, independent predictors of ISR were small reference diameter and calcific, ostial, or left anterior descending artery lesions.[69] Finally, the length of the stented segment increases the rate of restenosis in both BMS and DES,[69,89] with rates of BMS ISR almost doubling when comparing stent lengths less than 20 mm with stent lengths greater than 35 mm.[87]

PROCEDURE-RELATED FACTORS

In addition to lesion length, the number of implanted stents predicts increased risk of restenosis. Quantitative coronary angiographic analysis in 1349 patients found that the strongest independent, procedure-related predictors of BMS ISR were the use of multiple stents and a poststent minimal lumen diameter of less than 3 mm.[90]

There is also compelling evidence that stent underexpansion is a significant contributor to the development of adverse events, regardless of the stent type.[28,91,92] Minimum stent area as measured by IVUS is a consistent and powerful predictor for both angiographic and clinical restenosis.[93] Finally, incomplete stent coverage caused by nonoverlapping stents in series or by stent fracture has been implicated in ISR.[28,39,46,94]

Clinical Presentation

Restenosis after balloon angioplasty was generally considered to manifest as recurrent exertional angina.[95-97] Although there may be clinically silent cases of ISR, most cases result in recurrent symptoms, including unstable angina and myocardial infarction. This situation leads to repeat coronary revascularization, increased medical costs, and substantial increases in patient morbidity.[98]

BARE METAL STENT RESTENOSIS

Two early, small studies reported that most patients with restenosis after PCI presented with unstable angina or acute coronary syndrome.[99,100] Subsequently, two retrospective analyses of patients with

BMS ISR admitted for ischemia-driven PCI varied in their findings.[98,101] Chen and associates,[98] studying a sample of 984 patients from the Cleveland Clinic PCI database, found that the main clinical presentation was exertional angina (64.1%), with smaller percentages of patients experiencing unstable angina (26.4%) or acute myocardial infarction (9.5%). In contrast, Bainey and colleagues[101] reported that in 744 patients from the Alberta Provincial Project for Outcome Assessment in Coronary Artery Disease (APPROACH) database, unstable angina and non–ST segment elevation myocardial infarction were the leading clinical presentations (52.2%) compared with stable angina (25.3%) and ST segment elevation myocardial infarction (18.5%). Two prospective studies have added insight into the clinical features of BMS ISR.[102,103] Pate and coworkers[102] found that of 363 consecutive patients undergoing clinically driven catheterization for BMS ISR, 51% of patients had an unstable presentation, including 15% with recent or acute ST segment elevation myocardial infarction. Steinberg and colleagues[103] showed similar rates of unstable clinical presentation in 2539 patients presenting with BMS ISR: unstable angina (46.6%), stable angina (27.5%), acute myocardial infarction (6.7%), and asymptomatic (19.2%).

The presentation of BMS ISR affects clinical outcomes. The PRESTO trial found that patients with ISR who presented with acute coronary syndrome had a higher incidence of recurrent major adverse cardiac events (MACEs) compared with patients with stable angina (35% vs. 22%, P < .001) and a greater incidence of angiographic restenosis at 9-month follow-up (56% vs. 42%, P = .043).[104]

DRUG-ELUTING STENT RESTENOSIS

Most studies have found that ISR after DES implantation is more likely to manifest as stable angina than acute coronary syndromes. A study of 1958 patients with BMS ISR and 190 patients with DES ISR reported that 78.1% presented with unstable angina, 1.8% presented with acute myocardial infarction, and 20.1% presented with stable angina.[105] Compared with patients with BMS ISR, patients with DES ISR presented more frequently with stable angina (30.9% vs. 19.1%) and myocardial infarction (4.3% vs. 1.6%). However, Rathore and associates[71] found no significant differences in the clinical presentation between patients with BMS ISR (n = 487) and patients with SES ISR (n = 351), and most patients in this study had stable angina or were asymptomatic. Stable angina was the prevailing clinical presentation reported in a study of 163 patients with ISR after SES and PES implantation.[106] Similarly, Appleby and colleagues[107] found that patients with DES ISR (43 patients with SES and 26 patients with PES) were most likely to present with chronic stable angina (78%) and that only a small percentage presented with non–ST segment elevation myocardial infarction (17%) or ST segment elevation myocardial infarction (4%). Finally, 60% to 70% of patients with DES ISR either had stable angina or were asymptomatic in two retrospective analyses.[108,109]

TIMEFRAME FOR DEVELOPMENT OF IN-STENT RESTENOSIS

Patients typically present with ISR approximately 5 months after PCI with BMS.[99-101] Patients present later with ISR after PCI with DES; the mean time for patients with DES to have treatment for ISR ranges from 7½ to 13 months after PCI.[108,109] Early ISR (<3 months after the index procedure) has been associated with more extensive and aggressive subsequent restenosis recurrence.[110] The elution of antiproliferative drugs may slow the biologic response to injury and account for differences observed in regard to timing of presentation between DES and BMS ISR.

Although DES are associated with lower rates of restenosis compared with BMS, continuous neointimal growth and late restenosis have also been reported after DES. Serial IVUS analyses up to 2 years after PCI in 161 patients enrolled in the TAXUS II study demonstrated a slight increase in late neointimal hyperplasia formation in

PES compared with BMS.[111] A subsequent serial IVUS study reported that neointimal volume continued to increase numerically 2 to 4 years after SES implantation, although this difference did not reach statistical significance.[112] Similarly, results from the 2-year angiographic and IVUS follow-up from the SPIRIT II trial showed minor late neointimal increases in the EES group.[113] The reason for this finding is unclear, but delayed healing after DES placement, persistent and late biologic action of the drug, and a hypersensitivity reaction to the durable polymer have been postulated.

🔹 Evaluation

Early detection and treatment of restenosis are of paramount clinical importance. In addition to standard noninvasive stress tests, novel techniques for the evaluation of patients after revascularization have emerged. This section describes the use of computed tomography coronary angiography (CTA), the "gold standard" of invasive coronary angiography, and other adjuvant anatomic and functional imaging techniques for further evaluation of ISR.

NONINVASIVE EVALUATION OF IN-STENT RESTENOSIS

CTA has been shown to be a valuable imaging modality for the assessment of coronary artery disease. At the present time, 64-row CTA is the most widely used system, but 265-row and 320-row CTA have been introduced, enabling faster image acquisition. Owing to a high negative predictive value, CTA is particularly valuable in the exclusion of coronary artery disease in patients with a low-to-intermediate pretest probability.[114] Another indication for CTA is screening for ISR in selected patients with prior PCI.[114] The primary reasons for impaired image quality and compromised stent assessment for the evaluation of ISR by 64-row CTA are high-density artifacts generated by the metallic stent struts, motion artifacts related to patient respiration or chest movement, misalignment of slices because of heart rate variation or premature beats, and blooming effects resulting from vessel calcification.[115] The incidence of nonevaluable stents in 18 studies ranged from 0% to 19.5%, and in a meta-analysis of 14 studies using 64-row CTA evaluating 1398 stents, pooled estimates of the sensitivity and specificity for the detection of ISR (including 11% nonevaluable stents) were 79% and 81%, respectively.[116] The diagnostic value of CTA in the assessment of ISR is limited in heavily calcified arteries, intermediate or small sized arteries or stents (<3 mm), stents with thick struts (≥140 μm), and regions of stent overlap.[117,118] Newer stents with cobalt-chromium platforms produce fewer metal artifacts than other materials.[119] Given the lack of stent strut blooming effect with fully bioabsorbable stents, the potential future use of this stent technology may allow more precise assessment of ISR using CTA.

INVASIVE EVALUATION OF IN-STENT RESTENOSIS

Coronary angiography is regarded as the "gold standard" for the assessment of coronary restenosis severity and is used in most large randomized trials to define restenosis. IVUS has significantly increased the understanding of the restenotic process by depicting all layers of the coronary vessel, in addition to the lumen. Besides pathophysiologic evidence, IVUS provides valuable anatomic information, and IVUS measurement of minimal lumen area has been associated with the presence of functional ischemia.[120-122] By elucidating the underlying mechanisms of ISR, IVUS can be used to guide subsequent interventions. Accurate mechanistic comparisons of minor degrees of neointimal hyperplasia among different DES are ideally performed with IVUS or OCT because of its higher spatial resolution.[123,124] OCT is able to visualize the lumen outline of the vessel more accurately, but it has limited tissue penetration and cannot provide much information on the vessel area beyond the stent struts.

Although quantitative coronary angiography is a standard method for evaluating lesion severity, the complementary measurement of

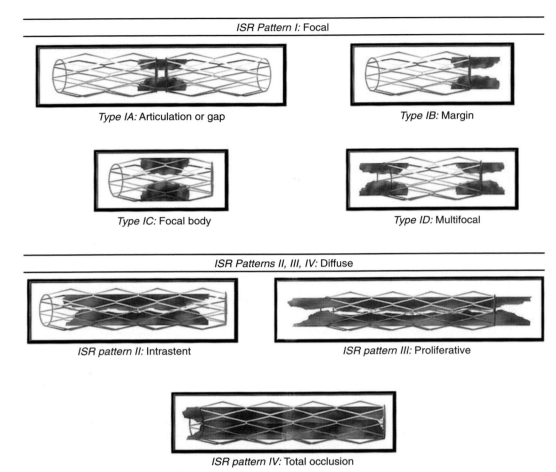

Figure 8-2   Mehran classification of in-stent restenosis *(ISR)*. Pattern I contains four types (IA-ID). Patterns II through IV are defined according to geographic position of ISR in relation to the previously implanted stent. (From Mehran R, Dangas G, Abizaid AS, et al. Angiographic patterns of in-stent restenosis: classification and implications for long-term outcome. *Circulation.* 1999;100:1872-1878.)

fractional flow reserve can provide information on the functional significance of a lesion.[125] Determination of fractional flow reserve by pressure-wire measurements provides a reliable method to evaluate angiographic intermediate lesions.[126-128]

PATTERNS OF IN-STENT RESTENOSIS

Angiography not only determines the presence of ISR and the degree of vessel compromise, but it also reveals different morphologic patterns of restenosis. Early studies demonstrated that patients with diffuse ISR (lesion length >10 mm) have a poorer clinical and angiographic outcome after repeat intervention compared with patients with focal ISR (lesion length <10 mm).[129-131] A more recent study reported that patients with DES ISR are at an increased risk for adverse events, in particular, repeat revascularization, and that the initial pattern of restenosis is the most important predictor of recurrent restenosis or the need for subsequent revascularization.[108]

Mehran and colleagues[130] first described the different patterns of ISR in 1999 and proposed a classification based on these angiographic patterns that has been widely adopted: pattern I refers to focal ISR; pattern II, to diffuse ISR within the stent; pattern III, to proliferative ISR, where the angiographic narrowing extends beyond the stent margins; and pattern IV, to ISR manifesting as a total occlusion (Figure 8-2). The clinical implication of the Mehran classification was reflected by increased need for repeat TLR at 1 year with increased severity of ISR: 19%, 35%, 50%, and 83% for patterns I, II, III, and IV, respectively. The ACC/AHA angiographic lesion classification is also of value: class B2 or C restenotic lesions are not only more difficult to treat and achieve optimal immediate angiographic results but also have higher repeat restenosis rates and poorer long-term clinical outcomes.[131]

ISR patterns appear to differ according to stent type (Table 8-2). Although the predominant restenosis pattern in BMS is nonfocal, most DES cases are focal.[71,94,109,132-136] However, the angiographic pattern of restenosis may differ according to the severity of the underlying lesion. In studies using SES and PES, the randomized SIRIUS and TAXUS IV trials reported a higher incidence of focal ISR lesion morphology compared with observational studies in which lesion type was mainly nonfocal. A potential explanation for this discrepancy might be differences in lesion complexity, with the randomized trials having lower rates of complex target lesions than the observational studies.

🔹 Prognosis

Although patients with ISR have multiple comorbidities and complex lesion characteristics, PCI for ISR is independently associated with increased rates of restenosis and repeat TVR even after adjustment for such factors by multivariate analysis.[71,78,137] Although multiple studies have suggested that ISR is a benign process, one report identified ISR as a predictor of long-term mortality.[137-139] The clinical presentation of ISR appears to influence outcome. The prognosis for patients with asymptomatic ISR is favorable compared with patients presenting with ischemic symptoms.[140-142] In contrast, the

TABLE 8-2	Morphologic Patterns of Sirolimus-Eluting, Paclitaxel-Eluting, and Bare Metal Stent In-Stent Restenosis								
	SES			PES			BMS		
Study	focal (%)	nonfocal (%)	n	focal (%)	nonfocal (%)	n	focal (%)	nonfocal (%)	n
Randomized Trials									
SIRIUS	83.9	16.1	31				43.0	57.0	128
TAXUS IV[53]				62.5	37.5	16	30.8	69.2	65
Observational Studies									
Lemos et al[94]	75.0	25.0	20						
Colombo et al[132]	100.0	0	14						
Iakovou et al[134]				50.0	50.0	98			
Corbett et al[135]	71.3	29.7	150	51.7	48.3	149			
Park et al[106]	76.3	23.7	97	51.3	48.7	80			
Kitahara et al[136]	79.0	21.0	124						
Rathore et al[71]	47.0	53.0	487				19.3	80.7	351

BMS, Bare metal stent; PES, paclitaxel-eluting stent; SES, sirolimus-eluting stent.
Modified from Dangas GD, Claessen BE, Caixeta A, et al. In-stent restenosis in the drug-eluting stent era. *J Am Coll Cardiol.* 2010;56:1897-1907.

presentation of ISR with biomarker-positive acute coronary syndrome is associated with an increased risk of further adverse events after ISR treatment.[71,104]

Treatment

PREVENTIVE THERAPY

Many drugs have been used systemically to inhibit neointimal hyperplasia in animal models, but translation of these approaches to humans in randomized clinical trials has mostly been unsuccessful. For example, the antiinflammatory drug tranilast (Rizaben) reduced ISR in a porcine model but not in humans.[143,144] In addition, clinical studies of other oral agents, including the angiotensin II receptor antagonist valsartan and numerous different statins, have not shown clear evidence of efficacy in the prevention of ISR.[145,146]

Cilostazol

Cilostazol is a phosphodiesterase III inhibitor with antiplatelet and antiproliferative effects in addition to its vasodilatory action. It has been approved for the treatment of ischemic symptoms (i.e., intermittent claudication) in individuals with peripheral artery disease. In the Drug-Eluting stenting followed by Cilostazol treatment reduces LAte REstenosis in patients with Long native coronary lesions (DECLARE-LONG II) study, patients who had undergone PCI with a long ZES (≥30 mm) were randomly assigned to 8 months of cilostazol or placebo in addition to standard dual antiplatelet therapy with aspirin and clopidogrel.[147] Cilostazol was associated with a 43% relative reduction in the incidence of ISR (10.8% vs. 19.1%, P = .02) and a 48% reduction in ischemic TLR at 12 months (5.2% vs. 10.0%, P = .04).[147]

In the Drug-Eluting stenting followed by Cilostazol treatment reduces LAte REstenosis in patients with Diabetes (DECLARE-DIABETES) study, cilostazol was associated with a relative risk reduction of 49% in ISR at 6 months in diabetic patients who underwent implantation of first-generation DES. After multivariate analysis, cilostazol was a strong predictor of reduced restenosis and TLR.[148] Cilostazol was also associated with a 36% reduction in the relative risk of binary restenosis at 6 months after PCI with BMS and was an independent predictor of the absence of restenosis at 6 months.[149]

A meta-analysis that included 10 randomized trials with a total enrollment of greater than 2000 patients reported a significant reduction in late luminal loss at 6 months with triple antiplatelet therapy (i.e., the addition of cilostazol) compared with dual antiplatelet therapy.[150] This association was evident both in patients treated with BMS and in patients treated with DES.[150] The risk of binary angiographic restenosis at 6 months was significantly reduced in the cilostazol group regardless of stent type. The reduction in TLR was particularly robust in patients receiving DES (odds ratio, 0.40, 95% confidence interval, 0.26-0.62; P < .001).

There were no differences between dual (without cilostazol) and triple (with cilostazol) antiplatelet therapy in regard to mortality, myocardial infarction, subacute stent thrombosis, and major bleeding at a follow-up of 6 to 9 months in the DECLARE-LONG II trial or by meta-analysis.[147,150] There was no increased risk of bleeding with cilostazol, although the incidence of skin rash (5% to 8%) and cilostazol discontinuation were common. There has been no large, dedicated, randomized controlled trial to date comparing dual versus triple antiplatelet therapy with cilostazol for the reduction of restenosis after stent-based PCI. Cilostazol is not approved for this indication in the United States at the present time.

Pioglitazone

In diabetic patients, oral pioglitazone appears to reduce rates of ISR and TVR after PCI with BMS. A meta-analysis of six randomized controlled trials showed significantly lower rates of ISR and TVR with pioglitazone compared with placebo (ISR, 18% vs. 40%, P < .01; TVR, 13% vs. 31%, P < .01).[151] However, only studies that exclusively enrolled diabetic patients demonstrated a statistically significant reduction in the incidence of ISR and TVR with pioglitazone. The potential mechanism by which pioglitazone could decrease restenosis may be multifactorial, involving a combination of direct antiproliferative, antiinflammatory, and pro-apoptotic effects.[151] Reduced insulin levels secondary to insulin sensitization and antithrombotic effects secondary to inhibition of fibrin formation may also play a role. Pioglitazone also improves endothelial dysfunction after SES implantation in nondiabetic patients.[152]

TREATMENT OF IN-STENT RESTENOSIS

Although the pathophysiology of restenosis is similar for BMS and DES, the efficacy of different types of treatment differs between stent types.

Treatment of Bare Metal Stent Restenosis

Although balloon angioplasty was initially considered the first-line treatment option for BMS ISR, this approach has a recurrence rate of more than 40%.[153] Reuse of BMS appears to increase the risk of restenosis even further.[153] In a single-center study of 931 patients, DES for the treatment of BMS ISR was associated with a significantly lower risk of major adverse cardiovascular events at a median follow-up of 3.2 years after adjustment for baseline characteristics (hazard ratio 0.63; 95% confidence interval, 0.42-0.95; P = .03).[154] Other interventional procedures, including rotational or directional coronary atherectomy, excimer laser angioplasty, and cutting balloon, do not offer significant additional efficacy.[155,156]

Several randomized trials have demonstrated the efficacy of vascular brachytherapy after balloon angioplasty for the treatment of BMS ISR.[157,158] However, there are late adverse effects after brachytherapy, including restenosis (i.e., a late "catch-up" phenomenon) and late thrombosis, necessitating prolonged dual antiplatelet therapy.[159-161]

The efficacy of DES for BMS ISR has been assessed in several trials. The Intracoronary Stenting and Angiographic Results: Drug Eluting Stents for In-Stent Restenosis (ISAR DESIRE) trial randomly assigned 300 patients with BMS ISR to treatment with SES, PES, or balloon angioplasty. SES and PES led to significantly lower rates of angiographic restenosis compared with balloon angioplasty (14.3%, 21.7%, and 44.6%, P < .001 for SES and PES compared with balloon angioplasty) and significantly less TVR (8%, 19%, and 33%). The Restenosis Intrastent: Balloon Angioplasty Versus Elective Sirolimus-Eluting Stenting II (RIBS-II) trial assessed the effectiveness of SES compared with balloon angioplasty for the first ISR after BMS and found that SES provided superior 1-year clinical and angiographic outcomes compared with balloon angioplasty (survival free of MACE, 88% vs. 64%, P < .004; TVR, 11% vs. 30%, P < .003).[120] Long-term follow-up at 4 years demonstrated sustained clinical efficacy of DES implantation for BMS ISR, with low rates of TLR and stent thrombosis.[162]

The Sirolimus-eluting Stent Versus Vascular Brachytherapy for In-Stent Restenosis (SISR) and TAXUS V ISR studies were randomized clinical trials that directly compared the safety and efficacy of brachytherapy and DES for the treatment of BMS ISR.[163-166] TAXUS V ISR randomly assigned 396 patients with ischemic symptoms and ISR lesions in native coronary arteries to treatment with brachytherapy or PES. Quantitative coronary angiography at 9 months demonstrated significantly greater late luminal loss, smaller minimal lumen diameter, and higher binary restenosis rates with brachytherapy compared with PES.[166] At 2-year follow-up, clinical restenosis was significantly reduced with PES, although the rates of death, myocardial infarction, and target vessel thrombosis were similar between treatments.[163] The SISR trial randomly assigned 384 patients with ischemic symptoms and BMS ISR to either brachytherapy or PCI with SES. SES treatment resulted in superior 6-month angiographic and 9-month clinical outcomes compared with brachytherapy (minimal lumen diameter, 1.80 vs. 1.52 mm, P < .001; target vessel failure, 21.6% vs. 12.4%, P = .02).[164] At 5-year follow-up, there were no significant differences in safety or efficacy outcomes between the two treatment strategies.[167] Despite the similar safety and efficacy of these two approaches, the ease of use of DES, combined with the unfavorable procedural logistics with brachytherapy such as the need for expensive equipment and the complexity of the procedure, has contributed to the decreased use of brachytherapy for this indication.

Treatment of Drug-Eluting Stent Restenosis

The optimal treatment for DES restenosis is uncertain. Potential options include conventional, cutting, scoring, or drug-eluting balloon angioplasty; BMS implantation; DES implantation (of the same or different type); vascular brachytherapy; and bypass surgery. However, the variable causes of DES restenosis pose difficulty in determining the optimal treatment strategy. A few randomized trials and a series of observational studies have been performed to evaluate clinical and angiographic outcomes after PCI for DES restenosis. Most of these studies enrolled small numbers of patients, used a wide variety of treatment modalities, and reported inconsistent findings, hindering any definitive conclusion about the best treatment approach.*

DES implantation is currently the most common treatment modality for DES restenosis because of its superior performance in clinical trials for de novo lesions and its ease of use.[175] Several observational studies have reported clinical outcomes of repeat DES placement compared with other therapies for the treatment of DES restenosis. Kim and associates[181] reported that repeat SES implantation significantly reduced 6-month restenosis rates compared with conventional treatment (4% in the SES group vs. 35% in the cutting balloon angioplasty or brachytherapy group). Mishkel and colleagues[184] observed that in 108 patients with SES or PES failure, the 1-year TLR rate was lowest when using a different DES compared with the same DES or conventional treatment with cutting balloon angioplasty, BMS, or brachytherapy (19%, 29%, and 37%, respectively). In a small randomized trial of patients with SES or PES failure, retreatment with SES had a trend toward lower TLR compared with stand-alone balloon angioplasty (5.9% vs. 13.1%, P = not significant [NS]).[191] Use of IVUS or optical coherence tomography to identify the pattern and underlying mechanism of ISR may be helpful in selecting the appropriate treatment modality.[192]

Same Drug-Eluting Stent or Different Drug-Eluting Stent

One possible cause of DES restenosis is drug resistance. Placing a stent that elutes a different drug may be more effective than a stent that elutes the originally used drug. The Intracoronary Stenting and Angiographic Results: Drug Eluting Stents for In-Stent Restenosis 2 (ISAR-DESIRE 2) trial randomly assigned 450 patients with SES restenosis to treatment with the same or different DES.[174] No significant differences between groups were observed with respect to in-stent late luminal loss at angiographic follow-up at 6 to 8 months or in the 1-year clinical endpoints of TLR, death or myocardial infarction, and stent thrombosis.

Vascular Brachytherapy

The use of brachytherapy for the treatment of DES restenosis has been investigated in observational studies.[186,187] In a retrospective study, 61 patients treated with brachytherapy for DES failure had similar rates of TVR but a significantly lower rate of MACE at 8 months compared with a consecutive series of 50 patients treated with repeat DES (9.8% vs. 24%, P = .044).[186] Bonello and colleagues[187] reported a TLR rate of 11% and a MACE rate of 26% at 1 year in 99 patients with DES failure who were treated with brachytherapy.

Drug-Eluting Balloon Catheters

Drug-coated balloon catheters may be an alternative option for the treatment of ISR. Initial clinical trials demonstrated the efficacy of a balloon coated with a paclitaxel-iopromide mixture in inhibiting restenosis. In the Treatment of In-Stent Restenosis by Paclitaxel Coated PTCA Balloons (PACCOCATH-ISR) trial, 52 patients were randomly assigned to paclitaxel-coated or uncoated balloon treatment of ISR. The paclitaxel-coated balloon significantly reduced the incidence of angiographic and clinical repeat restenosis.[193] The Paclitaxel Eluting PTCA Balloon in Coronary Artery Disease II (PEPCAD II) trial randomly assigned 131 patients to receive the second-generation paclitaxel-eluting balloon catheter SeQuent Please (B. Braun, Melsungen, Germany) or the Taxus Liberté PES for the treatment of BMS ISR.[194] Compared with PES, the drug-eluting balloon was associated with significantly reduced in-segment late luminal loss and binary restenosis at 6 months (7% vs. 20%) and reduced MACEs at 12 months (9% vs. 22%), mainly driven by reduced TLR. The PEPCAD DES trial randomly assigned 110 patients with DES restenosis to paclitaxel-coated balloon angioplasty or uncoated balloon angioplasty. The average lesion length was approximately 11.4 mm, and approximately two thirds of the target lesions were focal restenoses according to the Mehran criteria. At 6-month follow-up, paclitaxel-coated balloon angioplasty was superior to uncoated balloon angioplasty with respect to late lumen loss (0.43 ± 0.61 mm vs. 1.03 ± 0.77 mm, P < .001); binary angiographic

---

*References 71, 106, 160, 169, 170, 172, 173, 175, 190.

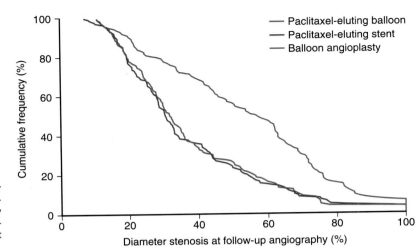

Figure 8-3 Cumulative frequency distribution curves for diameter stenosis by treatment group at 6- to 8-month angiographic follow-up in the ISAR-DESIRE 3 trial. Angioplasty with a paclitaxel-eluting balloon was non-inferior to paclitaxel-eltuing stent implantation in patients with drug-eluting stent restenosis.

restenosis (17.2% vs. 58.1%, $P < .001$); and the clinical endpoint of cardiac death, myocardial infarction, or TVR (16.7% vs. 50.0%, $P < .001$).[195]

The Intracoronary Stenting and Angiographic Results: Drug-Eluting Stent In-Stent Restenosis 3 Treatment Approaches (ISAR-DESIRE 3) trial[196] randomly allocated 402 patients with restenosis of a limus-eluting stent to treatment with the Sequent Please paclitaxel-eluting balloon, PES implantation, or standard balloon angioplasty. The primary endpoint was diameter stenosis at follow-up angiography at 6 to 8 months (Figure 8-3). Both the paclitaxel-eluting balloon and PES were superior to standard balloon angioplasty, and the paclitaxel-eluting balloon was non-inferior to PES. Late luminal loss was similar with the paclitaxel-eluting balloon and PES (0.37 +/− 0.59 mm and 0.34 +/− 0.61 mm). Rates of death, myocardial infarction, or target lesion thrombosis did not differ between treatment groups.

Conclusion

DES are superior to BMS because they reduce the risk of restenosis across all coronary lesions and patient subsets. Several randomized trials have reported binary restenosis rates after DES implantation of less than 10%. However, the rate of restenosis increases when treating complex lesions. Next-generation DES show promise for further decreasing the occurrence of restenosis after PCI through the use of novel antiproliferative drugs, improved stent platforms with thinner stent struts, more favorable stent geometries, better biocompatible or biodegradable polymers, and nonpolymeric DES surfaces. For BMS ISR, the treatment of choice is DES. However, the optimal therapeutic approach for DES restenosis is less clear. Further studies are warranted to understand better the pathology of ISR after newer generation DES implantation and to establish the optimal strategies for prevention and treatment of ISR.

REFERENCES

1. Serruys PW, de Jaegere P, Kiemeneij F, et al. A comparison of balloon-expandable-stent implantation with balloon angioplasty in patients with coronary artery disease. Benestent Study Group. *N Engl J Med* 1994;331:489-495.
2. Fischman DL, Leon MB, Baim DS, et al. A randomized comparison of coronary-stent placement and balloon angioplasty in the treatment of coronary artery disease. Stent Restenosis Study Investigators. *N Engl J Med* 1994;331:496-501.
3. Stone GW, Ellis SG, Cox DA, et al. One-year clinical results with the slow-release, polymer-based, paclitaxel-eluting TAXUS stent: the TAXUS-IV trial. *Circulation* 2004;109:1942-1947.
4. Moses JW, Leon MB, Popma JJ, et al. Sirolimus-eluting stents versus standard stents in patients with stenosis in a native coronary artery. *N Engl J Med* 2003;349:1315-1323.
5. Cutlip DE, Chauhan MS, Baim DS, et al. Clinical restenosis after coronary stenting: perspectives from multicenter clinical trials. *J Am Coll Cardiol* 2002;40:2082-2089.
6. Cutlip DE, Windecker S, Mehran R, et al. Clinical end points in coronary stent trials: a case for standardized definitions. *Circulation* 2007;115:2344-2351.
7. Hoffmann R, Mintz GS, Dussaillant GR, et al. Patterns and mechanisms of in-stent restenosis: a serial intravascular ultrasound study. *Circulation* 1996;94:1247-1254.
8. Farb A, Sangiorgi G, Carter AJ, et al. Pathology of acute and chronic coronary stenting in humans. *Circulation* 1999;99:44-52.
9. Kastrati A, Schomig A, Dietz R, et al. Time course of restenosis during the first year after emergency coronary stenting. *Circulation* 1993;87:1498-1505.
10. Barlis P, Regar E, Serruys PW, et al. An optical coherence tomography study of a biodegradable vs. durable polymer-coated limus-eluting stent: a LEADERS trial sub-study. *Eur Heart J* 2010;31:165-176.
11. Mintz GS, Popma JJ, Pichard AD, et al. Arterial remodeling after coronary angioplasty: a serial intravascular ultrasound study. *Circulation* 1996;94:35-43.
12. Mitra AK, Agrawal DK. In stent restenosis: bane of the stent era. *J Clin Pathol* 2006;59:232-239.
13. Virmani R, Kolodgie FD, Farb A, et al. Drug eluting stents: are human and animal studies comparable? *Heart* 2003;89:133-138.
14. Dzavik V. New frontiers and unresolved controversies in percutaneous coronary intervention. *Am J Cardiol* 2003;91:27A-33A.
15. Komatsu R, Ueda M, Naruko T, et al. Neointimal tissue response at sites of coronary stenting in humans: macroscopic, histological, and immunohistochemical analyses. *Circulation* 1998;98:224-233.
16. Isner JM, Kearney M, Bortman S, et al. Apoptosis in human atherosclerosis and restenosis. *Circulation* 1995;91:2703-2711.
17. Schwartz RS, Holmes Jr DR, Topol EJ. The restenosis paradigm revisited: an alternative proposal for cellular mechanisms. *J Am Coll Cardiol* 1992;20:1284-1293.
18. O'Sullivan JF, Martin K, Caplice NM. Microribonucleic acids for prevention of plaque rupture and in-stent restenosis: "a finger in the dam." *J Am Coll Cardiol* 2011;57:383-389.
19. Costa MA, Simon DI. Molecular basis of restenosis and drug-eluting stents. *Circulation* 2005;111:2257-2273.
20. Topol EJ, Serruys PW. Frontiers in interventional cardiology. *Circulation* 1998;98:1802-1820.
21. Lincoff AM, Topol EJ, Ellis SG. Local drug delivery for the prevention of restenosis: fact, fancy, and future. *Circulation* 1994;90:2070-2084.
22. Alvarado Y, Mita MM, Vemulapalli S, et al. Clinical activity of mammalian target of rapamycin inhibitors in solid tumors. *Targeted Oncol* 2011;6:69-94.
23. Yusuf RZ, Duan Z, Lamendola DE, et al. Paclitaxel resistance: molecular mechanisms and pharmacologic manipulation. *Curr Cancer Drug Targets* 2003;3:1-19.
24. Huang S, Houghton PJ. Mechanisms of resistance to rapamycins. *Drug Resist Updat* 2001;4:378-391.
25. Koster R, Vieluf D, Kiehn M, et al. Nickel and molybdenum contact allergies in patients with coronary in-stent restenosis. *Lancet* 2000;356:1895-1897.
26. Nebeker JR, Virmani R, Bennett CL, et al. Hypersensitivity cases associated with drug-eluting coronary stents: a review of available cases from the Research on Adverse Drug Events and Reports (RADAR) project. *J Am Coll Cardiol* 2006;47:175-181.

27. Mintz GS. Features and parameters of drug-eluting stent deployment discoverable by intravascular ultrasound. *Am J Cardiol* 2007;100:26M-35M.
28. Fujii K, Mintz GS, Kobayashi Y, et al. Contribution of stent underexpansion to recurrence after sirolimus-eluting stent implantation for in-stent restenosis. *Circulation* 2004;109: 1085-1088.
29. de Jaegere P, Mudra H, Figulla H, et al. Intravascular ultrasound-guided optimized stent deployment: immediate and 6 months clinical and angiographic results from the Multicenter Ultrasound Stenting in Coronaries Study (MUSIC Study). *Eur Heart J* 1998;19:1214-1223.
30. Cook S, Wenaweser P, Togni M, et al. Incomplete stent apposition and very late stent thrombosis after drug-eluting stent implantation. *Circulation* 2007;115:2426-2434.
31. Balakrishnan B, Tzafriri AR, Seifert P, et al. Strut position, blood flow, and drug deposition: implications for single and overlapping drug-eluting stents. *Circulation* 2005;111: 2958-2965.
32. Hwang CW, Levin AD, Jonas M, et al. Thrombosis modulates arterial drug distribution for drug-eluting stents. *Circulation* 2005;111:1619-1626.
33. Doi H, Maehara A, Mintz GS, et al. Classification and potential mechanisms of intravascular ultrasound patterns of stent fracture. *Am J Cardiol* 2009;103:818-823.
34. Chakravarty T, White AJ, Buch M, et al. Meta-analysis of incidence, clinical characteristics and implications of stent fracture. *Am J Cardiol* 2010;106:1075-1080.
35. Aoki J, Nakazawa G, Tanabe K, et al. Incidence and clinical impact of coronary stent fracture after sirolimus-eluting stent implantation. *Catheter Cardiovasc Interv* 2007;69:380-386.
36. Lee MS, Jurewitz D, Aragon J, et al. Stent fracture associated with drug-eluting stents: clinical characteristics and implications. *Catheter Cardiovasc Interv* 2007;69:387-394.
37. Umeda H, Gochi T, Iwase M, et al. Frequency, predictors and outcome of stent fracture after sirolimus-eluting stent implantation. *Int J Cardiol* 2009;133:321-326.
38. Park SM, Kim JY, Hong BK, et al. Predictors of stent fracture in patients treated with closed-cell design stents: sirolimus-eluting stent and its bare-metal counterpart, the BX velocity stent. *Coron Artery Dis* 2011;22:40-44.
39. Nakazawa G, Finn AV, Vorpahl M, et al. Incidence and predictors of drug-eluting stent fracture in human coronary artery a pathologic analysis. *J Am Coll Cardiol* 2009;54: 1924-1931.
40. Cha IH, Kim SH, Lim SY, et al. A case of a zotarolimus-eluting stent fracture in the left anterior descending artery in a patient undergoing hemodialysis. *Chonnam Med J* 2011;47: 57-59.
41. Costa MA, Angiolillo DJ, Tannenbaum M, et al. Impact of stent deployment procedural factors on long-term effectiveness and safety of sirolimus-eluting stents (final results of the multicenter prospective STLLR trial). *Am J Cardiol* 2008;101: 1704-1711.
42. Schampaert E, Cohen EA, Schluter M, et al. The Canadian study of the sirolimus-eluting stent in the treatment of patients with long de novo lesions in small native coronary arteries (C-SIRIUS). *J Am Coll Cardiol* 2004;43:1110-1115.
43. Schofer J, Schluter M, Gershlick AH, et al. Sirolimus-eluting stents for treatment of patients with long atherosclerotic lesions in small coronary arteries: double-blind, randomised controlled trial (E-SIRIUS). *Lancet* 2003;362:1093-1099.
44. Barbato E, Marco J, Wijns W. Direct stenting. *Eur Heart J* 2003;24:394-403.
45. Kereiakes DJ, Wang H, Popma JJ, et al. Periprocedural and late consequences of overlapping Cypher sirolimus-eluting stents: pooled analysis of five clinical trials. *J Am Coll Cardiol* 2006;48:21-31.
46. Tahara S, Bezerra HG, Sirbu V, et al. Angiographic, IVUS and OCT evaluation of the long-term impact of coronary disease severity at the site of overlapping drug-eluting and bare-metal stents: a substudy of the ODESSA trial. *Heart* 2010;96: 1574-1578.
47. Kastrati A, Mehilli J, Dirschinger J, et al. Intracoronary stenting and angiographic results: strut thickness effect on restenosis outcome (ISAR-STEREO) trial. *Circulation* 2001; 103:2816-2821.
48. Pache J, Kastrati A, Mehilli J, et al. Intracoronary stenting and angiographic results: strut thickness effect on restenosis outcome (ISAR-STEREO-2) trial. *J Am Coll Cardiol* 2003;41: 1283-1288.
49. Morton AC, Crossman D, Gunn J. The influence of physical stent parameters upon restenosis. *Pathol Biol* 2004;52: 196-205.
50. Kastrati A, Mehilli J, Dirschinger J, et al. Restenosis after coronary placement of various stent types. *Am J Cardiol* 2001;87: 34-39.
51. Trikalinos TA, Alsheikh-Ali AA, Tatsioni A, et al. Percutaneous coronary interventions for non-acute coronary artery disease: a quantitative 20-year synopsis and a network meta-analysis. *Lancet* 2009;373:911-918.
52. Pache J, Dibra A, Mehilli J, et al. Drug-eluting stents compared with thin-strut bare stents for the reduction of restenosis: a prospective, randomized trial. *Eur Heart J* 2005;26:1262-1268.
53. Stone GW, Ellis SG, Cox DA, et al. A polymer-based, paclitaxel-eluting stent in patients with coronary artery disease. *N Engl J Med* 2004;350:221-231.
54. Garg S, Serruys PW. Coronary stents: current status. *J Am Coll Cardiol* 2010;56(10 Suppl):S1-42.
55. Fajadet J, Wijns W, Laarman GJ, et al. Randomized, double-blind, multicenter study of the Endeavor zotarolimus-eluting phosphorylcholine-encapsulated stent for treatment of native coronary artery lesions: clinical and angiographic results of the ENDEAVOR II trial. *Circulation* 2006;114:798-806.
56. Kandzari DE, Leon MB, Popma JJ, et al. Comparison of zotarolimus-eluting and sirolimus-eluting stents in patients with native coronary artery disease: a randomized controlled trial. *J Am Coll Cardiol* 2006;48:2440-2447.
57. Leon MB, Mauri L, Popma JJ, et al. A randomized comparison of the ENDEAVOR zotarolimus-eluting stent versus the TAXUS paclitaxel-eluting stent in de novo native coronary lesions 12-month outcomes from the ENDEAVOR IV trial. *J Am Coll Cardiol* 2010;55:543-554.
58. Leon MB, Nikolsky E, Cutlip DE, et al. Improved late clinical safety with zotarolimus-eluting stents compared with paclitaxel-eluting stents in patients with de novo coronary lesions: 3-year follow-up from the ENDEAVOR IV (Randomized Comparison of Zotarolimus- and Paclitaxel-Eluting Stents in Patients With Coronary Artery Disease) trial. *JACC Cardiovasc Interv* 2010;3:1043-1050.
59. Kandzari DE, Mauri L, Popma JJ, et al. Late-term clinical outcomes with zotarolimus- and sirolimus-eluting stents: 5-year follow-up of the ENDEAVOR III (A Randomized Controlled Trial of the Medtronic Endeavor Drug [ABT-578] Eluting Coronary Stent System Versus the Cypher Sirolimus-Eluting Coronary Stent System in De Novo Native Coronary Artery Lesions). *JACC Cardiovasc Interv* 2011;4:543-550.
60. Stone GW, Rizvi A, Newman W, et al. Everolimus-eluting versus paclitaxel-eluting stents in coronary artery disease. *N Engl J Med* 2010;362:1663-1674.
61. Kedhi E, Joesoef KS, McFadden E, et al. Second-generation everolimus-eluting and paclitaxel-eluting stents in real-life practice (COMPARE): a randomised trial. *Lancet* 2010;375: 201-209.
62. Baber U, Mehran R, Sharma SK, et al. Impact of the everolimus-eluting stent on stent thrombosis: a meta-analysis of 13 randomized trials. *J Am Coll Cardiol* 2011;58:1569-1577.
63. van't Hof AW, de Boer MJ, Suryapranata H, et al. Incidence and predictors of restenosis after successful primary coronary angioplasty for acute myocardial infarction: the importance of age and procedural result. *Am Heart J* 1998;136:518-527.
64. Goldberg SL, Loussararian A, De Gregorio J, et al. Predictors of diffuse and aggressive intra-stent restenosis. *J Am Coll Cardiol* 2001;37:1019-1025.
65. Berenguer A, Mainar V, Bordes P, et al. Incidence and predictors of restenosis after sirolimus-eluting stent implantation in high-risk patients. *Am Heart J* 2005;150:536-542.
66. Alfonso F, Hernandez R, Banuelos C, et al. Initial results and long-term clinical and angiographic outcome of coronary stenting in women. *Am J Cardiol* 2000;86:1380-1383, A5.
67. Mehilli J, Kastrati A, Bollwein H, et al. Gender and restenosis after coronary artery stenting. *Eur Heart J* 2003;24: 1523-1530.
68. Kuchulakanti PK, Torguson R, Canos D, et al. Impact of treatment of coronary artery disease with sirolimus-eluting stents on outcomes of diabetic and nondiabetic patients. *Am J Cardiol* 2005;96:1100-1106.
69. Lemos PA, Hoye A, Goedhart D, et al. Clinical, angiographic, and procedural predictors of angiographic restenosis after sirolimus-eluting stent implantation in complex patients: an evaluation from the Rapamycin-Eluting Stent Evaluated At Rotterdam Cardiology Hospital (RESEARCH) study. *Circulation* 2004;109:1366-1370.
70. Moussa I, Leon MB, Baim DS, et al. Impact of sirolimus-eluting stents on outcome in diabetic patients: a SIRIUS (SIRolImUS-coated Bx Velocity balloon-expandable stent in the treatment of patients with de novo coronary artery lesions) substudy. *Circulation* 2004;109:2273-2278.
71. Rathore S, Kinoshita Y, Terashima M, et al. A comparison of clinical presentations, angiographic patterns and outcomes of in-stent restenosis between bare-metal stents and drug eluting stents. *EuroIntervention* 2010;5:841-846.
72. Sangiorgi G, Romagnoli E, Biondi-Zoccai G, et al. Percutaneous coronary implantation of sirolimus-eluting stents in unselected patients and lesions: clinical results and multiple outcome predictors. *Am Heart J* 2008;156:871-878.
73. Lee CW, Park DW, Lee BK, et al. Predictors of restenosis after placement of drug-eluting stents in one or more coronary arteries. *Am J Cardiol* 2006;97:506-511.
74. Roy P, Okabe T, Pinto Slottow TL, et al. Correlates of clinical restenosis following intracoronary implantation of drug-eluting stents. *Am J Cardiol* 2007;100:965-969.
75. Hermiller JB, Raizner A, Cannon L, et al. Outcomes with the polymer-based paclitaxel-eluting TAXUS stent in patients with diabetes mellitus: the TAXUS-IV trial. *J Am Coll Cardiol* 2005;45:1172-1179.
76. Kastrati A, Dibra A, Mehilli J, et al. Predictive factors of restenosis after coronary implantation of sirolimus- or paclitaxel-eluting stents. *Circulation* 2006;113:2293-2300.
77. Abizaid A, Kornowski R, Mintz GS, et al. The influence of diabetes mellitus on acute and late clinical outcomes following coronary stent implantation. *J Am Coll Cardiol* 1998;32: 584-589.
78. Mittal S, Weiss DL, Hirshfeld Jr JW, et al. Comparison of outcome after stenting for de novo versus restenotic narrowings in native coronary arteries. *Am J Cardiol* 1997;80: 711-715.
79. Elezi S, Kastrati A, Pache J, et al. Diabetes mellitus and the clinical and angiographic outcome after coronary stent placement. *J Am Coll Cardiol* 1998;32:1866-1873.
80. Singh M, Gersh BJ, McClelland RL, et al. Clinical and angiographic predictors of restenosis after percutaneous coronary intervention: insights from the Prevention of Restenosis With Tranilast and Its Outcomes (PRESTO) trial. *Circulation* 2004;109:2727-2731.
81. Patti G, Nusca A, Di Sciascio G. Meta-analysis comparison (nine trials) of outcomes with drug-eluting stents versus bare-metal stents in patients with diabetes mellitus. *Am J Cardiol* 2008;102:1328-1334.
82. Frobert O, Lagerqvist B, Carlsson J, et al. Differences in restenosis rate with different drug-eluting stents in patients with and without diabetes mellitus: a report from the SCAAR (Swedish Angiography and Angioplasty Registry). *J Am Coll Cardiol* 2009;53:1660-1667.
83. Halkin A, Selzer F, Marroquin O, et al. Clinical outcomes following percutaneous coronary intervention with drug-eluting vs. bare-metal stents in dialysis patients. *J Invas Cardiol* 2006;18:577-583.
84. Hassani SE, Chu WW, Wolfram RM, et al. Clinical outcomes after percutaneous coronary intervention with drug-eluting stents in dialysis patients. *J Invas Cardiol* 2006;18:273-277.
85. Elezi S, Kastrati A, Neumann FJ, et al. Vessel size and long-term outcome after coronary stent placement. *Circulation* 1998;98: 1875-1880.
86. Serruys PW, Kay IP, Disco C, et al. Periprocedural quantitative coronary angiography after Palmaz-Schatz stent implantation predicts the restenosis rate at six months: results of a meta-analysis of the BElgian NEtherlands Stent study (BENESTENT) I, BENESTENT II Pilot, BENESTENT II and MUSIC trials. Multicenter Ultrasound Stent In Coronaries. *J Am Coll Cardiol* 1999;34:1067-1074.
87. Kobayashi Y, De Gregorio J, Kobayashi N, et al. Stented segment length as an independent predictor of restenosis. *J Am Coll Cardiol* 1999;34:651-659.
88. Kasaoka S, Tobis JM, Akiyama T, et al. Angiographic and intravascular ultrasound predictors of in-stent restenosis. *J Am Coll Cardiol* 1998;32:1630-1635.
89. Mercado N, Boersma E, Wijns W, et al. Clinical and quantitative coronary angiographic predictors of coronary restenosis: a comparative analysis from the balloon-to-stent era. *J Am Coll Cardiol* 2001;38:645-652.
90. Kastrati A, Schomig A, Elezi S, et al. Predictive factors of restenosis after coronary stent placement. *J Am Coll Cardiol* 1997;30:1428-1436.
91. Castagna MT, Mintz GS, Leiboff BO, et al. The contribution of "mechanical" problems to in-stent restenosis: an intravascular ultrasonographic analysis of 1090 consecutive in-stent restenosis lesions. *Am Heart J* 2001;142:970-974.
92. Doi H, Maehara A, Mintz GS, et al. Impact of post-intervention minimal stent area on 9-month follow-up patency of paclitaxel-eluting stents: an integrated intravascular ultrasound analysis from the TAXUS IV, V, and VI and TAXUS ATLAS Workhorse, Long Lesion, and Direct Stent Trials. *JACC Cardiovasc Interv* 2009;2:1269-1275.
93. Honda Y, Fitzgerald PJ, Yock PG. Intravascular ultrasound. 5th edition ed. In: Topol EJ, ed. *Textbook of Interventional Cardiology*. 5th ed. Philadelphia: Saunders; 2007.
94. Lemos PA, Saia F, Ligthart JM, et al. Coronary restenosis after sirolimus-eluting stent implantation: morphological description and mechanistic analysis from a consecutive series of cases. *Circulation* 2003;108:257-260.
95. Mata LA, Bosch X, David PR, et al. Clinical and angiographic assessment 6 months after double vessel percutaneous coronary angioplasty. *J Am Coll Cardiol* 1985;6:1239-1244.
96. Serruys PW, Strauss BH, Beatt KJ, et al. Angiographic follow-up after placement of a self-expanding coronary-artery stent. *N Engl J Med* 1991;324:13-17.
97. Gruentzig AR, King 3rd SB, Schlumpf M, et al. Long-term follow-up after percutaneous transluminal coronary angioplasty: the early Zurich experience. *N Engl J Med* 1987;316: 1127-1132.
98. Chen MS, John JM, Chew DP, et al. Bare-metal stent restenosis is not a benign clinical entity. *Am Heart J* 2006;151: 1260-1264.
99. Walters DL, Harding SA, Walsh CR, et al. Acute coronary syndrome is a common clinical presentation of in-stent restenosis. *Am J Cardiol* 2002;89:491-494.
100. Bossi I, Klersy C, Black AJ, et al. In-stent restenosis: long-term outcome and predictors of subsequent target lesion revascularization after repeat balloon angioplasty. *J Am Coll Cardiol* 2000;35:1569-1576.
101. Bainey KR, Norris CM, Graham MM, et al. Clinical in-stent restenosis with bare-metal stents: is it truly a benign phenomenon? *Int J Cardiol* 2008;128:378-382.
102. Pate GE, Lee M, Humphries K, et al. Characterizing the spectrum of in-stent restenosis: implications for contemporary treatment. *Can J Cardiol* 2006;22:1223-1229.
103. Steinberg DH, Pinto Slottow TL, Buch AN, et al. Impact of in-stent restenosis on death and myocardial infarction. *Am J Cardiol* 2007;100:1109-1113.

104. Assali AR, Moustapha A, Sdringola S, et al. Acute coronary syndrome may occur with in-stent restenosis and is associated with adverse outcomes (the PRESTO trial). *Am J Cardiol* 2006;98:729-733.
105. De Labriolle A, Bonello L, Lemesle G, et al. Clinical presentation and outcome of patients hospitalized for symptomatic in-stent restenosis treated by percutaneous coronary intervention: comparison between drug-eluting stents and bare-metal stents. *Arch Cardiovasc Dis* 2009;102:209-217.
106. Park CB, Hong MK, Kim YH, et al. Comparison of angiographic patterns of in-stent restenosis between sirolimus- and paclitaxel-eluting stent. *Int J Cardiol* 2007;120:387-390.
107. Appleby CE, Khattar RS, Morgan K, et al. Drug eluting stents for the treatment of bare-metal in-stent restenosis: long-term outcomes in real world practice. *EuroIntervention* 2011;6: 748-753.
108. Latib A, Mussardo M, Ielasi A, et al. Long-term outcomes after the percutaneous treatment of drug-eluting stent restenosis. *JACC Cardiovasc Interv* 2011;4:155-164.
109. Lee MS, Pessegueiro A, Zimmer R, et al. Clinical presentation of patients with in-stent restenosis in the drug-eluting stent era. *J Invas Cardiol* 2008;20:401-403.
110. Sharma SK, Duvvuri S, Dangas G, et al. Rotational atherectomy for in-stent restenosis: acute and long-term results of the first 100 cases. *J Am Coll Cardiol* 1998;32:1358-1365.
111. Aoki J, Colombo A, Dudek D, et al. Peristent remodeling and neointimal suppression 2 years after polymer-based, paclitaxel-eluting stent implantation: insights from serial intravascular ultrasound analysis in the TAXUS II study. *Circulation* 2005; 112:3876-3883.
112. Aoki J, Abizaid AC, Serruys PW, et al. Evaluation of four-year coronary artery response after sirolimus-eluting stent implantation using serial quantitative intravascular ultrasound and computer-assisted grayscale value analysis for plaque composition in event-free patients. *J Am Coll Cardiol* 2005;46: 1670-1676.
113. Claessen BE, Beijk MA, Legrand V, et al. Two-year clinical, angiographic, and intravascular ultrasound follow-up of the XIENCE V everolimus-eluting stent in the treatment of patients with de novo native coronary artery lesions: the SPIRIT II trial. *Circ Cardiovas Interv* 2009;2:339-347.
114. Schroeder S, Achenbach S, Bengel F, et al. Cardiac computed tomography: indications, applications, limitations, and training requirements: report of a Writing Group deployed by the Working Group Nuclear Cardiology and Cardiac CT of the European Society of Cardiology and the European Council of Nuclear Cardiology. *Eur Heart J* 2008; 29:531-556.
115. Andreini D, Pontone G, Mushtaq S, et al. Multidetector computed tomography coronary angiography for the assessment of coronary in-stent restenosis. *Am J Cardiol* 2010;105: 645-655.
116. Sun Z, Jiang W. Diagnostic value of multislice computed tomography angiography in coronary artery disease: a meta-analysis. *Eur J Radiol* 2006;60:279-286.
117. Schuijf JD, Pundziute G, Jukema JW, et al. Evaluation of patients with previous coronary stent implantation with 64-section CT. *Radiology* 2007;245:416-423.
118. Haraldsdottir S, Gudnason T, Sigurdsson AF, et al. Diagnostic accuracy of 64-slice multidetector CT for detection of in-stent restenosis in an unselected, consecutive patient population. *Eur J Radiol* 2010;76:188-194.
119. Oncel D, Oncel G, Tastan A, et al. Evaluation of coronary stent patency and in-stent restenosis with dual-source CT coronary angiography without heart rate control. *AJR Am J Roentgenol* 2008;191:56-63.
120. Alfonso F, Perez-Vizcayno MJ, Hernandez R, et al. A randomized comparison of sirolimus-eluting stent with balloon angioplasty in patients with in-stent restenosis: results of the Restenosis Intrastent: Balloon Angioplasty Versus Elective Sirolimus-Eluting Stenting (RIBS-II) trial. *J Am Coll Cardiol* 2006;47:2152-2160.
121. Alfonso F, Suarez A, Perez L, et al. Intravascular ultrasound in patients with challenging in-stent restenosis: importance of precise stent visualization. *J Interv Cardiol* 2006;19:153-159.
122. Alfonso F, Goicolea J, Hernandez R, et al. Restenosis after coronary stenting presenting a "double lumen" morphology: value of intravascular ultrasound to recognize the true lumen and guide coronary intervention. *J Invas Cardiol* 1998;10: 177-180.
123. Barlis P, Schmitt JM. Current and future developments in intracoronary optical coherence tomography imaging. *EuroIntervention* 2009;4:529-533.
124. Brezinski ME, Tearney GJ, Weissman NJ, et al. Assessing atherosclerotic plaque morphology: comparison of optical coherence tomography and high frequency intravascular ultrasound. *Heart* 1997;77:397-403.
125. Lopez-Palop R, Pinar E, Lozano I, et al. Utility of the fractional flow reserve in the evaluation of angiographically moderate in-stent restenosis. *Eur Heart J* 2004;25:2040-2047.
126. Bech GJ, De Bruyne B, Pijls NH, et al. Fractional flow reserve to determine the appropriateness of angioplasty in moderate coronary stenosis: a randomized trial. *Circulation* 2001;103: 2928-2934.
127. Pijls NH, De Bruyne B, Peels K, et al. Measurement of fractional flow reserve to assess the functional severity of coronary-artery stenoses. *N Engl J Med* 1996;334:1703-1708.
128. Kruger S, Koch KC, Kaumanns I, et al. Use of fractional flow reserve versus stress perfusion scintigraphy in stent restenosis. *Eur J Intern Med* 2005;16:429-431.
129. Alfonso F, Perez-Vizcayno MJ, Hernandez R, et al. Long-term outcome and determinants of event-free survival in patients treated with balloon angioplasty for in-stent restenosis. *Am J Cardiol* 1999;83:1268-1270.
130. Mehran R, Dangas G, Abizaid AS, et al. Angiographic patterns of in-stent restenosis: classification and implications for long-term outcome. *Circulation* 1999;100:1872-1878.
131. Alfonso F, Cequier A, Angel J, et al. Value of the American College of Cardiology/American Heart Association angiographic classification of coronary lesion morphology in patients with in-stent restenosis: insights from the Restenosis Intra-stent Balloon angioplasty versus elective Stenting (RIBS) randomized trial. *Am Heart J* 2006;151:681e1-681e9.
132. Colombo A, Orlic D, Stankovic G, et al. Preliminary observations regarding angiographic pattern of restenosis after rapamycin-eluting stent implantation. *Circulation* 2003;107: 2178-2180.
133. Popma JJ, Leon MB, Moses JW, et al. Quantitative assessment of angiographic restenosis after sirolimus-eluting stent implantation in native coronary arteries. *Circulation* 2004;110: 3773-3780.
134. Iakovou I, Schmidt T, Ge L, et al. Angiographic patterns of restenosis after paclitaxel-eluting stent implantation. *J Am Coll Cardiol* 2005;45:805-806.
135. Corbett SJ, Cosgrave J, Melzi G, et al. Patterns of restenosis after drug-eluting stent implantation: insights from a contemporary and comparative analysis of sirolimus- and paclitaxel-eluting stents. *Eur Heart J* 2006;27:2330-2337.
136. Kitahara H, Kobayashi Y, Takebayashi H, et al. Angiographic patterns of restenosis after sirolimus-eluting stent implantation. *Circ J* 2009;73:508-511.
137. Lee MS, Yang T, Lasala JM, et al. Two-year clinical outcomes of paclitaxel-eluting stents for in-stent restenosis in patients from the ARRIVE programme. *EuroIntervention* 2011;7: 314-322.
138. Lasala JM, Cox DA, Lewis SJ, et al. Expanded use of the TAXUS Express stent: two-year safety insights from the 7,500 patient ARRIVE Registry programme. *EuroIntervention* 2009; 5:67-77.
139. Applegate RJ, Sacrinty MT, Kutcher MA, et al. "Off-label" stent therapy 2-year comparison of drug-eluting versus bare-metal stents. *J Am Coll Cardiol* 2008;51:607-614.
140. Hernandez RA, Macaya C, Iniguez A, et al. Midterm outcome of patients with asymptomatic restenosis after coronary balloon angioplasty. *J Am Coll Cardiol* 1992;19:1402-1409.
141. Kimura T, Yokoi H, Nakagawa Y, et al. Three-year follow-up after implantation of metallic coronary-artery stents. *N Engl J Med* 1996;334:561-566.
142. Alcocer A, Moreno R, Hernandez R, et al. Clinical variables related with in-stent restenosis late regression after bare-metal coronary stenting. *Arch Cardiol Mexico* 2006;76: 390-396.
143. Ishiwata S, Verheye S, Robinson KA, et al. Inhibition of neointima formation by tranilast in pig coronary arteries after balloon angioplasty and stent implantation. *J Am Coll Cardiol* 2000;35:1331-1337.
144. Holmes Jr DR, Savage M, LaBlanche JM, et al. Results of Prevention of REStenosis with Tranilast and its Outcomes (PRESTO) trial. *Circulation* 2002;106:1243-1250.
145. Peters S, Gotting B, Trummel M, et al. Valsartan for prevention of restenosis after stenting of type B2/C lesions: the VAL-PREST trial. *J Invas Cardiol* 2001;13:93-97.
146. Walter DH, Schachinger V, Elsner M, et al. Effect of statin therapy on restenosis after coronary stent implantation. *Am J Cardiol* 2000;85:962-968.
147. Lee SW, Park SW, Kim YH, et al. A randomized, double-blind, multicenter comparison study of triple antiplatelet therapy with dual antiplatelet therapy to reduce restenosis after drug-eluting stent implantation in long coronary lesions: results from the DECLARE-LONG II (Drug-Eluting Stenting Followed by Cilostazol Treatment Reduces Late Restenosis in Patients with Long Coronary Lesions) trial. *J Am Coll Cardiol* 2011;57: 1264-1270.
148. Lee SW, Park SW, Kim YH, et al. Drug-eluting stenting followed by cilostazol treatment reduces late restenosis in patients with diabetes mellitus the DECLARE-DIABETES Trial (A Randomized Comparison of Triple Antiplatelet Therapy with Dual Antiplatelet Therapy After Drug-Eluting Stent Implantation in Diabetic Patients). *J Am Coll Cardiol* 2008;51:1181-1187.
149. Douglas Jr JS, Holmes Jr DR, Kereiakes DJ, et al. Coronary stent restenosis in patients treated with cilostazol. *Circulation* 2005;112:2826-2832.
150. Tamhane U, Meier P, Chetcuti S, et al. Efficacy of cilostazol in reducing restenosis in patients undergoing contemporary stent based PCI: a meta-analysis of randomised controlled trials. *EuroIntervention* 2009;5:384-393.
151. Patel D, Walitt B, Lindsay J, et al. Role of pioglitazone in the prevention of restenosis and need for revascularization after bare-metal stent implantation: a meta-analysis. *JACC Cardiovasc Interv* 2011;4:353-360.
152. Kitahara H, Kobayashi Y, Iwata Y, et al. Effect of pioglitazone on endothelial dysfunction after sirolimus-eluting stent implantation. *Am J Cardiol* 2011;108:214-219.
153. Elezi S, Kastrati A, Hadamitzky M, et al. Clinical and angiographic follow-up after balloon angioplasty with provisional stenting for coronary in-stent restenosis. *Catheter Cardiovasc Interv* 1999;48:151-156.
154. Singh IM, Filby SJ, El Sakr F, et al. Drug-eluting stents versus bare-metal stents for treatment of bare-metal in-stent restenosis. *Catheter Cardiovasc Interv* 2010;76:257-262.
155. Radke PW, Kaiser A, Frost C, et al. Outcome after treatment of coronary in-stent restenosis: results from a systematic review using meta-analysis techniques. *Eur Heart J* 2003;24: 266-273.
156. Albiero R, Silber S, Di Mario C, et al. Cutting balloon versus conventional balloon angioplasty for the treatment of in-stent restenosis: results of the restenosis cutting balloon evaluation trial (RESCUT). *J Am Coll Cardiol* 2004;43:943-949.
157. Waksman R, Raizner AE, Yeung AC, et al. Use of localised intracoronary beta radiation in treatment of in-stent restenosis: the INHIBIT randomised controlled trial. *Lancet* 2002;359: 551-557.
158. Leon MB, Teirstein PS, Moses JW, et al. Localized intracoronary gamma-radiation therapy to inhibit the recurrence of restenosis after stenting. *N Engl J Med* 2001;344:250-256.
159. Costa MA, Sabate M, van der Giessen WJ, et al. Late coronary occlusion after intracoronary brachytherapy. *Circulation* 1999;100:789-792.
160. Baierl V, Baumgartner S, Pollinger B, et al. Three-year clinical follow-up after strontium-90/yttrium-90 beta-irradiation for the treatment of in-stent coronary restenosis. *Am J Cardiol* 2005;96:1399-1403.
161. Waksman R, Ajani AE, White RL, et al. Five-year follow-up after intracoronary gamma radiation therapy for in-stent restenosis. *Circulation* 2004;109:340-344.
162. Liistro F, Fineschi M, Grotti S, et al. Long-term effectiveness and safety of sirolimus stent implantation for coronary in-stent restenosis results of the TRUE (Tuscany Registry of sirolimus for unselected in-stent restenosis) registry at 4 years. *J Am Coll Cardiol* 2010;55:613-616.
163. Ellis SG, O'Shaughnessy CD, Martin SL, et al. Two-year clinical outcomes after paclitaxel-eluting stent or brachytherapy treatment for bare-metal stent restenosis: the TAXUS V ISR trial. *Eur Heart J* 2008;29:1625-1634.
164. Holmes Jr DR, Teirstein P, Satler L, et al. Sirolimus-eluting stents vs vascular brachytherapy for in-stent restenosis within bare-metal stents: the SISR randomized trial. *JAMA* 2006; 295:1264-1273.
165. Holmes Jr DR, Teirstein PS, Satler L, et al. 3-year follow-up of the SISR (Sirolimus-Eluting Stents Versus Vascular Brachytherapy for In-Stent Restenosis) trial. *JACC Cardiovasc Interv* 2008;1:439-448.
166. Stone GW, Ellis SG, O'Shaughnessy CD, et al. Paclitaxel-eluting stents vs vascular brachytherapy for in-stent restenosis within bare-metal stents: the TAXUS V ISR randomized trial. *JAMA* 2006;295:1253-1263.
167. Alli OO, Teirstein PS, Satler L, et al. Five-year follow-up of the Sirolimus-Eluting Stents vs Vascular Brachytherapy for Bare-metal In-Stent Restenosis (SISR) trial. *Am Heart J* 2012;163:438-445.
168. Degertekin M, Regar E, Tanabe K, et al. Sirolimus-eluting stent for treatment of complex in-stent restenosis: the first clinical experience. *J Am Coll Cardiol* 2003;41:184-189.
169. Radke PW, Kobella S, Kaiser A, et al. Treatment of in-stent restenosis using a paclitaxel-eluting stent: acute results and long-term follow-up of a matched-pair comparison with intracoronary beta-radiation therapy. *Eur Heart J* 2004;25:920-925.
170. Tanabe K, Serruys PW, Grube E, et al. TAXUS III Trial: in-stent restenosis treated with stent-based delivery of paclitaxel incorporated in a slow-release polymer formulation. *Circulation* 2003;107:559-564.
171. Kastrati A, Mehilli J, von Beckerath N, et al. Sirolimus-eluting stent or paclitaxel-eluting stent vs balloon angioplasty for prevention of recurrences in patients with coronary in-stent restenosis: a randomized controlled trial. *JAMA* 2005;293: 165-171.
172. Alfonso F, Perez-Vizcayno MJ, Cruz A, et al. Treatment of patients with in-stent restenosis. *EuroIntervention* 2009;5(Suppl D):D70-D78.
173. Lee SS, Price MJ, Wong GB, et al. Early- and medium-term outcomes after paclitaxel-eluting stent implantation for sirolimus-eluting stent failure. *Am J Cardiol* 2006;98:1345-1348.
174. Lloyd-Jones D, Adams R, Carnethon M, et al. Heart disease and stroke statistics—2009 update: a report from the American Heart Association Statistics Committee and Stroke Statistics Subcommittee. *Circulation* 2009;119:480-486.
175. Mehilli J, Byrne RA, Tiroch K, et al. Randomized trial of paclitaxel- versus sirolimus-eluting stents for treatment of coronary restenosis in sirolimus-eluting stents: the ISAR-DESIRE 2 (Intracoronary Stenting and Angiographic Results: Drug Eluting Stents for In-Stent Restenosis 2) study. *J Am Coll Cardiol* 2010;55:2710-2716.
176. Habara S, Mitsudo K, Kadota K, et al. Effectiveness of paclitaxel-eluting balloon catheter in patients with sirolimus-eluting stent restenosis. *JACC Cardiovasc Interv* 2011;4: 149-154.
177. Solinas E, Dangas G, Kirtane AJ, et al. Angiographic patterns of drug-eluting stent restenosis and one-year outcomes after treatment with repeated percutaneous coronary intervention. *Am J Cardiol* 2008;102:311-315.

178. Steinberg DH, Gaglia Jr MA, Pinto Slottow TL, et al. Outcome differences with the use of drug-eluting stents for the treatment of in-stent restenosis of bare-metal stents versus drug-eluting stents. *Am J Cardiol* 2009;103:491-495.

179. Cosgrave J, Melzi G, Biondi-Zoccai GG, et al. Drug-eluting stent restenosis: the pattern predicts the outcome. *J Am Coll Cardiol* 2006;47:2399-2404.

180. Garg S, Smith K, Torguson R, et al. Treatment of drug-eluting stent restenosis with the same versus different drug-eluting stent. *Catheter Cardiovasc Interv* 2007;70:9-14.

181. Kim YH, Lee BK, Park DW, et al. Comparison with conventional therapies of repeated sirolimus-eluting stent implantation for the treatment of drug-eluting coronary stent restenosis. *Am J Cardiol* 2006;98:1451-1454.

182. Lee SS, Price MJ, Wong GB, et al. Early- and medium-term outcomes after paclitaxel-eluting stent implantation for sirolimus-eluting stent failure. *Am J Cardiol* 2006;98:1345-1348.

183. Lemos PA, van Mieghem CA, Arampatzis CA, et al. Post-sirolimus-eluting stent restenosis treated with repeat percutaneous intervention: late angiographic and clinical outcomes. *Circulation* 2004;109:2500-2502.

184. Mishkel GJ, Moore AL, Markwell S, et al. Long-term outcomes after management of restenosis or thrombosis of drug-eluting stents. *J Am Coll Cardiol* 2007;49:181-184.

185. Moussa ID, Moses JW, Kuntz RE, et al. The fate of patients with clinical recurrence after sirolimus-eluting stent implantation (a two-year follow-up analysis from the SIRIUS trial). *Am J Cardiol* 2006;97:1582-1584.

186. Torguson R, Sabate M, Deible R, et al. Intravascular brachytherapy versus drug-eluting stents for the treatment of patients with drug-eluting stent restenosis. *Am J Cardiol* 2006;98:1340-1344.

187. Bonello L, Kaneshige K, De Labriolle A, et al. Vascular brachytherapy for patients with drug-eluting stent restenosis. *J Interv Cardiol* 2008;21:528-534.

188. Chatani K, Muramatsu T, Tsukahara R, et al. Predictive factors of re-restenosis after repeated sirolimus-eluting stent implantation for SES restenosis and clinical outcomes after percutaneous coronary intervention for SES restenosis. *J Interv Cardiol* 2009;22:354-361.

189. Singh IM, Filby SJ, Sakr FE, et al. Clinical outcomes of drug-eluting versus bare-metal in-stent restenosis. *Catheter Cardiovasc Interv* 2010;75:338-342.

190. Tagliareni F, La Manna A, Saia F, et al. Long-term clinical follow-up of drug-eluting stent restenosis treatment: retrospective analysis from two high volume catheterisation laboratories. *EuroIntervention* 2010;5:703-708.

191. Chevalier B. *The Intra-Drug Eluting Stent (DES) Restenosis Study (CRISTAL). Presented at Transcatheter Cardiovascular Therapeutics conference,* Washington, DC, 2008.

192. Spanos V, Stankovic G, Tobis J, et al. The challenge of in-stent restenosis: insights from intravascular ultrasound. *Eur Heart J* 2003;24:138-150.

193. Scheller B, Hehrlein C, Bocksch W, et al. Treatment of coronary in-stent restenosis with a paclitaxel-coated balloon catheter. *N Engl J Med* 2006;355:2113-2124.

194. Unverdorben M, Vallbracht C, Cremers B, et al. Paclitaxel-coated balloon catheter versus paclitaxel-coated stent for the treatment of coronary in-stent restenosis. *Circulation* 2009; 119:2986-2994.

195. Rittger H, Brachmann J, Sinha A-M, et al. A randomized, multicenter, single-blinded trial comparing paclitaxel-coated balloon angioplasty with plain balloon angioplasty in drug-eluting stent restenosis: the PEPCAD-DES Study. *J Am Coll Cardiol* 2012;59:1377-1382.

196. Byrne RA, Neumann FJ, Mehilli J, et al. Paclitaxel-eluting balloons, paclitaxel-eluting stents, and balloon angioplasty in patients with restenosis after implantation of a drug-eluting stent (ISAR-DESIRE 3): a randomised, open-label trial. *Lancet* 2013;381:461-467.

197. Morice MC, Serruys PW, Sousa JE, et al. A randomized comparison of a sirolimus-eluting stent with a standard stent for coronary revascularization. *N Engl J Med* 2002;346:1773-1780.

198. Morice MC, Serruys PW, Barragan P, et al. Long-term clinical outcomes with sirolimus-eluting coronary stents: five-year results of the RAVEL trial. *J Am Coll Cardiol* 2007;50: 1299-1304.

199. Weisz G, Leon MB, Holmes Jr DR, et al. Five-year follow-up after sirolimus-eluting stent implantation results of the SIRIUS (Sirolimus-Eluting Stent In De-Novo Native Coronary Lesions) Trial. *J Am Coll Cardiol* 2009;53:1488-1497.

200. Ardissino D, Cavallini C, Bramucci E, et al. Sirolimus-eluting vs uncoated stents for prevention of restenosis in small coronary arteries: a randomized trial. *JAMA* 2004;292:2727-2734.

201. Menozzi A, Solinas E, Ortolani P, et al. Twenty-four months clinical outcomes of sirolimus-eluting stents for the treatment of small coronary arteries: the long-term SES-SMART clinical study. *Eur Heart J* 2009;30:2095-2101.

202. Sabate M, Jimenez-Quevedo P, Angiolillo DJ, et al. Randomized comparison of sirolimus-eluting stent versus standard stent for percutaneous coronary revascularization in diabetic patients: the diabetes and sirolimus-eluting stent (DIABETES) trial. *Circulation* 2005;112:2175-2183.

203. Jimenez-Qeuvedo P. *Four years follow-up of DIABETES trial. Presented at i2 Summit/American College of Cardiology Scientific Sessions,* Orlando, FL, 2009.

204. Colombo A, Drzewiecki J, Banning A, et al. Randomized study to assess the effectiveness of slow- and moderate-release polymer-based paclitaxel-eluting stents for coronary artery lesions. *Circulation* 2003;108:788-794.

205. Silber S, Colombo A, Banning AP, et al. Final 5-year results of the TAXUS II trial: a randomized study to assess the effectiveness of slow- and moderate-release polymer-based paclitaxel-eluting stents for de novo coronary artery lesions. *Circulation* 2009;120:1498-1504.

206. Ellis SG, Stone GW, Cox DA, et al. Long-term safety and efficacy with paclitaxel-eluting stents: 5-year final results of the TAXUS IV clinical trial (TAXUS IV-SR: Treatment of De Novo Coronary Disease Using a Single Paclitaxel-Eluting Stent). *JACC Cardiovasc Interv* 2009;2:1248-1259.

207. Stone GW, Ellis SG, Cannon L, et al. Comparison of a polymer-based paclitaxel-eluting stent with a bare-metal stent in patients with complex coronary artery disease: a randomized controlled trial. *JAMA* 2005;294:1215-1223.

208. Ellis SG, Cannon L, Mann T, et al. Final 5-year outcomes from the TAXUS V de novo trial: long-term safety and effectiveness of the paclitaxel-eluting TAXUS stent in complex lesions [abstract]. *Am J Cardiol* 2009;104:135D.

209. Dawkins KD, Grube E, Guagliumi G, et al. Clinical efficacy of polymer-based paclitaxel-eluting stents in the treatment of complex, long coronary artery lesions from a multicenter, randomized trial: support for the use of drug-eluting stents in contemporary clinical practice. *Circulation* 2005;112:3306-3313.

210. Grube E, Dawkins K, Guagliumi G, et al. TAXUS VI final 5-year results: a multicentre, randomised trial comparing polymer-based moderate-release paclitaxel-eluting stent with a bare-metal stent for treatment of long, complex coronary artery lesions. *EuroIntervention* 2009;4:572-577.

211. Fajadet J, Wijns W, Laarman GJ, et al. Long-term follow-up of the randomised controlled trial to evaluate the safety and efficacy of the zotarolimus-eluting driver coronary stent in de novo native coronary artery lesions: five year outcomes in the ENDEAVOR II study. *EuroIntervention* 2010;6: 562-567.

212. Morice MC, Colombo A, Meier B, et al. Sirolimus- vs paclitaxel-eluting stents in de novo coronary artery lesions: the REALITY trial: a randomized controlled trial. *JAMA* 2006; 295:895-904.

213. Windecker S, Remondino A, Eberli FR, et al. Sirolimus-eluting and paclitaxel-eluting stents for coronary revascularization. *N Engl J Med* 2005;353:653-662.

214. Raber L, Wohlwend L, Wigger M, et al. Five-year clinical and angiographic outcomes of a randomized comparison of sirolimus-eluting and paclitaxel-eluting stents: results of the Sirolimus-Eluting Versus Paclitaxel-Eluting Stents for Coronary Revascularization LATE trial. *Circulation* 2011;123: 2819-2828.

215. Dibra A, Kastrati A, Mehilli J, et al. Paclitaxel-eluting or sirolimus-eluting stents to prevent restenosis in diabetic patients. *N Engl J Med* 2005;353:663-670.

216. Mehilli J, Dibra A, Kastrati A, et al. Randomized trial of paclitaxel- and sirolimus-eluting stents in small coronary vessels. *Eur Heart J* 2006;27:260-266.

217. Serruys PW, Ruygrok P, Neuzner J, et al. A randomised comparison of an everolimus-eluting coronary stent with a paclitaxel-eluting coronary stent: the SPIRIT II trial. *EuroIntervention* 2006;2:286-294.

218. Garg S, Serruys PW, Miquel-Hebert K. Four-year clinical follow-up of the XIENCE V everolimus-eluting coronary stent system in the treatment of patients with de novo coronary artery lesions: the SPIRIT II trial. *Catheter Cardiovasc Interv* 2011;77:1012-1017.

219. Stone GW, Midei M, Newman W, et al. Comparison of an everolimus-eluting and a paclitaxel-eluting stent in patients with coronary artery disease: a randomized trial. *JAMA* 2008;299:1903-1913.

220. Applegate RJ, Yaqub M, Hermiller JB, et al. Long-term (three-year) safety and efficacy of everolimus-eluting stents compared to paclitaxel-eluting stents (from the SPIRIT III Trial). *Am J Cardiol* 2011;107:833-840.

221. Windecker S, Serruys PW, Wandel S, et al. Biolimus-eluting stent with biodegradable polymer versus sirolimus-eluting stent with durable polymer for coronary revascularisation (LEADERS): a randomised non-inferiority trial. *Lancet* 2008; 372:1163-1173.

222. Stefanini GG, Kalesan B, Serruys PW, et al. Long-term clinical outcomes of biodegradable polymer biolimus-eluting stents versus durable polymer sirolimus-eluting stents in patients with coronary artery disease (LEADERS): 4 year follow-up of a randomised non-inferiority trial. *Lancet* 2011;378: 1940-1948.

CHAPTER 9

Intravascular Ultrasound–Guided Coronary Stent Implantation

RICARDO A. COSTA | MATTHEW J. PRICE

KEY POINTS

- Intravascular ultrasound performed after percutaneous coronary intervention can identify significant predictors of stent thrombosis, including stent underexpansion, inflow/outflow disease, and dissection.

- Postintervention in-stent cross-sectional area as measured by intravascular ultrasound is significantly associated with the risk of restenosis.

- Stent underexpansion is more commonly seen in early drug-eluting stent thrombosis, whereas in case-control studies, incomplete stent apposition is more frequently observed in late and very late drug-eluting stent thrombosis.

- In randomized clinical trials in the bare metal stent era, intravascular ultrasound–directed stent implantation resulted in a significantly larger postprocedure minimal lumen diameter and a significant reduction in the rate of repeat revascularization and major adverse cardiovascular events, without an effect on myocardial infarction or mortality.

- Observational registries in the drug-eluting stent era suggest a potential clinical benefit with intravascular ultrasound guidance, but these results must be interpreted in the context of possible unmeasured confounders.

Introduction

Percutaneous coronary intervention (PCI) has substantially evolved since its introduction in 1977, achieving high rates of safety and efficacy, and is currently the predominant mode of revascularization for obstructive coronary artery disease.[1] Intravascular ultrasound (IVUS) has a higher resolution than angiography and provides tomographic cross-sectional views of the intravascular milieu and quantitative measurements of various vascular parameters that cannot be obtained by angiography. IVUS has been of fundamental importance in the development of interventional cardiology, providing unique insights into the understanding of coronary atherosclerosis and helping to refine percutaneous interventional procedures. A seminal contribution of this intravascular imaging modality was the pioneering work of Colombo and colleagues,[2] which fundamentally changed the technique of coronary stent implantation. After high-pressure balloon dilation of underexpanded stents guided by IVUS observation, final in-stent minimal lumen area increased 26% from 6.5 ± 2.0 mm^2 to 8.8 ± 2.5 mm^2, whereas the mean stent expansion (tightest in-stent lumen area relative to the reference area) increased from $49 \pm 13\%$ to $66 \pm 13\%$ ($P < .0001$), resulting in remarkably low rates of acute (0.6%) and subacute (0.3%) thrombosis without the need for systemic postprocedural anticoagulation. This observation was crucial to establishing the widespread application of metallic stents for the percutaneous treatment of coronary artery disease. In addition, IVUS has been shown to be an important tool to identify the mechanisms of bare metal stent (BMS) and drug-eluting stent (DES) failure and to understand the progression of, and the impact of different treatment modalities on, the natural history of atherosclerosis. In this chapter, we discuss the role of IVUS guidance for BMS and DES implantation, with special emphasis on the contribution of this imaging tool to the understanding of the mechanisms behind stent failure (i.e., restenosis and thrombosis).

Criteria for Optimal Stent Implantation

Randomized clinical trials of the efficacy of IVUS to guide stent implantation have used various criteria to define an optimal result (Table 9-1). The Multicenter Ultrasound Stents in Coronaries (MUSIC) study was the first trial to define prospectively specific IVUS criteria for optimal stent implantation.[3] In this study, optimal stent deployment was based on three IVUS parameters: complete apposition, adequate stent expansion, and symmetric stent expansion (see Table 9-1). Although all three criteria were achieved in 81% of the patients in the MUSIC trial, this definition of optimal stent deployment was subsequently shown to be very stringent and difficult to achieve in practice. The MUSIC criteria were fulfilled in only 50% of patients in the Strategy for Intracoronary Ultrasound-guided PTCA and Stenting (SIPS) trial,[4] 56% of patients in the Optimization with Intracoronary Ultrasound to Reduce Stent Restenosis (OPTICUS) trial,[5] and 64% of patient in the study by Gaster and colleagues.[6] The Restenosis after Intravascular Ultrasound Stenting (RESIST) trial[7] used a less complex criterion to define optimal stent expansion: minimal stent cross-sectional area greater than 80% of the average proximal and distal reference lumen cross-sectional area. This criterion was met by 80% of the IVUS-guided stenting group and by only 59% of the angiography-guided group, although despite this difference, a clinical benefit with IVUS was not observed.

In the Thrombocyte activity evaluation and effects of Ultrasound guidance in Long Intracoronary stent Placement (TULIP) study,[8] optimal stent implantation for more complex and long lesions was defined as (1) complete stent apposition, (2) in-stent minimal lumen diameter 80% or greater of the mean proximal and distal reference lumen diameters, and (3) in-stent minimal lumen area greater than or equal to the distal reference lumen area. Despite this complexity, these criteria were achieved by 89% of the patients assigned to the IVUS-guided group and translated into a significant reduction in the 12-month target lesion revascularization (TLR) and major adverse cardiac event (MACE) rates compared with the group guided by angioplasty alone. The Angiography Versus Intravascular Ultrasound Directed (AVID) trial[9] used the following criteria: (1) in-stent minimal lumen area should be 90% or more of the distal vessel lumen area, (2) there should be complete stent apposition to the vessel wall, and (3) all dissections with exposure of the media layer should be covered by stent placement. Only 48% of the vessels in the IVUS-guided group fulfilled these criteria for optimal stent implantation, and of the patients in the IVUS-guided group who did not initially meet the criteria, only 37% received further management, emphasizing a very low rate of operator response to the IVUS findings. It is challenging in general to apply these IVUS criteria in long lesions and tapering vessels, where a mismatch between the proximal and distal references may be accentuated, increasing the risk of acute complications such as dissections or perforations in the distal stent

TABLE 9-1	Intravascular Ultrasound Criteria for Stent Optimization
Study	*Criteria*
MUSIC	**Apposition:** Complete apposition of stent over its entire length against vessel wall **MLA:** In-stent MLA ≥90% of average reference lumen area or ≥100% of lumen area of reference segment with lowest lumen area and in-stent lumen area of proximal stent entrance ≥90% of proximal reference area; in the setting of in-stent lumen area >9.0 mm: In-stent MLA ≥80% of average reference lumen area or ≥90% of lumen area of reference segment with lowest lumen area **Symmetry:** Symmetric stent expansion defined by MLD/maximal lumen diameter ≥0.7 mm
RESIST	**CSA:** Intrastent CSA >80% of average proximal and distal reference lumen CSA
TULIP	**Apposition:** Complete stent apposition **MLD:** In-stent MLD ≥80% of mean proximal and distal reference lumen diameters **MLA:** In-stent MLA greater than or equal to distal reference lumen area
AVID	**Apposition:** Complete stent apposition to vessel wall **MLA:** In-stent MLA ≥90% of distal vessel lumen area **Dissections:** All dissections with exposure of media layer should be covered by stent placement
PRAVIO	**CSA:** In-stent CSA >70% of optimal post-dilation balloon CSA, defined as calculated CSA of a balloon with diameter equal to average media-to-media distance across segment of interest

AVID, Angiography Versus Intravascular Ultrasound Directed; *CSA,* cross-sectional area; *MLA,* minimal lumen area; *MLD,* minimal lumen diameter; *MUSIC,* Multicenter Ultrasound Stents in Coronaries; *PRAVIO,* Preliminary Investigation to the Angiographic Versus IVUS Optimization; *RESIST,* Restenosis after Intravascular Ultrasound Stenting; *TULIP,* Thrombocyte activity evaluation and effects of Ultrasound guidance in Long Intracoronary stent Placement.

edge. The Preliminary Investigation to the Angiographic Versus IVUS Optimization (PRAVIO) criteria attempt to address this limitation by incorporating the change in media-to-media dimensions across the stented segment (see Table 9-1).

🔷 Intravascular Ultrasound–Guided Implantation of Bare Metal Stents

IMPACT OF INTRAVASCULAR ULTRASOUND ON BARE METAL STENT RESTENOSIS AND TARGET LESION REVASCULARIZATION

Percent residual diameter stenosis and minimal lumen diameter achieved after PCI have been identified as major angiographic determinants of restenosis, emphasizing the importance of the acute gain after the procedure in relation to the need for repeat revascularization.[10,11] In a large cohort of 1706 patients (2343 lesions) treated with BMS, longer total stent length (odds ratio [OR], 1.26 for every 10-mm increase in total stent length), smaller reference lumen diameter (OR, 0.43 for every 1-mm increase in reference lumen diameter), and smaller final minimal lumen diameter (OR, 0.55 for every 1-mm increase in the final minimal lumen diameter) were identified as strong predictors of in-stent restenosis. In lesions treated with IVUS guidance, IVUS stent lumen cross-sectional area was a better independent predictor than the angiographic parameters (OR, 0.81 for every 1-mm^2 increase in the stent lumen cross-sectional area).[12]

Clinical Trials of Intravascular Ultrasound–Guided Percutaneous Coronary Intervention with Bare Metal Stents

Given the observation that use of IVUS improves final stent dimensions, several studies assessed whether IVUS-guided stent implantation improves clinical outcomes compared with standard,

angiographically guided PCI. Albiero and associates[13] were the first to assess the outcomes of IVUS-guided PCI compared with quantitative coronary angiography–guided PCI to optimize implantation of the Palmaz-Schatz stent. In this study, the investigators compared 173 patients treated in their institution under IVUS guidance with a matched population of 173 patients from a different hospital that received a Palmaz-Schatz stent implanted under quantitative coronary angiography guidance only. Compared with the angiography-guided group, the IVUS-guided group demonstrated a larger minimal lumen diameter immediately after stenting and at 6-month follow-up. In the early phase of the study, more stringent IVUS criteria for optimal stent expansion and a more aggressive dilation strategy with larger diameter balloons were used; among these patients, the IVUS-guided group displayed a significantly lower rate of 6-month binary angiographic restenosis (9.2% vs. 22.3%, P = .04). However, when a less aggressive approach to the IVUS findings was used in the late phase of the study, no difference in 6-month angiographic restenosis was detected (22.7% vs. 23.7%, P = 1.0). Although this was an observational, nonrandomized, and retrospective study, it provided the first evidence that IVUS-guided PCI could reduce restenosis and need of repeat revascularization. Similar results regarding the effect of IVUS guidance on final stent dimensions were reproduced by other groups.[14]

The landmark MUSIC study[3] was the first to define specific IVUS criteria for optimal stent deployment (see Table 9-1). In this study, all three criteria for optimal stent expansion were met in 81% of the patients, and low 6-month restenosis and TLR rates of 9.7% and 5.7% were observed after BMS implantation. The RESIST trial[7] was the first randomized trial to assess the impact of IVUS-guided stent implantation on clinical outcomes. After successful stent implantation, 155 patients were randomly assigned to either no further balloon dilation or additional dilation until the IVUS criterion for stent expansion was achieved, defined in this case as in-stent minimal lumen area 80% or greater of the reference lumen area. Although a significantly larger mean stent cross-sectional area was observed after the procedure in the group assigned to IVUS-guided balloon dilation (7.16 ± 2.48 mm vs. 7.95 ± 2.21 mm, P = .04), a nonsignificant 6.3% absolute reduction in the restenosis rate was observed at 6-month follow-up (28.8% vs. 22.5%, P =.25). However, the small sample size and event rates provided only 40% power to detect a statistically significant difference in the rates of restenosis between study arms, and a potential beneficial effect of IVUS guidance could not be excluded.

The Can Routine Ultrasound Influence Stent Expansion (CRUISE) study[15] was a prospective, multicenter, nonrandomized IVUS substudy of the Stent Anti-Thrombotic Regimen Study (STARS)[16] in which the use of IVUS or angiography was assigned on a center-by-center basis. Nine centers were assigned to stent deployment under IVUS guidance, and seven centers were assigned to angiography guidance with documented (but blinded) IVUS at the conclusion of the procedure. The study enrolled 525 patients, of whom 499 had completed quantitative coronary angiography, IVUS, and clinical follow-up at 9 months. The IVUS-guided group had a larger postprocedural minimal lumen diameter by quantitative coronary angiography (2.9 ± 0.4 mm vs. 2.7 ± 0.5 mm, P < .001) and a larger minimal lumen area by IVUS (7.78 ± 1.72 mm^2 vs. 7.06 ± 2.13 mm^2, P < .001). At 9-month follow-up, these differences translated into a statistically significant 44% relative reduction in the rate of target vessel revascularization (TVR) (8.5% vs. 15.3%, P < .05). The OPTICUS study[5] randomly assigned 550 patients to IVUS-guided (n = 273) or angiography-guided (n = 277) stent implantation. The primary endpoints were angiographic binary restenosis, minimal lumen diameter, and percent diameter stenosis as determined by quantitative coronary angiography at 6-month follow-up; secondary endpoints included the rate of MACE. At 6-month follow-up, there were no differences between the two groups with respect to the rate of binary restenosis (24.5% vs. 22.8%, P = .68), minimal lumen diameter (1.95 ± 0.72 mm vs. 1.91 ± 0.68 mm, P = .52), and percent diameter stenosis (34.8 ± 20.6% vs. 36.8 ± 19.6%, P = .29). Likewise, IVUS guidance did not reduce the rate of MACE (relative risk, 1.07; 95% confidence interval [CI], 0.75-1.52; $P = .71$) or the need for repeat revascularization (relative risk, 1.04; 95% CI, 0.64-1.67; $P = .87$) at 12 months.

Similar results were observed in a predefined, observational IVUS substudy of the Prevention of Restenosis with Tranilast and its Outcomes (PRESTO) trial,[17] in which 796 patients who underwent IVUS during the PCI procedure (IVUS group) were compared with 8274 patients who did not undergo IVUS (angiography group). Patients in the IVUS group had similar rates of death, myocardial infarction, and ischemia-driven TVR at 9 months compared with the angiography group (relative risk, 1.10; 95% CI, 0.91-1.34) despite having a larger postprocedure minimal lumen diameter and smaller percent diameter stenosis.

The AVID trial is the largest randomized study yet performed to assess the effect of IVUS-guided stent placement on target lesion revascularization.[9] After an optimal angiographic result was achieved following stent placement (defined as <10% residual stenosis), 800 patients were randomly assigned to either angiography-guided or IVUS-guided therapy; blinded IVUS was performed in the angiography group. IVUS guidance resulted in a larger postprocedure in-stent minimal lumen area (7.55 ± 2.82 mm^2 vs. 6.90 ± 2.43 mm^2, $P = .001$), but at 12 months only a trend toward a lower TLR rate was observed (8.1% vs. 12.0%, $P = .08$). However, IVUS guidance significantly reduced the 12-month TLR rate for lesions with a distal reference diameter greater than 2.5 mm (4.3% vs. 10.1%, $P = .01$) and lesions with 70% or greater diameter stenosis before PCI (3.1% vs. 14.2%, $P = .002$).

The TULIP trial compared IVUS-guided with angiography-guided stent implantation for long lesions (>20 mm) in 144 randomly assigned patients.[8] At 6-month follow-up, IVUS resulted in significantly larger minimal lumen diameter (1.82 ± 0.53 mm vs. 1.51 ± 0.71 mm, $P = .042$), significantly less TLR (4% vs. 14%, $P = .037$), and significantly fewer MACE (6% vs. 20%, $P = .01$) compared with angiography, suggesting that IVUS-guided stent implantation may be beneficial in selected patients and lesions at higher risk for restenosis.

A major limitation of the aforementioned studies is their small sample size. Also, in some cases, studies did not define clear IVUS parameters to guide stent expansion, or in studies that did provide such parameters, they were not achieved in many subjects (see the section on IVUS-guided implantation of BMS).

Meta-analyses

Studies examining clinical outcomes with IVUS-guided or angiography-guided PCI enrolled relatively small numbers of patients and were underpowered on their own to definitively assess the role of IVUS-guided PCI on clinical endpoints. A meta-analysis of nine studies that compared IVUS-guided with angiography-guided stenting, five of which were randomized trials (RESIST,[7] OPTICUS,[5] AVID,[9] TULIP,[8] and SIPS[4]), included 2972 patients.[18] At 6 months, the rate of the composite endpoint of death and nonfatal myocardial infarction was similar for either strategy (4.1% for angiography-guided stenting vs. 4.5% for IVUS-guided stenting). However, IVUS-guided stenting demonstrated significant reduction in overall MACE (OR, 0.79; 95% CI, 0.64-0.98; $P = .03$), driven by a 38% reduction in TVR (OR, 0.62; 95% CI, 0.49-0.78; $P < .001$). In addition, patients with IVUS-guided stenting had significantly less binary restenosis (OR, 0.75; 95% CI, 0.60-0.94; $P = .01$). Parise and coworkers[19] conducted a meta-analysis restricted to randomized studies comparing IVUS-guided with angiography-guided PCI with BMS (Figure 9-1). Seven studies (five multicenter and two single-center) comprising 2193 patients were included, with a follow-up period ranging from 6 months to 2½ years. In contrast to the earlier meta-analysis, this study incorporated the Direct Stenting versus Optimal Angioplasty (DIPOL) study,[20] the study by Gaster and colleagues,[6,21] the final results of the AVID trial,[9] and the long-term follow-up of the RESIST study.[22] IVUS guidance was associated with a significantly larger postprocedure angiographic minimal lumen diameter (mean difference 0.12 mm;

95% CI, 0.06-0.1 per 8 mm; $P < .0001$), a significant reduction in revascularization (OR, 0.66; 95% CI, 0.48-0.91; $P = .004$), and a significant reduction in overall MACE (OR, 0.69; 95% CI, 0.49-0.97; $P = .03$). Use of IVUS had no significant effect on the incidence of mortality or myocardial infarction.

IMPACT OF INTRAVASCULAR ULTRASOUND ON BARE METAL STENT THROMBOSIS

High rates of acute and subacute stent thrombosis were initially a substantial limitation of coronary stenting, with an incidence ranging from 10% to 20%.[23-26] Aggressive systemic antiplatelet and anticoagulant therapy was required after stent implantation, increasing the risk of bleeding complications.[10,11] A seminal study by Colombo and coworkers[2] reported a high prevalence of stent underexpansion and malapposition by IVUS despite a good angiographic result, providing critical insights into the potential mechanisms underpinning the phenomenon of stent thrombosis. High-pressure stent deployment along with dual antiplatelet therapy with aspirin and ticlopidine dramatically reduced the rate of stent thrombosis to an incidence of approximately 0.9% in the modern BMS era.[27]

Predictors of Stent Thrombosis

In a pooled analysis of six randomized stent trials involving 6186 patients and 6219 treated vessels, the variables most significantly associated with stent thrombosis were persistent dissection National Heart, Lung, and Blood Institute grade B or higher after stenting (OR, 3.7; 95% CI, 1.9-7.7), total stent length (OR, 1.3; 95% CI, 1.2-1.5 per 10 mm), and final minimal lumen diameter within the stent (OR, 0.4; 95% CI, 0.2-0.7 per 1 mm).[27] Several IVUS characteristics have been associated with BMS thrombosis. The Predictors and Outcomes of Stent Thrombosis (POST)[28] was a retrospective, multicenter registry that aimed to investigate whether IVUS provided additional predictive information regarding acute and subacute stent thrombosis. The registry included 53 patients presenting with stent thrombosis after PCI who had undergone IVUS examination at the end of the index procedure. At least one abnormal IVUS feature (stent underexpansion, malapposition, inflow/outflow disease, dissection, or thrombus) were identified by IVUS in 94% of cases, whereas angiography detected an abnormality in only 32%. In another study, 27 patients presenting with subacute stent thrombosis who had undergone IVUS during the index procedure were compared with a matched control group without stent thrombosis. At least one IVUS abnormality (dissection, thrombus, and tissue protrusion through stent struts leading to lumen compromise) was present in 78% of the patients with stent thrombosis compared with 33% of the matched control group ($P = .0002$); multiple abnormalities were found in 48% of the group with stent thrombosis compared with 3% of the matched control group ($P < .0001$).[29] These observations suggest that structural or mechanical variables are the predominant etiologic factors involved in acute and subacute stent thrombosis. Although no study has investigated whether the routine use of IVUS can affect the rate of BMS thrombosis, it seems reasonable to posit that IVUS, by identifying these mechanical and procedural abnormalities, may prompt their subsequent treatment and potentially play an important role in PCI safety.

COST-EFFECTIVENESS OF INTRAVASCULAR ULTRASOUND DURING PERCUTANEOUS CORONARY INTERVENTION WITH BARE METAL STENTS

The cost-effectiveness of IVUS-guided PCI is an important issue. IVUS use requires a learning curve, increases procedural time, and results in greater resource utilization. A cost-effectiveness analysis of the RESIST study demonstrated an 18% increase in the medical costs in the periprocedural phase ($2934 \pm 670€$ s vs. $2481 \pm 911€$) with the use of IVUS to optimize stent implantation, mainly as a result of the cost of IVUS catheters and the need for a greater number of balloon catheters.[22] However, the cumulative medical costs at 18 months were

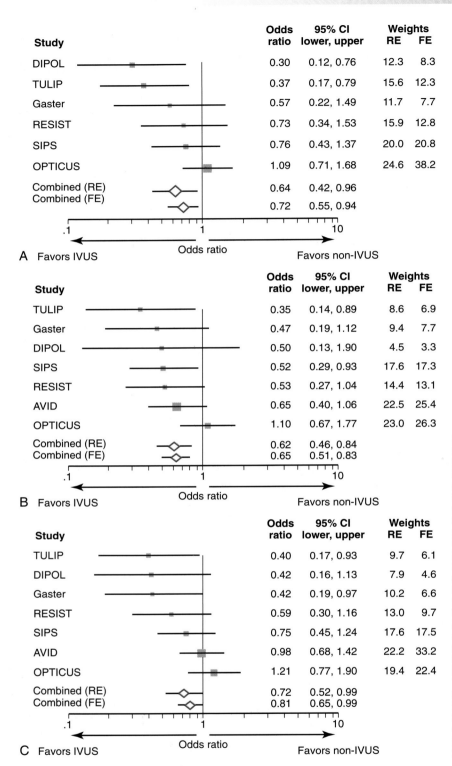

Figure 9-1 Impact of intravascular ultrasound *(IVUS)* versus angiography guidance of percutaneous coronary intervention with bare metal stents. **A,** Odds ratio plots with 95% confidence intervals *(CI)* for rates of 6-month angiographic restenosis among six randomized studies with angiography follow-up and reporting restenosis. IVUS guidance was associated with a significantly lower rate of 6-month angiographic restenosis. Combined estimates from both random effects *(RE)* and fixed effects *(FE)* models are shown. **B,** Odds ratio plots with 95% CI for rates of repeat revascularization from seven randomized studies with follow-up ranging from 6 months to 2½ years. IVUS guidance was associated with a significant reduction in revascularization. **C,** Odds ratio plots with 95% CI for rates of MACE from seven randomized studies. IVUS guidance was associated with significant reduction in MACE. *AVID,* Angiography vs Intravascular Ultrasound; *DIPOL,* Direct Stenting vs Optimal Angioplasty study; *OPTICUS,* Optimization with Intracoronary Ultrasound to Reduce Stent Restenosis; *RESIST,* Restenosis after IVUS-Guided Stenting; *SIPS,* Strategy of Intravascular Ultrasound-Guided PTCA and Stenting; *TULIP,* Thrombocyte Activity Evaluation and Effects of Ultrasound Guidance in Long Intracoronary Stent Placement. (Adapted from Parise H, Maehara A, Stone GW, et al. Meta-analysis of randomized studies comparing intravascular ultrasound versus angiographic guidance of percutaneous coronary intervention in pre-drug-eluting stent era. *Am J Cardiol.* 2011;107:374-382.)

only slightly higher in the IVUS-guided group (4679 ± 1471€ vs. 4535 ± 2020€), driven by a lower rate of repeat revascularization. Gaster and colleagues[6] used an activity-based costing method to estimate the incremental costs of IVUS-guided procedures and costs of reinterventions in 108 patients randomly assigned to IVUS-guided or angiography-guided PCI. The initial cost of IVUS guidance was increased as a result of the extra procedure time, IVUS catheter cost, and use of slightly more balloon catheters and stents. However, at 6

months, the total cost was lower in the IVUS-guided group because these patients had an improved clinical outcome with less angina, lower rates of reintervention, and fewer hospitalization days. Overall, these increased clinical benefits outweighed the initial cost increase. At 2½ years of follow-up, the cost-effectiveness of IVUS guidance was accentuated; more patients in the IVUS-guided group were free from MACE at 2½ years compared with the angiography-guided group (78% vs. 59%, P = .04), and the cumulative cost was significantly lower in the IVUS-guided group compared with the angiography-guided group ($P = .01$) in addition to the mean cost per day ($P = .01$).[21] In a prospective, prespecified economic analysis of the SIPS[30] trial, in-hospital costs were numerically higher in the group randomly assigned to PCI under IVUS guidance ($\$5245 \pm 2256$/patient vs. $\$4776 \pm 2961$/patient, $P = .15$). Total costs over the 2-year period numerically favored the IVUS-guided group ($\$15,947 \pm 8545$/patient vs. $\$16,103 \pm 9954$/patient, $P = .89$), resulting from a significantly greater 2-year MACE-free survival (80% vs. 69%, $P < .04$) and slightly lower 2-year costs for cardiac hospitalizations in the IVUS group, whereas costs for medications and indirect costs were similar. Overall, the incremental cost-effectiveness ratio for IVUS guidance was $\$1417$/MACE-free survival gained.

Adjunctive IVUS examination before PCI may help optimize the procedure results and minimize the elevated initial procedure costs. Careful IVUS examination of the target lesion site before PCI allows accurate measurement of the vessel dimensions, qualitative assessment of the underlying plaque (e.g., calcified plaques), and better definition of the most "normal-looking" reference segments. Such a strategy may provide the operator additional information to select adjunctive devices and appropriately sized balloon catheters and stents efficiently.

🔶 Intravascular Ultrasound–Guided Implantation of Drug-Eluting Stents

IMPACT OF INTRAVASCULAR ULTRASOUND ON DRUG-ELUTING STENT RESTENOSIS

The introduction of DES has markedly reduced the incidence of clinical and angiographic restenosis by 60% to 80% compared with BMS in pivotal randomized trials.[31-33] Nonetheless, DES do not completely abolish restenosis, which occurs at a rate of 3% to 20%, depending on patient and lesion characteristics and DES type.[34] In the BMS era, "the bigger, the better" concept dominated the approach to PCI by providing a large postprocedure lumen to compensate for subsequent late loss resulting from neointimal growth.[35,36] This concept was initially abandoned with DES because of neointimal suppression and consequent diminshed late lumen loss. However, stent underexpansion represents the main mechanism of DES restenosis and the need for repeat revascularization.[37] In the IVUS substudy of the Sirolimus-Eluting Stent in De-Novo Native Coronary Lesions (SIRIUS) trial,[38] the optimal immediate postintervention minimum stent cross-sectional area to predict adequate stent patency (defined as a minimal lumen area $>4.0\ mm^2$) at 8-month follow-up was $5.0\ mm^2$ (Figure 9-2). The positive predictive value for this cutoff point was 90%, suggesting that sirolimus-eluting stent (SES) failure in the SIRIUS trial was mostly a result of stent underexpansion. In a large study with serial 6-month angiographic follow-up of 449 patients with 543 native coronary lesions treated with SES, the only independent predictors of angiographic restenosis by a multivariate logistic regression analysis were postprocedural minimum stent cross-sectional area by IVUS (OR, 0.586; 95% CI, 0.387-0.888; $P = .012$) and IVUS-measured stent length (OR, 1.029; 95% CI, 1.002-1.056; $P = .035$). The final minimal stent cross-sectional area and stent length by IVUS that best separated restenosis from nonrestenosis were $5.5\ mm^2$ and 40 mm.[39] In a pooled analysis from IVUS substudies of the TAXUS IV, V, and VI and TAXUS ATLAS Workhorse, Long Lesion, and Direct Stent randomized trials that comprised 1580 patients, multivariate logistic regression analysis identified postintervention IVUS minimum stent cross-sectional area as the independent predictor of subsequent in-stent restenosis with both paclitaxel-eluting stents and BMS ($P = .0002$ for both). The optimal thresholds for postintervention IVUS minimum stent cross-sectional area that best predicted stent patency at 9-month follow-up were $5.7\ mm^2$ for paclitaxel-eluting stents and $6.4\ mm^2$ for BMS (see Figure 9-2).[40]

These observations are supported by findings from studies of patients with DES failure. In an IVUS analysis of 33 patients

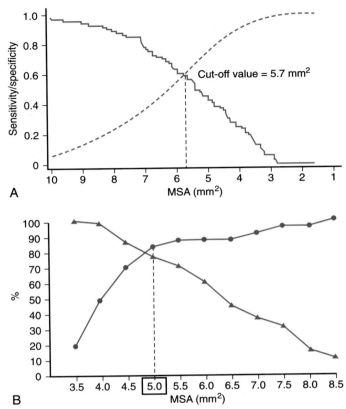

Figure 9-2 Sensitivity and specificity of minimal stent area *(MSA)* to predict angiographic in-stent restenosis for paclitaxel-eluting stents **(A)** and sirolimus-eluting stents **(B)** derived from randomized clinical trials. The vertical axis represents the amount of sensitivity or specificity, and the horizontal axis represents MSA according to IVUS postprocedure. Curves represent sensitivity or specificities across the range of MSAs. For both stent platforms, postintervention IVUS MSA was an independent predictor of subsequent in-stent restenosis, with similar optimal thresholds for predicting stent patency at 9 months follow-up. (Adapted from Sonoda S, Morino Y, Ako J, et al. Impact of final stent dimenon long-term results following sirolimus-eluting stent implantation: serial intravascular ultrasound analysis from the SIRIUS trial. *J Am Coll Cardiol* 2004;43:1959-1963; and Doi H, Maehara A, Mintz GS, et al. Impact of post-intervention minimal stent area on 9-month follow-up patency of paclitaxel-eluting stents: an integrated intravascular ultrasound analysis from the TAXUS IV, V, and VI and TAXUS ATLAS Workhorse, Long Lesion, and Direct Stent Trials. *JACC Cardiovasc Interv* 2009;2:1269-1275.)

presenting with target vessel failure after SES (4 with thrombosis, 26 with in-stent restenosis, 4 with a new stenosis >5 mm proximal to the stent, and 1 with suspected stent embolization), a minimum SES area less than $5.0\ mm^2$ was observed in 67% (in particular, in 67% of cases with in-stent restenosis).[41] Consistent with these observations, in a study of 209 patients and 319 lesions treated with at least one SES under IVUS guidance, the TLR rate was only 1.3%, and in all cases the final minimum stent cross-sectional area was less than $6.0\ mm^2$.[42] Kang and associates[43] identified 76 lesions with both angiography-defined and IVUS-defined in-stent restenosis after SES, paclitaxel-eluting stents, and zotarolimus-eluting stents (i.e., >50% diameter stenosis by angiography and minimal lumen area $<4.0\ mm^2$ by IVUS). Stent underexpansion, defined as minimal stent cross-sectional area less than $5.0\ mm^2$, was observed in 32 lesions (42%), whereas significant neointimal hyperplasia (% area >50% of stent) was seen in 71 lesions (93%). Total stent length negatively correlated with minimal stent area ($r = -0.613$, $P < .001$) and with vessel area ($r = -0.416$, $P < .001$), stent area ($r = -0.436$, $P < .001$), and percent neointimal hyperplasia area ($r = -0.229$, $P = .047$) at the minimum lumen site but not with the minimal lumen area itself ($r = -0.084$,

$P = .472$). Receiver operator characteristic curve analysis demonstrated that total stent length equal to 28 mm was the cutoff point that best separated a minimal stent area less than 5.0 mm^2 from a minimal stent area 5.0 mm^2 or greater, with 70% sensitivity and 61% specificity. Compared with focal or multifocal patterns of restenosis, a diffuse pattern (significant neoinimal hyperplasia length >10 mm) was most commonly observed with longer total stent lengths and had a higher rate of stent underexpansion (39% for diffuse pattern vs. 22% for multifocal and 6% for focal, $P = .004$). No differences were observed in the angiography or IVUS patterns of restenosis among the three DES types studied. However, significant neointimal hyperplasia greater than 10 mm in length was seen more frequently in lesions treated with paclitaxel-eluting stents and zotarolimus-eluting stents compared with lesions treated with SES (32% vs. 33% vs. 9%, $P = .038$). In addition, paclitaxel-eluting stents displayed a similar rate of underexpansion at the minimum lumen site compared with SES and zotarolimus-eluting stents (14% vs. 27% vs. 20%, $P = .461$) but had a higher rate of significant neointimal hyperplasia (100% vs. 79% vs. 87%, $P = .037$). These observations support the proposition that underexpansion associated with longer stent length is an important preventable mechanism of in-stent restenosis.

The utility of a single cutoff value to predict stent patency and define optimal stent implantation should be interpreted with caution because the studies that defined a cutoff of 5.0 to 5.5 mm^2 enrolled patients who were at predominantly low to moderate risk for restenosis with regard to lesion complexity. This particular cutoff value may not be applicable to long lesions, lesions with small reference vessel diameters, and lesions with overlapping stents. Acknowledging these limitations, a new criterion for stent optimization was proposed in the PRAVIO trial, which incorporates vessel remodeling (allowing for plaque compression and further expansion of the media layer), integrates vessel dimensions along the entire treated segment, and is more applicable to long lesions and tapering vessels. The maximum and minimum diameters of the media-to-media dimension of the vessel are measured along the stented area at the proximal, mid-lesion, distal, and any other points of interest; these diameters are averaged, and this value is used to select the optimal post-dilating balloon. A value for optimal stent expansion is defined as a final stent cross-sectional area greater than 70% of the calculated cross-sectional area of the chosen balloon. For example, if the average vessel size is determined to be 3.0 mm, a 3.0-mm noncompliant balloon, which has a calculated cross-sectional area of 7.07 mm^2, is used to post-dilate the stented segment, and optimal stent expansion by IVUS is achieved if the stent cross-sectional area is greater than 4.95 mm^2. In the setting of tapered vessels, the optimization balloon diameter may be determined based on the media-to-media distance within the given segment.[44] In the PRAVIO trial, a significant positive correlation was observed between optimized balloon size and final stent cross-sectional area ($R = 0.66$, $P < .0001$), and the final minimal lumen diameter was significantly larger in the IVUS-guided group compared with the angiography-guided group (3.09 ± 0.50 mm^2 vs. 2.67 ± 0.54 mm^2, $P < .0001$).[44]

Other Mechanisms of Drug-Eluting Stent Restenosis

Incomplete lesion coverage is a recognized cause of DES restenosis. In a quantitative IVUS analysis of the randomized SIRIUS trial that sought to identify predictors of edge stenosis after DES implantation, a larger percentage of plaque area at the reference segment was associated with edge stenosis in the DES cohort, indicating that inadequate lesion coverage may contribute to edge stenosis.[45] These results suggest that using IVUS to select stent length to ensure full lesion coverage may improve DES efficacy. Uneven distribution of stent struts might also affect the amount of neointima after DES implantation, presumably as a consequence of a nonuniform drug delivery to the vessel wall. In a case-control IVUS study, the site of minimal lumen area in restenotic lesions had a larger maximum interstrut angle (135 ± 39 degrees vs. 72 ± 23 degrees, $P < .01$) and fewer stent struts (4.9 ± 1.0 vs. 6.0 ± 0.5, $P < .01$) compared with nonrestenotic lesions,

even when normalized for the number of stent cells. The number of visualized stent struts normalized for the number of stent cells and the maximum interstrut angle were the only independent IVUS predictors of neointimal hyperplasia cross-sectional area and in-stent minimal lumen area ($P < .01$ for both variables).[46] Optimizing stent expansion or implanting another DES may counteract underdosing from nonuniform stent strut distribution. Stent fracture, leading to local drug underdosing, has also been proposed as a mechanism for focal DES restenosis.[47-49]

Nominal Balloon Inflation Pressure and Predicted Minimal Stent Diameter

Stent manufacturers routinely provide compliance charts; these are developed to predict minimum stent diameter from nominal balloon inflation pressure. However, these charts are based on in vitro measurements in air or water and do not reflect the actual conditions intrinsic to a diseased coronary vessel. DES achieve only 75 ± 10% of the predicted minimum stent diameter and 66 ± 17% of the predicted minimum stent cross-sectional area, and 24% of SES and 28% of paclitaxel-eluting stents did not achieve a minimum stent cross-sectional area of 5 mm^2.[50] Similar findings were reported with BMS.[51]

Drug-Eluting Stent Treatment of Bare Metal In-Stent Restenosis

Stent underexpansion is a frequent cause of DES failure after treatment of BMS restenosis. In a series of 48 in-stent restenotic lesions treated with SES, 9 of the 11 recurrent lesions had a minimum stent cross-sectional area less than 5.0 mm^2 compared with only 5 of the nonrecurrent group ($P = .003$).[52] The mechanisms of recurrent in-stent restenosis after DES and vascular brachytherapy differ. Vascular brachytherapy failures were caused by significant, recurrent, and diffuse proliferation of neointimal hyperplasia in the setting of adequate stent expansion, whereas DES failures were caused by only modest and focal neointimal hyperplasia in the setting of stent underexpansion.[53]

IMPACT OF INTRAVASCULAR ULTRASOUND ON STENT THROMBOSIS

Early Drug-Eluting Stent Thrombosis

Several case-control studies have explored the relationship between procedure-related factors and early (i.e., acute and subacute) stent thrombosis after DES implantation. IVUS-defined stent underexpansion and inflow/outflow disease at the time of the index procedure have been consistently identified as critical variables associated with subsequent thrombotic events. In a study aiming to determine the predictors of stent thrombosis after SES implantation, Fujii and associates[54] compared 15 patients who developed stent thrombosis at a median of 14 days after successful SES implantation with 45 matched control patients without evidence of thrombosis. Minimum stent cross-sectional area (4.3 ± 1.6 mm^2 vs. 6.2 ± 1.9 mm^2, $P < .001$) and stent expansion (0.65 ± 0.18 mm^2 vs. 0.85 vs. 0.14 mm^2, $P < .001$) were significantly smaller in the stent thrombosis group. The presence of a significant residual reference segment stenosis was also more common in the stent thrombosis group compared with the matched control group (67% vs. 9%, $P < .001$). Multivariate logistic regression analysis identified stent underexpansion ($P = .03$) and significant residual reference segment stenosis ($P = .02$) as independent predictors of stent thrombosis. Similar results were reported by another study evaluating the IVUS predictors for DES thrombosis in 13 patients with 14 DES thromboses compared with a matched control group of 27 patients. Compared with the control group, a smaller minimum stent cross-sectional area was seen in the stent thrombosis group (4.6 ± 1.1 mm^2 vs. 5.6 ± 1.7 mm^2, $P = .0489$), and 11 of 14 patients in the stent thrombosis group had minimum stent cross-sectional area 5.0 mm^2 or less compared with 12 of 30 patients in the control group ($P = .0392$). In addition, the stent thrombosis group had a larger proximal reference plaque burden (66 ± 8% vs. 56 ± 10%, $P = .002$) and a tendency toward similar findings in the distal edge.[55] In an IVUS substudy of the Harmonizing Outcomes with Revascularization and Stents in Acute Myocardial Infarction (HORIZONS-AMI) study, smaller final lumen area and inflow/outflow disease (residual stenosis or dissection) but not acute malapposition were related to early stent thrombosis after acute myocardial infarction intervention. All patients with early stent thrombosis displayed at least one of the following characteristics on IVUS: minimum lumen area less than 5 mm², edge dissection, residual stenosis (lumen area <4.0 mm² with >70% plaque burden within 10 mm of the stent edge), or tissue protrusion (narrowing the lumen to <4 mm²).[56]

Late and Very Late Stent Thrombosis

The pathophysiology of late stent thrombosis is still not completely understood and may be multifactorial in origin. Delayed arterial healing[57-59] along with several clinical and procedural risk factors[60,61] have been associated with increased risk of late stent thrombosis. Late stent malapposition is consistently seen at the time of very late stent thrombosis in case-control studies using IVUS. In a single-center study, Cook and colleagues[62] compared the IVUS findings of 13 patients presenting with very late stent thrombosis after DES (>1 year after implantation) with a control group of 144 patients who had IVUS examination performed 8 months after DES implantation but without stent thrombosis. At the time of presentation, patients with very late stent thrombosis had a higher rate of incomplete stent apposition (77% vs. 12%, $P < .001$) and significantly larger maximal malapposition area (8.3 ± 7.5 mm² vs. 4.0 ± 3.8 mm², $P = .03$) compared with controls. Subsequently, the same group reported the results of 10 patients with 11 very late stent thromboses who underwent thrombus aspiration and IVUS examination during emergency PCI for the thrombotic event. Incomplete stent apposition was present in 73% of these stents, and there was evidence of outward vessel remodeling (remodeling index of 1.6 ± 0.3). Eosinophil counts were increased within the thrombus aspirates, correlated with the cross-sectional area at the sites of incomplete stent apposition.[63] Whether stent malapposition was early (i.e., at the time of the index procedure) or late acquired (i.e., developed after the procedure as a result of mechanisms such as vessel remodeling or thrombus dissolution) cannot be determined in these studies because IVUS was unavailable at the time of the index procedure.

In a registry of 557 patients treated with SES or paclitaxel-eluting stents who were studied with serial IVUS at baseline and 6-month follow-up, late acquired incomplete apposition, although not infrequent, was not associated with DES thrombosis.[64] Late acquired incomplete stent apposition was identified in 82 patients (12.1% overall; 71 lesions [13.2%] after SES and 14 lesions [8.4%] after paclitaxel-eluting stents, $P = .12$). Signs of vessel remodeling were observed, represented by an increase in the external elastic membrane area that was significantly greater than the increase in plaque area. Independent predictors for late incomplete stent apposition were total stent length, primary stenting in acute myocardial infarction, and chronic total occlusion lesions. At 10-month mean clinical follow-up, late acquired incomplete stent apposition was not associated with major adverse cardiovascular events. On serial IVUS at 2-year follow-up, malapposition detected at 6 months continuously progressed, and new areas of malapposition developed, all related to ongoing positive remodeling.[65] Siqueira and colleagues[66] studied 195 patients after implantation of SES or paclitaxel-eluting stents with serial IVUS examinations at baseline and 6-month to 8-month follow-up and a longer clinical follow-up (median 24.3 months). Late acquired incomplete stent apposition was identified in 10 patients, and another 13 patients (6.6%) had persistent incomplete stent apposition; 9 out of 10 cases of late incomplete stent apposition occurred within the stent, whereas all cases of persistent incomplete stent apposition occurred at stent edges. Two patients with late acquired incomplete stent apposition had angiographically documented very late stent thrombosis manifested as acute ST segment elevation

myocardial infarction, whereas none of the patients with persistent incomplete stent apposition experienced stent thrombosis. In a prospective study of 194 patients, the presence of incomplete stent apposition as assessed by IVUS 8 months after DES implantation was associated with a higher rate of myocardial infarction and very late stent thrombosis during long-term follow-up (hazard ratio [HR], 23.2; 95% CI, 2.65-2.03; $P < .001$).[67] Although these case-control studies show a consistent relationship between malapposition and very late stent thrombosis at the time of presentation, incidentally detected late stent malapposition during routine follow-up studies of DES-treated patients is not associated with an increased frequency of subsequent events. For example, in the TAXUS experience, neither routinely detected acute incomplete stent apposition nor late incomplete stent apposition was associated with MACE over 2-year follow-up.[68]

CLINICAL IMPACT OF INTRAVASCULAR ULTRASOUND GUIDANCE FOR DRUG-ELUTING STENT IMPLANTATION

Because the mechanical and structural characteristics that are predictive of DES restenosis and thrombosis for the most part can be identified by IVUS at the time of the index procedure, the potential benefit of IVUS-guided stent optimization is intuitive. Several registries and initial randomized clinical trials have explored the potential efficacy of IVUS in reducing DES failure.

Observational Registries

Roy and coworkers[69] explored the impact of IVUS guidance on DES outcomes and, in particular, definite stent thrombosis by comparing 884 patients treated with DES under IVUS guidance with a propensity score–matched group of 884 patients treated with a DES under only angiographic guidance. During the in-hospital phase, patients treated with DES under IVUS guidance had a significantly lower rate of Q-wave myocardial infarction (0.1% vs. 0.9%, $P = .02$), whereas the rates of all-cause mortality were similar between the groups. The rate of definite stent thrombosis was significantly higher in the angiography-guided group at 30 days (1.4% vs. 0.5%, $P = .046$) and 12 months (2.0% vs. 0.7%, $P = .014$), driven primarily by differences in subacute stent thrombosis. Although there were no significant differences in MACE at 12 months, the rate of TLR at 12 months tended to be lower in the IVUS group (5.1% vs. 7.2%, $P = .07$). IVUS guidance was identified as an independent predictor of freedom from cumulative stent thrombosis at 12 months (adjusted HR, 0.5; 95% CI, 0.1-0.8, $P = .02$).

In a prospective registry that included 8371 patients who underwent PCI guided by IVUS (n = 4627) or angiography (n = 3744), the unadjusted 3-year cumulative survival rate was significantly greater in patients undergoing IVUS-guided PCI (96.4 ± 0.3% vs. 93.6 ± 0.4%, $P < .001$); patients undergoing IVUS-guided PCI had a significantly lower adjusted risk of mortality at 3-year follow-up (adjusted HR, 0.627; 95% CI, 0.50-0.79; $P < .001$). The risk of mortality was significantly reduced with IVUS in the patients receiving DES (HR, 0.46; 95% CI, 0.33-0.66; $P < .001$) but not in patients receiving BMS (HR, 0.82; 95% CI, 0.60-1.10; $P = .185$). Overall, the risks of myocardial infarction, TVR, and stent thrombosis were not associated with IVUS guidance.[70] Similarly, in the Revascularization for Unprotected Left Main Coronary Artery Stenosis: Comparison of Percutaneous Coronary Angioplasty versus Surgical Revascularization (MAIN-COMPARE) registry, the 3-year incidence of mortality was lower with IVUS guidance compared with angiography guidance in patients treated with DES (HR, 0.39; 95% CI, 0.15-1.02; $P = .055$).[71] In the Comprehensive Assessment of Sirolimus-eluting stents in Complex lesions (MATRIX) registry, 1504 consecutive and unselected patients treated with SES were prospectively included, of whom 631 patients (42%) underwent IVUS-guided SES implantation. IVUS guidance was associated with a reduction in both early (30 days) and long-term (up to 2 years) events, with significant adjusted differences in death or myocardial infarction, MACE, mortality, and myocardial infarction favoring IVUS guidance.[72]

Randomized Trials

The HOME DES IVUS trial was the first randomized study comparing the effect of IVUS guidance (n = 105 patients) versus angiographic guidance (n = 105 patients) for DES implantation on the long-term outcome of patients with complex coronary disease and a high clinical risk profile.[73] The IVUS criteria for optimal stent deployment were as follows: (1) full apposition of the stent to the vessel wall, (2) minimal stent cross-sectional area 5.0 mm^2 or greater or minimal cross-sectional area greater than 90% of distal reference lumen cross-sectional area for small vessels, and (3) no edge dissections. The rate of achievement of these criteria was not reported. At 18 months, no differences between the IVUS-guided and angiography-guided groups were observed in the rates of MACE (11% vs. 12%, P = not significant [NS]) or stent thrombosis (3.8% vs. 5.7%, P = NS). The Angiography Versus IVUS Optimization (AVIO) trial randomly assigned 284 patients with complex lesions (longer than 28 mm, chronic total occlusions, bifurcations, small vessels, and requiring at least four stents) to DES implantation under IVUS or angiography guidance.[74] The criterion for optimal stent expansion was previously tested in the PRAVIO study[44] but was achieved in only 75 lesions (41.2%) of the patients in the IVUS group. The primary endpoint of postprocedure in-lesion minimal lumen diameter, as determined by quantitative coronary angiography, was significantly larger in the IVUS-guided group compared with the angiography-guided group (2.70 ± 0.46 mm vs. 2.51 ± 0.46 mm, P = .0002), but the rates of MACE at 9 months were similar (14.1% vs. 16.9%, P = .42) between groups, as were the rates of cardiac death (0% vs. 1.4%), myocardial infarction (7.0% vs. 8.5%), and TLR (7.0% vs. 5.0%). Only one definite stent thrombosis was identified in the IVUS-guided group, and no stent thrombosis occurred in the angiography-guided DES implantation.

Findings of large prospective registries appear to support a clinical benefit for IVUS-guided DES implantation, although unmeasured confounders could partly explain the observed differences in outcomes between IVUS and angiography guidance. To date, randomized trials have been underpowered to address definitively the clinical utility of IVUS guidance, given their small sample size, low event rates, and infrequent achievement of stent optimization despite IVUS use.

🔹 Guideline Recommendations

The 2011 American College of Cardiology Foundation/American Heart Association Task Force on Practice Guidelines/Society of Cardiovascular Angiography and Interventions Guideline for Percutaneous Coronary Intervention made several recommendations regarding the use of IVUS for the diagnosis and treatment of coronary stenosis (Table 9-2).[75] In particular, the guidelines state that IVUS may be considered for guidance of coronary stent implantation, particularly in cases of left main coronary artery stenting (class IIb, level of evidence B).

🔹 Conclusion

Studies using IVUS after stent implantation have identified key mechanical and structural characteristics associated with BMS and DES restenosis and thrombosis. Stent underexpansion, derived from the minimal lumen area within the stented segment, is significantly associated with a higher risk of restenosis and early stent thrombosis. Lack of lesion coverage, edge dissection, and inflow/outflow disease also have been associated with DES failure. Late incomplete stent

TABLE 9-2	Recommendations Regarding Intravascular Ultrasound in the 2011 ACCF/AHA/SCAI Guideline for Percutaneous Coronary Intervention	
Class	**Recommendations**
I	None
IIa	IVUS is reasonable for assessment of angiographically indeterminant left main coronary artery disease (LOE: B) IVUS and coronary angiography are reasonable 4-6 weeks and 1 year after cardiac transplantation to exclude donor coronary artery disease, detect rapidly progressive cardiac allograft vasculopathy, and provide prognostic information (LOE: B) IVUS is reasonable to determine the mechanism of stent restenosis (LOE: C)
IIb	IVUS may be reasonable for assessment of non–left main coronary arteries with angiographically intermediate coronary stenosis (50%-70% diameter stenosis) (LOE: B) IVUS may be considered for guidance of coronary stent implantation, particularly in cases of left main coronary artery stenting (LOE: B) IVUS may be reasonable to determine mechanism of stent thrombosis (LOE: C)
III (no benefit)	IVUS for routine lesion assessment is not recommended when revascularization with percutaneous coronary intervention or coronary artery bypass grafting is not being contemplated (LOE: C)

Data from Levine GN, Bates ER, Blankenship JC, et al 2011 ACCF/AHA/ SCAI Guideline for Percutaneous Coronary Intervention: a report of the American College of Cardiology Foundation/ American Heart Association Task Force on Practice Guidelines and the Society for Cardiovascular Angiography and Interventions. *Circulation* 2011;124:e574-e651.
ACCF/AHA/SCAI, American College of Cardiology Foundation/American Heart Association Force on Practice Guidelines/Society for Cardiovascular Angiography and Interventions; *IVUS*, intravascular ultrasound; *LOE*, level of evidence.

apposition is a common finding in patients with late and very late DES thrombosis in case-control studies, although the absolute risk of thrombosis with late acquired incomplete stent apposition is unclear because a significant relationship between thrombosis and this phenomenon has not been observed in prospective studies using routine serial IVUS. Given that mechanical and structural characteristics that in large part determine stent failure can be identified by IVUS and addressed by the operator, a strategy of IVUS-guided stent optimization has been proposed to improve clinical outcomes after stenting. Several prospective, randomized trials of IVUS-guided versus angiography-guided stent implantation were performed in the BMS era that used various criteria for optimal stent deployment. Although for the most part these trials did not demonstrate clinical benefit with IVUS, the trials were limited by the frequent failure to achieve adequate stent expansion in the patients randomly assigned to IVUS guidance. Despite this limitation, a treatment benefit was observed in the TULIP trial, which enrolled patients with angiographically complex disease, and in the AVID trial among patients with vessels 2.5 mm or greater in diameter and patients with high-grade stenosis before stenting. Meta-analysis of randomized trials showed a reduction in angiographic restenosis, repeat revascularization, and MACE, without an effect on myocardial infarction or death. In the DES era, a potential mortality benefit with IVUS-guided stent implantation was detected in observational registries, but these findings must be interpreted within the context of possibly unmeasured confounders. An appropriately powered randomized clinical trial to determine whether IVUS-directed PCI reduces stent thrombosis would be challenging to complete, given the infrequent incidence of this highly morbid complication.

REFERENCES

1. Roger VL, Go AS, Lloyd-Jones DM, et al. Heart disease and stroke statistics—2011 update: a report from the American Heart Association. *Circulation* 2011;123:e18-e209.
2. Colombo A, Hall P, Nakamura S, et al. Intracoronary stenting without anticoagulation accomplished with intravascular ultrasound guidance. *Circulation* 1995;91:1676-1688.
3. de Jaegere P, Mudra H, Figulla H, et al. Intravascular ultrasound-guided optimized stent deployment: immediate and 6 months clinical and angiographic results from the Multicenter Ultrasound Stenting in Coronaries Study (MUSIC Study). *Eur Heart J* 1998;19:1214-1223.
4. Frey AW, Hodgson JM, Muller C, et al. Ultrasound-guided strategy for provisional stenting with focal balloon combination catheter: results from the randomized Strategy for Intracoronary Ultrasound-guided PTCA and Stenting (SIPS) trial. *Circulation* 2000;102:2497-2502.
5. Mudra H, di Mario C, de Jaegere P, et al. Randomized comparison of coronary stent implantation under ultrasound or angiographic guidance to reduce stent restenosis (OPTICUS Study). *Circulation* 2001;104:1343-1349.
6. Gaster AL, Slothuus U, Larsen J, et al. Cost-effectiveness analysis of intravascular ultrasound guided percutaneous coronary intervention versus conventional percutaneous coronary intervention. *Scand Cardiovasc J* 2001;35:80-85.
7. Schiele F, Meneveau N, Vuillemenot A, et al. Impact of intravascular ultrasound guidance in stent deployment on 6-month restenosis rate: a multicenter, randomized study comparing two strategies—with and without intravascular ultrasound guidance. RESIST Study Group. REStenosis after Ivus guided STenting. *J Am Coll Cardiol* 1998;32:320-328.
8. Oemrawsingh PV, Mintz GS, Schalij MJ, et al. Intravascular ultrasound guidance improves angiographic and clinical outcome of stent implantation for long coronary artery stenoses: final results of a randomized comparison with angiographic guidance (TULIP Study). *Circulation* 2003;107:62-67.
9. Russo RJ, Silva PD, Teirstein PS, et al. A randomized controlled trial of angiography versus intravascular ultrasound-directed bare-metal coronary stent placement (the AVID Trial). *Circ Cardiovasc Interv* 2009;2:113-123.
10. Serruys PW, de Jaegere P, Kiemeneij F, et al. A comparison of balloon-expandable-stent implantation with balloon angioplasty in patients with coronary artery disease. Benestent Study Group. *N Engl J Med* 1994;331:489-495.
11. Fischman DL, Leon MB, Baim DS, et al. A randomized comparison of coronary-stent placement and balloon angioplasty in the treatment of coronary artery disease. Stent Restenosis Study Investigators. *N Engl J Med* 1994;331:496-501.
12. Kasaoka S, Tobis JM, Akiyama T, et al. Angiographic and intravascular ultrasound predictors of in-stent restenosis. *J Am Coll Cardiol* 1998;32:1630-1635.
13. Albiero R, Rau T, Schluter M, et al. Comparison of immediate and intermediate-term results of intravascular ultrasound versus angiography-guided Palmaz-Schatz stent implantation in matched lesions. *Circulation* 1997;96:2997-3005.
14. Blasini R, Neumann FJ, Schmitt C, et al. Comparison of angiography and intravascular ultrasound for the assessment of lumen size after coronary stent placement: impact of dilation pressures. *Cathet Cardiovasc Diagn* 1997;42:113-119.
15. Fitzgerald PJ, Oshima A, Hayase M, et al. Final results of the Can Routine Ultrasound Influence Stent Expansion (CRUISE) study. *Circulation* 2000;102:523-530.
16. Leon MB, Baim DS, Popma JJ, et al. A clinical trial comparing three antithrombotic-drug regimens after coronary-artery stenting. Stent Anticoagulation Restenosis Study Investigators. *N Engl J Med* 1998;339:1665-1671.
17. Orford JL, Denktas AE, Williams BA, et al. Routine intravascular ultrasound scanning guidance of coronary stenting is not associated with improved clinical outcomes. *Am Heart J* 2004;148:501-506.
18. Casella G, Klauss V, Ottani F, et al. Impact of intravascular ultrasound-guided stenting on long-term clinical outcome: a meta-analysis of available studies comparing intravascular ultrasound-guided and angiographically guided stenting. *Catheter Cardiovasc Interv* 2003;59:314-321.
19. Parise H, Maehara A, Stone GW, et al. Meta-analysis of randomized studies comparing intravascular ultrasound versus angiographic guidance of percutaneous coronary intervention in pre-drug-eluting stent era. *Am J Cardiol* 2011;107:374-382.
20. Gil RJ, Pawlowski T, Dudek D, et al. Comparison of angiographically guided direct stenting technique with direct stenting and optimal balloon angioplasty guided with intravascular ultrasound: the multicenter, randomized trial results. *Am Heart J* 2007;154:669-675.
21. Gaster AL, Slothuus Skjoldborg U, Larsen J, et al. Continued improvement of clinical outcome and cost effectiveness following intravascular ultrasound guided PCI: insights from a prospective, randomised study. *Heart* 2003;89:1043-1049.
22. Schiele F, Meneveau N, Seronde MF, et al. Medical costs of intravascular ultrasound optimization of stent deployment: results of the multicenter randomized "REStenosis after Intravascular ultrasound STenting" (RESIST) study. *Int J Cardiovasc Intervent* 2000;3:207-213.
23. Sigwart U, Puel J, Mirkovitch V, et al. Intravascular stents to prevent occlusion and restenosis after transluminal angioplasty. *N Engl J Med* 1987;316:701-706.
24. de Feyter PJ, DeScheerder I, van den Brand M, et al. Emergency stenting for refractory acute coronary artery occlusion during coronary angioplasty. *Am J Cardiol* 1990;66:1147-1150.
25. Schatz RA, Baim DS, Leon M, et al. Clinical experience with the Palmaz-Schatz coronary stent: initial results of a multicenter study. *Circulation* 1991;83:148-161.
26. Serruys PW, Strauss BH, Beatt KJ, et al. Angiographic follow-up after placement of a self-expanding coronary-artery stent. *N Engl J Med* 1991;324:13-17.
27. Cutlip DE, Baim DS, Ho KK, et al. Stent thrombosis in the modern era: a pooled analysis of multicenter coronary stent clinical trials. *Circulation* 2001;103:1967-1971.
28. Uren NG, Schwarzacher SP, Metz JA, et al. Predictors and outcomes of stent thrombosis: an intravascular ultrasound registry. *Eur Heart J* 2002;23:124-132.
29. Cheneau E, Leborgne L, Mintz GS, et al. Predictors of subacute stent thrombosis: results of a systematic intravascular ultrasound study. *Circulation* 2003;108:43-47.
30. Mueller C, Hodgson JM, Schindler C, et al. Cost-effectiveness of intracoronary ultrasound for percutaneous coronary interventions. *Am J Cardiol* 2003;91:143-147.
31. Morice MC, Serruys PW, Sousa JE, et al. A randomized comparison of a sirolimus-eluting stent with a standard stent for coronary revascularization. *N Engl J Med* 2002;346:1773-1780.
32. Moses JW, Leon MB, Popma JJ, et al. Sirolimus-eluting stents versus standard stents in patients with stenosis in a native coronary artery. *N Engl J Med* 2003;349:1315-1323.
33. Stone GW, Ellis SG, Cox DA, et al. A polymer-based, paclitaxel-eluting stent in patients with coronary artery disease. *N Engl J Med* 2004;350:221-231.
34. Dangas GD, Claessen BE, Caixeta A, et al. In-stent restenosis in the drug-eluting stent era. *J Am Coll Cardiol* 2010;56:1897-1907.
35. Kuntz RE, Safian RD, Carrozza JP, et al. The importance of acute luminal diameter in determining restenosis after coronary atherectomy or stenting. *Circulation* 1992;86:1827-1835.
36. Kuntz RE, Gibson CM, Nobuyoshi M, et al. Generalized model of restenosis after conventional balloon angioplasty, stenting and directional atherectomy. *J Am Coll Cardiol* 1993;21:15-25.
37. Mintz GS. Features and parameters of drug-eluting stent deployment discoverable by intravascular ultrasound. *Am J Cardiol* 2007;100:26M-35M.
38. Sonoda S, Morino Y, Ako J, et al. Impact of final stent dimensions on long-term results following sirolimus-eluting stent implantation: serial intravascular ultrasound analysis from the SIRIUS trial. *J Am Coll Cardiol* 2004;43:1959-1963.
39. Hong MK, Mintz GS, Lee CW, et al. Intravascular ultrasound predictors of angiographic restenosis after sirolimus-eluting stent implantation. *Eur Heart J* 2006;27:1305-1310.
40. Doi H, Maehara A, Mintz GS, et al. Impact of post-intervention minimal stent area on 9-month follow-up patency of paclitaxel-eluting stents: an integrated intravascular ultrasound analysis from the TAXUS IV, V, and VI and TAXUS ATLAS Workhorse, Long Lesion, and Direct Stent Trials. *JACC Cardiovasc Interv* 2009;2:1269-1275.
41. Takebayashi H, Kobayashi Y, Mintz GS, et al. Intravascular ultrasound assessment of lesions with target vessel failure after sirolimus-eluting stent implantation. *Am J Cardiol* 2005;95:498-502.
42. Cheneau E, Pichard AD, Satler LF, et al. Intravascular ultrasound stent area of sirolimus-eluting stents and its impact on late outcome. *Am J Cardiol* 2005;95:1240-1242.
43. Kang SJ, Mintz GS, Park DW, et al. Mechanisms of in-stent restenosis after drug-eluting stent implantation: intravascular ultrasound analysis. *Circ Cardiovasc Interv* 2011;4:9-14.
44. Gerber RT, Latib A, Ielasi A, et al. Defining a new standard for IVUS optimized drug eluting stent implantation: the PRAVIO study. *Catheter Cardiovasc Interv* 2009;74:348-356.
45. Sakurai R, Ako J, Morino Y, et al. Predictors of edge stenosis following sirolimus-eluting stent deployment (a quantitative intravascular ultrasound analysis from the SIRIUS trial). *Am J Cardiol* 2005;96:1251-1253.
46. Takebayashi H, Mintz GS, Carlier SG, et al. Nonuniform strut distribution correlates with more neointimal hyperplasia after sirolimus-eluting stent implantation. *Circulation* 2004;110:3430-3434.
47. Lemos PA, Saia F, Ligthart JM, et al. Coronary restenosis after sirolimus-eluting stent implantation: morphological description and mechanistic analysis from a consecutive series of cases. *Circulation* 2003;108:257-260.
48. Sianos G, Hofma S, Ligthart JM, et al. Stent fracture and restenosis in the drug-eluting stent era. *Catheter Cardiovasc Interv* 2004;61:111-116.
49. Lee MS, Jurewitz D, Aragon J, et al. Stent fracture associated with drug-eluting stents: clinical characteristics and implications. *Catheter Cardiovasc Interv* 2007;69:387-394.
50. de Ribamar Costa Jr J, Mintz GS, Carlier SG, et al. Intravascular ultrasound assessment of drug-eluting stent expansion. *Am Heart J* 2007;153:297-303.
51. de Ribamar Costa Jr J, Mintz GS, Carlier SG, et al. Intravascular ultrasonic assessment of stent diameters derived from manufacturer's compliance charts. *Am J Cardiol* 2005;96:74-78.
52. Fujii K, Mintz GS, Kobayashi Y, et al. Contribution of stent underexpansion to recurrence after sirolimus-eluting stent implantation for in-stent restenosis. *Circulation* 2004;109:1085-1088.
53. Kim SW, Mintz GS, Escolar E, et al. An intravascular ultrasound analysis of the mechanisms of restenosis comparing drug-eluting stents with brachytherapy. *Am J Cardiol* 2006;97:1292-1298.
54. Fujii K, Carlier SG, Mintz GS, et al. Stent underexpansion and residual reference segment stenosis are related to stent thrombosis after sirolimus-eluting stent implantation: an intravascular ultrasound study. *J Am Coll Cardiol* 2005;45:995-998.
55. Okabe T, Mintz GS, Buch AN, et al. Intravascular ultrasound parameters associated with stent thrombosis after drug-eluting stent deployment. *Am J Cardiol* 2007;100:615-620.
56. Choi SY, Witzenbichler B, Maehara A, et al. Intravascular ultrasound findings of early stent thrombosis after primary percutaneous intervention in acute myocardial infarction: a Harmonizing Outcomes with Revascularization and Stents in Acute Myocardial Infarction (HORIZONS-AMI) substudy. *Circ Cardiovasc Interv* 2011;4:239-247.
57. Joner M, Finn AV, Farb A, et al. Pathology of drug-eluting stents in humans: delayed healing and late thrombotic risk. *J Am Coll Cardiol* 2006;48:193-202.
58. Finn AV, Nakazawa G, Joner M, et al. Vascular responses to drug eluting stents: importance of delayed healing. *Arterioscler Thromb Vasc Biol* 2007;27:1500-1510.
59. Finn AV, Joner M, Nakazawa G, et al. Pathological correlates of late drug-eluting stent thrombosis: strut coverage as a marker of endothelialization. *Circulation* 2007;115:2435-2441.
60. Iakovou I, Schmidt T, Bonizzoni E, et al. Incidence, predictors, and outcome of thrombosis after successful implantation of drug-eluting stents. *JAMA* 2005;293:2126-2130.
61. Kuchulakanti PK, Chu WW, Torguson R, et al. Correlates and long-term outcomes of angiographically proven stent thrombosis with sirolimus- and paclitaxel-eluting stents. *Circulation* 2006; 113(8):1108-1113.
62. Cook S, Wenaweser P, Togni M, et al. Incomplete stent apposition and very late stent thrombosis after drug-eluting stent implantation. *Circulation* 2007;115:2426-2434.
63. Cook S, Ladich E, Nakazawa G, et al. Correlation of intravascular ultrasound findings with histopathological analysis of thrombus aspirates in patients with very late drug-eluting stent thrombosis. *Circulation* 2009;120:391-399.
64. Hong MK, Mintz GS, Lee CW, et al. Late stent malapposition after drug-eluting stent implantation: an intravascular ultrasound analysis with long-term follow-up. *Circulation* 2006;113:414-419.
65. Kang SJ, Mintz GS, Park DW, et al. Late and very late drug-eluting stent malapposition: serial 2-year quantitative IVUS analysis. *Circ Cardiovasc Interv* 2010;3:335-340.
66. Siqueira DA, Abizaid AA, de Ribamar Costa J, et al. Late incomplete apposition after drug-eluting stent implantation: incidence and potential for adverse clinical outcomes. *Eur Heart J* 2007;28:1304-1309.
67. Cook S, Eshtehardi P, Kalesan B, et al. Impact of incomplete stent apposition on long-term clinical outcome after drug-eluting stent implantation. *Eur Heart J* 2012;33:1334-1343.
68. Steinberg DH, Mintz GS, Mandinov L, et al. Long-term impact of routinely detected early and late incomplete stent apposition: an integrated intravascular ultrasound analysis of the TAXUS IV, V, and VI and TAXUS ATLAS workhorse, long lesion, and direct stent studies. *JACC Cardiovasc Interv* 2010;3:486-494.
69. Roy P, Steinberg DH, Sushinsky SJ, et al. The potential clinical utility of intravascular ultrasound guidance in patients undergoing percutaneous coronary intervention with drug-eluting stents. *Eur Heart J* 2008;29:1851-1857.
70. Hur SH, Kang SJ, Kim YH, et al. Impact of intravascular ultrasound-guided percutaneous coronary intervention on long-term clinical outcomes in a real world population. *Catheter Cardiovasc Interv* 2011 Jul 29. doi: 10.1002/ccd.23279. [Epub ahead of print]
71. Park SJ, Kim YH, Park DW, et al. Impact of intravascular ultrasound guidance on long-term mortality in stenting for unprotected left main coronary artery stenosis. *Circ Cardiovasc Interv* 2009;2:167-177.
72. Claessen BE, Mehran R, Mintz GS, et al. Impact of intravascular ultrasound imaging on early and late clinical outcomes following percutaneous coronary intervention with drug-eluting stents. *JACC Cardiovasc Interv* 2011;4:974-981.
73. Jakabcin J, Spacek R, Bystron M, et al. Long-term health outcome and mortality evaluation after invasive coronary treatment using drug eluting stents with or without the IVUS guidance: randomized control trial. HOME DES IVUS. *Catheter Cardiovasc Interv* 2010;75:578-583.
74. Colombo A. AVIO: *a prospective, randomized trial of intravascular ultrasound-guided compared to angiography-guided stent implantation in complex coronary lesions. Presented TCT 2010: Transcatheter Cardiovascular Therapeutics 22nd Annual Scientific Symposium,* Washington, DC; 2010.
75. Levine GN, Bates ER, Blankenship JC, et al. 2011 ACCF/AHA/SCAI Guideline for Percutaneous Coronary Intervention: a report of the American College of Cardiology Foundation/American Heart Association Task Force on Practice Guidelines and the Society for Cardiovascular Angiography and Interventions. *Circulation* 2011;124:e574-e651.

CHAPTER 10

Optical Coherence Tomography: Stent Implantation and Evaluation

HIROSADA YAMAMOTO | MARCO A. COSTA

KEY POINTS

- Optical coherence tomography uses light in the near-infrared spectrum, providing substantially greater axial and lateral resolution compared with intravascular ultrasound.

- Frequency-domain optical coherence tomography allows for rapid imaging acquisition with a small volume of contrast (<15 mL) and has eliminated the need for balloon occlusion.

- Several imaging artifacts can occur during performance of optical coherence tomography, including attenuation from blood; sew-up artifact; the "merry-go-round," "sunflower," and "fold-over" effects; and "blooming" of stent struts owing to image saturation.

- The sharp delineation of the lumen contour allows for easy image interpretation and fully automated lumen area measurement as well as the evaluation of stent struts, with excellent interobserver and intraobserver reliability.

- Edge dissections and tissue prolapse are frequently detected by optical coherence tomography after stent implantation, and the clinical sequelae of these findings require prospective evaluation.

- Optical coherence tomography is especially sensitive compared with intravascular ultrasound in the evaluation of stent struts, including malapposition and tissue coverage.

- Optical coherence tomography is likely to become the intravascular imaging technique of choice for the evaluation of acute and longer-term results of bioresorbable polymeric stents.

Introduction

Intravascular imaging plays an important role in percutaneous coronary intervention (PCI). Intravascular optical coherence tomography (OCT) is a catheter-based invasive imaging modality that uses infrared light rather than ultrasound. In 1991, the addition of transverse scanning (B-scan) enabled two-dimensional imaging of the retina.[1] Fujimoto named this technique OCT, and it rapidly expanded to numerous biomedical and clinical applications. In this chapter, we describe basic OCT physical principles, image acquisition, and the evaluation of stent implantation and follow-up.

Basic Principles of Optical Coherence Tomography

The light source of intravascular OCT uses a bandwidth in the near-infrared spectrum. Although longer wavelengths provide deeper tissue penetration, the optimal choice of wavelength in an arterial vessel is also determined by tissue absorption characteristics and the refractive index of the interface between the catheter and vessel wall. Current OCT systems use a central wavelength of approximately 1300 nm, providing up to 3 mm of penetration, depending on tissue properties.

AXIAL AND LATERAL RESOLUTION

The OCT image is formed by the backscattering of light from the vessel wall (i.e., the time it takes for emitted light to travel between the target tissue and back to the lens), producing an echo time delay with a measurable signal intensity or magnitude. Multiple axial scans (A-lines) are continuously acquired as the image wire rotates; a full revolution creates a complete cross-section of the vessel. The axial resolution of OCT (minimum distance in the beam direction that can be identified as separate echoes) ranges from 12 to 18 μm and is substantially greater than the 150- to 200-μm axial resolution of intravascular ultrasound (IVUS). Similarly, with catheter-based OCT, the lateral resolution (ability to discern two adjacent objects [i.e., perpendicular to the imaging beam]) is typically 20 to 90 μm compared with 150 to 300 μm for IVUS.

TIME-DOMAIN AND FREQUENCY-DOMAIN OPTICAL COHERENCE TOMOGRAPHY

Two different technologies can be used to obtain OCT images: time-domain OCT, the first generation technique, and the newer frequency-domain OCT (Figure 10-1). Both systems use a reference arm and an interferometer to detect echo time delays of light. The interferometer uses a beam splitter, dividing the light into a measurement arm (tissue sample) and a reference arm. The reference arm in time-domain OCT is mechanically scanned by a moving mirror to produce a time-varying time delay. In frequency-domain OCT, because the light source is frequency swept, the interference of the two light beams (tissue and reference) oscillates according to the frequency difference. In both systems, the interference of the signal ultimately provides amplitude and frequency data. Frequency-domain OCT has the advantage of an improved signal-to-noise ratio allowing extremely fast-scanning laser systems to increase imaging speed, while delivering comparable or improved image quality compared with the earlier time-domain systems.

Optical Coherence Tomography–Guided Coronary Intervention

IMAGE ACQUISITION

The first commercially available OCT system was the LightLab M2x OCT Imaging System (LightLab, Westford, Massachusetts). In this time-domain OCT system, images are recorded by an ImageWire (LightLab), which is a general purpose, single-mode, fiberoptic wire that rotates inside a fluid-filled polymer tube (Figure 10-2). A microlens assembly at the distal end is approximately 1 mm in length and 125 μm in diameter (i.e., similar to the fiber itself). This assembly focuses and reflects the light beam at approximately 80 degrees from the fiber's axis to allow circumferential imaging of the vessel. The wire is attached to an automated pullback engine integrated with the console. The external diameter of the ImageWire is 0.019 inch, and it is fused to a short segment of a standard 0.014-inch guide wire at the distal end. In contrast to IVUS, OCT requires clearing or flushing of blood from the vessel lumen during imaging because any residual red blood cells cause significant signal attenuation. The occlusive technique is strongly recommended when a time-domain OCT system is used. With this approach, coronary blood flow is interrupted by the

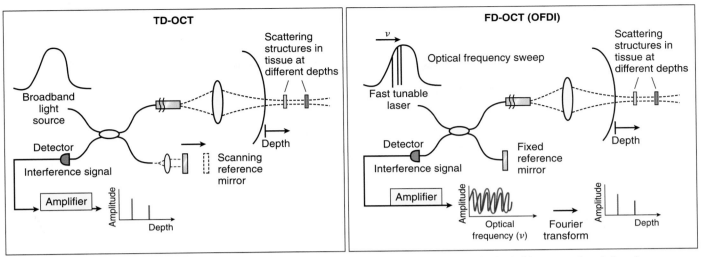

Figure 10-1 Schemes of time-domain OCT *(TD-OCT)* and frequency-domain OCT *(FD-OCT)*. *OFDI,* Optical frequency domain imaging.

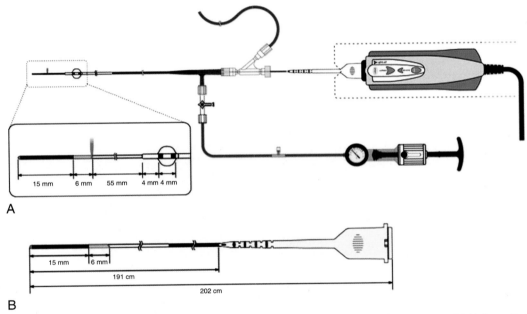

Figure 10-2 Representative images of a time-domain OCT system. **A,** Constructed time-domain OCT catheter system with Helios occlusion balloon catheter and ImageWire. **B,** Overview of an Imagewire.

gentle inflation of an occlusion balloon proximal to the segment to be imaged. A crystalloid solution (usually Ringer lactate) is flushed through the endhole of an over-the-wire low-pressure occlusion balloon catheter (Helios; Goodman, Nagoya, Japan) at a flow rate of 0.5 to 1.0 mL/sec. The vessel occlusion time should be adjusted according to patient condition and electrocardiogram changes (e.g., ST segment elevation or QRS duration) with the infusion set to stop automatically after a maximum of 30 seconds to avoid hemodynamic instability or arrhythmias. A power injector is recommended for injection of the flush solution at a constant rate.[2] This occlusive technique has several limitations. First, size mismatch between the balloon and vessel may lead to inadequate clearing of the lumen, resulting in insufficient image quality. Second, ostial and proximal lesions (<15 mm from ostium) cannot be assessed because of the presence of the occlusive balloon. To overcome these limitations, nonocclusive techniques without proximal balloon occlusion have been proposed.[3] For a nonocclusive technique, iodinated contrast agent is

recommended both for its low arrhythmogenic potential and for its high viscosity.

The frequency-domain OCT system (C7 XR Imaging System; LightLab) is commercially available in Asia, the European Union, and North and South America (Figure 10-3, A). The optical fiber is encapsulated within a rotating torque wire built within a rapid-exchange 2.6F catheter compatible with a 6F guide (Figure 10-3, B and C). The frequency-domain OCT catheter is first positioned over a regular coronary guide wire, distal to the region of interest. The imaging starting point can be identified by the most proximal radiopaque marker, which rests 10 mm distal to the starting position of the OCT beam. Imaging is performed during injection of contrast medium to ensure complete blood clearance. The infusion rate of contrast medium is usually set to 3 to 6 mL/sec for the left coronary artery and 3 to 5 mL/sec for the right coronary artery, depending on vessel runoff and size. The pullback can start automatically when blood clearance is recognized or can be manually activated. The

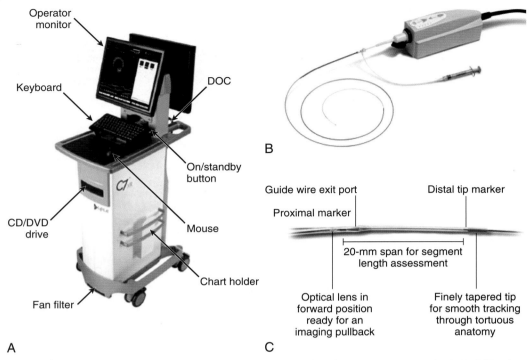

Figure 10-3 Representative images of a frequency-domain OCT (FD-OCT) system. **A,** Representative FD-OCT console. **B,** FD-OCT catheter (Dragonfly). **C,** The tip of an FD-OCT catheter.

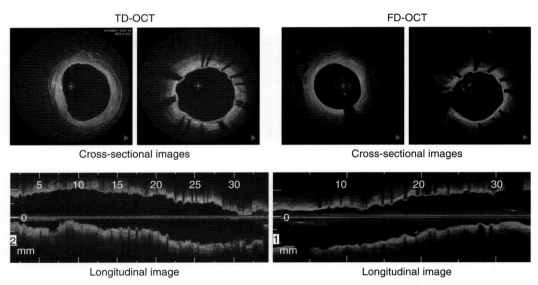

Figure 10-4 Representative images of time-domain OCT *(TD-OCT)* and frequency-domain OCT *(FD-OCT)*. *Left,* Longitudinal and cross-sectional images of TD-OCT. *Right,* Longitudinal and cross-sectional images of FD-OCT. A high pullback speed minimizes heart motion artifacts on the FD-OCT longitudinal image.

pullback speed can reach 20 to 40 mm/sec. An acquisition speed of 20 mm/sec enables the acquisition of 200 cross-sectional image frames over 4 to 6 cm of coronary artery segments in 3.5 seconds with a total infused volume of less than 15 mL of contrast medium per pullback. This capability of frequency-domain OCT may represent a powerful advantage for its use in PCI, allowing quick evaluation of the stent and of the landing zones. However, in contrast to the time-domain OCT system, the frequency-domain OCT catheter is a rapid-exchange system, and as a result the guide wire shadow hides a part of the lumen image (Figure 10-4).

Vessel and Stent Assessment

OCT provides accurate assessment of the target lumen geometry and extent and severity of disease. The fundamental parameters to guide interventional procedures include minimal luminal area, plaque rupture, thrombus, reference luminal diameter and area, percentage lumen obstruction, stent apposition, stent expansion, minimal stent cross-sectional area, plaque prolapse, and dissection (Figures 10-5 and 10-6).[4] These parameters are based on the evaluation of the lumen-wall or lumen-wall-stent interface. Although the clinical impact of OCT-detected plaque protrusion and stent-edge dissections

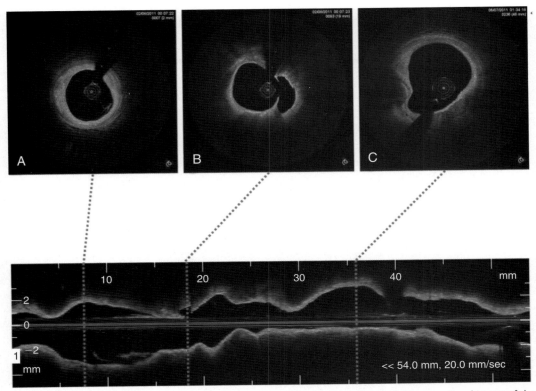

Figure 10-5 Preprocedure frequency-domain OCT image in a patient with acute coronary syndrome. **A,** Cross-sectional image of the distal reference of lesion. **B,** Culprit site of lesion depicting plaque rupture and its thin-cap thickness (30 μm). **C,** Cross-sectional image of the proximal reference of lesion.

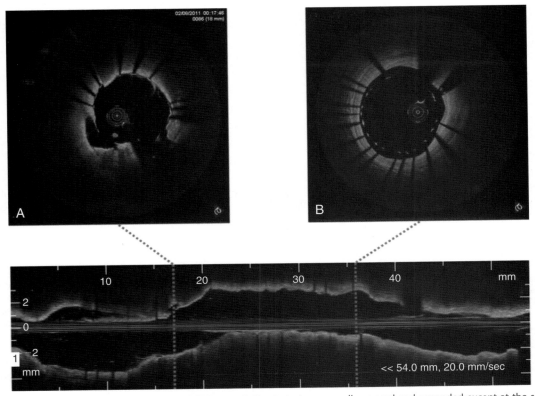

Figure 10-6 Post–stent implantation frequency-domain OCT image. **A,** Stent struts were well apposed and expanded except at the site of the ruptured plaque ("cavity"). **B,** Cross-sectional image of the proximal site of the stent. Many malapposed stent struts were observed.

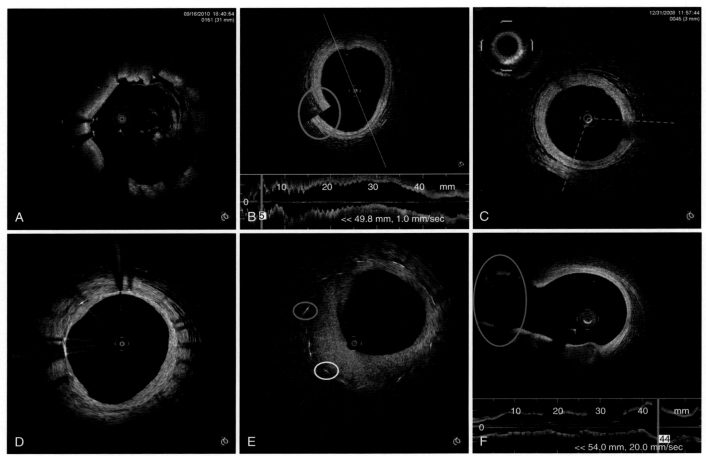

Figure 10-7   Most frequently observed artifacts. **A,** Incomplete blood displacement, resulting in light attenuation. **B,** Sew-up artifact, the result of rapid wire or vessel movement along one frame formation, causing misalignment of the image. *Red circle* indicates sew-up site. **C,** Air bubbles, formed inside the catheter, produce an attenuated image along the corresponding arc. Detail reveals the bubbles (bright structures) between 4 o'clock and 7 o'clock. **D,** Saturation artifact. Some scan lines have a streaked appearance. **E,** Eccentric wire can distort stent reflection orientation. The struts align toward the imaging wire and are elongated. *Red circle* indicates "merry-go-round" artifact; *white circle* indicates normal blooming. **F,** Fold-over artifact *(red circle)* (frequency-domain OCT system). Longitudinal view demonstrates that the cross-section is located at the level of a side branch *(red line)*.

is unknown, prior pathology and IVUS studies have suggested the risk of stent thrombosis associated with malapposition.[5]

Safety of Optical Coherence Tomography

Barlis and colleagues[6] evaluated the safety of time-domain OCT in 468 patients from six centers. Approximately half of patients underwent time-domain OCT using a nonocclusive technique. Procedure-related complications occurred in only 2.1% of cases, and there were no major adverse cardiac events during or within 24 hours after OCT examination. In our own series, including 155 consecutive frequency-domain OCT imaging pullbacks, there were no episodes of vasospasm, distal embolization, thrombosis, arrhythmias, or chest pain noted during or after the procedure.

Imaging Artifacts

Several imaging artifacts are common to both OCT and IVUS, whereas other artifacts are unique to OCT imaging systems.[7] Most of these artifacts do not substantially compromise clinical interpretation of the image if they are restricted to a few discontinuous frames, although they may render imprecise the assessment of plaque characteristics or measurements. Important artifacts to consider during stent evaluation include the following:

1. *Residual blood.* If red cell density is high, the OCT light beam becomes attenuated and unfocused (Figure 10-7, A), and this reduces the brightness of the vessel wall. The presence of diluted blood does not appear to affect area measurements if the lumen surface can be clearly defined.
2. *Sew-up artifact.* This artifact is the result of rapid artery or imaging wire movement in imaging formation of one frame, leading to single point misalignment of the lumen border (Figure 10-7, B). The faster speed of frequency-domain OCT has significantly minimized the frequency and impact of sew-up artifacts compared with the earlier time-domain OCT systems.
3. *Bubble artifact.* This artifact occurs when small air bubbles are formed in the silicon lubricant used to reduce friction between the sheath and the revolving optic fiber in time-domain OCT systems. It can attenuate the signal along a region of the vessel wall, and images with this artifact are unsuitable for tissue characterization (Figure 10-7, C).
4. *Artifacts related to eccentric wire position.* Eccentricity of the OCT wire in the vessel lumen can influence many aspects of the image interpretation. This phenomenon is likely secondary to imaging sweep speed; it is more pronounced with an eccentric imaging wire position, leading to longer distance between each A-line

and consequently decreasing the lateral resolution, and has been dubbed the "merry-go-round" effect (Figure 10-7, *E*). In addition, the reflection from metallic stent struts align toward the imaging wire as a by-product of rotational scanning, akin to sunflowers aligning to the sun, resulting in the "sunflower" effect.[8] This artifact is pronounced with eccentric wire position because it can display strut reflections almost perpendicular to the lumen surface in oblique regions from the wire. The larger size of the frequency-domain OCT catheter has minimized these artifacts.

5. *Saturation artifact.* This phenomenon occurs when light reflected from a highly specular surface (e.g., stent struts) produces signals with amplitudes that exceed the dynamic range of the data acquisition system (Figure 10-7, *D*). This artifact should be kept in mind when defining the stent surface. Our group measured the average "normal" blooming of a stainless steel stent from 2250 struts in 471 cross-sectional OCT images.[9] The mean blooming thickness was 37 ± 8 μm. These values are important particularly for malapposition quantification because the blooming thickness value needs to be considered in addition to stent and polymer thickness when assessing the distance from the inner stent surface to the lumen border.

6. *Nonuniform rotational distortion.* This artifact is the result of variation in the rotational speed of the spinning optical fiber. It is usually produced by vessel tortuosity or by an imperfection in the torque wire or sheath interfering with smooth rotation of the optical fiber, which can result in focal image loss or shape distortion.

7. *Foldover artifact.* This artifact is more specific to the new generation of frequency-domain OCT. It is the consequence of "phase wrapping" or "aliasing" along the Fourier transformation when structure signals are reflected from outside the system's field of view. This artifact typically occurs when imaging side branches or large vessels (Figure 10-7, *F*).

🔹 Stent Analysis and Evaluation

The high spatial resolution of OCT, combined with the blood-free environment, provides substantial advantages for the study of coronary stents compared with technology such as IVUS.[7] Detailed stent strut evaluations can be performed, in vivo, with high interobserver and intraobserver reliabilities.[10] OCT can define important parameters of baseline stent implantation, such as the measurement of stent area and diameters, the detection of dissections, and stent strut malapposition. OCT enables detailed evaluation of tissue coverage during follow-up.[11] Intravascular OCT may become the modality of choice for stent analysis in both clinical practice and research studies.

Z-OFFSET

The Z-offset is a manually adjustable image calibration that is important for accurate measurement. The Z-offset is the zero-point setting of the system and corrects for the difference in the optical path length between the sample and reference arm.[7] Within the frequency-domain OCT system, the semitransparent catheter around the optic fiber is more suitable for direct calibration. When calibrating the image, it is assumed that the calibration uniformly affects the entire image, provided that the wire is centrally located in the lumen. It is important to ensure that the Z-offset is corrected on individual cross-sections selected by operators to guide PCI in the catheterization laboratory. We found that a 1% change in the magnitude of the ideal Z-offset can result in a 6% to 7% error in diameter and a 12% to 14% error in area measurements.[7] Small changes in magnitude can also amplify the contour distortion, which may result in misjudgment of the image. This is mostly true in cases in which the imaging wire in time-domain OCT systems is located in an eccentric position.[8]

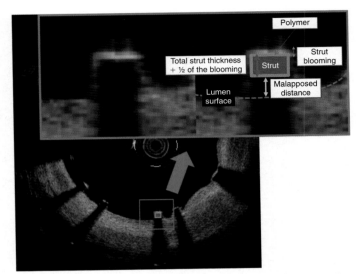

Figure 10-8 Malapposition quantification. The cross-sectional image illustrates various levels of stent strut protrusion. The strut located at 6 o'clock is malapposed (see detail). Malapposition is defined when the measured distance from the surface of the blooming to the lumen contour is higher than the total thickness of the stent strut + polymer + one half of the blooming. (The stent surface theoretically should be located at one half the distance of the blooming thickness.)

ASSESSMENT OF OPTICAL COHERENCE TOMOGRAPHY STENT IMAGES AT THE LEVEL OF A SINGLE FRAME

Stent Strut Appearance by Optical Coherence Tomography

Stent struts have a unique feature in OCT. Most commercially available stents, whether bare metal or drug-eluting, have a metallic frame. Light fully reflects on the surface of stent struts creating a hyperbright signal, referred to as "blooming" (Figure 10-8). Because of the inability of light to pass through metal, a shadow can also be seen behind the blooming artifact. The operator must be aware of this phenomenon to avoid overcalling the presence of stent malapposition. Both features (blooming and shadowing) help in the identification of individual struts, a step needed for the qualitative and quantitative analysis of OCT images.

Stent Expansion and Malapposition

The evaluation of stent expansion is particularly important in the clinical setting because underexpansion has been associated with stent failure. Incomplete stent apposition is also correlated to the development of stent thrombosis.[5,12] Stent strut malapposition is defined as the lack of contact between stent struts and the underlying vessel wall in a nonbifurcated segment (Figure 10-9, *A*). Since OCT can show only the echolucent surface of the strut because of limited penetration through the metal, strut and polymer thickness should be considered in determining apposition for each type of stent design. Malapposition is confirmed when the distance from the surface of the blooming to the lumen contour is higher than the total thickness of the stent strut plus polymer plus one half of the blooming (because the stent surface should theoretically be located at one half the distance of the blooming thickness) (see Figure 10-8). The thickness of the stent strut and polymer according to the device manufacturer must be known for each particular stent type for accurate malapposition assessment.

OCT is more sensitive and accurate for stent malapposition detection compared with IVUS. Although the concept of OCT evaluation is similar to that of IVUS on a cross-sectional level, the blood-free

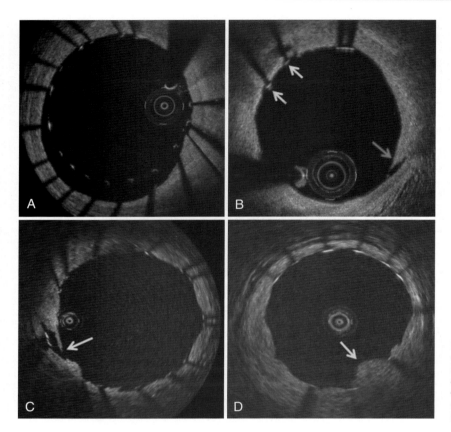

Figure 10-9 OCT findings at stent implantation. **A,** Under-expanded stent with malapposed struts. **B,** Edge dissection. Dissection flap *(red arrow)* and stent struts *(yellow arrows)* are observed. **C,** Dissection in stented segment. There is disruption of the luminal vessel surface between stent struts *(yellow arrow).* **D,** Tissue prolapse between stent struts *(yellow arrow).*

environment obtained with OCT creates a sharp interface between the vessel wall and stent strut.[13] The stent contour can be traced using the detected stent struts as anchor points and interpolating the tracing in areas with absences of stent struts. Fully automated stent segmentation algorithms are currently being developed.

Dissections

Edge dissection is defined as a disruption of the luminal vessel surface in the edge segment, within 5 mm proximal and distal to the stented region (Figure 10-9, *B*). Dissection within the stented segment is a disruption of the luminal vessel surface, with a visible dissection flap in the segment covered by the stent struts (Figure 10-9, *C*). Endothelial integrity is important in preventing thrombus deposition, and data from pathology have linked the disruption of vessel continuity to stent thrombosis.[14] In 73 consecutive patients evaluated by OCT imaging immediately after stent implantation, edge and intrastent dissections were observed in 26.3% and 87.5% of vessels imaged; however, these were not associated with clinical events during the hospitalization.[15] These rates are significantly higher compared with rates of edge dissections detected by IVUS (10.7% in one study[16]). In our series, stent edge dissection was observed in 32.5% of target vessels. The clinical significance of edge dissections identified by OCT needs to be addressed by prospective trials; however, many of these dissections are left untreated and appear to be benign.

Tissue Prolapse

The protrusion of tissue between adjacent stent struts toward the lumen without disruption of the continuity of the luminal vessel surface is called tissue prolapse (Figure 10-9, *D*). Data obtained from IVUS studies have noted tissue prolapse rates ranging from 16.6% to 35% after stent implantation.[17] Given the improved assessment of the

stent segment by OCT, this imaging technology is able to detect some amount of tissue prolapse in almost all stented segments.[15] This finding is similar to observations on postmortem evaluation.[18] Similar to edge dissections, the clinical impact of OCT-detected tissue prolapse immediately after stenting needs to be investigated more thoroughly.

ASSESSMENT OF OPTICAL COHERENCE TOMOGRAPHY STENT IMAGES AT THE LEVEL OF THE STENT STRUT

Stent Strut Classification

Stent struts are classified on OCT into four main categories: covered-embedded, covered-protruding (disturbing lumen contour but covered), uncovered-apposed, and uncovered-malapposed (Figure 10-10).[19] A semiautomatic stent contour algorithm can be used to apply 360 radial cords for detailed quantification of neointimal hyperplasia thickness at every degree of the cross-section. Strut coverage is qualitatively assessed for the presence of any tissue that resembles neointimal hyperplasia.

Determining Malapposition

If a strut is classified as uncovered, the distance between the superficial reflection and the lumen contour is subsequently measured to assess for malapposition. A stent strut is classified as malapposed if the measured distance is greater than the nominal thickness of the stent strut. The real position of the inner surface of the stent strut falls in the center of the blooming. Two methodologies have been used for quantitative strut level assessment. The first method consists of measuring the distance from the center of the blooming to the vessel

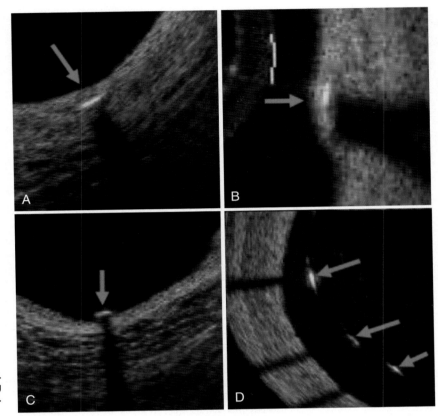

Figure 10-10 Stent strut coverage OCT classification. **A,** Covered-embedded strut *(arrow).* **B,** Covered-protruding strut *(arrow).* **C,** Uncovered-apposed strut *(arrow).* **D,** Uncovered-malapposed strut *(arrows).*

wall.[20,21] The second method consists of measuring the distance from the inner surface of the blooming to the vessel wall and correcting for half of the thickness of the blooming (18 μm).[8] We favor the latter method because of its high interobserver agreement and less variability because defining the center of the bright strut reflection is prone to error.[22]

SPECIAL SITUATIONS

Bifurcations

The evaluation of bifurcated segments demands special attention because the struts located in the ostium of the side branch are floating and not apposed to the vessel wall. The longitudinal reconstruction of the vessel may help in defining the limits of the bifurcation. Kyono and coworkers[23] proposed a methodology for bifurcation assessment that takes into consideration the opening angle of the side branch ostium in cross-sectional OCT images. To evaluate the axial tissue distribution after stent implantation, these investigators divided the segment of interest into three distinct regions. Using this methodology, they reported a variable pattern of strut coverage in the bifurcation among different stent technologies.

Overlap

Overlapping stents are readily identified by OCT as a two-layer segment; however, a precise classification of the layers in a two-dimensional image is impossible. The Optical Coherence Tomography for DES Safety (ODESSA) study was the first prospective trial using OCT to assess overlapping stents in human coronary arteries.[22] Among 250 stented segments with no detectable neointimal

hyperplasia by IVUS, 20 segments had neointimal coverage ranging from 67% to 100% by OCT.[24] In contrast to the relatively uniform lack of neointimal hyperplasia detected by IVUS, OCT revealed a highly heterogeneous response to DES, which varied even within the same cross-sectional image.

🔹 Future Considerations

OCT possesses the necessary properties (image speed, resolution, accuracy, and ease of use) to become the standard invasive imaging modality in the cardiac catheterization laboratory. OCT is likely to play a critical role in assessment of biodegradable polymeric stents, such as the everolimus-eluting bioresorbable vascular scaffold (Abbott Vascular, Santa Clara, California),[25] given the limited ability of IVUS to image polymeric materials, especially measuring of the stent length at baseline post-procedure and findings on follow-up.[26] In this situation, quantitative coronary angiography incurs systematic underestimation, and solid-state IVUS incurs random error. Bioresorbable vascular scaffold struts are seen as "boxes" with clear delineation by OCT of strut borders at implantation, allowing assessment of stent integrity, apposition, eccentricity, and stent degradation and neointima formation at follow-up. Faster laser sources enable extremely high imaging pullback speeds at high frame rates and may ultimately make three-dimensional OCT reconstruction part of routine image interpretation (Figure 10-11). Further developments in software to allow automated identification of the site of minimal lumen area, lesion length, and reference vessel diameter are critical to expedite and facilitate guidance of PCI based on OCT images. As a light-based technology, OCT will continue to evolve quickly, and ongoing hardware and software development will make the method even more attractive for clinicians.

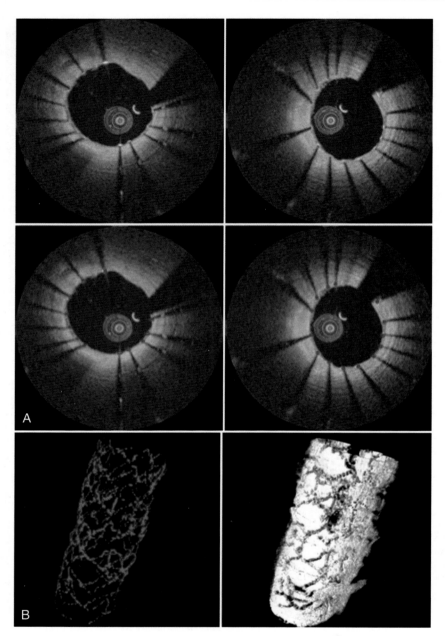

Figure 10-11 Automatic stent detection from OCT pull-back sequences. **A,** Representative frames from a pullback *(top row)* and corresponding detected stents overlaid on original data *(red, bottom row).* **B,** After serial two-dimensional detection, stents are reconstructed in three dimensions by stacking up the detected stents. A surface rendering of the stent is shown on the *left,* which is fused with a volume rendering of the original OCT data to create the three-dimensional reconstruction shown on the *right.*

REFERENCES

1. Brezinski ME, Tearney GJ, Bouma BE, et al. Optical coherence tomography for optical biopsy: properties and demonstration of vascular pathology. *Circulation* 1996;93:1206-1213.
2. Prati F, Regar E, Mintz GS, et al. Expert review document on methodology, terminology, and clinical applications of optical coherence tomography: physical principles, methodology of image acquisition, and clinical application for assessment of coronary arteries and atherosclerosis. *Eur Heart J* 2010;31:401-415.
3. Prati F, Cera M, Ramazzotti V, et al. Safety and feasibility of a new non-occlusive technique for facilitated intracoronary optical coherence tomography (OCT) acquisition in various clinical and anatomical scenarios. *EuroIntervention* 2007;3: 365-370.
4. Bouma BE, Tearney GJ, Yabushita H, et al. Evaluation of intracoronary stenting by intravascular optical coherence tomography. *Heart* 2003;89:317-320.
5. Cook S, Wenaweser P, Togni M, et al. Incomplete stent apposition and very late stent thrombosis after drug-eluting stent implantation. *Circulation* 2007;115:2426-2434.
6. Barlis P, Gonzalo N, Di Mario C, et al. A multicentre evaluation of the safety of intracoronary optical coherence tomography. *EuroIntervention* 2009;5:90-95.
7. Bezerra HG, Costa MA, Guagliumi G, et al. Intracoronary optical coherence tomography: a comprehensive review clinical and research applications. *JACC Cardiovasc Interv* 2009;2: 1035-1046.
8. Suzuki N, Guagliumi G, Bezerra HG, et al. The impact of an eccentric intravascular ImageWire during coronary optical coherence tomography imaging. *EuroIntervention* 2011;6: 963-969.
9. Guagliumi G, Costa MA, Sirbu V, et al. Strut coverage and late malapposition with paclitaxel-eluting stents compared with bare metal stents in acute myocardial infarction: optical coherence tomography substudy of the Harmonizing Outcomes with Revascularization and Stents in Acute Myocardial Infarction (HORIZONS-AMI) Trial. *Circulation* 2011;123:274-281.
10. Gonzalo N, Garcia-Garcia HM, Serruys PW, et al. Reproducibility of quantitative optical coherence tomography for stent analysis. *EuroIntervention* 2009;5:224-232.

11. Templin C, Meyer M, Müller MF, et al. Coronary optical frequency domain imaging (OFDI) for in vivo evaluation of stent healing: comparison with light and electron microscopy. *Eur Heart J* 2010;31:1792-1801.

12. Colombo A, Hall P, Nakamura S, et al. Intracoronary stenting without anticoagulation accomplished with intravascular ultrasound guidance. *Circulation* 1995;91:1676-1688.

13. Yamaguchi T, Terashima M, Akasaka T, et al. Safety and feasibility of an intravascular optical coherence tomography image wire system in the clinical setting. *Am J Cardiol* 2008;101: 562-567.

14. Farb A, Burke AP, Kolodgie FD, et al. Pathological mechanisms of fatal late coronary stent thrombosis in humans. *Circulation* 2003;108:1701-1706.

15. Gonzalo N, Serruys PW, Okamura T, et al. Optical coherence tomography assessment of the acute effects of stent implantation on the vessel wall: a systematic quantitative approach. *Heart* 2009;95:1913-1919.

16. Fujii K, Carlier SG, Mintz GS, et al. Stent underexpansion and residual reference segment stenosis are related to stent thrombosis after sirolimus-eluting stent implantation: an intravascular ultrasound study. *J Am Coll Cardiol* 2005;45:995-998.

17. Futamatsu H, Sabate M, Angiolillo DJ, et al. Characterization of plaque prolapse after drug-eluting stent implantation in diabetic patients: a three-dimensional volumetric intravascular ultrasound outcome study. *J Am Coll Cardiol* 2006;48:1139-1145.

18. Farb A, Sangiorgi G, Carter AJ, et al. Pathology of acute and chronic coronary stenting in humans. *Circulation* 1999;99: 44-52.

19. Mehanna EA, Attizzani GF, Kyono H, et al. Assessment of coronary stent by optical coherence tomography, methodology and definitions. *Int J Cardiovasc Imaging* 2011;27:259-269.

20. Ishigami K, Uemura S, Morikawa Y, et al. Long-term follow-up of neointimal coverage of sirolimus-eluting stents—evaluation with optical coherence tomography. *Circ J* 2009;73:2300-2307.

21. Miyoshi N, Shite J, Shinke T, et al. Comparison by optical coherence tomography of paclitaxel-eluting stents with sirolimus-eluting stents implanted in one coronary artery in one procedure—6-month follow-up. *Circ J* 2010;74:903-908.

22. Guagliumi G, Musumeci G, Sirbu V, et al. Optical coherence tomography assessment of in vivo vascular response after implantation of overlapping bare-metal and drug-eluting stents. *JACC Cardiovasc Interv* 2010;3:531-539.

23. Kyono H, Guagliumi G, Sirbu V, et al. Optical coherence tomography (OCT) strut-level analysis of drug-eluting stents (DES) in human coronary bifurcations. *EuroIntervention* 2010;6: 69-77.

24. Bezerra H, Guagliumi G, Valescchi O, et al. Unraveling the lack of neointimal hyperplasia detected by intravascular ultrasound using optical coherence tomography: lack of spatial resolution or a true biological effect? *J Am Coll Cardiol* 2009;53(Suppl A): 90A.

25. Onuma Y, Serruys PW, Perkins LE, et al. Intracoronary optical coherence tomography and histology at 1 month and 2, 3, and 4 years after implantation of everolimus-eluting bioresorbable vascular scaffolds in a porcine coronary artery model: an attempt to decipher the human optical coherence tomography images in the ABSORB trial. *Circulation* 2010;122: 2288-2300.

26. Gutierrez-Chico JL, Serruys PW, Girasis C, et al. Quantitative multi-modality imaging analysis of a fully bioresorbable stent: a head-to-head comparison between QCA, IVUS and OCT. *Int J Cardiovasc Imaging* 2012;28:467-478.

CHAPTER 11

Fractional Flow Reserve–Guided Percutaneous Coronary Intervention

WILLIAM F. FEARON

Measuring fractional flow reserve (FFR) has become an indispensable tool for guiding percutaneous coronary intervention (PCI). Although the coronary angiogram is the reference standard for diagnosing coronary artery disease (CAD), it has limited accuracy for identifying ischemia-producing lesions when there is intermediate angiographic narrowing. Noninvasive stress imaging techniques correlate well with angiographic single-vessel CAD; however, in patients with multivessel CAD, noninvasive imaging is less accurate. For these reasons, an invasive method for identifying ischemia-producing lesions, such as FFR, is critical to optimally guide decisions regarding PCI. The aims of this chapter are to review the concept of FFR, examine the studies demonstrating the safety of deferring PCI based on FFR, evaluate the role of FFR in specific lesion subsets, outline the benefit of FFR in guiding PCI in patients with multivessel CAD, and discuss the limitations of FFR.

Concept and Definition of Fractional Flow Reserve

FFR is defined as the maximum flow down a vessel in the presence of a stenosis compared with the maximum flow in the theoretical absence of the stenosis.[1] In other words, it is the fraction of expected blood flow reaching a particular myocardial territory. The calculation of FFR is based on the assumption that during maximal coronary vasodilation, resistance is minimized and constant. In that setting, myocardial flow becomes proportional to myocardial pressure and distal coronary pressure is a reflection of the maximum myocardial flow in the presence of a stenosis. In a normal epicardial coronary vessel, there is very little resistance to flow and the distal coronary pressure is equal to the proximal coronary or aortic pressure. Therefore, in a diseased vessel, the proximal pressure is a reflection of what the distal pressure would be in the hypothetical absence of the epicardial disease. Thus, FFR can be determined by measuring the distal coronary pressure during maximal hyperemia and dividing it by the simultaneously measured proximal coronary pressure. FFR has a number of unique aspects that make it an especially useful invasive index (Box 11-1).

FFR is measured by using a 0.014-inch coronary guidewire with a miniaturized, high-fidelity pressure sensor mounted 3 cm from the tip of the wire at the junction of the radiopaque and radiolucent segments. Currently, there are two manufacturers of the pressure wire (St. Jude Medical, Little Canada, Minnesota; Volcano Therapeutics, San Diego, California), each of which has its own console that analyzes and displays the pressure recordings. Both wires can be integrated into and displayed directly on the catheterization laboratory pressure monitor system.

After the administration of 50 to 70 units/kg of heparin and 100 to 200 μg of intracoronary nitroglycerin to dilate the epicardial coronary vessel maximally, a coronary pressure wire is connected to a commercially available analyzer and calibrated outside the body. Typically, the pressure wire is advanced through a guiding catheter and the pressure sensor is positioned near the ostium of the left or right coronary artery, where the pressure signal from the wire is equalized to the pressure signal from the catheter. The wire is then advanced to the distal third of the vessel, beyond the stenosis of interest. Maximal coronary hyperemia is induced generally with a bolus of intracoronary adenosine (>100 μg) or intravenous (IV) adenosine (140 μg/kg/min infusion). A variety of pharmacologic agents can be used to measure FFR; their characteristics are outlined in Table 11-1.

FFR is measured as the mean distal pressure measured with the wire divided by the mean proximal coronary or aortic pressure as measured with the guide catheter. In the presence of diffuse disease or sequential stenoses, the wire can be pulled slowly back to the ostium of the coronary during maximal hyperemia to determine whether there is a focal area responsible for the bulk of the pressure gradient in the case of diffuse disease, or to determine which lesion is most responsible for the gradient in the case of sequential stenoses (Figure 11-1). In this way, FFR is not only a vessel-specific method for identifying ischemia, but is also lesion-specific.[2] This concept explains why many believe that FFR is a more accurate determinant of ischemic heart disease than noninvasive stress imaging.[3]

Deferring Percutaneous Coronary Intervention Based on Fractional Flow Reserve

FFR was first validated in patients with intermediate single-vessel CAD. In a landmark study by Pijls and colleagues, 45 patients with chest pain and intermediate single-vessel CAD underwent three different noninvasive stress tests.[4] If any one of these was positive for ischemia, the patient was defined as having ischemia. FFR was measured in all patients and was less than 0.75 in all 21 patients with ischemia. In 21 of 24 patients with an FFR of 0.75 or higher, all three noninvasive tests were negative for ischemia, giving FFR a specificity of 100% and a sensitivity of 88% at a cutoff value of 0.75. None of the deferred patients required revascularization during 14 months of follow-up.

This study established 0.75 as the cutoff value for defining an ischemia-producing lesion. Subsequent studies have demonstrated a gray zone extending from 0.75 to 0.80. If the FFR is below 0.75, one can be sure that significant ischemia is present. If the FFR is above

0.80, one can be sure that significant ischemia is not present. If the FFR is between 0.75 and 0.80, one should use clinical judgment to guide the decision regarding revascularization. For example, if the FFR is in the gray zone and the patient has typical symptoms with a focal, proximal LAD lesion, one might favor PCI. On the other hand, if the patient has more diffuse disease or less typical symptoms, one might consider optimal medical therapy.

Another landmark study, which provided further support for deferring PCI based on FFR, was the DEFER trial.[5] In this study, 325 patients with intermediate CAD who were referred for PCI had their FFR measured. If the FFR was less than 0.75, the patients underwent PCI with angioplasty or bare metal stents, as planned. The 181 patients in whom FFR was 0.75 or higher were randomized to the performance of PCI or deferral of PCI. At 2-year follow-up, the event-free survival (death, myocardial infarction, repeat revascularization, and procedural complication prolonging hospitalization) was numerically higher, although not statistically significant, in the deferral group as compared with the performance group (89% vs. 83%, $P = 0.27$). These findings have been extended out to 5-year follow-up and continue to demonstrate similar, if not better, outcomes when lesions that are not hemodynamically significant are managed medically instead of with PCI.[6] The death and MI rate at 5 years was 3.3% in the deferral group compared with 7.9% in the performance group ($P = 0.21$).

Subsequent studies, performed by numerous different investigators and in a wide range of patients, have consistently shown that deferring PCI in patients with CAD and an FFR more than 0.75 to 0.80 is safe and results in excellent patient outcomes.[7]

Fractional Flow Reserve in Specific Lesion Subsets

FFR can be particularly helpful in guiding the decision regarding the need for PCI in a number of lesion subsets, such as intermediate left main disease, ostial and bifurcation disease, tandem lesions, and diffuse disease.

LEFT MAIN DISEASE

The angiographic determination of significant left main disease has been shown to be particularly inaccurate. A number of single-center studies have demonstrated the safety of measuring FFR to guide the decision regarding revascularization when intermediate left main

disease exists.[8] The largest of these studies evaluated 213 patients with equivocal left main disease in whom FFR was measured.[9] If the FFR was less than 0.80, the patient underwent revascularization; if it was 0.80 or higher, revascularization of the left main was deferred. The 5-year, event-free survival estimates were similar between both groups, supporting the role of FFR in this setting. Of note, 23% of the left main lesions that had a diameter stenosis of less than 50% were physiologically significant, highlighting the fact that flow down a vessel supplying a large amount of myocardium can be compromised by a modest luminal narrowing.

Although a number of reports have demonstrated the usefulness of measuring FFR to assess intermediate left main disease, the effect of downstream epicardial disease in the left anterior descending (LAD)

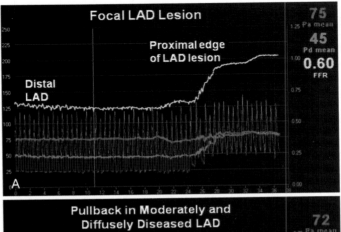

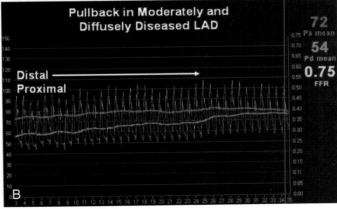

Figure 11-1   A, Fractional flow reserve *(FFR)* tracing of a pressure wire pullback in a vessel with a focal lesion demonstrates the sudden loss of the pressure gradient as the sensor is pulled proximal to the lesion. **B,** An FFR tracing of a pressure wire pullback in a vessel with diffuse disease demonstrates the gradual loss of the pressure gradient as the wire is pulled more proximally in the vessel. *LAD,* Left anterior descending (artery).

> **BOX 11-1   UNIQUE ASPECTS OF FRACTIONAL FLOW RESERVE**
>
> Normal value of 1.0 in all patients and vessels
> Independent of the microvasculature
> Specific for the epicardial vessel
> Not affected by hemodynamic changes
> Accounts for collateral flow
> Reproducible

TABLE 11-1	Hyperemic Agents				
Agent	**Administration**	**Peak Effect**	**Side Effects**	**Comments**	
Adenosine (or ATP)	IV at 140 µg/kg/min	Duration of infusion	Dyspnea, chest pain	Reference standard	
Adenosine (or ATP)	IC at 40-100 µg	15 sec	Transient arteriovenous block	Does not allow pullback	
Papaverine	IC at 10-20 mg	60 sec	Torsades de pointes	Not used commonly	
Nitroprusside	IC at 0.3-0.9 µg/kg	30 sec	Hypotension	Not well studied	
Dobutamine	IV at 20-50 µg/kg/min	Duration of infusion	Tachycardia	Slow onset	
Regadenoson	IV bolus of 0.4 mg	2-3 min	Dyspnea, chest pain, headache	Not well studied with FFR	

ATP, Adenosine triphosphate; *FFR,* fractional flow reserve; *IC,* intracoronary; *IV,* intravenous.

or left circumflex (LCX) artery on the FFR assessment of the left main remains unclear. Disease in the LAD will certainly affect FFR assessment of the left main when the pressure wire is in the distal LAD. Even if the pressure wire is positioned proximal to the LAD disease, but distal to the left main, prior studies have highlighted the impact of the distal lesion on FFR assessment of the proximal lesion. However, in theory, LAD disease might also affect the FFR assessment of the left main when the pressure wire is positioned in a nondiseased LCX because the LAD stenosis could impair maximal flow across the left main and potentially elevate the measured FFR falsely. Preliminary data have suggested that this is only the case when there is severe proximal LAD disease; in most cases, FFR of the left main can be reliably assessed with the pressure wire in the unobstructed downstream vessel. If both the LAD and LCX are significantly diseased, it will not be possible to assess the significance of the left main lesion using FFR without first stenting the downstream disease.

BIFURCATION SIDE BRANCHES

Ostial and bifurcation lesions can also be difficult to assess angiographically. FFR has been evaluated in the setting of ostial side branch lesions compromised by a main branch stent (so-called jailed side branches) and has demonstrated that surprisingly few angiographically significant lesions are functionally significant (Figure 11-2).[10] This finding is opposite to what is seen in left main disease; because many of these jailed side branches supply a small amount of myocardium, a very significant narrowing is necessary to result in myocardial ischemia. Basing the decision of further PCI in the setting of jailed side branches has been shown to be safe, as in other settings.

SERIAL LESIONS

In the setting of tandem or serial lesions, measuring FFR can be particularly helpful. The first step should be to place the pressure wire in the distal vessel beyond both lesions and measure FFR with IV adenosine. If it is above the ischemic threshold, one can safely defer intervention. If it is below the ischemic threshold, one should slowly pull the pressure wire back during maximal hyperemia and identify which lesion is responsible for most of the pressure gradient. If PCI is to be performed, this lesion should be stented first. Because maximal flow across the remaining lesion will now be greater after removal of the first lesion, it is critical to remeasure FFR to determine whether the second lesion is now functionally significant (Figure 11-3). Complex formulas have been derived to predict the FFR across each lesion before performing PCI, but because these equations require inflating a balloon in the vessel to measure the coronary wedge pressure, they are not applicable to the clinical setting.[11]

DIFFUSE DISEASE

Because atherosclerosis is a diffuse process, it is not uncommon to find diffuse angiographic disease in a coronary artery. Although the vessel may not have any area of critical narrowing, the impact of the moderate diffuse disease can result in myocardial ischemia. Measuring FFR can be particularly helpful in this setting because it will identify the ischemia. Also, by performing a slow pullback of the pressure wire during maximal hyperemia, one can distinguish diffuse disease, which will not respond well to PCI from more focal disease, which will respond well. Occasionally, angiographically normal-appearing vessels can have occult atherosclerosis, which can be detected by FFR assessment.[12]

◈ Fractional Flow Reserve in Multivessel Disease

The Fractional Flow Reserve versus Angiography for Multivessel Evaluation (FAME) trial was an important study comparing two strategies for deciding on which lesions to perform PCI.[13] Patients who

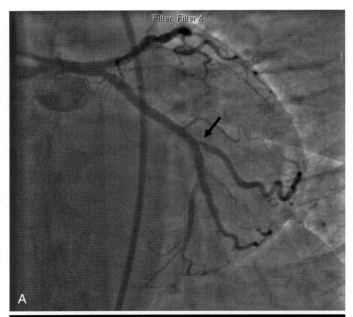

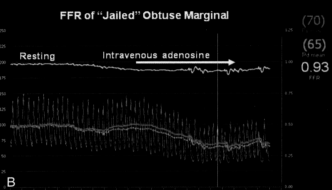

Figure 11-2   A, Angiogram of a left coronary artery after stenting of the left circumflex, resulting in compromise of the ostium of the obtuse marginal branch *(arrow).* **B,** A fractional flow reserve *(FFR)* tracing with the pressure wire in the obtuse marginal branch demonstrates a nonischemic FFR of 0.93, despite the significant angiographic appearance.

had coronary narrowing of at least 50% in two or more major epicardial vessels that the investigator deemed warranted PCI, based on the angiographic appearance and the patient's clinical information, were included in the study. The operator identified the lesions requiring PCI and the patient was randomized to one of two strategies. If the patient was randomized to the angiography-guided strategy, the operator performed PCI on the identified lesions in the usual fashion. If the patient was randomized to the FFR-guided strategy, the operator first performed FFR measurement across the identified lesions and only performed PCI if the FFR was 0.80 or lower.

A number of important findings stemmed from this study. First, the 509 patients randomized to FFR-guided PCI received one third fewer stents compared with the 496 patients randomized to the angiography-guided strategy, despite the fact that in both groups, roughly three lesions were identified per patient. Importantly, there was no difference in procedure time between the two strategies; although measuring FFR does add some time to the procedure, it saves time by eliminating unnecessary extra PCI. In the FAME trial, it also significantly decreased the amount of contrast agent administered to the FFR-guided PCI patients.

The primary endpoint of the FAME trial was the 1-year composite of death, myocardial infarction, and need for repeat revascularization.

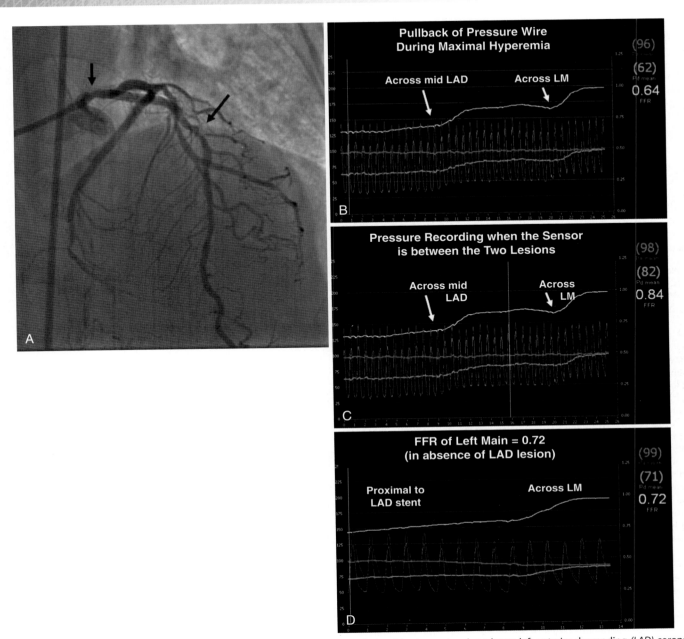

Figure 11-3   A, Angiogram demonstrating a moderate left main *(LM)* coronary lesion *(short arrow)* and moderate left anterior descending *(LAD)* coronary lesion *(long arrow).* **B,** Pressure pullback recording showing the two focal step-ups in pressure gradient as the sensor is pulled from the distal LAD artery to the ostium of the left coronary artery. **C,** When the pressure sensor is between the two lesions, before treatment of the distal lesion, the ratio between the pressure wire pressure and the guiding catheter pressure is 0.84. **D,** After stenting of the distal lesion, the flow across the proximal lesion is now greater so that with the sensor in the same location as in **C,** the ratio is now 0.72. *FFR,* Fractional flow reserve.

This was significantly lower in patients randomized to FFR-guided PCI compared with those randomized to angiography-guided PCI (13.2% vs. 18.3%; *P* = 0.02). In addition, the rates of death and myocardial infarction were significantly lower in the FFR-guided patients (7.3% vs. 11.1%; *P* = 0.04). There was no significant difference in the percentage of patients free from angina at 1 year.

The difference in the primary endpoint was not driven by a large difference in any single component; each was decreased by 30% to 40% in the FFR-guided PCI patients (Figure 11-4). In addition, the difference in myocardial infarction was not driven by small periprocedural enzyme leaks, which occurred in a similar number in each group.

These findings have now been extended out to 2 years, at which point there continued to be a separation of the curves comparing the rate of the composite endpoint, and the percentage of patients with death or myocardial infarction continued to be significantly lower in the FFR-guided PCI patients (8.4% vs. 12.9%; *P* = 0.02).[14] Importantly, the myocardial infarction and revascularization rates in the 513 angiographically significant–appearing lesions, which were deferred based on an FFR more than 0.80, were only 0.2% and 3.2%, respectively. These data add strong support to previous studies demonstrating the safety of treating hemodynamically nonsignificant lesions medically, despite their angiographic appearance.

Why an FFR-guided PCI strategy results in improved outcomes likely has to do with the risk of PCI and the differences in the risk of adverse events stemming from hemodynamically significant lesions as compared with nonsignificant ones. Every time a stent is placed, there

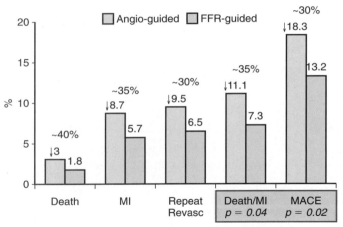

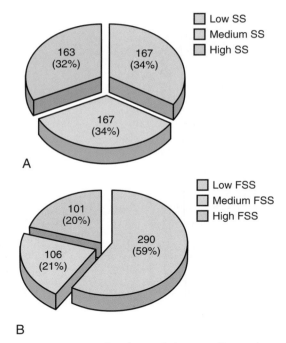

Figure 11-4 Chart reflecting the adverse event rates at 1 year in patients enrolled in the FAME trial. *FFR,* Fractional flow reserve; *MACE,* major adverse cardiac events; *MI,* myocardial infarction; *Revasc,* revascularization. (From Tonino PAL, De Bruyne B, Pijls NHJ, et al. Fractional flow reserve versus angiography for guiding PCI in patients with multivessel coronary disease [FAME study]. *N Engl J Med.* 2009;360:213-224.)

Figure 11-5 Proportions of study population according to the tertiles of classic SYNTAX score *(SS)* **(A)** and those of fractional flow reserve-guided SYNTAX score *(FSS)* **(B)**. (From Nam CW, Mangiacapra F, Entjes R, et al; FAME Study Investigators. Functional SYNTAX score for risk assessment in multivessel coronary artery disease. *J Am Coll Cardiol.* 2011;58:1211-1218.)

are acute risks and longer term risks, such as stent thrombosis and restenosis. In general, these risks are outweighed by the benefit of relieving ischemia when PCI is performed on an ischemia-producing lesion. However, as noted, the risk of an adverse event from a nonsignificant lesion receiving medical treatment is extremely low and generally is not outweighed by the risk of performing PCI.

Another important finding from the FAME trial was the inadequacy of angiography for identifying ischemia-producing lesions. A substudy has shown that approximately 35% of lesions between 50% and 70% narrowed are hemodynamically significant, whereas 20% of lesions between 70% and 90% are not significant based on FFR.[15] Thus, the angiogram alone is insufficient to provide information about the hemodynamic significance of lesions between 50% and 90% narrowed. If one performs PCI on all these lesions, as was done in the angiography-guided PCI arm of FAME, a number of unnecessary stents will be placed and unnecessary risk incurred. On the other hand, if one were to decide arbitrarily not to treat lesions less than 70% narrowed, a number of ischemia-producing lesions would be left unrevascularized, likely resulting in increased symptoms and perhaps adverse events. Historically, we have been taught to perform anatomic complete revascularization, whereby all angiographically significant—appearing lesions are treated. FAME has shown us the importance of following a functionally complete revascularization strategy, whereby ischemia-producing lesions are treated with PCI and nonischemia-producing lesions are treated medically.

The additional information obtained from FFR may have important implications on treatment decisions in patients with multivessel disease. The Synergy Between Percutaneous Coronary Intervention With TAXUS and Cardiac Surgery (SYNTAX) score, an angiography-based grading system, has been advocated as a means for deciding whether a patient with multivessel coronary disease would have a better outcome with coronary artery bypass graft (CABG) surgery or with PCI.[16] This approach is based on data showing that patients with more complex coronary disease resulting in a high SYNTAX score tend to have better outcomes when randomized to coronary artery bypass grafting instead of PCI in the SYNTAX study.[17] However, the SYNTAX score is limited by the fact that it is based on the coronary angiogram. With FFR, we have a greater appreciation regarding the inability to determine whether a stenosis is functionally significant when basing that decision on the angiogram alone.

Recently, a functional SYNTAX score was proposed in which only lesions with an FFR less than 0.80 are scored when calculating the SYNTAX score and functionally insignificant lesions are neglected.[18]

The functional SYNTAX score was calculated in the FFR-guided patients in the FAME study and compared with the traditional SYNTAX score. Roughly one third of the higher risk patients moved to a lower risk group after calculating the functional SYNTAX score (Figure 11-5). In addition, the functional SYNTAX score was a better predictor of outcomes compared with the SYNTAX score. The functional SYNTAX score will need to be tested prospectively, but it may be a more accurate method for determining the best treatment option and prognosis in patients with multivessel coronary disease.

A final important component to the FFR-guide strategy tested in the FAME study was the economic aspect. Measuring FFR adds costs to a procedure, both for the wire and hyperemic agent. In a formal analysis incorporating equipment costs as well as follow-up costs in the FAME study, the FFR-guided strategy saved more than $2000/patient at 1 year ($14,315 vs. $16,700; P < 0.001).[19] A bootstrap simulation showed that the FFR-guided strategy was a cost-saving measure in over 90% of cases and cost-effective in over 99% (Figure 11-6). It is unusual in medicine for a new strategy not only to improve outcomes, but also to save resources.

Limitations of Fractional Flow Reserve

There are a few potential pitfalls to measuring FFR that can result in a false-positive or false-negative FFR result (Table 11-2). First, a pressure wire can have drift in the pressure reading, resulting in a falsely high or low FFR. This is detected when the pressure wire is pulled back to the ostium of the vessel after measuring FFR and a difference between the guiding catheter pressure recording and pressure wire recording is noted. If this occurs, the wire can be re-equalized and FFR measured again, or the FFR measurement can be adjusted to account for the drift.

Coronary vasospasm can cause a moderate but not functionally significant lesion to have an ischemic FFR. This is one of the reasons why nitroglycerin should be administered before measuring FFR. Another situation responsible for a falsely low FFR can occur in a tortuous vessel, in which the pressure wire straightens it out, resulting

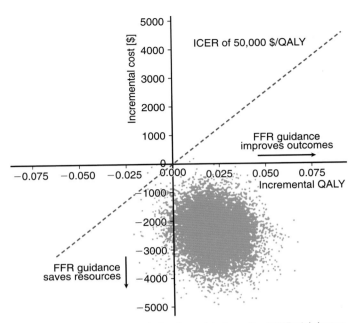

Figure 11-6. Bootstrap simulation from data from the FAME trial demonstrating that an FFR-guided strategy is cost-effective in over 99% and cost saving in over 90% of cases. *FFR,* Fractional flow reserve; *ICER,* incremental cost-effectiveness ratio; *QALY,* quality-adjusted life-year. (From Fearon WF, Bornschein B, Tonino PA, et al; Fractional Flow Reserve Versus Angiography for Multivessel Evaluation [FAME] Study Investigators. Economic evaluation of fractional flow reserve-guided percutaneous coronary intervention in patients with multivessel disease. *Circulation.* 2010;122:2545-2550.)

TABLE 11-2	Common Pitfalls Using Fractional Flow Reserve (FFR)
Reading	*Pitfall*
Falsely high or low FFR	Pressure sensor drift
Falsely low FFR	Coronary vasospasm Pseudostenosis caused by pressure wire in torturous coronary vessel
Falsely high FFR	Inadequate hyperemia caused by one of the following: side hole guide catheter when using intracoronary adenosine; lack of guide catheter engagement with coronary ostium when using intracoronary adenosine; insufficient adenosine dose; administration of adenosine through small, peripheral vein Deep seating of coronary guide catheter

in an accordion effect and pseudolesions. This commonly occurs if one places a pressure wire down an LAD via an internal mammary bypass graft, in which case the stiffer shaft of the wire leads to kinking of the internal mammary graft and a falsely low FFR.

The primary pitfall resulting in a falsely high FFR is caused by inadequate hyperemia. Achieving maximal hyperemia is critical to performing an accurate assessment of FFR. With intracoronary adenosine, this can be as a result of low doses being administered or poor technique. If the guide catheter is not well engaged, or if the guide catheter has side holes, the adenosine may spill out into the aorta and

not go down the coronary artery. Guide catheters with side holes should not be used when measuring FFR with intracoronary adenosine. On the other hand, if the guide catheter is too deeply seated and not withdrawn after the administration of adenosine, the aortic pressure can be ventricularized, resulting in less difference between the proximal and distal coronary pressures. If IV adenosine is administered in a small peripheral vein, it might be metabolized before it reaches the heart.

A patient undergoing a stress imaging study may experience exercise-induced vasoconstriction at the site of a moderate coronary stenosis, which in combination results in a significant stenosis and myocardial ischemia. In the catheterization laboratory, FFR is measured after the pharmacologic induction of maximal hyperemia, thereby simulating stress but without the vasoconstriction. In theory, this may result in a higher FFR compared with what might have been measured after exercise. Fortunately, this situation does not appear to be common clinically but is one of the reasons for the application of the gray zone with FFR between 0.75 and 0.80.

Patients presenting with ST segment elevation myocardial infarction represent a particular subset in which FFR application is limited. The measurement of FFR is based on the assumption that microvascular resistance is minimized and held constant. In the setting of an ST segment elevation myocardial infarction, there is acute microvascular dysfunction, some of which results in myocardial infarction and some of which is transient. In the acute setting, the microvascular stunning will lead to a lower maximal achievable flow down the culprit vessel, smaller gradient, and higher FFR across any given stenosis. With time, the microvasculature may recover, maximum achievable flow may increase, and a larger gradient with a lower FFR may be measured. Fortunately, in the setting of ST segment elevation myocardial infarction, the culprit vessel and culprit lesion are usually readily identified based on the electrocardiogram and coronary angiogram so that FFR is not necessary. Occasionally, one will see a moderate stenosis proximal or distal to an acute occlusion in a patient presenting with ST segment elevation myocardial infarction; it is important to remember this limitation if one is going to assess the significance of the moderate stenosis after treating the culprit lesion. Exactly how long one has to wait before relying on FFR in the culprit vessel of a patient with a myocardial infarction likely is variable. De Bruyne and associates have measured FFR down the culprit vessel in 57 patients who were all at least 6 days post–myocardial infarction.[20] They found that FFR could still accurately differentiate patients with ischemic myocardial perfusion scans from those with nonischemic ones. Samady and coworkers have measured FFR in 48 acute coronary syndrome patients, 36 of whom had an ST segment elevation myocardial infarction at least 3 days before measurement.[21] In this setting, they found that FFR down the culprit vessel correlated well with myocardial perfusion scans and myocardial contrast echocardiography.

FFR in nonculprit vessels of patients presenting with ST segment elevation myocardial infarction has been shown to be reliable in the acute setting.[22] In addition, FFR has been shown to be reliable in patients presenting with non–ST segment elevation myocardial infarction, either in the culprit vessel or nonculprit vessel.[23]

FFR has not been well validated in patients with cardiomyopathy or significant left ventricular hypertrophy. In the case of the latter, the mass of myocardium outgrows the vasculature, and ischemia may occur at a lower threshold, meaning that a higher FFR cutoff value might be warranted. FFR in bypass grafts has not been well studied, but with the sensor positioned in the native vessel beyond the anastomosis of the bypass graft, FFR should theoretically remain accurate.

REFERENCES

1. Pijls NHJ, van Son JAM, Kirkeeide RL, et al. Experimental basis of determining maximum coronary, myocardial and collateral blood flow by pressure measurements for assessing functional stenosis severity before and after percutaneous transluminal coronary angioplasty. *Circulation* 1993;86:1354-1367.

2. Kern MJ, Lerman A, Bech JW, et al. Physiological assessment of coronary artery disease in the cardiac catheterization laboratory. A scientific statement from the American Heart Association Committee on Diagnostic and Interventional Cardiac Catheterization, Council on Clinical Cardiology. *Circulation* 2006;114:1321-1341.

3. Ragosta M, Bishop AH, Lipson LC, et al. Comparison between angiography and fractional flow reserve versus single-photon emission computed tomographic myocardial perfusion imaging for determining lesion significance in patients with multivessel coronary disease. *Am J Cardiol* 2007;99:896-902.

4. Pijls NH, De Bruyne B, Peels K, et al. Measurement of fractional flow reserve to assess the functional severity of coronary-artery stenoses. *N Engl J Med* 1996;334:1703-1708.

5. Bech GJ, De Bruyne B, Pijls NH, et al. Fractional flow reserve to determine the appropriateness of angioplasty in moderate coronary stenosis: a randomized trial. *Circulation* 2001;103:2928-2934.

6. Pijls NH, van Schaardenburgh P, Manoharan G, et al. Percutaneous coronary intervention of functionally nonsignificant stenosis: 5-year follow-up of the DEFER Study. *J Am Coll Cardiol* 2007;49:2105-2111.

7. Kern MJ, Samady H. Current concepts of integrated coronary physiology in the catheterization laboratory. *J Am Coll Cardiol* 2010;55:173-185.

8. Lindstaedt M. Patient stratification in left main coronary artery disease—rationale from a contemporary practice. *Int J Card* 2008;130:326-334.

9. Hamilos M, Muller O, Cuisset T, et al. Long-term clinical outcome after fractional flow reserve-guided treatment in patients with angiographically equivocal left main coronary artery stenosis. *Circulation* 2009;120:1505-1512.

10. Koo BK, Kang HJ, Youn TJ, et al. Physiologic assessment of jailed side branch lesions using fractional flow reserve. *J Am Coll Cardiol* 2005;46:633-637.

11. Pijls NHJ, De Bruyne B, Bech GJW, et al. Coronary pressure measurement to assess the hemodynamic significance of serial stenoses within one coronary artery: validation in humans. *Circulation* 2000;102:2371-2377.

12. De Bruyne B, Hersbach F, Pijls NH, et al. Abnormal epicardial coronary resistance in patients with diffuse atherosclerosis but "normal" coronary angiography. *Circulation* 2001;104:2401-2406.

13. Tonino PAL, De Bruyne B, Pijls NHJ, et al. Fractional flow reserve versus angiography for guiding PCI in patients with multivessel coronary disease (FAME study). *N Engl J Med* 2009;360:213-224.

14. Pijls NH, Fearon WF, Tonino PA, et al; FAME Study Investigators. Fractional flow reserve versus angiography for guiding percutaneous coronary intervention in patients with multivessel coronary artery disease: 2-year follow-up of the FAME (Fractional Flow Reserve Versus Angiography for Multivessel Evaluation) study. *J Am Coll Cardiol* 2010;56:177-184.

15. Tonino PA, Fearon WF, De Bruyne B, et al. Angiographic versus functional severity of coronary artery stenoses in the FAME study fractional flow reserve versus angiography in multivessel evaluation. *J Am Coll Cardiol* 2010;55:2816-2821.

16. European Association for Percutaneous Cardiovascular Interventions; Wijns W, Kolh P, Danchin N, et al. Guidelines on myocardial revascularization: the Task Force on Myocardial Revascularization of the European Society of Cardiology (ESC) and the European Association for Cardio-Thoracic Surgery (EACTS). *Eur Heart J* 2010;31:2501-2555.

17. Serruys PW, Morice MC, Kappetein AP, et al; SYNTAX Investigators. Percutaneous coronary intervention versus coronary-artery bypass grafting for severe coronary artery disease. *N Engl J Med* 2009;360:961-972.

18. Nam CW, Mangiacapra F, Entjes R, et al; FAME Study Investigators. Functional SYNTAX score for risk assessment in multivessel coronary artery disease. *J Am Coll Cardiol* 2011;58:1211-1218.

19. Fearon WF, Bornschein B, Tonino PA, et al; Fractional Flow Reserve Versus Angiography for Multivessel Evaluation (FAME) Study Investigators. Economic evaluation of fractional flow reserve-guided percutaneous coronary intervention in patients with multivessel disease. *Circulation* 2010;122:2545-2550.

20. De Bruyne B, Pijls NH, Bartunek J, et al. Fractional flow reserve in patients with prior myocardial infarction. *Circulation* 2001;104:157-162.

21. Samady H, Lepper W, Powers ER, et al. Fractional flow reserve of infarct-related arteries identifies reversible defects on noninvasive myocardial perfusion imaging early after myocardial infarction. *J Am Coll Cardiol* 2006;47:2187-2193.

22. Ntalianis A, Sels JW, Davidavicius G, et al. Fractional flow reserve for the assessment of nonculprit coronary artery stenoses in patients with acute myocardial infarction. *JACC Cardiovasc Interv* 2010;3:1274-1281.

23. Sels JW, Tonino PA, Siebert U, et al. Fractional flow reserve in unstable angina and non-ST-segment elevation myocardial infarction experience from the FAME (Fractional flow reserve versus Angiography for Multivessel Evaluation) study. *JACC Cardiovasc Interv* 2011;4:1183-1189.

CHAPTER 12

Optimal Antithrombotic Therapy

DOMINICK J. ANGIOLILLO

In the last decades, percutaneous coronary interventions (PCIs) have experienced exponential development. This is attributed to advancements in the design of materials and techniques that have proven to be safe and efficacious in improving outcomes in patients undergoing PCI and to the introduction of better antithrombotic therapies. The development of antithrombotic agents has occurred as a result of the improved understanding of the thrombotic and hemostatic processes involved in atherothrombotic disease. This has led to the development of safer and more efficacious antiplatelet and anticoagulant treatment strategies. Translational investigations in the field have also helped develop the concept of individualized antithrombotic treatment strategies in patients undergoing PCI. The aim of this chapter is to review currently available antiplatelet and anticoagulant therapies and their incorporation into optimal treatment strategies for patients undergoing PCI with coronary stents.

Pathophysiology of Atherothrombosis

The rupture or erosion of an atheromatous plaque and subsequent thrombus formation can lead to an acute coronary syndrome, which may have different clinical expressions, including unstable angina, non–ST elevation myocardial infarction, and ST elevation myocardial infarction. The exposure of subendothelial collagen after a plaque rupture or erosion allows platelet adhesion at the site of vessel injury; this is followed by the activation and aggregation of platelets. In addition, exposure of tissue factor triggers the extrinsic pathway of the coagulation cascade (Figure 12-1).[1,2] This is a dynamic process that results in thrombus formation, which has four phases:

1. Initiation and formation of the platelet plug. This is composed of three stages: initiation phase, involving platelet adhesion; extension phase, including activation, additional recruitment, and aggregation; and perpetuation phase, characterized by platelet stimulation and stabilization of clot.
2. Propagation of the clotting process. This is mainly driven by the sequential activation of coagulation factors, resulting in significant stepwise response amplification to the activation of thrombin (factor II), which has a central role in the conversion of fibrinogen in fibrin, forming the hemostatic plug. In addition, thrombin also promotes platelet activation and aggregation via protease-activated receptors (PARs).
3. Termination of clotting by antithrombotic control mechanisms.
4. Removal of the clot by fibrinolysis.

Advances in the understanding of the complex mechanisms regulating these processes have been pivotal for the development of antithrombotic therapies inhibiting platelets (antiplatelet therapies) and coagulation factors (anticoagulant therapies) used for the prevention of recurrent atherothrombotic events in patients undergoing PCI.

Antiplatelet Therapy

Three different families of antiplatelet agents are approved for the treatment and/or prevention of recurrent events in patients with coronary artery disease (CAD) undergoing PCI. These include cyclooxygenase (COX) inhibitors, adenosine diphosphate (ADP) $P2Y_{12}$ receptor antagonists, and glycoprotein (GP) IIb/IIIa inhibitors. Table 12-1 summarizes the dosing recommendations for these drugs.

CYCLOOXYGENASE INHIBITOR: ASPIRIN

Mechanisms of Action

Aspirin is an irreversible inhibitor of COX activity of prostaglandin H (PGH) synthase 1 and synthase 2, also referred to as COX-1 and COX-2, respectively.[3] These isozymes catalyze the conversion of arachidonic acid (AA) to PGH_2, which serves as a substrate for the generation of several prostanoids, including thromboxane A2 (TXA2) and prostacyclin (PGI_2). TXA2, an amplifier of platelet activation and vasoconstrictor, is mainly derived from platelet COX-1 and is highly sensitive to inhibition by aspirin, whereas vascular PGI2, a platelet inhibitor and vasodilator, is derived largely from COX-2 and is less susceptible to inhibition by low doses of aspirin (Figure 12-2). Only high doses of aspirin can inhibit COX-2, which has antiinflammatory and analgesic effects, whereas low doses of aspirin are sufficient to inhibit COX-1 activity, leading to antiplatelet effects. Aspirin is

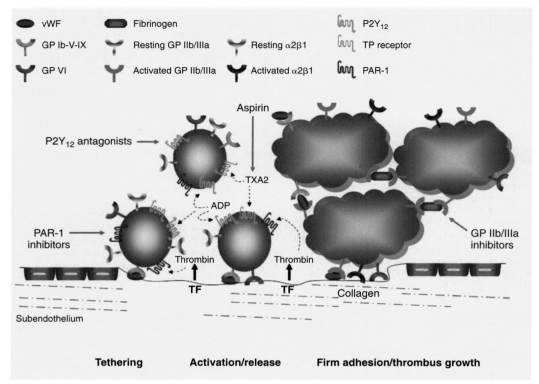

Figure 12-1 Platelet-mediated thrombosis. The interaction between glycoprotein *(GP)* Ib and von Willebrand factor *(vWF)* mediates platelet tethering, enabling subsequent interaction between GP VI and collagen. This triggers the shift of integrins to a high-affinity state and the release of adenosine diphosphate *(ADP)* and thromboxane A2 *(TXA2)*, which bind to the $P2Y_{12}$ and thromboxane receptors *(TP)*, respectively. Tissue factor triggers thrombin formation locally, which contributes to platelet activation via binding to the platelet protease-activated receptor *(PAR-1)*. (From Angiolillo DJ, Ueno M, Goto S. Basic principles of platelet biology and clinical implications. *Circ J* 2010;74:597-607.)

TABLE 12-1	Recommended Doses and Need for Renal Adjustment of Clinically Approved Antiplatelet Drugs			
Drug	*Recommended Dose*	*Renal Adjustment*	*Renal Dosing*	
COX-1 Inhibitors				
Aspirin	81-325 mg daily	Yes	Avoid in patients with severe renal impairment.	
$P2Y_{12}$ inhibitors				
Clopidogrel	For patients undergoing PCI with stenting—300-600-mg loading dose, 75-mg daily maintenance dose For patients undergoind PCI after fibrinolytic therapy—300 mg within 24 hr and 600 mg > 24 hr after receiving fibrinolytic therapy	No	NA	
Prasugrel	60-mg loading dose, 10-mg daily maintenance dose	No	NA	
Ticagrelor	180-mg loading dose, 90-mg twice daily maintenance dose	No	NA	
Glycoprotein IIb/IIIa Antagonists				
Abciximab	IV bolus of 0.25 mg/kg, followed by 0.125 µg/kg/min (max, 10 µg/min); after PCI, continue for 12 hr	No	NA	
Eptifibatide	IV bolus of 180 µg/kg followed by maintenance dose of 2.0 µg/kg/min. Continue infusion for 18 to 24 hr. In case of PCI, IV bolus of 180 µg/kg administered immediately before initiation of the procedure followed by maintenance dose of 2.0 µg/kg/min and second 180-µg/kg bolus 10 min after first bolus. Infusion should be continued until hospital discharge or for up to 18 to 24 hr, whichever comes first. A minimum of 12 hr of infusion is recommended.		If creatinine clearance is < 50 mL/min, adjust maintenance dose to 1 µg/kg/min. In case of PCI, if creatinine clearance < 50 mL/min, IV bolus of 180 µg/kg administered immediately before initiation of the procedure, immediately followed by continuous infusion of 1.0 µg/min and second 180-µg/kg bolus administered 10 min after the first.	
Tirofiban	IV bolus of 0.4 µg/kg for 30 min followed by maintenance dose of 0.1 µg/kg/min. Continue infusion for 18 to 24 hr. In case of PCI, IV bolus, 10 µg/kg in 3 min, followed by 0.1 µg/kg/min for minimum of 12 hr and up to 18-24 hr (standard dose regimen); or IV bolus, 25 µg/kg in 3 min followed by 0.1 µg/kg/min for minimum of 12 hr and up to 18-24 hr (high-bolus regimen)		If creatinine clearance < 50 mL/min, adjust maintenance dose to IV bolus of 0.2 µg/kg for 20 min followed by maintenance dose of 0.05 µg/kg/min.	

COX, Cyclooxygenase; *IV,* intravenous; *NA,* not applicable; *PCI,* percutaneous coronary intervention.

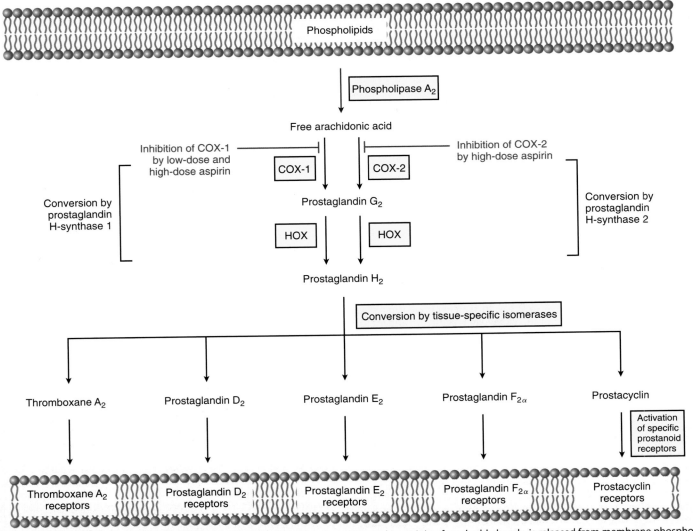

Figure 12-2 Mechanism of action of aspirin. Arachidonic acid, a 20-carbon fatty acid containing four double bonds, is released from membrane phospholipids by several forms of phospholipase A_2, which are activated by diverse stimuli. Arachidonic acid is converted by cytosolic prostaglandin H synthases, which have both cyclooxygenase *(COX)* and hydroperoxidase *(HOX)* activity, to the unstable intermediates prostaglandin G_2 and prostaglandin H_2, respectively. The synthases are also termed *cyclooxygenases* and exist in two forms, COX-1 and COX-2. Low-dose aspirin selectively inhibits COX-1, whereas high-dose aspirin inhibits both COX-1 and COX-2. Prostaglandin H_2 is converted by tissue-specific isomerases to multiple prostanoids. These bioactive lipids activate specific cell membrane receptors of the superfamily of G-protein–coupled receptors, such as the thromboxane receptor, prostaglandin D_2 receptors, prostaglandin E_2 receptors, prostaglandin $F_{2\alpha}$ receptors, and the prostacyclin receptor. (From Patrono C, García Rodríguez LA, Landolfi R, et al. Low-dose aspirin for the prevention of atherothrombosis. *N Engl J Med* 2005;353:2373-2383.)

rapidly absorbed in the upper gastrointestinal tract and detectable platelet inhibition is detected within 60 minutes after drug intake. The plasma half-life of aspirin is approximately 20 minutes and peak plasma levels are achieved within 30 to 40 minutes. However, enteric-coated aspirin delays absorption and peak plasma levels are achieved approximately 3 to 4 hours after ingestion. Because platelets have a minimal capability for protein synthesis and aspirin induces an irreversible COX-1 blockade, COX-mediated TXA2 synthesis is prevented for the entire life span of the platelet ($\approx$7 to 10 days).[3]

Indications

Aspirin is the mainstay of antiplatelet therapy for the secondary prevention of recurrent ischemic events in patients with various clinical manifestations of CAD, including stable CAD, all acute coronary syndrome subsets, and those undergoing coronary revascularization (percutaneous or surgical).[4-6] In high-risk patients, particularly those

with ACS and undergoing PCI, aspirin should be given as promptly as possible at an initial dose of 162 to 325 mg.[4,5] However, the optimal maintenance dose of aspirin for the prevention of cardiovascular events has been the subject of controversy. Registry data have shown that oral aspirin doses of 75 to 150 mg/day are as effective as higher doses for the long-term prevention of ischemic events.[3] Importantly, higher doses of aspirin (>150 mg) do not offer greater protection from recurrent ischemic events, whereas bleeding events, in particular gastrointestinal bleeding, are significantly increased.[3] These findings are in line with the Clopidogrel optimal loading dose Usage to Reduce Recurrent EveNTs-Organization to Assess Strategies in Ischemic Syndromes (CURRENT/OASIS-7) trial, which did not show significant differences in efficacy between patients randomized to high-dose (325 mg) and low-dose (100 mg) aspirin. Based on these findings, the most updated PCI guidelines state that it is reasonable to consider 81 mg/day as a maintenance regimen.[5]

Side Effects

The side effects of aspirin are primarily gastrointestinal, dose-related, and ameliorated by using low doses (75 to 162 mg/day). Aspirin use can lead to gastric erosions, hemorrhage, and ulcers that can contribute to anemia.[3] The increased risk of extracranial bleeding is approximately 60%. In the CURRENT-OASIS 7 trial, although there were no differences in major bleeds between the two aspirin doses, a trend toward an increased rate of gastrointestinal bleeds in the high-dose group (0.38% vs. 0.24%; $P = 0.051$) was observed.[7] However, this trial was only 30 days, and longer durations of high-dose aspirin would likely have increased the risk of adverse events.

There are other interactions and side effects related to aspirin that merit attention. Some nonsteroidal antiinflammatory drugs (NSAIDs), such as naproxen and ibuprofen, by competing for the COX-1 active site, may interfere with the action of aspirin when administered concomitantly, resulting in attenuation of its antiplatelet effects.[3] This may contribute to reducing aspirin's cardioprotective effects; thus, the prescription of NSAIDs should be under careful consideration in PCI patients. Three types of aspirin sensitivity have been described: respiratory sensitivity (asthma and/or rhinitis), cutaneous sensitivity (urticaria and/or angioedema), and systemic sensitivity (anaphylactoid reaction).[8] The prevalence of aspirin-exacerbated respiratory tract disease is approximately 10% and, for aspirin-induced urticaria, the prevalence varies from 0.07% to 0.2%. In patients presenting with allergy or intolerance to aspirin, clopidogrel is the treatment of choice.[6] Desensitization using escalating doses of oral aspirin is also a therapeutic option.

P2Y$_{12}$ INHIBITORS

ADP is one of the main platelet-activating factors. Platelet ADP signaling pathways are mediated by the P2Y$_1$ and P2Y$_{12}$ receptors, which play a key role in platelet activation and aggregation processes.[1,2] The P2Y$_1$ and P2Y$_{12}$ receptors are G-protein–coupled receptors and are both required for platelet aggregation. ADP-stimulated effects are mediated mainly by P2Y$_{12}$ receptor activation, which leads to sustained platelet aggregation and stabilization of the platelet aggregate, whereas P2Y$_1$ is responsible for an initial weak and transient phase of platelet aggregation and change in platelet shape. Inhibition of the P2Y$_{12}$ signaling pathway is crucial, particularly in the setting of PCI, as noted in seminal studies with ticlopidine, a first-generation thienopyridine. The combination of aspirin and ticlopidine was shown to be associated with better outcomes, in particular the prevention of thrombotic complications, than aspirin monotherapy or aspirin plus warfarin in patients undergoing coronary stenting.[9] This is likely explained by the fact that arterial thrombotic complications are primarily platelet-mediated, therefore supporting the role of enhanced platelet inhibition. Importantly, ticlopidine in combination with aspirin is associated with more enhanced platelet inhibition, which is attributed to a synergistic effect achieved by inhibiting COX-1– and P2Y$_{12}$-mediated signaling. However, ticlopidine has two major disadvantages. First, ticlopidine has a limited safety profile, with appreciable rates of agranulocytosis, rash, and gastrointestinal effects. Second, ticlopidine achieves antiplatelet effects slowly given that the drug cannot be administered with a sufficient loading dose because of the risk of toxicity. These factors have led to the development of a second-generation thienopyridine, clopidogrel, to overcome these limitations.

Clopidogrel has shown to have a more favorable safety profile compared with ticlopidine, and therefore has become the thienopyridine of choice in the setting of PCI.[10] Clopidogrel has been evaluated in a large number of clinical trials, supporting its role in the setting of acute coronary syndrome and PCI (Table 12-2). However, clopidogrel also presents limitations, the most important of which is its broad range in regard to interindividual antiplatelet drug effects.[11] In particular, a considerable number of patients persist with high platelet reactivity despite clopidogrel therapy, exposing them to an increased risk of recurrent ischemic events, including stent thrombosis.[12,13] This

has led to the development of newer generation P2Y$_{12}$ receptor inhibitors. These include prasugrel, a third-generation thienopyridine, and ticagrelor, the first drug in a new class called cyclopentyltriazolopyrimidine (CPTP) (Table 12-3).

Mechanisms of Action

Clopidogrel

Thienopyridines are oral prodrugs and thus need to be metabolized by the hepatic cytochrome P450 (CYP) system to form an active metabolite that irreversibly inhibits the P2Y$_{12}$ receptor (Figure 12-3). Clopidogrel is a second-generation thienopyridine, which requires a two-step oxidation by the CYP system to generate an active metabolite.[14] However, approximately 85% of the prodrug is hydrolyzed by esterases to an inactive carboxylic acid derivative and only approximately 15% of the prodrug is metabolized by the CYP system into an active metabolite. Multiple CYP enzymes are involved in this process—CYP3A4, CYP3A5, CYP2C9, and CYP1A2 isoenzymes are involved in one oxidation step, whereas CYP2B6 and CYP2C19 are involved in both steps. Although clopidogrel has a half-life of only 8 hours, it has an irreversible effect on platelets and thus is active throughout its life span (7 to 10 days).

Prasugrel

Prasugrel is a third-generation thienopyridine, which has a more efficient metabolism than clopidogrel.[15] After oral ingestion, the prodrug is hydrolyzed by carboxyesterases, mainly in the intestine, which gives rise to a thiolactone intermediate that is then converted to the active metabolite by a one-step oxidation by the hepatic CYP450 system (see Figure 12-3). CYP isoenzymes involved in this process include CYP3A, CYP2B6, CYP2C9, and CYP2C19. Therefore prasugrel's active metabolite is generated more rapidly and effectively than that of clopidogrel.[16] This more favorable pharmacokinetic profile translates into better pharmacodynamic effects, showing more potent platelet inhibition, lower interindividual variability, and a faster onset of antiplatelet activity compared with clopidogrel, even when the latter is used at high doses (≥600 mg).[17] A 60-mg loading dose of prasugrel achieves 50% platelet inhibition by 30 minutes and 80% to 90% inhibition by 1 to 2 hours.[16,17] Similar to other thienopyridines, prasugrel is characterized by irreversible effects on platelets and thus is active throughout the platelets' life span (7 to 10 days).[12]

Ticagrelor

Ticagrelor is the first nonthienopyridine that is part of a new class of P2Y$_{12}$ inhibitors (CPTP) approved for clinical use.[18] Ticagrelor is an orally administered, direct-acting, reversible inhibitor of the P2Y$_{12}$ receptor (see Figure 12-3). Although ticagrelor has direct-acting effects (no metabolism required), approximately 30% of its effects are attributed to a metabolite generated by the CYP system, in particular by the CYP3A4 isoenzyme. Ticagrelor is rapidly absorbed and exerts its effects on P2Y$_{12}$-mediated signaling, acting as a noncompetitive ADP antagonist and inhibiting platelet inhibition via allosteric modulation of the receptor. Also, ticagrelor has shown faster, more potent, and less variable platelet inhibition than clopidogrel. A 180-mg loading dose of ticagrelor achieves 80% to 90% platelet inhibition by 1 to 2 hours. Ticagrelor has a half-life of 7 to 12 hours, requiring twice-daily dosing. Although the slope of offset of ticagrelor effects is rapid, approximately 5 days are needed after ticagrelor withdrawal to return to baseline platelet function.

Indications, Timing of Treatment, Dosing, and Duration of Therapy

Clopidogrel

Adding clopidogrel to aspirin has shown to be particularly beneficial in the settings of PCI and across the spectrum of acute coronary syndrome manifestations (see Table 12-2). Current acute coronary syndrome and PCI guidelines recommend treatment with a P2Y$_{12}$ receptor inhibitor as soon as possible.[4,5] The trade-off of starting

TABLE 12-2	Phase 3 Trials of Clopidogrel Therapy*						
Trial Name[†]	N	Patients	Treatment (mg/day)	Primary Endpoint	Event Rate (Active Treatment vs. Control %)	P value
CAPRIE	19,185	Previous stroke, MI, or symptomatic PAD	Clopidogrel vs. ASA	Ischemic stroke, MI, or vascular death at 1 yr	5.3% vs. 5.8%	.043
CURE	12,562	NSTE ACS, unstable angina	Clopidogrel + ASA vs. ASA	CV death, nonfatal MI, and stroke at 1 yr	9.3% vs. 11.4%	<.001
CREDO	2,116	ACS with PCI	Clopidogrel + ASA vs. ASA	CV death, MI, or stroke at 1 yr	8.5% vs. 11.5%	.02
PCI-CURE	2,658	NSTE ACS with PCI	Clopidogrel + ASA vs. ASA	CV death, MI, or revascularization within 30 days	4.5% vs. 6.4%	.03
CLARITY	3,491	STEMI	Clopidogrel + ASA + FA vs. ASA + FA	Occluded infarct-related artery, death or recurrent MI before angiography	15.0% vs. 21.7%	<.001
COMMIT	45,852	STEMI	Clopidogrel + ASA vs. ASA	CV death, reinfarction, or stroke at 28 days	9.2% vs. 10.1%	.002
CHARISMA	15,603	CVD or multiple risk factors	Clopidogrel + ASA vs. ASA	MI, stroke, or CV death at 28 months	6.8% vs. 7.3%	.22
CURRENT-OASIS 7	25,087	ACS with planned early invasive management with intended PCI	Double-dose clopidogrel + ASA vs. low-dose clopidogrel + ASA	CV death, MI, or stroke at 30 days	4.2% vs. 4.4% (overall cohort)	.37

Note: Clopidogrel was given as a loading dose of 300 mg and then 75 mg daily in CURE, CREDO, PCI-CURE, CLARITY, COMMIT, CHARISMA. Clopidogrel, 75 mg daily, was administered in CAPRIE. In CURRENT/OASIS 7, double-dose clopidogrel was defined as a 600-mg loading dose and 150 mg once daily for 7 days, followed by 75 mg once daily. Standard-dose clopidogrel was defined as a 300-mg loading dose, followed by 75 mg once daily. Patients were also randomized to receive low-dose (75-100 mg per day) or high-dose (300- 325 mg per day) aspirin.
*For acute coronary syndrome, percutaneous coronary intervention, and secondary prevention of atherothrombotic disease.
†CAPRIE: Clopidogrel vs Aspirin in Patients at Risk of Ischemic Events trial; CURE: Clopidogrel in Unstable Angina to Prevent Recurrent Events trial; CREDO: Clopidogrel for the Reduction of Events During Observation trial; CLARITY: Clopidogrel as Adjunctive Reperfusion Therapy trial; COMMIT: Clopidogrel and Metoprolol in Myocardial Infarction trial; CHARISMA: Clopidogrel for High Atherothrombotic Risk and Ischemic Stabilization, Management, and Avoidance trial; CURRENT-OASIS-7: Clopidogrel Optimal Loading Dose Usage to Reduce Recurrent Events/Optimal Antiplatelet Strategy for Intervention trial.
ACS, Acute coronary syndrome; ASA, aspirin; CV, cardiovascular; CVD, cardiovascular disease; FA, fibrinolytic agent; MI, myocardial infarction; PAD, peripheral artery disease; PCI, percutaneous coronary intervention; NSTE, non–ST segment elevation; STEMI, ST elevation myocardial infarction.

TABLE 12-3	Currently Available and Investigational P2Y$_{12}$ Receptor Inhibitors				
Agent	Class	Mechanism of Action	Mode of Administration	Frequency of Administration	Approval or Development Status
Ticlopidine	Thienopyridine (first generation)	Prodrug Irreversible	Oral	Daily	Approved 1991
Clopidogrel	Thienopyridine (second generation)	Prodrug Irreversible	Oral	Daily	Approved 1997
Prasugrel	Thienopyridine (third generation)	Prodrug Irreversible	Oral	Daily	Approved 2009
Ticagrelor (AZD6140)	Cyclopentyltria- zolopyrimidine	Direct-acting Reversible	Oral	Twice daily	Approved 2011
Cangrelor	ATP analogue	Direct-acting Reversible	IV	N/A	Phase 3 CHAMPION-PLATFORM and CHAMPION-PCI completed in 2009; additional trials ongoing
Elinogrel (PRT060128)	Quinazolinedione	Direct-acting Reversible	IV and oral	Twice daily	Phase 2 trials completed in 2009

ATP, Adenosine triphosphate; IV, intravenous.

therapy before knowing the coronary anatomy is that patients will need to wait at least 5 to 7 days after drug suspension if surgical revascularization is needed to minimize the risk of bleeding complications. Most data on clopidogrel pretreatment in patients undergoing PCI have been derived from studies using a 300-mg loading dose of clopidogrel. These included the Clopidogrel in Unstable Angina to Prevent Recurrent Events (PCI-CURE), Clopidogrel for the Reduction of Events During Observation (CREDO), and Clopidogrel as Adjunctive Reperfusion Therapy (PCI-CLARITY) trials.[19-21] These trials, however, differed in clinical settings and timing of pretreatment. The CREDO trial was the only one of these trials designed exclusively for patients undergoing PCI. A post hoc analysis of this

study has shown that a benefit of clopidogrel pretreatment is achieved only if it occurred 12 to 15 hours before PCI.[22] In a meta-analysis of these three randomized trials, clopidogrel pretreatment before PCI was shown to be beneficial and safe, regardless of whether a GP IIb/IIIa inhibitor was used at the time of PCI.[23] These data have been challenged by the introduction into clinical practice of high loading dose regimens of clopidogrel, questioning whether pretreatment can be obviated if a 600-mg loading dose is used. However, only small trial data have suggested that 600 mg given at the time of PCI can obviate the need for pretreatment in PCI patients.[24]

The approved loading and maintenance doses of clopidogrel are 300 and 75 mg, respectively. Since these doses were derived from

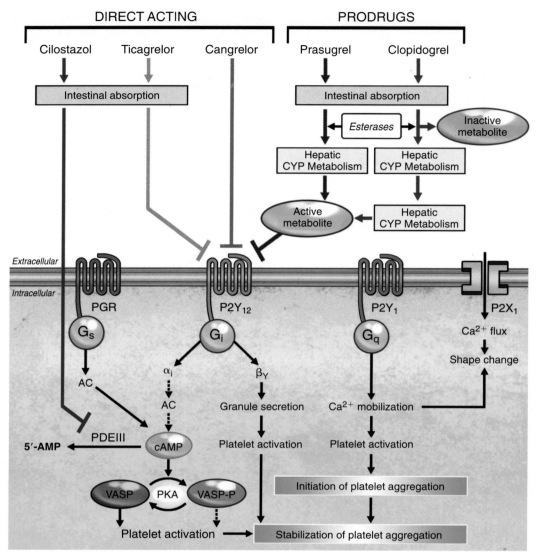

Figure 12-3 **Therapeutic options for optimizing platelet inhibition in clopidogrel-poor metabolizers.** Clopidogrel is a prodrug, which after intestinal absorption undergoes two-step hepatic oxidation by cytochrome P450 *(CYP)* enzymes (CYP3A, CYP2C9, and CYP1A2 are involved in one step; CYP2B6 and CYP2C19 are involved in both steps) to generate an active metabolite that inhibits platelet activation and aggregation processes through irreversible blockade of the P2Y$_{12}$ receptor. Approximately 85% of clopidogrel is hydrolyzed prehepatically by esterases into an inactive compound; thus, only 15% is available for hepatic metabolism. Genetic polymorphisms encoding for proteins and enzymes at various levels that modulate clopidogrel metabolism can affect platelet inhibitory effects—intestinal absorption, P-glycoprotein (encoded by ABCB1 gene); hepatic metabolism, CYP enzymes (particularly CYP2C19 loss of function alleles); and platelet membrane receptors (e.g., P2 receptors). Increasing the clopidogrel dose is not consistently associated with enhanced platelet inhibition in poor metabolizers, which may be achieved by other strategies. Prasugrel, like clopidogrel, is also an oral prodrug with a similar intestinal absorption process. However, in contrast to clopidogrel, esterases are part of prasugrel's activation pathway, and prasugrel is oxidized more efficiently to its active metabolite via a single CYP-dependent step. Direct-acting antiplatelet agents (e.g., cangrelor, ticagrelor, cilostazol) have reversible effects and do not require hepatic metabolism for pharmacodynamic activity. Ticagrelor and cilostazol are administered orally and, after intestinal absorption, inhibit platelet activation by direct blockade of the P2Y$_{12}$ receptor and phosphodiesterase III *(PDE-III)*, respectively. Cangrelor is administered via IV and directly inhibits the P2Y$_{12}$ receptor, bypassing intestinal absorption. Genetic polymorphisms of target proteins and enzymes (intestine, liver, platelet membrane) modulating clopidogrel-mediated platelet inhibition do not affect the pharmacodynamic activity of prasugrel, cilostazol, ticagrelor, and cangrelor, which ultimately inhibit platelet activation and aggregation processes by modulating intraplatelet levels of cyclic adenosine monophosphate *(cAMP)* and phosphorylation of vasodilator-stimulated phosphoprotein *(VASP-P)*. *AC,* Adenylyl cyclase; *ADP,* adenosine diphosphate; *ATP,* adenosine triphosphate; *G$_i$,* inhibitory regulative G-protein; *G$_q$,* class of G protein that activates phospholipase C; *G$_s$,* stimulative regulative G-protein; *PGE$_1$,* prostaglandin E$_1$; *PGR,* prostaglandin receptor; *PKA,* protein kinase; *solid black arrows,* activation; *dotted black arrows,* inhibition. (From Angiolillo DJ, Ueno M. Optimizing platelet inhibition in clopidogrel poor metabolizers: therapeutic options and practical considerations. *JACC Cardiovasc Interv* 2011;4:411-414.)

pharmacodynamic studies showing levels of platelet inhibition that paralleled those achieved by ticlopidine, for which higher doses were not applicable in clinical practice because of potential toxicity, several pharmacodynamic and clinical investigations have assessed the impact of higher clopidogrel dosing regimens.[11] Studies have shown that clopidogrel loading doses of 600 mg or higher are associated with

more prompt and potent platelet inhibition than 300 mg. This has been associated with a greater reduction in ischemic events, mainly driven by a reduction in periprocedural myocardial infarction.[12,13] Accordingly, practice guidelines support the use of the 600-mg loading dose in the setting of PCI.[5] Pharmacodynamic studies have also assessed a 150-mg clopidogrel maintenance dose, which is also associated with more potent platelet inhibition compared with 75 mg. However, limited clinical data have supported its routine use. The CURRENT-OASIS 7 trial evaluated the efficacy and safety of double-dose clopidogrel (600-mg loading dose followed by 150 mg daily for 7 days) versus the standard dose (300 mg after 75 mg) in patients with acute coronary syndrome.[7] Although in the overall study population there was no significant difference in the primary endpoint (composite of cardiovascular death, myocardial infarction, or stroke) at 30 days between patients receiving double-dose versus standard-dose clopidogrel, in PCI patients the double-dose clopidogrel was associated with a significant reduction in the primary endpoint and in rates of stent thrombosis compared with the standard-dose regimen.[25]

In patients presenting with an acute coronary syndrome, clopidogrel 75 mg daily, should be given for at least 12 months, irrespective of the type of treatment management (medical, PCI, coronary artery bypass grafting [CABG]). In the setting of PCI, clopidogrel 75 mg daily, should also be given for at least 12 months after drug-eluting stent (DES) implantation and for a minimum of 1 month (ideally, up to 12 months) with use of a bare metal stent (BMS).[5] Guidelines have recommended continuation of therapy beyond 12 months in DES-treated patients, depending on patient risk, and should be considered on an individualized basis. Shorter durations, however, may also be considered if patients are at increased risk of bleeding.

Current recommendations on the duration of dual antiplatelet therapy are not based on prospective randomized data. Registry data have shown conflicting results, with some suggesting that shorter durations of clopidogrel therapy (e.g., 6 months) are as effective as a longer duration of therapy (e.g., 12 months), whereas others have suggested a continuing benefit of prolonging clopidogrel therapy beyond 1 year in DES-treated patients.[5] In a post hoc analysis from the Clopidogrel for High Atherothrombotic Risk and Ischemic Stabilization, Management and Avoidance (CHARISMA) trial, patients with a history of a prior myocardial infarction achieved a 24% relative risk reduction in ischemic events with prolonged therapy of up to 3 years.[26] This has also raised the question of whether prolonging dual antiplatelet therapy may be dependent on the clinical setting, in which patients with acute coronary syndrome may potentially derive continuing benefit from prolonged treatment. However, prospective randomized trials are warranted to define this. Recent studies have suggested that the duration of dual antiplatelet therapy may depend on the type of DES being used. Encouraging data have been generated from the use of second-generation DES, which have shown to present a more favorable safety profile compared with earlier generation DES. In the Efficacy of Xience/promus vs. Cypher in rEducing Late Loss after stENTing (EXCELLENT) trial, 6-month dual antiplatelet therapy was shown to be noninferior to a 12-month regimen with regard to the risk of target vessel failure at 12 months after DES implantation.[27] Noninferiority was shown to be significant only in the everolimus-eluting stent subgroup but not in the sirolimus-eluting group. Recent reports from the Synergy Between Stent and Drugs to Avoid Ischemic Recurrences After Percutaneous Coronary Intervention (PRODIGY) trial have shown that 2 years of dual antiplatelet therapy after coronary stenting is not more effective than 6 months of treatment for reducing ischemic events but doubled the rate of major bleeding.[28] A series of ongoing, large-scale, clinical trials are addressing the optimal duration of dual antiplatelet therapy.[5]

Prasugrel

Prasugrel is indicated to reduce the rate of thrombotic cardiovascular events, including stent thrombosis, in patients with acute coronary syndrome who are to be managed with PCI. The recommended dose of prasugrel is a 60-mg loading dose and a 10-mg maintenance dose. A dose modification (5-mg maintenance dose) is recommended for low-weight patients (<60 kg) by the U.S. Food and Drug Administration (FDA) and European Medical Agency (EMA). The EMA recommends a 5-mg maintenance dose also for older patients (>75 years), whereas the FDA recommends consideration of a 10-mg maintenance dose for older patients at high risk for ischemia, such those with a history of diabetes or prior myocardial infarction. Treatment is recommended for up to 15 months.

Prasugrel was extensively studied in the Trial to Assess Improvement in Therapeutic Outcomes by Optimizing Platelet Inhibition with Prasugrel (TRITON) trial, which showed that prasugrel plus aspirin was significantly more effective than clopidogrel plus aspirin for preventing short- and long-term (up to 15 months) ischemic events (composite of cardiovascular death, nonfatal myocardial infarction, or nonfatal stroke) in patients with moderate- to high-risk acute coronary syndrome, with and without ST segment elevation, and undergoing PCI.[29] These events were mainly driven by a reduction in the incidence of myocardial infarction. Patients with diabetes mellitus and those with ST elevation myocardial infarction derived the greatest absolute ischemic benefit from prasugrel therapy, without any increase in major bleeding events, although there were no significant interactions between the treatment effects of prasugrel and the presence or absence of these two characteristics. There was also a marked reduction in early (<30 days) and late (>30 days, up to 15 months) stent thrombosis rates with prasugrel therapy, observed in patients treated with BMS and those treated with DES, and reduced rates of urgent target vessel revascularization. However, prasugrel was associated with a significantly higher risk for major bleeding, including life-threatening bleeding, compared with clopidogrel.

Prasugrel needs to be withheld for 7 days in patients requiring surgery. Although in the TRITON trial patients needed to have their coronary anatomy known prior to treatment with prasugrel, except for patients undergoing primary PCI in whom pretreatment was allowed, the FDA allows clinicians to pretreat with prasugrel if CABG surgery is deemed unlikely. However, to date, there are no data on the benefits of prasugrel pretreatment in the setting of unstable angina or non–ST elevation myocardial infarction. The ACCOAST trial, which randomly assigned invasively managed patients with non–ST elevation myocardial infarction to prasugrel pre-treatment or at the time of PCI, was halted prematurely because of safety concerns.[29a]

Ticagrelor

Ticagrelor is indicated for the prevention of atherothrombotic events in patients with acute coronary syndrome (unstable angina, non–ST elevation myocardial infarction, or ST elevation myocardial infarction), including patients managed medically and those managed with PCI or CABG. This indication is derived from the Platelet Inhibition and Outcomes (PLATO) trial, which assessed the efficacy and safety of 1-year treatment with ticagrelor plus aspirin versus clopidogrel plus aspirin in patients with and without ST elevation acute coronary syndrome.[30] Ticagrelor has shown better short- and long-term outcomes (composite of cardiovascular death, nonfatal myocardial infarction, or nonfatal stroke). There was also a significant reduction in cardiovascular death and overall death in ticagrelor-treated patients. In the PLATO trial, pretreatment with clopidogrel was allowed. Treatment with ticagrelor should be initiated with a single 180-mg loading dose and then continued at 90 mg, twice daily. Treatment is recommended for up to 12 months. In a predefined subgroup analysis of patients enrolled in the PLATO trial showed a borderline significant interaction with enrollment geographic area ($P = 0.05$), which suggested an attenuation of the treatment efficacy of ticagrelor in patients recruited in North America. It has been suggested that this may be attributed to the use of a higher aspirin dose regimen (e.g., 325 mg), which was more prevalent in North America, that may have limited the efficacy of ticagrelor.[30a] Therefore, low aspirin maintenance doses (i.e., <100 mg) are recommended for ticagrelor-treated patients.

Side Effects

Bleeding complications remain the primary concern in patients treated with $P2Y_{12}$ receptor inhibitors. Bleeding events are increased with dual antiplatelet therapy compared with aspirin alone. In clopidogrel-treated patients, the risk of bleeding has been attributed to the dose of aspirin used; in particular, higher doses of aspirin

(>200 mg) were associated with an increased risk of bleeding.[31] Ticagrelor should be used with low-dose aspirin (<100 mg) because higher doses may limit its efficacy.[32] Prasugrel has not been shown to be affected by aspirin doses. Spontaneous bleeding is increased with the more potent novel P2Y[12] receptor antagonists prasugrel and ticagrelor.[29,30] With both agents, the risk of spontaneous bleeding increases over time; these drugs are contraindicated in patients at high risk of bleeding. In particular, in low-weight patients, there was no net clinical benefit of prasugrel because of the increased bleeding risk, suggesting the need for dose modifications in these settings. However, the safety of the 5-mg dose has not been prospectively studied—this dose is derived from pharmacokinetic findings. In older patients with diabetes or prior myocardial infarction, the benefits may outweigh the risks, supporting the use of prasugrel at standard dosing in older patients with these risk factors. Patients with prior stroke or a transient ischemic attack (TIA) had net clinical harm from prasugrel, which should be avoided in these patients. Ticagrelor was not associated with a significant increase in overall bleeding events compared with clopidogrel; however, it was associated with a higher rate of spontaneous non–CABG-related major bleeding, including more cases of fatal intracranial bleeding, although overall fatal bleeding was not increased.[30] Ticagrelor is therefore contraindicated in patients at high risk of bleeding, in those with a history of prior intracranial hemorrhage, and in those with severe hepatic dysfunction.

Other rare complications of thienopyridines are neutropenia with ticlopidine (0.1%) and the potentially fatal thrombotic thrombocytopenic purpura, which has been shown mainly with clopidogrel.[10] Other adverse nonbleeding events have shown to be higher with ticagrelor versus clopidogrel, including dyspnea, ventricular pauses, and increases in serum uric acid and serum creatinine levels, which have been associated with higher rates of treatment discontinuation.[30]

Drug-regulating agencies have mandated a boxed warning for clopidogrel based on pharmacodynamic studies showing a drug interaction between proton pump inhibitors (mainly omeprazole and esomeprazole), as well as the presence of reduced antiplatelet effects among patient carriers of loss of function CYP2C19 alleles.[33,34] These drug interactions and genetic modulating effects have not been shown with prasugrel and ticagrelor. Prasugrel and ticagrelor, however, need to be used with caution in patients treated with drugs associated with increased bleeding potential, including fibrinolytics and oral anticoagulant therapy.[29] In patients treated with ticagrelor, coadministration of strong CYP3A4 inhibitors is not recommended, and the concomitant use of strong CYP3A4 inducers or CYP3A4 substrates with narrow therapeutic indices is discouraged.[30]

GLYCOPROTEIN IIB/IIIA INHIBITORS

Mechanisms of Action

The GP IIb/IIIa receptor is an integrin, a heterodimer consisting of noncovalently associated alpha and beta subunits, the alpha-2b and beta-3 subunits.[35] By competing with fibrinogen and von Willebrand factor (vWF) for GP IIb/IIIa binding, GP IIb/IIIa antagonists interfere with platelet cross linking and platelet-derived thrombus formation.[36] Since the GP IIb/IIIa receptor represents the final common pathway leading to platelet aggregation, these agents are very potent platelet inhibitors. Only parenteral forms are available for clinical use, since trials of the oral GP IIb/IIIa inhibitors demonstrated lack of benefit, including increased mortality.

There are three parenteral GP IIb/IIIa antagonists approved for clinical use—abciximab, eptifibatide, and tirofiban. Abciximab is a large chimeric monoclonal antibody with a high binding affinity that results in a prolonged pharmacologic effect.[35] It is a monoclonal antibody that is a Fab (fragment antigen binding) fragment of a chimeric human-mouse genetic reconstruction of 7E3. The specific binding site of abciximab is the beta-3 subunit. Its plasma half-life is biphasic, with an initial half-life of less than 10 minutes and a second-phase half-life of approximately 30 minutes. However, because of its high affinity for the GP IIb/IIIa receptor, it has a biologic half-life of 12 to 24 hours

and, because of its slow clearance from the body, it has a functional half-life up to 7 days. Platelet-associated abciximab can be detected for more than 14 days after treatment discontinuation.

Eptifibatide and tirofiban, also termed *small-molecule agents*, do not induce an immune response and have a lower affinity for the GP IIb/IIIa receptor. Eptifibatide is a reversible and highly selective heptapeptide with a rapid onset and short plasma half-life of 2 to 2.5 hours. After discontinuation of the infusion, the recovery of platelet aggregation occurs within 4 hours.[35] Tirofiban is a tyrosine-derived nonpeptide inhibitor that functions as a mimic of the RGD amino acid sequence and is highly specific for the GP IIb/IIIa receptor. Tirofiban has a rapid onset and short duration of action, with a plasma half-life of approximately 2 hours. Similarly to eptifibatide, tirofiban has significant recovery of platelet aggregation within 4 hours of completion of infusion.

Indications

Numerous clinical trials have been conducted over the past decades to elucidate the appropriate indications for the use of GP IIb/IIIa inhibitors. Currently, these agents are indicated only in the setting of PCI.[4,5] However, clinical trials have shown no benefit to the use of these agents in the setting of patients with stable CAD undergoing elective PCI if pretreated with clopidogrel.[37] However, GP IIb/IIIa inhibitors have shown to be of benefit in the setting of acute coronary syndrome patients undergoing PCI.[38] Among patients with unstable angina or non–ST elevation myocardial infarction undergoing PCI, guidelines have advised that high-risk patients, especially those with positive cardiac biomarkers, should receive a GP IIb/IIIa antagonist.[4,5,38] The small-molecule agents eptifibatide and tirofiban may be started 1 to 2 days before and continued during the procedure, but abciximab is recommended only in the setting of PCI. However, recent clinical trials have failed to show any benefit with the routine use of upstream compared with ad hoc GP IIb/IIIa inhibition in acute coronary syndrome patients undergoing PCI; therefore, this upstream strategy is no longer recommended.[39] Abciximab has been extensively evaluated in the setting of patients with ST elevation myocardial infarction undergoing primary PCI. In the prethienopyridine era, abciximab was associated with a significant reduction in the rate of reinfarction and mortality rates at 30 days.[35] However, more recent data have argued against upstream GP IIb/IIIa inhibitor use in patients pretreated with P2Y[12] inhibitors undergoing primary PCI. No renal adjustment is required for abciximab dosing. Epifibatide and tirofiban are renally excreted and therefore require dose adjustments in patients with renal dysfunction (epifibatide, 1 µg/kg/min with creatinine clearance < 50 mL/min; tirofiban dose reduction by 50% with creatinine clearance < 30 mL/min).[5]

Side Effects

The primary adverse effect of GP IIb/IIIa receptor antagonists is bleeding.[35] The risk of bleeding complications has limited the use of GP IIb/IIIa receptor antagonists, which are now reserved for high thrombotic risk settings. Bleeding complications with GP IIb/IIIa receptor antagonists are increased in older patients and in those with chronic kidney disease. This has been frequently attributed to overdosing, underscoring the need for dose adjustments in these settings. In addition, adjusting heparin dosing (50 to 70 IU/kg) is pivotal to reduce bleeding complications in patients treated with GP IIb/IIIa receptor antagonists undergoing PCI. Thrombocytopenia is also an undesirable side effect of GP IIb/IIIa receptor antagonists, in particular abciximab. Although the overall incidence is relatively low, the effects may be life-threatening. Thrombocytopenia with abciximab (as defined by a platelet count < 100,000/liter) occurs in 2.5% to 6% of patients and severe thrombocytopenia (platelet count < 50,000/liter) occurred in 0.4% to 1.6% of patients in clinical trials. This complication is less common with eptifibatide and tirofiban. In cases of severe thrombocytopenia, the immediate cessation of therapy is the main approach. Thrombocytopenia in patients undergoing PCI is associated with more ischemic events, bleeding complications, and transfusions. The platelet count typically falls within hours of GP IIb/IIIa administration. Readministration of abciximab, but not eptifibatide and tirofiban, is associated with a slightly increased risk of thrombocytopenia; its use should thus be avoided or changed for another small-molecule agent. Treatment with GP IIb/IIIa inhibitors can also cause pseudothrombocytopenia, which occurs as a result of artifactual platelet clumping in vitro, with an incidence as high as 2.1% with the use of abciximab. A smear to examine for the presence of clumped platelets directly may be required for an accurate diagnosis.

Anticoagulant Therapy

The role of anticoagulant therapy is to block the activity of coagulation factors. The understanding of the role of coagulation factors in thrombosis has led to the development of anticoagulant agents that target specific elements of the coagulation cascade (Figure 12-4). The blockade of coagulation factors in the acute setting of acute coronary syndrome and PCI patients is pivotal because procoagulant factors are associated with enhanced platelet reactivity, thus increasing thrombotic risk. Table 12-4 summarizes the dosing recommendations for these anticoagulant drugs.

INDIRECT THROMBIN INHIBITORS: UNFRACTIONATED HEPARIN AND LOW-MOLECULAR-WEIGHT HEPARIN

Mechanisms of Action

Unfractionated Heparin

Indirect thrombin inhibitors include unfractionated heparin (UFH) and low-molecular weight heparins (LMWHs), which require a cofactor to exert their effects fully.[40] UFH is a heterogeneous mixture of variable molecular weight (2 to 30 kDa) polysaccharide molecules. UFH has two structural components that are pivotal in determining its function: (1) a unique pentasaccharide sequence, mainly responsible for factor Xa inhibition; and (2) saccharide chain lengths more than 18 units long, needed to achieve thrombin inhibition. The pentasaccharide sequence is required for the binding of UFH to antithrombin (AT), thereby increasing the potency of AT by up to 1000-fold. This UFH-AT complex inactivates factors IIa, Xa, IXa, XIa, and

XIIa. Factors IIa (also known as thrombin) and Xa are the most sensitive to the UFH effects, although thrombin is approximately 10 times more susceptible than factor Xa.

UFH is cleared via two different processes. The primary elimination pathway is a rapid but saturable depolymerization in endothelial cells and macrophages, and the second slower pathway is via nonsaturable renal clearance. These kinetics confer a nonlinear response at therapeutic doses, with the intensity and duration of effect rising disproportionately with increasing dose. This makes the periodic adjustment of dosage mandatory, using the activated time of thromboplastin. Moreover, the anticoagulant effect of UFH is lost within a few hours after withdrawal; this can lead to a risk of reactivation of the coagulation process, known as heparin rebound, and thereby a transiently increased risk of thrombosis.[40] In addition to its anticoagulant activity, UFH has various other biologic effects because of its heterogeneous binding properties to a variety of cells and proteins. The most clinically significant nonanticoagulant effect of UFH is its potential to induce immune-mediated platelet activation, resulting in a phenomenon known as *heparin-induced thrombocytopenia*.

Low-Molecular-Weight Heparins

LMWHs are produced through the depolymerization of the polysaccharide chains of UFH, producing fragments ranging from 2 to 10 kDa.[41] These shorter chain lengths contain the unique pentasaccharide sequence necessary to bind to AT (<18 saccharides), but these lengths are too short to form the ternary complex cross linking AT and thrombin. Thus, the primary effects of LMWHs are mostly on factor Xa inhibition (e.g., the ratio of enoxaparin's anti-Xa to anti-IIa activity is 4:1). LMWHs have reduced binding to plasma proteins and cells compared with UFH, thereby providing a more favorable and predictable pharmacokinetic profile. After subcutaneous injection, LMWHs have a bioavailability higher than 90% and a predictable anticoagulant response; they do not require monitoring because of their more rapid and predictable absorption. Anti-Xa levels peak 3 to 5 hours after a subcutaneous dose of LMWH.[27] The elimination half-life of LMWHs is largely dose-independent and occurs 3 to 6 hours after a subcutaneous dose, being cleared by the kidney and leading to prolonged anti-Xa effect and linear accumulation of anti-Xa activity in patients with a creatinine clearance lower than 30 mL/min. LMWHs also produce fewer platelet agonist effects and are less often associated with heparin-induced thrombocytopenia.

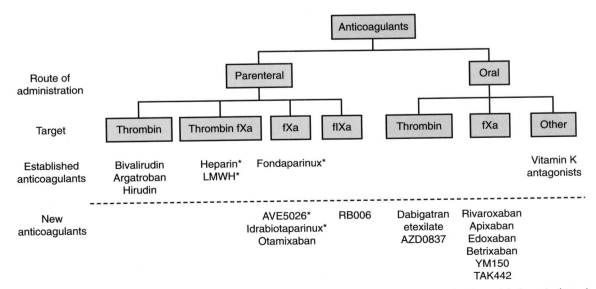

Figure 12-4 **Classification of established anticoagulants and new anticoagulants.** AVE5026 is an ultralow-molecular-weight heparin that primarily inhibits fXa and has minimal activity against thrombin. Anticoagulants with asterisks indirectly inhibit coagulation by interacting with antithrombin. *FxIa,* Factor Ixa. (From Eikelboom, JW, Weitz Jl. New anticoagulants. *Circulation* 2010;121:1523-1532.)

TABLE 12-4	Recommended Doses and Need for Renal Adjustment of Clinically Approved Anticoacoagulant Drugs			
Anticoacoagulant Drugs	*Recommended Dose*	*Renal Adjustment*	*Renal Dosing*	
Indirect Thrombin Inhibitors				
UFH	For patients undergoing PCI who have received prior anticoagulant therapy and for whom IV GPI is planned—additional UFH as needed (e.g., 2000-5000 U) to achieve ACT of 200-250 sec For patients undergoing PCI who have received prior anticoagulant therapy and for whom no IV GPI is planned—additional UFH as needed (e.g., 2000-5000 U) to achieve ACT of 250-300 sec for HemoTec, 300-350 sec for Hemocron For patients undergoing PCI who have not received prior anticoagulant therapy and for whom IV GPI is planned—50- to 70-U/kg bolus to achieve ACT of 200-250 sec For patients undergoing PCI who have not received prior anticoagulant therapy and for whom no IV GPI is planned—70-100 U/kg bolus to achieve target ACT of 250-300 sec for HemoTec, 300-350 sec for Hemocron	No	NA	
Enoxaparin	IV dose of 30-mg bolus followed by SC dose of 1 mg/kg/12 hr During PCI, for patients who have already received enoxaparin, if last SC dose was administered 8 to 12 hr earlier, then PCI; or if only one SC dose of enoxaparin has been administered, IV dose of 0.3 mg/kg of enoxaparin should be given If last SC dose was administered within the prior 8 hr, no additional enoxaparin should be given before PCI During PCI, for patients who have not received prior anticoagulant therapy—0.5- to 0.75-mg/kg IV bolus	Yes	If creatinine clearance < 30 mL/min, extend dosing interval of maintenance dose to 1 mg/kg/24 hr.	
Direct Thrombin Inhibitor				
Bivalirudin	For patients who have received UFH, wait 30 min, then give 0.75-mg/kg IV bolus, then 1.75 mg/kg/hr IV infusion For patients who have not received prior anticoagulant therapy—0.75-mg/kg bolus, then 1.75 mg/kg/hr IV infusion	Yes	No reduction in bolus dose needed for any degree of renal impairment. Patients with moderate renal impairment (30-59 mL/min) should receive infusion of 1.75 mg/kg/hr. If creatinine clearance < 30 mL/min, reduction of infusion rate to 1.0 mg/kg/hr should be considered. If patient is on hemodialysis, infusion should be reduced to 0.25 mg/kg/hr.	
Direct Factor X Inhibitor				
Fondaparinux	2.5 SC daily	Yes	In patients with moderate renal impairment (30-50 mL/min), fondaparinux dose should be reduced by 50%. Avoid administration in patients with creatinine clearance < 30 mL/min.	

ACT, Activated clotting time; *GPI,* glycoprotein inhibitor; *IV,* intravenous; *NA,* not applicable; *PCI,* percutaneous coronary intervention; *SC,* subcutaneous; *UFH,* unfractionated heparin.

Indications

Unfractionated Heparin

UFH has been used in the management of acute coronary syndrome and PCI patients for many years, and its benefit when added to platelet inhibitors has been clearly established.[4,5] In addition, many of the platelet inhibitor trials have been conducted with the coadministration of heparin. This has established heparin as a class IA therapy when used with platelet inhibitors. In the setting of PCI without GP IIb/IIIa inhibitors, UFH is recommended at a dose of 70 to 100 IU/kg; a dose of 50 to 70 IU/kg is recommended for patients undergoing PCI with the use of GP IIb/IIIa inhibitor.

Low-Molecular-Weight Heparins

Although many different LMWH preparations have been developed, enoxaparin is the most widely studied in clinical trials of unstable angina and non–ST elevation myocardial infarction, ST elevation myocardial infarction, and PCI. For patients in whom an invasive strategy is selected, enoxaparin (1 mg/kg subcutaneously twice daily) has established efficacy for patients in whom an invasive or conservative strategy is selected. Careful attention is needed to adjust the LMWH dose appropriately in patients with renal insufficiency (1.0 mg/kg subcutaneously every 24 hours for patients with an estimated creatinine clearance < 30 mL/min). If LMWH has been started as the upstream anticoagulant, it should be continued without stacking of UFH. If patients undergo PCI, enoxaparin can be administered in several ways:

1. The first dosing regimen option is 1 mg/kg subcutaneously twice daily; when this route is used, it is important to ensure that the last dose of subcutaneous LMWH is administered within 8 hours of the procedure and that at least two subcutaneous doses of LMWH are given before the procedure to ensure a steady state.
2. If the last dose of enoxaparin was given 8 to 12 hours before PCI, a 0.3-mg/kg IV bolus enoxaparin is recommended at the time of PCI.
3. The third dosing regimen option is 1 mg/kg enoxaparin given IV (if no GP IIb/IIIa inhibitor is used) or 0.75 mg/kg (if a GP IIb/IIIa inhibitor is used) at the time of PCI.[4,5] For elective PCI, an IV dose of 0.5 mg/kg was found to be safe in the SafeTy and Efficacy of Enoxaparin in PCI patients, an internationaL randomized Evaluation (STEEPLE) study.[42]

Overall, enoxaparin is a good alternative to UFH in PCI settings. In patients undergoing primary PCI, the largest evidence derives from the Acute Myocardial Infarction Treated with Primary Angioplasty and Intravenous Enoxaparin or Unfractionated Heparin to Lower Ischemic and Bleeding Events at Short- and Long-term Follow-up (ATOLL) trial. Although enoxaparin did not achieve a reduction in the primary ischemic endpoint, it did significantly reduce some clinical ischemic outcomes in comparison with UFH, without differences in bleeding or procedural success.[43]

Side Effects

Bleeding remains an undesirable effect of indirect thrombin inhibitors; its risk varies according to the dosage used and risk profile of the population. The risk of bleeding increases with higher heparin dosages, concomitant use of antiplatelet drugs or oral anticoagulants, and increasing patient age (>70 years). Patients with renal dysfunction have increased risk of bleeding with LMWHs, underscoring the importance of adjusted dosing in these patients.[4,5] Reversal of the anticoagulant effect of UFH can be achieved rapidly with a 1-mg IV bolus of protamine to neutralize 100 IU of UFH; however, the degree to which the anti-Xa activity of LMWH is neutralized by protamine is variable and uncertain. Another adverse effect described with heparin is the development of heparin-induced thrombocytopenia, which usually occurs between 5 and 15 days after the initiation of therapy. In the setting of heparin-induced thrombocytopenia, a direct antithrombin drug must be selected. Patients treated with LMWH can develop heparin-induced thrombocytopenia, and these drugs are not recommended for use in patients with documented or suspected heparin-induced thrombocytopenia. Less commonly, the long-term use of heparin can be associated with the development of osteoporosis and rare allergic reactions.[40]

DIRECT THROMBIN INHIBITORS

Mechanisms of Action

Direct thrombin inhibitors (DTIs) exert their anticoagulant effects by binding directly to thrombin. In turn, this inhibits thrombin activity and thrombin-mediated activation of other coagulation factors (e.g., fibrin from fibrinogen), as well as thrombin-induced platelet aggregation.[44] Importantly, DTIs inhibit clot-bound and free thrombin, thereby providing a potential rationale for clinical use in the setting of acute coronary syndrome and PCI. Several DTIs, including lepirudin, argatroban, and bivalirudin, have been approved for use. Lepirudin and argatroban are indicated only for the treatment of heparin-induced thrombocytopenia, whereas bivalirudin is used as a first-line anticoagulant in the setting of acute coronary syndrome and PCI.

Bivalirudin

Bivalirudin is a 20–amino acid polypeptide and is a synthetic version of hirudin. Its amino terminal D-Phe-Pro-Arg-Pro domain, which interacts with the active site of thrombin, is linked via four Gly residues to a dodecapeptide analogue of the carboxy terminal of hirudin (thrombin exosite). Bivalirudin forms a 1:1 stoichiometric complex with thrombin, but once bound, the amino terminal of bivalirudin is cleaved by thrombin, thereby restoring thrombin activity (Figure 12-5).[44] Bivalirudin is not immunogenic, although antibodies against hirudin can cross-react with bivalirudin, with unknown clinical consequences. Bivalirudin has a half-life of 25 minutes; proteolysis, hepatic metabolism, and renal excretion contribute to its clearance. The half-life of bivalirudin is prolonged with severe renal impairment; therefore, a dosage adjustment is required in dialysis-dependent patients. Patients with moderate renal impairment (30 to 59 mL/min) should receive an infusion of 1.75 mg/kg/hr. If the creatinine clearance is less than 30 mL/min, reduction of the infusion rate to 1 mg/kg/hr should be considered. If a patient is on hemodialysis, the infusion rate should be reduced to 0.25 mg/kg/hr. The infusion may be continued for 4 hours after the procedure at the discretion of the operator.

Indications. Bivalirudin is currently approved for use during PCI as an alternative to the use of UFH. The benefit of bivalirudin as an anticoagulant in patients undergoing PCI has been demonstrated across the spectrum of CAD manifestations (stable CAD, unstable angina non–ST elevation myocardial infarction, and ST elevation myocardial infarction). In the PCI setting, bivalirudin has been tested in comparison with UFH with and without abciximab in several trials, showing noninferiority in terms of ischemic events, with significantly less bleeding complications. This has been confirmed in several studies, particularly in patients with unstable angina and non–ST-elevation myocardial infarction.[45,46] The benefits of bivalirudin are enhanced in patients at greater risk of bleeding, including older patients, diabetics, and patients with chronic kidney disease. Recently, in the Harmonizing Outcomes with Revascularization and Stents in Acute Myocardial Infarctions (HORIZONS-AMI) trial, bivalirudin reduced cardiac mortality and all-cause mortality among ST elevation myocardial infarction patients compared with UFH with abciximab at 3-year follow-up.[47,47a]

FACTOR XA INHIBITORS

Fondaparinux

Fondaparinux is a synthetic analogue of the AT-binding pentasaccharide sequence found in UFH. Fondaparinux is a selective factor Xa inhibitor that binds reversibly to AT, producing an irreversible conformational change at the reactive site of AT that enhances its reactivity with factor Xa. Fondaparinux is rapidly absorbed and has a bioavailability of 100% after subcutaneous injection. Steady levels of fonadaparinux are achieved after three or four doses. The elimination of this anticoagulant is mainly renal, with a half-life of 17 hours, and therefore the use of fondaparinux is contraindicated in those with severe renal impairment. Fondaparinux produces a predictable anticoagulant response and exhibits linear pharmacokinetics when given in subcutaneous doses of 2 to 8 mg or in IV doses ranging from 2 to 20 mg that result in anti-Xa activity approximately seven times that of LMWHs.[48]

The OASIS-5 trial demonstrated the noninferiority of fondaparinux in combined death, myocardial infarction, or refractory ischemia at 9 days, which was achieved with significantly lower major bleeding in comparison with enoxaparin among patients with unstable angina non–ST elevation myocardial infarction.[49] Moreover, a reduction in mortality at 6 months was also observed. In the group of patients who underwent PCI, there was evidence for more catheter-related thrombus formation with fondaparinux, indicating that anticoagulation with fondaparinux alone is insufficient for PCI; adjunctive UFH at therapeutic doses should be used, as confirmed in the OASIS-8 trial.[50] In the OASIS-6 trial, patients with ST elevation myocardial infarction who underwent primary PCI had no significant benefit with fondaparinux and had more catheter-related thrombi, more coronary complications, and a trend toward higher mortality and/or myocardial infarction compared with UFH.[51]

Indications

Based on a dose-ranging study of fondaparinux versus enoxaparin in the setting of unstable angina and non–ST elevation myocardial infarction, fondaparinux 2.5 mg daily was shown to have the best efficacy and safety profile when compared with 4-, 8-, and 12-mg doses of fondaparinux and with enoxaparin, 1 mg/kg twice daily.[49] In patients with moderate renal impairment (30 to 50 mL/min), the fondaparinux dose should be reduced by 50%. Coagulation monitoring is not recommended. Fondaparinux is recommended for unstable angina and non–ST elevation myocardial infarction acute coronary syndrome patients for whom an early conservative or delayed invasive strategy of management is considered. For patients treated with upstream fondaparinux and undergoing PCI, additional IV boluses of UFH should be given at the time of the procedure, as well as additional IV doses of fondaparinux (2.5 mg if also receiving a GP IIb/IIIa inhibitor and 5 mg if not). Fondaparinux should not be used in

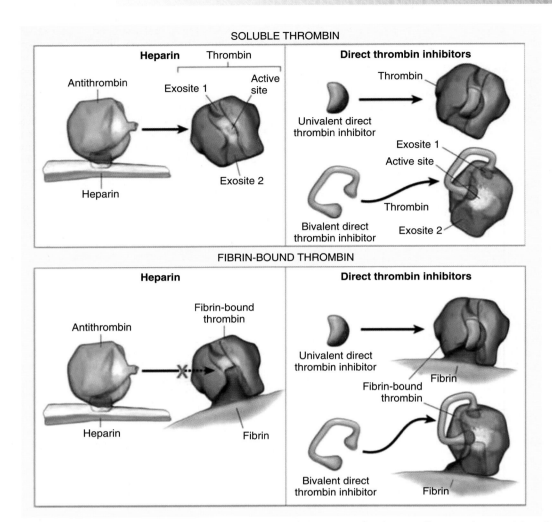

Figure 12-5 **Mechanism of action of direct thrombin inhibitors compared with heparin.** In the absence of heparin, the rate of thrombin inactivation by antithrombin is relatively low, but after conformational change induced by heparin, antithrombin irreversibly binds to and inhibits the active site of thrombin. Thus, the anticoagulant activity of heparin originates from its ability to generate a ternary heparin-thrombin-antithrombin complex. The activity of direct thrombin inhibitors is independent of the presence of antithrombin and is related to the direct interaction of these drugs with the thrombin molecule. Although bivalent direct thrombin inhibitors simultaneously bind the exosite 1 and the active site, the univalent drugs in this class interact only with an active site of the enzyme. *Lower panel,* The heparin-antithrombin complex cannot bind fibrin-bound thrombin, whereas given their mechanism of action, direct thrombin inhibitors can bind to and inhibit the activity of not only soluble thrombin, but also thrombin bound to fibrin, as is the case in a blood clot. (From Di Nisio M, Middeldorp S, Buller HR. Direct thrombin inhibitors. *N Engl J Med* 2005;353:1028-1040.)

patients with acute ST elevation myocardial infarction undergoing primary PCI .[4,5]

Individualizing Antitplatelet and Antithrombotic Therapy

Over the past decade, an overwhelming number of studies have been conducted in patients on aspirin and clopidogrel therapy, supporting the contention that recurrent events after PCI and acute coronary syndrome may at least partly be attributed to the broad variability in individual antiplatelet drug response. Most studies have shown that levels of on-treatment platelet reactivity, which represent the absolute level of platelet reactivity during treatment, rather than a change (absolute or relative), to be a better measure of risk of a future adverse event.[13] In particular, platelet function studies have shown that patients with persistently high on-treatment platelet reactivity, despite aspirin and clopidogrel therapy, have an increased risk of recurrent ischemic events, including stent thrombosis, whereas patients with low levels of platelet reactivity have an increased risk of bleeding.[52]

Numerous definitions have been used in the literature to define the pharmcodynamic effect of antiplatelet drugs. These include resistance, nonresponders, hyporesponders, and hyperresponders.[11,13] In the strictest sense, the terms *resistance* or *nonresponders* imply complete failure of an antiplatelet drug to inhibit the target of its action. However, these terms imply an all or none effect, whereas most pharmacodynamic studies demonstrate a broad range of effects, thus supporting the concept of response variability in which some patients may have lower (hyporesponders) or higher (hyperresponders) than anticipated antiplatelet effects. These terms are laboratory-based definitions, which imply that a platelet function test be performed. Because thrombotic events involve multiple signaling pathways, it is incorrect to attribute ischemic outcomes to a specific drug response profile without laboratory testing of the antiplatelet agent in the affected patient.

ASPIRIN RESPONSE

The term *aspirin resistance* has been considered to be the failure of aspirin to inhibit COX-1.[53] Laboratory methods to assess aspirin response are divided into COX-1–specific and COX-1–nonspecific methods.[39] COX-1–specific methods include the measurement of serum TXB2 or agonist-induced TXB2 in platelet-rich plasma and AA-induced platelet aggregation. Examples of systems that measure AA-induced aggregation are light transmittance aggregometry, impedance aggregometry (whole blood), VerifyNow Aspirin test, thromboelastography, and the Multiplate Analyzer. However, the COX-1–specific assays have several limitations; for example, serum TXB2 measurement may be affected by nonplatelet sources, such as leukocytes. Moreover, leukocyte COX-2 activity may play a role in the response of platelet to AA. COX-1–nonspecific methods include PFA-100, urine biomarker 11-dehydrothromboxane B2 (11-dh-TXB2) levels, and light transmittance aggregometry with agonists other than AA, including ADP, epinephrine, or collagen. Although all these tests have the ability to assess the effects of aspirin on the platelet phenotype, they share the common limitation that the results are influenced by multiple variables and thus are not necessarily reflective of the true status of COX-1 blockade. Therefore, there is a broad variability in the results obtained with the use of these tests, which explains why the prevalence of resistance reported by investigators varies considerably (from 5.5% to 61%). When using COX-1–specific tests, such as light transmittance aggregometry following AA stimuli, aspirin resistance is infrequent (≈1%).[54] Numerous studies and meta-analyses using various laboratory assays have supported the poor prognostic implications of inadequate aspirin-induced effects; however, which of the multitude of tests to assess aspirin effects best predicts outcomes remains unknown.[55]

CLOPIDOGREL RESPONSE

Clopidogrel specifically inhibits the $P2Y_{12}$ receptor, and numerous pharmacodynamic studies have shown a broad variability in individual response to this agent.[11,13] ADP activates platelets through both the $P2Y_1$ and $P2Y_{12}$ receptors, so the results obtained by light transmittance aggregometry are not fully reflective of levels of clopidogrel-mediated $P2Y_{12}$ blockade. Other tests used to evaluate clopidogrel effects include the platelet vasodilator-stimulated phosphoprotein (VASP-P) test, VerifyNow $P2Y_{12}$ assay, Innovance PFA P2Y system, PFA-100, thromboelastography with platelet mapping, and flow cytometric measurements of platelet membrane receptors and selectins. Numerous studies have reported that the pharmacologic variability in antiplatelet effects mediated by clopidogrel, as assessed by several platelet function assays, are a potential cause of thrombotic events, mainly after PCI. Most of these studies have demonstrated that levels of on-treatment platelet reactivity are the best risk predictor of thrombotic events. Cutoff values of on-treatment platelet reactivity associated with recurrent ischemic events may vary somewhat in these studies. This may be attributed not only to differences in the assay used, but also to the patient populations studied, clinical setting, and definitions of ischemic endpoints.

Dual Antiplatelet Drug Response

Recent studies have found that some patients may be nonresponders to both aspirin and clopidogrel, with a prevalence from 6% to 10%, depending on the platelet function test used.[53] Studies that have specifically assessed the response profile to both aspirin and clopidogrel have demonstrated that these patients are at highest risk of a recurrent thrombotic event, particularly stent thrombosis.[56] Although the underlying mechanisms of dual nonresponsiveness are unknown, one hypothesis is that different pathways involved in platelet reactivity can modulate each other and sometimes lead to the development of a global hyperreactive platelet phenotype.

Hyperresponsiveness

Recent studies have linked an enhanced response to antiplatelet drugs, mainly clopidogrel, with an increased risk for bleeding.[52] Bleeding has emerged as an important predictor of long-term mortality, even more than a recurrent myocardial infarction.[57] Several studies

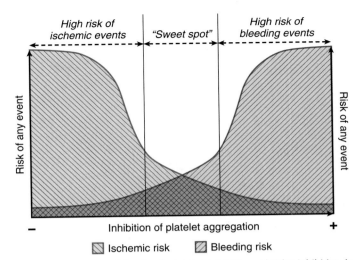

Figure 12-6   Optimal levels of platelet inhibition. Platelet inhibition is related to the risk of ischemic and bleeding events. In particular, low levels of platelet inhibition increase the risk of recurrent ischemic events, whereas high inhibition increases the risk of bleeding. Therefore, the objective of antiplatelet therapies should be to inhibit platelet function to such an extent that the risk of ischemic and bleeding outcomes is minimized. This optimal range of platelet inhibition (therapeutic window) or so-called sweet spot, may be tailored to specific populations or clinical scenarios with different ischemic and bleeding risks. (From Ferreiro JL, Sibbing D, Angiolillo DJ. Platelet function testing and risk of bleeding complications. *Thromb Haemost* 2010; 103:1128-1135.)

in patients undergoing CABG surgery have shown thromboelastography to be a good predictor for hemoglobin loss. Other tests have also been studied for predicting bleeding complications and the need for blood transfusion, particularly in patients taking clopidogrel who are undergoing CABG as well as PCI. However, other studies have failed to find any association between platelet reactivity and bleeding. Further studies are warranted to understand the range of platelet reactivity and the therapeutic window, which offers the greatest benefit in terms of safety and efficacy (i.e., levels of platelet reactivity that are not too low and not too high to promote bleeding and recurrent ischemic events, respectively; Figure 12-6).

Mechanisms of Antiplatelet Drug Response Variability

Several mechanisms leading to variability in response to aspirin or clopidogrel have been identified. This is a multifactorial process, including genetic, cellular, and clinical factors, as described in this section.[11,13,53]

GENETIC FACTORS

Aspirin

The most studied polymorphism affecting aspirin response is the PI^A polymorphism of the GP IIIa subunit.[58] This polymorphism is responsible for the Pro33-Leu amino acid change that has been associated with increased platelet reactivity, differences in aspirin-induced effects, and an increased risk of vascular thrombosis. Carriers of the phospholipase A2 (PLA2) allele have been shown to require a higher dose of aspirin to experience the same antiplatelet effect compared with PLA1 homozygous subjects.[58,59] Other polymorphisms of glycoproteins, such as the GP Ia C807T polymorphism, which has been associated with differences in enumeration of this collagen receptor, have been associated with increased platelet reactivity, although not consistently with differences in aspirin-induced effects.[60] Polymorphisms affecting the gene encoding COX-1 have been associated with the activity of this enzyme and influence aspirin dose requirements.[61] The COX-1 C50T polymorphism has been associated with higher TXB2 levels, a marker associated with thrombotic risk, before and after aspirin treatment in healthy subjects. Moreover, a functional polymorphism of the COX-2 (G-765C) enzyme has also been shown to affect aspirin-induced effects, as assessed by TXB2 levels after aspirin treatment.[62] Polymorphisms of the P2Y$_1$ receptor have also been investigated, but with controversial findings.[63]

Studies have focused on polymorphisms of the major enzymes involved in the metabolism of aspirin, including CYP2C9 and uridine 5'-diphospho (UDP) glucuronosyltransferase (UGT1A6), which is involved in aspirin hydroxylation and glucuronidation.[58,64] Although there is no polymorphism directly related to bleeding in aspirin-treated patients, CYP2C9*2 and CYP2C9*3 polymorphisms have been associated with an increased risk of gastrointestinal bleeding related to NSAIDs, mostly caused by gastrointestinal peptic ulcer, a frequent complication of aspirin.[65] Large-scale clinical studies are required to investigate the association between aspirin-induced ulcer and the genotypes of enzymes metabolizing aspirin, especially CYP2C9, because this polymorphism is related to clopidogrel metabolism and thus synergistic interactions may occur.

Other factors extrinsic to the platelet, such as hemostatic factors, may affect platelet function. Therefore, aspirin may have different degrees of efficacy according to hemostatic polymorphisms. For example, it has been shown that inhibition of factor XIII activation by aspirin may be influenced the Val34-Leu polymorphism, suggesting that low-dose aspirin may provide greater benefit with respect to myocardial infarction risk reduction in Leu34 carriers compared with noncarriers.[66]

Clopidogrel

Polymorphisms of genes codifying proteins involved in clopidogrel-mediated platelet inhibition have been studied according to the different stages that modulate the effects—absorption (e.g., ABCB1), hepatic metabolism (e.g., cytochrome P450 isoenzymes), and platelet reactivity (e.g., platelet membrane receptors).[58] ABCB1 encodes MDR1 (multidrug resistance transporter), an intestinal permeability (P)-glycoprotein involved in clopidogrel absorption. Its genetic variants (e.g., 3435C>T) have been associated with clopidogrel response and cardiovascular events in some studies but not confirmed in others.[67] Clopidogrel is a prodrug requiring two-step oxidation by the hepatic cytochrome P450 (CYP) system to generate an active metabolite.[11] CYP3A4, CYP3A5, CYP2C9, and CYP1A2 are involved in one step; CYP2B6 and CYP2C19 are involved in both steps. Patients with loss of function CYP2C19 alleles have reduced generation of clopidogrel active metabolite, resulting in less clopidogrel effect. Thus, these polymorphisms have been reported as possible determinants of clopidogrel response variability and adverse clinical outcomes. Patients can be divided according to the predicted affect of CYP2C19 genotype on the metabolizer status—extensive metabolizer, intermediate metabolizer, poor metabolizer, and ultrarapid metabolizer.[68] Loss of function alleles confer intermediate metabolizer and/or poor metabolizer status, whereas wild-type or gain of function alleles confer extensive metabolizer or ultrarapid metabolizer status. Several studies have demonstrated a relationship between loss of function allele carriage and diminished clopidogrel pharmacokinetic and pharmacodynamics as well as with clinical thrombotic outcomes, such as stent thrombosis or new myocardial infarction, particularly among PCI-treated patients.[69] More recent observations have suggested that the loss of function alleles may be more influential in the earlier phases of treatment (up to 30 days) but fail to have prognostic implications on long-term events.[70]

Carriers of gain of function alleles, associated with increased clopidogrel-mediated antiplatelet effects, have been associated with more benefit from clopidogrel treatment, but also an increased risk of bleeding events.[71] However, this relationship is not consistent among different studies. More recently, it has been suggested that the Q192R polymorphism of paraoxonase-1 (PON1) influences clopidogrel bioactivation, significantly modulates the pharmacokinetic and pharmacodynamic effects of clopidogrel, and has important clinical implications.[72] However, subsequent investigations have not confirmed these findings.[73]

Several other small pharmacogenetic studies have suggested that polymorphisms of genes encoding for platelet membrane receptors may be involved in the downstream effects of clopidogrel.[58] These include polymorphisms of P2YR$_{12}$, which encodes the P2Y$_{12}$ receptor; ITGB3, which encodes the platelet fibrinogen receptor GP IIb/IIIa; ITGA2, which encodes the platelet collagen receptor GP Ia; and the PAR-1 gene, which encodes the protease-activated receptor-1 for thrombin. However, study findings have not been consistent.

Genetics represents one of the many factors contributing to variability in individual response to an antiplatelet agent. For example, studies have suggested that the loss of function CYP2C19*2 polymorphism, which has most consistently been associated with clopidogrel effects and clinical outcomes, contributes only 5% to 12% to clopidogrel response variability. Current guidelines provide a class IIb (level of evidence C) recommendation for genetic testing, which should be performed only with the intent to modify therapy if a poor metabolizer status is identified.[4,5] The boxed warning for clopidogrel suggests considering alternative treatments for patients identified as poor metabolizers (i.e., those patients who carry two loss of function alleles [homozygotes for CYP2c19 loss of function alleles]). A recent study using escalating maintenance doses of clopidogrel (up to 300 mg daily) found that there was no impact on optimizing platelet function in poor metabolizers, whereas a maintenance dose of 225 mg was necessary to reach levels of platelet reactivity in patients who were carriers of only one loss of function allele similar to non-carriers.[74] Overall, these data suggest considering the use of prasugrel or ticagrelor, which are not affected by CYP2C19 genetic variation, as a more reliable strategy to optimize platelet inhibition, if needed. Routine genetic testing is not recommended, according to guidelines (class III recommendation).

CELLULAR FACTORS

Several cellular factors may influence the antiplatelet effects mediated by aspirin and clopidogrel. Among these, levels of reticulated platelets, young platelets characterized by increased reactivity, which are indicative of accelerated platelet turnover, have been shown to be associated with a reduced response to aspirin and clopidogrel.[11,13] Clinical conditions characterized by increased platelet turnover include patients with diabetes mellitus, acute coronary syndrome, and stroke and those undergoing CABG.

Upregulation of platelet activation signaling pathways can also mitigate antiplatelet drug effects. For example, even though aspirin may fully block the COX-1 enzyme, TXA2 production by the aspirin-insensitive COX-2 isoform in newly formed platelets or other cells can still stimulate thromboxane receptors (TPs), thus leading to reduced aspirin-induced effects.[53] Upregulation of platelet activation pathways occurs frequently in patients with diabetes mellitus.[75] Platelets are targets of the effects of insulin mediated by the IRS-1 receptor. Insulin binding with the platelet IRS-1 receptor induces a loss of G$_i$ activity, which in turn leads to an increase in cyclic adenosine monophosphate (cAMP) levels and reduces platelet reactivity. However, insulin reduces platelet reactivity in healthy volunteers but not in type 2 diabetes mellitus patients, who are affected by insulin resistance. Intracellular cAMP levels modulate the status of VASP-P, which is the main intracellular mediator of P2Y$_{12}$ signaling.[11] Therefore, loss of sensitivity to insulin in type 2 diabetes mellitus platelets reduces cAMP levels; it may be hypothesized that this leads to upregulation of the activity of the P2Y$_{12}$ signaling pathway, which may explain the reduced responsiveness to clopidogrel. Upregulation of other signaling pathways, such as thrombin-mediated platelet activation, is also key in hampering the platelet inhibitory effects of antiplatelet agents. Dysregulation of calcium metabolism is an important feature in platelets from patients with diabetes mellitus and obesity, which lead to a hyperreactive platelet phenotype through multiple mechanisms. Settings associated with increased oxidative stress leading to the excessive generation of potent oxidants, such as superoxide anions and hydrogen peroxide, also increase platelet activation. These can also be mediated by endothelial dysfunction.

CLINICAL FACTORS

The most important factor for achieving adequate antiplatelet effects is compliance.[11,13,53] Poor compliance to antiplatelet therapy is not only the cause of a reduced aspirin or clopidogrel response but also a risk factor for recurrent cardiovascular events. Among patients who are compliant to their prescribed antiplatelet regimen, other clinical factors have been identified that are associated with reduced pharmacodynamic effects of these drugs. Of these, clinical settings, such as diabetes mellitus, acute coronary syndrome, obesity, and chronic kidney disease, all associated with a hyperreactive platelet phenotype, have also been associated with reduced platelet inhibition of antiplatelet treatment. This may in part explain the increased risk of a recurrent ischemic event in these patients. Suboptimal dosing has also been suggested to contribute to inadequate platelet inhibition.

Drug interactions represent another common cause of reduced antiplatelet effects.[76] Competition of aspirin with other NSAIDs, such as ibuprofen, can prevent the irreversible acetylation and inactivation of COX-1 by aspirin, reducing its cardioprotective effects.[3] Drugs that are substrates or inhibit the different CYP isoforms involved in clopidogrel conversion into its active metabolite can also potentially interfere and lead to an impairment of its antiplatelet effects. These include drugs that are commonly used in patients with cardiovascular disease, such as lipophilic statins, coumadin derivatives, and calcium channel blockers. Much attention has been given to the clopidogrel drug interaction induced by proton pump inhibitors (PPIs).[51] These agents are commonly prescribed for patients on dual antiplatelet therapy because they are recommended to reduce the risk of bleeding complications.[4,5] However, a series of pharmacodynamic studies have shown that PPIs metabolized by CYP2C19, such as omeprazole, reduced the generation of clopidogrel's active metabolite and its effects on platelet function.[33] This interaction has not been shown for PPIs that do not interfere with CYP2C19, such as pantoprazole, suggesting that this interaction is a drug-specific effect, rather than a class effect. Although the clinical implications of this drug interaction remain controversial, drug-regulating authorities have prompted a black box warning for the concomitant use of PPIs interfering with CYP2C19 activity, such as omeprazole and clopidogrel. Most recently, however, the only prospective randomized trial assessing the clinical implications associated with concomitant clopidogrel and omeprazole use did not show any increase in ischemic events or significant reduction in bleeding.[77] Further studies are needed to elucidate fully the clinical implications of this and other drug interactions.

⬢ Optimizing Antiplatelet Drug Response

Variability in antiplatelet drug responses can translate into potentially severe and even fatal consequences; thus, efforts must be undertaken to find measures to overcome this problem. The most important approach is first to ensure patient compliance.[53] Furthermore, drug interactions also need to be considered as a potential cause of reduced pharmacodynamic effect, so any medications interfering with aspirin and clopidogrel effects need to be avoided. This may be challenging in the polypharmacy patient, who may be taking other medications that are commonly prescribed for the prevention of recurrent events. In addition to these important considerations, other strategies have been proposed to overcome inadequate antiplatelet drug response.[78] These include increased dosing, use of an additional antiplatelet agent, and use of novel antiplatelet drugs. The next section describes how these strategies can be used to improve the administration of pharmacodynamic measures and how current study results, applied

according to platelet function test or genetic test results, can affect clinical outcomes.

INCREASED DOSING

Increasing the dose of an antiplatelet agent may appear as an intuitive strategy to increase its inhibitory effects. Practice guidelines have defined the optimal dose range of aspirin to be from 75 to 325 mg for the prevention of recurrent ischemic events.[4,5] However, there is no evidence to support the contention that higher doses of aspirin within this dose range are associated with better outcomes compared with lower doses based on registry data and the CURRENT-OASIS 7 trial.[3] This was the first large-scale clinical trial to compare outcomes in patients randomized to high (325 mg) versus low (100 mg) doses of aspirin, which failed to show any ischemic benefit. On the contrary, higher aspirin doses are associated with an increased risk of bleeding complications. In line with these clinical observations, pharmacodynamic studies have not shown that higher doses of aspirin can improve response profiles when using COX-1–specific assays, such as AA-induced light transmittance aggregometry, although they may have an impact on aspirin-induced effects as assessed by less specific pharmacodynamic measures.[53] Because aspirin has a very limited bioavailability, another proposed strategy has been to administer aspirin twice daily rather than simply increasing the once-daily aspirin dose. This strategy has been suggested to overcome increased platelet turnover, which results in an increased proportion of non–aspirin-inhibited platelets during the daily dosing interval.[79] Large-scale clinical trials are warranted to support the safety and efficacy of this dosing regimen.

High clopidogrel dosing has been suggested as a strategy to optimize platelet inhibition. Numerous studies have shown that a high loading dose regimen of clopidogrel ($\geq$600 mg) can achieve a greater and faster degree of platelet inhibition compared with a standard 300-mg loading dose.[80,81] Moreover, these improved profiles achieved with 600 mg of loading dose have been associated with better clinical outcomes, mainly driven by reducing periprocedural myocardial infarction in patients undergoing PCI.[25,82] A high maintenance dose of clopidogrel (150 mg/day) is also associated with increased platelet inhibition compared with the standard 75-mg daily dose.[83,84] However, a high clopidogrel dosing regimen does not achieve optimal levels of platelet inhibition in most patients with inadequate response to standard dosing.[85,86] The CURRENT-OASIS 7 trial did not show any differences in the primary composite endpoint at 30 days in acute coronary syndrome patients randomized to a high clopidogrel dosing regimen (600-mg loading dose, 150-mg maintenance dose daily for 1 week, followed by 75 mg daily) versus a standard clopidogrel dosing regimen (300-mg loading dose, 75-mg maintenance dose daily; hazard ratio [HR], 0.94; 95% confidence interval [CI], 0.83-1.06; P = .30), with an increase in major bleeding (HR 1.24; 95% CI, 1.05-1.46; P = .01). However, this high dosing regimen reduced ischemic vent rates, including stent thrombosis, in patients undergoing PCI.

The efficacy of a high clopidogrel dosing regimen has been evaluated in studies of patients with high on-treatment platelet reactivity. Small trials, which identified patients with high platelet reactivity according to the VASP-P test, have shown that tailored, incremental, 600-mg loading doses of clopidogrel (up to 2400 mg) reduced on-treatment platelet reactivity below the defined threshold stent thrombosis compared with patients without a tailored strategy.[87,88] The Gauging Responsiveness with A VerifyNow Assay—Impact on Thrombosis and Safety (GRAVITAS) trial is to date the largest trial assessing the impact of tailored antiplatelet therapy on patients undergoing PCI.[89] In this study, patients undergoing drug-eluting stent implantation, who demonstrated high on-clopidogrel platelet reactivity 12 to 24 hours after PCI (defined by VerifyNow), were randomized to a high clopidogrel dosing regimen (600 mg followed by 150 mg daily for 6 months) versus standard clopidogrel therapy. Compared with standard therapy, high-dose clopidogrel achieved only a modest pharmacodynamic effect, did not reduced the rate of recurrent ischemic events (2.3% vs 2.3%; HR, 1.01; 95% CI, 0.58-1.75; P = .98), and did not increase Global Use of Strategies to Open Occluded Arteries (GUSTO) severe or moderate bleeding. Possible explanations of these neutral findings include the low event rates in the overall study, likely because of the low-risk profile of the study population, and the weak pharmacologic intervention—40% of patients treated with high clopidogrel dosing still presented with high on-treatment platelet reactivity (using the predefined cutoff point of >230 $P2Y_{12}$ Reactivity Unit [PRU]). A time-dependent analysis from GRAVITAS has suggested that a PRU lower than 208 at 12 to 24 hours after PCI is a better predictor of cardiovascular events.[90] These data underscore the need for more potent platelet-inhibiting strategies (e.g., prasugrel, ticagrelor) rather than increases in clopidogrel dosing to optimize platelet inhibition. Currently, platelet function testing carries a class IIb recommendation, level of evidence B in the unstable angina, non–ST elevation myocardial infarction guidelines, and level of evidence C in the PCI guidelines, suggesting that this test may be useful for selected patients at increased risk of future events if there is a plan to change treatment to prasugrel or ticagrelor.[4,5] Routine platelet function testing is not recommended (class III). Platelet function tests have not yet been widely implemented for several reasons, including the fact that there are many platelet function assays available, but there is no clear consensus as to which is the best. Setting a cutoff value to define patients with high platelet reactivity is challenging and there is currently limited evidence to indicate that alteration of therapy based on high platelet reactivity improves outcomes.[13]

Recent investigations have also considered the use of genotyping to define poor clopidogrel metabolizers, who are at increased risk of having inadequate platelet inhibition, to tailor antiplatetelet therapy.[78] Carriers of the CYP2C19*2 polymorphism have a higher prevalence of high on clopidogrel platelet reactivity. Repeated loading doses of 600 mg of clopidogrel have enabled 88% of these patients to reach levels of platelet reactivity, assessed by the VASP-P test, below a threshold associated with ischemic risk.[91] The recent CLopidogrel and respOnse Variability Investigation Study (CLOVIS-2) has shown that a 900-mg loading dose of clopidogrel can overcome a poor response in patients heterozygous for the CYP2C19*2 allele.[92] However, results from studies in the chronic phase of therapy have not been as promising, with only modest effects associated with high maintenance dosing. The Accelerated Platelet Inhibition by a Double Dose of Clopidogrel According to Gene Polymorphism (ACCEL-DOUBLE) study has shown that despite use of a high maintenance dose of 150 mg of clopidogrel, patient carriers of the CYP2C19*2 allele continue to show high platelet reactivity and an increased prevalence of high on-treatment platelet reactivity.[93] These findings are in line with recent trial data demonstrating that a clopidogrel maintenance dose regimen of 225 mg/day is needed to achieve optimal responses among carriers of the CYP2C19*2 allele.[74]

TRIPLE ANTIPLATELET THERAPY

Glycoprotein IIb/IIIa Inhibitors

The addition of a third antiplatelet agent (triple antiplatelet therapy) may be considered for acute and maintenance phase therapy in patients on aspirin and clopidogrel therapy as a strategy to enhance platelet inhibition. The use of a GP IIb/IIIa inhibitor in the acute setting achieves enhanced platelet inhibition in patients receiving aspirin and a loading dose of clopidogrel (irrespective of using 300 or 600 mg). Cuisset and associates have evaluated the effect of adding abciximab to dual antiplatelet therapy in clopidogrel nonresponders defined by light transmittance aggregometry referred to elective PCI. They showed a reduction in the rate of short-term cardiovascular events in abciximab-treated patients compared with conventional therapy.[94] Similarly, the Tailoring Treatment With Tirofiban in Patients Showing Resistance to Aspirin and/or Resistance to Clopidogrel (3T/2R) trial, which randomized aspirin and clopidogrel poor responders defined by the VerifyNow assay undergoing elective PCI

to receive tirofiban or placebo, showed an ischemic benefit over the short term (30 days) and long term (1 year) in the triple therapy group.[95]

Cilostazol

Other studies conducted in patients in the maintenance phase of dual antiplatelet therapy have evaluated the addition of cilostazol, a phosphodiesterase III inhibitor, to enhance platelet inhibition. Several pharmacodynamic studies have shown that adjunctive cilostazol therapy achieves greater levels of platelet inhibition compared with dual antiplatelet therapy alone.[78] In the Adjunctive Cilostazol vs. High Maintenance Dose Clopidogrel in Patients with Clopidogrel Resistance (ACCEL-RESISTANCE) study, adjunctive treatment with cilostazol reduced the rate of high on-treatment platelet reactivity and intensified platelet inhibition to a greater extent than high clopidogrel (150 mg) maintenance therapy.[96] This effect has been shown even in carriers of the CYP2C19 loss of function allele.[97] Importantly, triple antiplatelet therapy has been associated with better outcomes, including reduced stent thrombosis, in patients undergoing PCI treated with both bare metal and drug-eluting stents. Note that this ischemic benefit occurs without any increase in bleeding.[1] However, nonbleeding side effects, such as headache, palpitations, and gastrointestinal disturbances, are very common with cilostazol and often lead to treatment discontinuation.

NOVEL ANTIPLATELET DRUGS

The development and introduction into clinical practice of novel antiplatelet drugs represents another promising strategy to improve clinical outcomes in high-risk patients (Figure 12-7). These strategies are directed to various targets of platelet-mediated signaling and thus may have differential effects and implications.[1] Platelet signaling pathways that have been targeted most often include those mediated by thromboxane, thrombin, and $P2Y_{12}$ receptors. Novel thromboxane receptor inhibitors, some targeting not only the TP receptor but also thromboxane synthase, have the potential benefit of mitigating platelet activation mediated by non–COX-1 sources of thromboxane.

Several novel $P2Y_{12}$ receptor antagonists, some already clinically approved (e.g., prasugrel, ticagrelor), represent important advancements over clopidogrel and have been extensively described (see earlier). Both agents are associated with more potent platelet inhibition and less response variability compared with clopidogrel and achieve levels of on-treatment platelet reactivity below thresholds associated with adverse ischemic events in most patients.[15,18] The pharmacodynamic effects of prasugrel and ticagrelor are not modulated by the genetic polymorphisms and drug interactions affecting the clopidogrel response. Therefore, these agents may represent valid treatment alternatives for poor clopidogrel responders and metabolizers, defined by platelet function and genetic testing, respectively.[4,5] However, no large-scale studies have evaluated the clinical implications of this strategy, except for the Testing Platelet Reactivity In Patients Undergoing Elective Stent Placement on Clopidogrel to Guide Alternative Therapy With Prasugrel (TRIGGER-PCI) trial, which was conducted in stable CAD patients undergoing PCI with DES implantation. It was terminated for futility, because only one ischemic event occurred during interim analysis.[98] The potential ischemic benefit of these agents needs to be weighed against the bleeding risk associated with more potent $P2Y_{12}$ inhibition. Accordingly, other novel $P2Y_{12}$ receptor antagonists still under clinical investigation, such as cangrelor and elinogrel, warrant further investigation prior to being considered as an alternative strategy to clopidogrel.[99,100] Another pivotal platelet signaling pathway mediated by thrombin receptors is being evaluated with the PAR-1 receptor antagonists vorapaxar and atopaxar in patients with various manifestations of atherosclerotic disease.[101] Thrombin-mediated platelet signaling is among the most potent inducers of platelet activation. Therefore, PAR-1 receptor blockade, in addition to COX-1 and $P2Y_{12}$

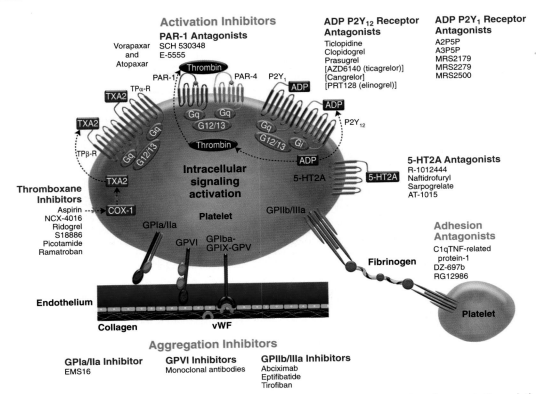

Figure 12-7   Sites of action of current and emerging antithrombotic drugs and antiplatelet agents. Platelet adherence to the endothelium occurs at sites of vascular injury through the binding of glycoprotein *(GP)* receptors to exposed extracellular matrix proteins (collagen and von Willebrand factor *[vWF]*). Platelet activation occurs via complex intracellular signaling processes and causes the production and release of multiple agonists, including thromboxane A2 *(TXA2)* and adenosine diphosphate *(ADP)*, and local production of thrombin. These factors bind to their respective G-protein–coupled receptors, mediating paracrine and autocrine platelet activation. Furthermore, they potentiate each other's actions (P2Y$_{12}$ signaling modulates thrombin generation). The major platelet integrin GP IIb/IIIa mediates the final common step of platelet activation by undergoing a conformational shape change and binding fibrinogen and vWF, leading to platelet aggregation. The net result of these interactions is thrombus formation mediated by platelet-platelet interactions with fibrin. Current and emerging therapies inhibiting platelet receptors, integrins, and proteins involved in platelet activation include the thromboxane inhibitors, ADP receptor antagonists, GP IIb/IIIa inhibitors, and novel protease-activated receptor *(PAR)* antagonists and adhesion antagonists. *COX,* Cyclooxygenase; *G$_i$,* inhibitory regulative G-protein; *G$_q$,* class of G protein that activates phospholipase C; *5-HT2A,* 5-hydroxytryptamine 2A receptor; *TP,* thromboxane receptor. Reversible-acting agents are indicated by brackets. (From Angiolillo DJ, Capodanno D, Goto S. Platelet thrombin receptor antagonism and atherothrombosis. *Eur Heart J* 2010;31:17-28.)

receptor-inhibiting strategies, has the potential to provide more comprehensive platelet blockade. However, clinical trial results thus far have shown an increased bleeding risk without any significant ischemic benefit.[102] Also, new oral anticoagulants (anti-II and anti-X) are also being tested as an adjunct to COX-1 and P2Y$_{12}$ receptor therapy (see Figure 12-4). Ongoing studies will provide more insights into the safety and efficacy of this approach.

DUAL ANTIPLATELET THERAPY IN PATIENTS ON CHRONIC ORAL ANTICOAGULATION

Approximately 5% of patients undergoing PCI also present with an indication for oral anticoagulation therapy.[103,104] The main reason for oral anticoagulant (OAC) therapy is atrial fibrillation, which is the most common cardiac arrhythmia. It is associated with considerable morbidity and mortality rates due to stroke and thromboembolic complications. Approximately 70% to 80% of all patients in atrial fibrillation have an indication for continuous OAC, and coronary artery disease coexists in 20% to 30% of these patients. These patients pose a significant treatment dilemma, because they require use of dual antiplatelet therapy to prevent recurrent atherothrombotic complications, including stent thrombosis, but also require anticoagulant therapy to prevent thromboembolic events. Aspirin plus clopidogrel is insufficient to prevent stroke compared with OAC alone. OAC is also insufficient to prevent stent thrombosis, likely because the

mechanisms of thrombus formation differ between those associated with atrial fibrillation and those associated with coronary artery disease and stent thrombosis. Coagulation factors play a central role in the development of thrombotic events during atrial fibrillation, whereas platelets are more important in the pathophysiology of atherothrombotic events. Thus, patients with atrial fibrillation who also undergo PCI with stent implantation have a higher risk for thrombotic events and stent thrombosis if they are not on both therapies concomitantly. The choice of antithrombotic medications for these patients is dependent on the balance between the risk of stroke and emboli, recurrent ischemic events, including stent thrombosis, and major bleeding. However, the recommendations given in guidelines do not offer specific answers to all the scenarios and are based on a low level of evidence.

Triple therapy with aspirin plus clopidogrel plus OAC is associated with a considerable risk of bleeding complications, which are known to be associated with increased morbidity and mortality, particularly after stent implantation. Therefore, the general principle for the use of triple therapy is to choose a treatment regimen that is tailored to the patient, taking into consideration the anticipated risk of an adverse event, particularly major bleeding.[103,104] Such risk varies over time, being the greatest in the first month for bleeding and stent thrombosis, and it remains constant over time for stroke and embolization. According to a North American consensus document, in patients at very low risk of stroke or emboli (CHADS$_2$ score = 0 to

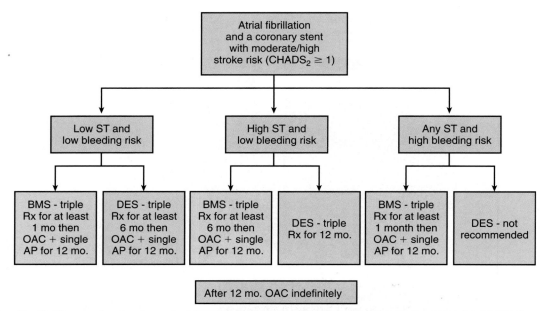

Figure 12-8 **Algorithm for the use of oral anticoagulant** *(OAC)* **therapy in stented patients requiring dual oral antiplatelet** *(AP)* **therapy.** Recommendations for the duration of triple therapy in patients with atrial fibrillation and a coronary stent (bare metal stent *[BMS]* or drug-eluting stent *[DES]*), with a moderate or high stroke risk (CHADS2 ≥ 1). *Rx,* Therapy; *ST,* stent thrombosis. (From Faxon DP, Eikelboom JW, Berger PB, et al. Antithrombotic therapy in patients with atrial fibrillation undergoing coronary stenting: a North American perspective: executive summary. *Circ Cardiovasc Interv* 2011;4:522-534.)

1), dual antiplatelet therapy (DAPT) without warfarin is probably preferable and is consistent with current guidelines (Figure 12-8).[5] In patients at higher risk of stroke (CHADS₂ score ≥ 2) who are not at a very high risk of bleeding, triple therapy should be given. In those at higher risk of stroke and bleeding, the duration of antiplatelet therapy should be reduced in proportion to the bleeding risk.

The duration of antithrombotic treatment also affects risk, as does the intensity of therapy. The risk of stent thrombosis is greatest in the first month after placement and it has been clearly demonstrated that DAPT is superior to aspirin alone, or the combination of one antiplatelet agent and warfarin.[9] Therefore, in all patients, regardless of subsequent management, there is a need for DAPT for at least 1 month. In patients with a BMS who are at low risk for stent thrombosis or in patients who are at high risk for bleeding, it may be reasonable to use triple therapy for 1 month followed by one antiplatelet agent and warfarin thereafter. Low-dose aspirin (<100 mg) should be used and concomitant NSAID use avoided. Furthermore, warfarin should be dose-adjusted and closely monitored to keep the international normalized ratio (INR) between 2 and 2.5 IU. In addition, the following factors should also be considered.

1. Vascular access and procedural characteristics. Radial access has gained considerable interest and is being increasingly used as the preferred vascular access site, given the reported lower risk of major bleeding. The choice of the procedural anticoagulant is an important consideration, with lower rates of bleeding reported with the use of bivalirudin and use of femoral closure devices and increased rates reproted with the use of GP IIb/IIIa agents.

2. Indications for PCI and stent selection. Careful consideration should be given to the necessity of PCI with stent placement because many stable angina patients can be managed on maximal medical therapy, thus avoiding the bleeding risks associated with triple therapy. When PCI is indicated, balloon angioplasty alone can at times achieve an acceptable result. In such patients, the risk of restenosis is higher; however, thienopyridine may not be required, resulting in a reduction in risk of bleeding that may outweigh the increased risk of restenosis. When stent placement is necessary during PCI and an oral anticoagulant is absolutely

required long term, placement of a BMS is generally preferred over a DES. Because the risk of stent restenosis is greatest in long lesions, small vessels, and patients with diabetes, the degree of benefit of a lower restenosis rate with DES in patients without these factors may be exceeded by the increased risk of bleeding with the longer duration of triple antithrombotic therapy. In patients requiring PCI with long lesions, small vessels, diabetes, in-stent restenosis, or other risk factors for restenosis, placement of a DES is not unreasonable. Although American College of Cardiology/American Heart Association (ACC/AHA) guidelines recommend 12 months of DAPT, preliminary data have indicated that stent thrombosis may be very low when DAPT is discontinued 6 months after the placement of a second-generation DES.[27]

3. Proton pump inhibitor use. Because 20% to 30% of the major bleeding events after PCI are gastrointestinal, the use of PPIs has been advocated.[5] Numerous studies have shown that these agents can reduce erosions, ulcers, and gastrointestinal bleeding. However, pharmacodynamic and pharmacokinetic studies have shown that PPIs that interfere with CYP2C19 activity reduce the ex vivo platelet inhibitory effects of clopidogrel. This has prompted a black box warning by drug-regulating authorities about the use of such drugs. It is important to note that this interaction is not class-specific but drug-specific, because it applies only to PPIs (e.g., omeprazole, esomeprazole) interfering with the activity of CYP2C19, which is key in transforming the clopidogrel prodrug into its active metabolite. The clinical implications for such drug-drug interactions are controversial because retrospective registry data and post hoc assessments of randomized trials have produced conflicting findings. Recent guidelines have supported the use of PPIs in patients at high risk of bleeding.[4] However, PPIs not interfering with CYP2C19 activity and clopidogrel-mediated effects (e.g., pantoprazole) should be considered.

4. Warfarin and one antiplatelet agent. The use of one antiplatelet agent in combination with warfarin is uncommon after PCI but is almost always prescribed after the initial use of triple therapy for 1 to 12 months. However, the antiplatelet agent that should

be used, aspirin or clopidogrel, is unclear. Since blockade of P2Y$_{12}$ receptor–mediated signaling with clopidogrel is associated with greater platelet inhibitory effects than COX-1 inhibition with aspirin, and the role of P2Y$_{12}$ receptor blockade on recurrent thrombotic events is established, clopidogrel might be

expected to be more effective at reducing stent thrombosis, but with increased bleeding. Clopidogrel is the preferred P2Y$_{12}$ receptor inhibitor; prasugrel and ticagrelor should not be given until the safety of triple therapy has been demonstrated, given the increased bleeding associated with these agents.

REFERENCES

1. Angiolillo DJ, Ueno M, Goto S. Basic principles of platelet biology and clinical implications. *Circ J* 2010;74:597-607.
2. Davì G, Patrono C. Platelet activation and atherothrombosis. *N Engl J Med* 2007;357:2482-2494.
3. Patrono C, García Rodríguez LA, Landolfi R, et al. Low-dose aspirin for the prevention of atherothrombosis. *N Engl J Med* 2005;353:2373-2383.
4. Wright RS, Anderson JL, Adams CD, et al. 2011 ACCF/AHA focused update of the guidelines for the management of patients with unstable angina/non-ST-elevation myocardial infarction (updating the 2007 guideline). A report of the American College of Cardiology/American Heart Association Task Force on practice guidelines developed in collaboration with the American College of Emergency Physicians, Society for Cardiovascular Angiography and Interventions, and Society of Thoracic Surgeons. *J Am Coll Cardiol* 2011;57: 1920-1959.
5. Levine GN, Bates ER, Blankenship JC, et al. 2011 ACCF/ AHA/SCAI Guideline for Percutaneous Coronary Intervention: executive summary. A report of the American College of Cardiology Foundation/American Heart Association Task Force on Practice Guidelines and the Society for Cardiovascular Angiography and Interventions. *J Am Coll Cardiol* 2011;58: 2550-2583.
6. Smith SC Jr, Benjamin EJ, Bonow RO, et al. AHA/ACCF secondary prevention and risk reduction therapy for patients with coronary and other atherosclerotic vascular disease: 2011 update. A guideline from the American Heart Association and American College of Cardiology Foundation endorsed by the World Heart Federation and the Preventive Cardiovascular Nurses Association. *J Am Coll Cardiol* 2011;58: 2432-2446.
7. Mehta SR, Bassand JP, Chrolavicius S, et al. Dose comparisons of clopidogrel and aspirin in acute coronary syndromes. CURRENT-OASIS 7 Investigators. *N Engl J Med* 2010;363: 930-942.
8. Rossini R, Angiolillo DJ, Musumeci G, et al. Aspirin desensitization in patients undergoing percutaneous coronary interventions with stent implantation. *Am J Cardiol* 2008;101: 786-789.
9. Leon MB, Baim DS, Popma JJ, et al. A clinical trial comparing three antithrombotic-drug regimens after coronary-artery stenting. Stent Anticoagulation Restenosis Study Investigators. *N Engl J Med* 1998;339:1665-1671.
10. Bertrand ME, Rupprecht HJ, Urban P, et al; CLASSICS Investigators. Double-blind study of the safety of clopidogrel with and without a loading dose in combination with aspirin compared with ticlopidine in combination with aspirin after coronary stenting: the clopidogrel aspirin stent international cooperative study (CLASSICS). *Circulation* 2000;102:624-629.
11. Angiolillo DJ, Fernandez-Ortiz A, Bernardo E, et al. Variability in individual responsiveness to clopidogrel: clinical implications, management, and future perspectives. *J Am Coll Cardiol* 2007;49:1505-1516.
12. Brar SS, ten Berg J, Marcucci R, et al. Impact of platelet reactivity on clinical outcomes after percutaneous coronary intervention: a collaborative meta-analysis of individual participant data. *J Am Coll Cardiol* 2011;58:1945-1954.
13. Bonello L, Tantry US, Marcucci R, et al; Working Group on High On-Treatment Platelet Reactivity. Consensus and future directions on the definition of high on-treatment platelet reactivity to adenosine diphosphate. *J Am Coll Cardiol* 2010;56: 919-933.
14. Tang M, Mukundan M, Yang J, et al. Antiplatelet agents aspirin and clopidogrel are hydrolyzed by distinct carboxylesterases, and clopidogrel is transesterificated in the presence of ethyl alcohol. *J Pharmacol Exp Ther* 2006;319:1467-1476.
15. Angiolillo DJ, Suryadevara S, Capranzano P, et al. Prasugrel: a novel platelet ADP P2Y12 receptor antagonist. A review on its mechanism of action and clinical development. *Expert Opin Pharmacother* 2008;9:2893-2900.
16. Brandt JT, Payne CD, Wiviott SD, et al. A comparison of prasugrel and clopidogrel loading doses on platelet function: magnitude of platelet inhibition is related to active metabolite formation. *Am Heart J* 2007;153:66.e9-e16.
17. Wiviott SD, Trenk D, Frelinger AL, et al. Prasugrel compared with high loading- and maintenance-dose clopidogrel in patients with planned percutaneous coronary intervention: the Prasugrel in Comparison to Clopidogrel for Inhibition of Platelet Activation and Aggregation-Thrombolysis in Myocardial Infarction 44 trial. *Circulation* 2007;116:2923-2932.
18. Capodanno D, Dharmashankar K, Angiolillo DJ. Mechanism of action and clinical development of ticagrelor, a novel platelet ADP P2Y12 receptor antagonist. *Expert Rev Cardiovasc Ther* 2010;8:151-158.
19. Mehta SR, Yusuf S, Peters RJ, et al; Clopidogrel in Unstable angina to prevent Recurrent Events trial (CURE) Investigators. Effects of pretreatment with clopidogrel and aspirin followed by long-term therapy in patients undergoing percutaneous coronary intervention: the PCI-CURE study. *Lancet* 2001;358:527-533.
20. Steinhubl SR, Berger PB, Mann JT 3rd, et al; CREDO Investigators. Clopidogrel for the Reduction of Events During Observation. Early and sustained dual oral antiplatelet therapy following percutaneous coronary intervention: a randomized controlled trial. *JAMA* 2002;288:2411-2420.
21. Sabatine MS, Cannon CP, Gibson CM, et al; Clopidogrel as Adjunctive Reperfusion Therapy (CLARITY)-Thrombolysis in Myocardial Infarction (TIMI) 28 Investigators. Effect of clopidogrel pretreatment before percutaneous coronary intervention in patients with ST-elevation myocardial infarction treated with fibrinolytics: the PCI-CLARITY study. *JAMA* 2005;294: 1224-1232.
22. Steinhubl SR, Berger PB, Brennan DM, et al. Optimal timing for the initiation of pre-treatment with 300 mg clopidogrel before percutaneous coronary intervention. *J Am Coll Cardiol* 2006;47:939-943.
23. Sabatine MS, Hamdalla HN, Mehta SR, et al. Efficacy and safety of clopidogrel pretreatment before percutaneous coronary intervention with and without glycoprotein IIb/IIIa inhibitor use. *Am Heart J* 2008;155:910-917.
24. Di Sciascio G, Patti G, Pasceri V, et al; ARMYDA-5 PRELOAD Investigators. Effectiveness of in-laboratory high-dose clopidogrel loading vs. routine pre-load in patients undergoing percutaneous coronary intervention: results of the ARMYDA-5 PRELOAD (Antiplatelet therapy for Reduction of MYocardial Damage during Angioplasty) randomized trial. *J Am Coll Cardiol* 2010;56:550-557.
25. Mehta SR, Tanguay JF, Eikelboom JW, et al; CURRENT-OASIS 7 trial investigators. Double-dose vs. standard-dose clopidogrel and high-dose vs. low-dose aspirin in individuals undergoing percutaneous coronary intervention for acute coronary syndromes (CURRENT-OASIS 7): a randomised factorial trial. *Lancet* 2010;376:1233-1243.
26. Bhatt DL, Flather MD, Hacke W, et al; CHARISMA Investigators. Patients with prior myocardial infarction, stroke, or symptomatic peripheral arterial disease in the CHARISMA trial. *J Am Coll Cardiol* 2007;49:1982-1988.
27. Gwon HC, Hahn JY, Park KW, et al. Six-month vs. 12-month dual antiplatelet therapy after implantation of drug-eluting stents: the Efficacy of Xience/Promus vs. Cypher to Reduce Late Loss After Stenting (EXCELLENT) randomized, multicenter study. *Circulation* 2012;125:505-513.
28. Valgimigli M. *Synergy between stent and drugs to avoid ischemic recurrences after percutaneous coronary intervention (PRODIGY) trial*. Hot line session. Presented at the European Society of Cardiology Congress, Paris, August 30, 2011.
29. Wiviott SD, Braunwald E, McCabe CH, et al; TRITON-TIMI 38 Investigators. Prasugrel vs. clopidogrel in patients with acute coronary syndromes. *N Engl J Med* 2007;357:2001-2015.
29a. Montalescot G, Bolognese L, Dudek D, et al. A comparison of prasugrel at the time of percutaneous coronary intervention or as pretreatment at the time of diagnosis in patients with non-ST-segment elevation myocardial infarction: design and rationale for the ACCOAST study. *Am Heart J*. 2011;161(4):650-656.
30. Wallentin L, Becker RC, Budaj A, et al; PLATO Investigators. Ticagrelor vs. clopidogrel in patients with acute coronary syndromes. *N Engl J Med* 2009;361:1045-1057.
30a. Mahaffey KW, Wojdyla DM, Carroll K, et al. Ticagrelor compared with clopidogrel by geographic region in the Platelet Inhibition and Patient Outcomes (PLATO) trial. *Circulation* 2011;124:544-554.
31. Peters RJ, Mehta SR, Fox KA, et al; Clopidogrel in Unstable angina to prevent Recurrent Events (CURE) Trial Investigators. Effects of aspirin dose when used alone or in combination with clopidogrel in patients with acute coronary syndromes: observations from the Clopidogrel in Unstable angina to prevent Recurrent Events (CURE) study. *Circulation* 2003;108: 1682-1687.
32. Mahaffey KW, Wojdyla DM, Carroll K, et al. Ticagrelor compared with clopidogrel by geographic region in the Platelet Inhibition and Patient Outcomes (PLATO) trial. *Circulation* 2011;124:544-554.
33. Angiolillo DJ, Gibson CM, Cheng S, et al. Differential effects of omeprazole and pantoprazole on the pharmacodynamics and pharmacokinetics of clopidogrel in healthy subjects: randomized, placebo-controlled, crossover comparison studies. *Clin Pharmacol Ther* 2011;89:65-74.
34. Simon T, Bhatt DL, Bergougnan L, et al. Genetic polymorphisms and the impact of a higher clopidogrel dose regimen on active metabolite exposure and antiplatelet response in healthy subjects. *Clin Pharmacol Ther* 2011;90:287-295.
35. Topol EJ, Byzova TV, Plow EF. Platelet GPIIb-IIIa blockers. *Lancet* 1999;353:227-231.
36. Hantgan RR, Nichols WL, Ruggeri ZM. Von Willebrand factor competes with fibrin for occupancy of GPIIb:IIIa on thrombin-stimulated platelets. *Blood* 1990;75:889-894.
37. Kastrati A, Mehilli J, Schuhlen H, et al. A clinical trial of abciximab in elective percutaneous coronary intervention after pretreatment with clopidogrel. *N Engl J Med* 2004;350: 232-238.
38. Kastrati A, Mehilli J, Neumann FJ, et al. Abciximab in patients with acute coronary syndromes undergoing percutaneous coronary intervention after clopidogrel pretreatment: the ISAR-REACT 2 randomized trial. *JAMA* 2006;295:1531-1538.
39. Giugliano RP, White JA, Bode C, et al; EARLY ACS Investigators. Early vs. delayed, provisional eptifibatide in acute coronary syndromes. *N Engl J Med* 2009;360:2176-2190.
40. Hirsh J, Anand SS, Halperin JL, et al. Mechanism of action and pharmacology of unfractionated heparin. *Arterioscler Thromb Vasc Biol* 2001;21:1094-1096.
41. Weitz JI. Low-molecular-weight heparins. *N Engl J Med* 1997; 337:688-698.
42. Montalescot G, White HD, Gallo R, et al; STEEPLE Investigators. Enoxaparin vs. unfractionated heparin in elective percutaneous coronary intervention. *N Engl J Med* 2006;355: 1058-1060.
43. Montalescot G, Zeymer U, Silvain J, et al; ATOLL Investigators. Intravenous enoxaparin or unfractionated heparin in primary percutaneous coronary intervention for ST-elevation myocardial infarction: the international randomised open-label ATOLL trial. *Lancet* 2011;378:693-703.
44. Di Nisio M, Middeldorp S, Buller HR. Direct thrombin inhibitors. *N Engl J Med* 2005;353:1028-1040.
45. Stone GW, McLaurin BT, Cox DA, et al; ACUITY Investigators. Bivalirudin for patients with acute coronary syndromes. *N Engl J Med* 2006;355:2203-2216.
46. Kastrati A, Neumann FJ, Schulz S, et al; ISAR-REACT 4 Trial Investigators. Abciximab and heparin vs. bivalirudin for non-ST-elevation myocardial infarction. *N Engl J Med* 2011;365: 1980-1989.
47. Stone GW, Witzenbichler B, Guagliumi G, et al. Bivalirudin during primary PCI in acute myocardial infarction. *N Engl J Med* 2008;358:2218-2230.
47a. Stone GW, Witzenbichler B, Guagliumi G, et al. Heparin plus a glycoprotein IIb/IIIa inhibitor versus bivalirudin monotherapy and paclitaxel-eluting stents versus bare-metal stents in acute myocardial infarction (HORIZONS-AMI): final 3-year results from a multicentre, randomised controlled trial. *Lancet* 2011;377(9784):2193-2204.
48. Paolucci F, Clavies MC, Donat F, et al. Fondaparinux sodium mechanism of action: identification of specific binding to purified and human plasma-derived proteins. *Clin Pharmacokinet* 2002;41(Suppl 2):11-18.
49. Yusuf S, Mehta SR, Chrolavicius S, et al. Comparison of fondaparinux and enoxaparin in acute coronary syndromes. *N Engl J Med* 2006;354:1464-1476.
50. Steg PG, Jolly SS, Mehta SR, et al. Low-dose vs standard-dose unfractionated heparin for percutaneous coronary intervention in acute coronary syndromes treated with fondaparinux: the FUTURA/OASIS-8 randomized trial. *JAMA* 2010;304: 1339-1349.
51. Yusuf S, Mehta SR, Chrolavicius S, et al. Effects of fondaparinux on mortality and reinfarction in patients with acute ST-segment elevation myocardial infarction: the OASIS-6 randomized trial. *JAMA* 2006;295:1519-1530.
52. Ferreiro JL, Sibbing D, Angiolillo DJ. Platelet function testing and risk of bleeding complications. *Thromb Haemost* 2010;103: 1128-1135.
53. Angiolillo DJ. Variability in responsiveness to oral antiplatelet therapy. *Am J Cardiol* 2009;103(Suppl):27A-34A.
54. Gurbel PA, Bliden KP, DiChiara J, et al. Evaluation of dose-related effects of aspirin on platelet function: results from the Aspirin-Induced Platelet Effect (ASPECT) study. *Circulation* 2007;115:3156-3164.

55. Snoep JD, Hovens MM, Eikenboom JC, et al. Association of laboratory-defined aspirin resistance with a higher risk of recurrent cardiovascular events: a systematic review and meta-analysis. *Arch Intern Med* 2007;167:1593-1159.

56. Gori AM, Marcucci R, Migliorini A, et al. Incidence and clinical impact of dual nonresponsiveness to aspirin and clopidogrel in patients with drug-eluting stents. *J Am Coll Cardiol* 2008;52: 734-739.

57. Pocock SJ, Mehran R, Clayton TC, et al. Prognostic modeling of individual patient risk and mortality impact of ischemic and hemorrhagic complications: assessment from the Acute Catheterization and Urgent Intervention Triage Strategy trial. *Circulation* 2010;121:43-51.

58. Marín F, González-Conejero R, Capranzano P, et al. Pharmacogenetics in cardiovascular antithrombotic therapy. *J Am Coll Cardiol* 2009;54:1041-1057.

59. Cooke GE, Bray PF, Hamlington JD, et al. PLA2 polymorphism and efficacy of aspirin. *Lancet* 1998;351:1253.

60. Corral J, González-Conejero R, Rivera J, et al. Role of the 807 C/T polymorphism of the alpha2 gene in platelet GP Ia collagen receptor expression and function—effect in thromboembolic diseases. *Thromb Haemost* 1999;81:951-956.

61. Halushka MK, Walker LP, Halushka PV. Genetic variation in cyclooxygenase 1: effects on response to aspirin. *Clin Pharmacol Ther* 2003;73:122-130.

62. Gonzalez-Conejero R, Rivera J, Corral J, et al. Biological assessment of aspirin efficacy on healthy individuals: heterogeneous response or aspirin failure? *Stroke* 2005;36:276-280.

63. Li Q, Chen BL, Ozdemir V, et al. Frequency of genetic polymorphisms of COX1, GpIIIa and P2Y1 in a Chinese population and association with attenuated response to aspirin. *Pharmacogenomics* 2007;8:577-586.

64. Bigler J, Whitton J, Lampe JW, et al. CYP2C9 and UGT1A6 genotypes modulate the protective effect of aspirin on colon adenoma risk. *Cancer Res* 2001;61:3566-3569.

65. Pilotto A, Seripa D, Franceschi M, et al. Genetic susceptibility to nonsteroidal anti-inflammatory drug–related gastroduodenal bleeding: role of cytochrome P450 2C9 polymorphisms. *Gastroenterology* 2007;133:465-471.

66. Undas A, Sydor WJ, Brummel K, et al. Aspirin alters the cardioprotective effects of the factor XIII Val34Leu polymorphism. *Circulation* 2003;107:17-20.

67. Mega JL, Close SL, Wiviott SD, et al. Genetic variants in ABCB1 and CYP2C19 and cardiovascular outcomes after treatment with clopidogrel and prasugrel in the TRITON-TIMI 38 trial: a pharmacogenetic analysis. *Lancet* 2010;376: 1312-1319.

68. Mega JL, Close SL, Wiviott SD, et al. Cytochrome P-450 polymorphisms and response to clopidogrel. *N Engl J Med* 2009; 360:354-362.

69. Mega JL, Simon T, Collet JP, et al. Reduced-function CYP2C19 genotype and risk of adverse clinical outcomes among patients treated with clopidogrel predominantly for PCI: a meta-analysis. *JAMA* 2010;304:1821-1830.

70. Wallentin L, James S, Storey RF, et al; PLATO investigators. Effect of CYP2C19 and ABCB1 single nucleotide polymorphisms on outcomes of treatment with ticagrelor vs. clopidogrel for acute coronary syndromes: a genetic substudy of the PLATO trial. *Lancet* 2010;376:1320-1328.

71. Sibbing D, Koch W, Gebhard D, et al. Cytochrome 2C19*17 allelic variant, platelet aggregation, bleeding events, and stent thrombosis in clopidogrel-treated patients with coronary stent placement. *Circulation* 2010;121:512-518.

72. Bouman HJ, Schömig E, van Werkum JW, et al. Paraoxonase-1 is a major determinant of clopidogrel efficacy. *Nat Med* 2011; 17:110-116.

73. Campo G, Ferraresi P, Marchesini J, et al. Relationship between paraoxonase Q192R gene polymorphism and on-clopidogrel platelet reactivity over time in patients treated with percutaneous coronary intervention. *J Thromb Haemost* 2011;9: 2106-2108.

74. Mega JL, Hochholzer W, Frelinger AL 3rd, et al. Dosing clopidogrel based on CYP2C19 genotype and the effect on platelet reactivity in patients with stable cardiovascular disease. *JAMA* 2011;306:2221-2228.

75. Ferreiro JL, Angiolillo DJ. Diabetes and antiplatelet therapy in acute coronary syndrome. *Circulation* 2011;123:798-813.

76. Bates ER, Lau WC, Angiolillo DJ. Clopidogrel-drug interactions. *J Am Coll Cardiol* 2011;57:1251-1263.

77. Bhatt DL, Cryer BL, Contant CF, et al; COGENT Investigators. Clopidogrel with or without omeprazole in coronary artery disease. *N Engl J Med* 2010;363:1909-1917.

78. Angiolillo DJ, Ueno M. Optimizing platelet inhibition in clopidogrel poor metabolizers: therapeutic options and practical considerations. *JACC Cardiovasc Interv* 2011;4:411-414.

79. Capodanno D, Patel A, Dharmashankar K, et al. Pharmacodynamic effects of different aspirin dosing regimens in type 2 diabetes mellitus patients with coronary artery disease. *Circ Cardiovasc Interv* 2011;4:180-187.

80. von Beckerath N, Taubert D, Pogatsa-Murray G, et al. Absorption, metabolization, and antiplatelet effects of 300-, 600-, and 900-mg loading doses of clopidogrel: results of the ISAR-CHOICE (Intracoronary Stenting and Antithrombotic Regimen: Choose Between 3 High Oral Doses for Immediate Clopidogrel Effect) trial. *Circulation* 2005;112:2946-2950.

81. Price MJ, Coleman JL, Steinhubl SR, et al. Onset and offset of platelet inhibition after high-dose clopidogrel loading and standard daily therapy measured by a point-of-care assay in healthy volunteers. *Am J Cardiol* 2006;98:681-684.

82. Patti G, Colonna G, Pasceri V, et al. Randomized trial of high loading dose of clopidogrel for reduction of periprocedural myocardial infarction in patients undergoing coronary intervention: results from the ARMYDA-2 (Antiplatelet therapy for Reduction of MYocardial Damage during Angioplasty) study. *Circulation* 2005;111:2099-2106.

83. von Beckerath N, Kastrati A, Wieczorek A, et al. A double-blind, randomized study on platelet aggregation in patients treated with a daily dose of 150 or 75 mg of clopidogrel for 30 days. *Eur Heart J* 2007;28:1814-1819.

84. Angiolillo DJ, Shoemaker SB, Desai B, et al. Randomized comparison of a high clopidogrel maintenance dose in patients with diabetes mellitus and coronary artery disease: results of the Optimizing Antiplatelet Therapy in Diabetes Mellitus (OPTIMUS) study. *Circulation* 2007;115:708-716.

85. Angiolillo DJ, Bernardo E, Palazuelos J, et al. Functional impact of high clopidogrel maintenance dosing in patients undergoing elective percutaneous coronary interventions. Results of a randomized study. *Thromb Haemost* 2008;99:161-168.

86. Angiolillo DJ, Costa MA, Shoemaker SB, et al. Functional effects of high clopidogrel maintenance dosing in patients with inadequate platelet inhibition on standard dose treatment. *Am J Cardiol* 2008;101:440-445.

87. Bonello L, Camoin-Jau L, Arques S, et al. Adjusted clopidogrel loading doses according to vasodilator-stimulated phosphoprotein phosphorylation index decrease rate of major adverse cardiovascular events in patients with clopidogrel resistance: a multicenter randomized prospective study. *J Am Coll Cardiol* 2008;51:1404-1411.

88. Bonello L, Camoin-Jau L, Armero S, et al. Tailored clopidogrel loading dose according to platelet reactivity monitoring to prevent acute and subacute stent thrombosis. *Am J Cardiol* 2009;103:5-10.

89. Price MJ, Berger PB, Teirstein PS, et al; GRAVITAS Investigators. Standard- vs high-dose clopidogrel based on platelet function testing after percutaneous coronary intervention: the GRAVITAS randomized trial. *JAMA* 2011;305:1097-1105.

90. Price MJ, Angiolillo DJ, Teirstein PS, et al. Platelet reactivity and cardiovascular outcomes after percutaneous coronary intervention: a time-dependent analysis of the Gauging Responsiveness with a VerifyNow P2Y12 assay: Impact on Thrombosis and Safety (GRAVITAS) trial. *Circulation* 2011; 124:1132-1137.

91. Bonello L, Armero S, Ait Mokhtar O, et al. Clopidogrel loading dose adjustment according to platelet reactivity monitoring in patients carrying the 2C19*2 loss of function polymorphism. *J Am Coll Cardiol* 2010;56:1630-1636.

92. Collet JP, Hulot JS, Anzaha G, et al; CLOVIS-2 Investigators. High doses of clopidogrel to overcome genetic resistance: the randomized crossover CLOVIS-2 (Clopidogrel and Response Variability Investigation Study 2). *JACC Cardiovasc Interv* 2011;4:392-402.

93. Jeong YH, Kim IS, Park Y, et al. Carriage of cytochrome 2C19 polymorphism is associated with risk of high post-treatment platelet reactivity on high maintenance-dose clopidogrel of 150 mg/day: results of the ACCEL-DOUBLE (Accelerated Platelet Inhibition by a Double Dose of Clopidogrel According to Gene Polymorphism) study. *JACC Cardiovasc Interv* 2010; 3:731-741.

94. Cuisset T, Frere C, Quilici J, et al. Glycoprotein IIb/IIIa inhibitors improve outcome after coronary stenting in clopidogrel nonresponders. *JACC Cardiovasc Interv* 2008;1:649-653.

95. Valgimigli M, Campo G, de Cesare N, et al; Tailoring Treatment with Tirofiban in Patients Showing Resistance to Aspirin and/or Resistance to Clopidogrel (3T/2R) Investigators. Intensifying platelet inhibition with tirofiban in poor responders to aspirin, clopidogrel, or both agents undergoing elective coronary intervention: results from the multicenter, prospective, randomized Tailoring Treatment with Tirofiban in Patients Showing Resistance to Aspirin and/or Resistance to Clopidogrel study. *Circulation* 2009;119:3215-3222.

96. Jeong YH, Lee SW, Choi BR, et al. Randomized comparison of adjunctive cilostazol vs. high maintenance dose clopidogrel in patients with high post-treatment platelet reactivity: results of the ACCEL-RESISTANCE (Adjunctive Cilostazol Vs. High Maintenance Dose Clopidogrel in Patients With Clopidogrel Resistance) randomized study. *J Am Coll Cardiol* 2009;53: 1101-1109.

97. Hwang SJ, Jeong YH, Kim IS, et al. Cytochrome 2C19 polymorphism and response to adjunctive cilostazol vs. high maintenance-dose clopidogrel in patients undergoing percutaneous coronary intervention. *Circ Cardiovasc Interv* 2010;3: 450-459.

98. Trenk D, Stone GW, Gawaz M, et al. A randomized trial of prasugrel versus clopidogrel in patients with high platelet reactivity on clopidogrel after elective percutaneous coronary intervention with implantation of drug-eluting stents: results of the TRIGGER-PCI (Testing Platelet Reactivity In Patients Undergoing Elective Stent Placement on Clopidogrel to Guide Alternative Therapy With Prasugrel) study. *J Am Coll Cardiol* 2012;59:2159-2164.

99. Ueno M, Ferreiro JL, Angiolillo DJ. Update on the clinical development of cangrelor. *Expert Rev Cardiovasc Ther* 2010;8: 1069-1077.

100. Ueno M, Rao SV, Angiolillo DJ. Elinogrel: pharmacological principles, preclinical and early phase clinical testing. *Future Cardiol* 2010;6:445-453.

101. Angiolillo DJ, Capodanno D, Goto S. Platelet thrombin receptor antagonism and atherothrombosis. *Eur Heart J* 2010;31: 17-28.

102. Tricoci P, Huang Z, Held C, et al; TRACER Investigators. Thrombin-receptor antagonist vorapaxar in acute coronary syndromes. *N Engl J Med* 2012;366:20-33.

103. Holmes DR Jr, Kereiakes DJ, Kleiman NS, et al. Combining antiplatelet and anticoagulant therapies. *J Am Coll Cardiol* 2009;54:95-109.

104. Faxon DP, Eikelboom JW, Berger PB, et al. Antithrombotic therapy in patients with atrial fibrillation undergoing coronary stenting: a North American perspective: executive summary. *Circ Cardiovasc Interv* 2011;4:522-534.

Specific Lesion Subsets

The Role of Drug-Eluting Stents or Cardiac Bypass Surgery in the Treatment of Multivessel Coronary Artery Disease

MATTHEW J. PRICE

KEY POINTS

- The results of many of the randomized trials comparing revascularization therapies are difficult to apply in current practice, because angioplasty or bare metal stents were used in patients undergoing percutaneous coronary intervention (PCI), internal mammary artery grafts were not uniformly used in those treated with coronary artery bypass grafting (CABG), three-vessel disease was infrequently present in the enrolled populations, and concomitant medical therapy has evolved over time.

- The risk of death or myocardial infarction appears similar between drug-eluting stents (DES) and CABG in observational nonrandomized studies, lending equipoise for randomized clinical trials comparing the safety and efficacy of PCI with CABG for the treatment of multivessel disease.

- In the SYNTAX trial, which enrolled patients with unprotected left main obstruction or three-vessel disease eligible for either revascularization strategy, PCI with paclitaxel-eluting stents was not noninferior to CABG for the endpoint of major adverse cardiovascular and cerebrovascular events (MACCE).

- The SYNTAX score is a risk model that includes several anatomic variables reflecting lesion complexity; in patients eligible for either procedure, higher SYNTAX scores are associated with a greater risk of MACCE after PCI, but are not associated with MACCE after CABG.

- CABG and PCI appear to provide comparable outcomes in patients with three-vessel disease and low SYNTAX scores (≦22).

- Current guidelines state that it is reasonable to prefer CABG over PCI in patients with complex three-vessel coronary artery disease (e.g., SYNTAX score >22) who are good candidates for surgery (class IIA, level of evidence B).

- The use of newer generation DES with decreased stent thrombosis rates and possibly less catch-up restenosis may further improve the relative efficacy of PCI compared with CABG, but this hypothesis remains to be proven.

- In the FREEDOM trial, CABG was superior to PCI with first-generation DES in diabetic patients with predominantly three-vessel disease, significantly reducing the rate of death and myocardial infarction while increasing the rate of stroke.

Coronary artery bypass grafting (CABG) has been the traditional approach to the treatment of multivessel coronary artery disease. The rapid evolution in catheter-based technology and advances in adjunctive pharmacotherapy have made the comparative efficacy of percutaneous coronary intervention (PCI) a moving target. Several large randomized trials were performed in the angioplasty and bare metal stent eras, but the patients enrolled in these trials, interventional treatments applied in the PCI patients, relatively infrequent use of internal mammary artery grafts during CABG, and their concomitant

medical therapy make the results of these trials challenging to apply to current practice (Table 13-1).[1-9] A collaborative, patient-level meta-analysis of 10 randomized clinical trials (6 using angioplasty and 4 using bare metal stents) involving 7812 patients in whom approximately one third had three-vessel disease has found that 5-year mortality is similar between PCI and CABG.[10] However, there was a significant interaction between the presence of diabetes and treatment effect, and CABG was associated with a lower risk of death among the 1233 diabetic patients. Furthermore, PCI with bare metal stents was associated with substantially more repeat revascularization than CABG as a result of restenosis from neointimal hyperplasia. CABG may possibly protect from late myocardial infarction by bypassing the at-risk coronary tree. Drug-eluting stents (DES) significantly reduce the risk of restenosis and target lesion revascularization compared with bare metal stents for simple and complex disease.[11-13] This, combined with more effective adjunctive acute and chronic pharmacotherapeutic strategies applied in current practice, raises the possibility that PCI with DES could provide equivalent, or even superior, outcomes compared with CABG for the treatment of multivessel disease. This chapter will review the current data comparing PCI with DES for this patient subset.

Observational Studies Comparing Drug-Eluting Stents with Cardiac Surgery

A large number of observational, nonrandomized studies have compared clinical outcomes after DES implantation with those after CABG. Given their nonrandomized nature, the results may be substantially influenced by selection bias. Many of these studies used various statistical techniques to adjust for variables that are unevenly distributed between treatment comparison groups, such as regression or propensity score analyses. However, despite these adjustments, observational data may still be limited in providing unbiased estimates of treatment effects as a result of unmeasured confounders, and the findings must be interpreted in this context. In addition, some patients may not be appropriate for either treatment strategy (e.g., prohibitive surgical risk, coronary anatomy simply not amenable to stenting). In the specific setting of revascularization strategy for multivessel disease, particular attention should be paid to the duration of follow-up, because differential efficacy between CABG and PCI may appear over longer-term follow-up. In a meta-analysis of 25 studies involving 34,278 patients with varying durations of follow-up, PCI was associated with a similar risk of mortality and myocardial infarction, significantly less stroke, but a greater risk of repeat revascularization and overall major adverse cardiovascular and cerebrovascular events (MACCEs).[14] Similarly, in the 11 studies involving 28,693 patients with multivessel disease, PCI was associated with a similar risk for myocardial infarction (relative risk [RR], 1.17; 95% confidence interval [CI], 0.92-1.49), but an increased risk for repeat revascularization

TABLE 13-1	Patient and Procedural Characteristics from Representative Randomized Clinical Trials of the Angioplasty and Bare Metal Stent Eras*								
	Frequency (%)								
Parameter	**BARI (N = 1829)**	**CABRI (N = 1054)**	**EAST (N = 392)**	**ERACI-II (N = 450)**	**GABI (N = 323)**	**MASS-II (N = 408)**	**RITA-1 (N = 1011)**	**SoS (N = 988)**	**ARTS (N = 1205)**
Diabetes	19	12	23	17	13	28	6	14	17
Hypertension	49	36	53	71	42	62	26	45	45
Hypercholesterolemia	44	44	40	61	63	79	NR	52	58
PVD	17	7	NR	23	8	0	NR	7	5
CHF	9	0	3	0	0	0	0	6	0
LV dysfunction	19	15	16	20	13	3	26	20	17
3VD	41	43	40	49	38	56	12	42	29
Proximal LAD disease	37	61	72	51	28	95	56	46	NR
Stent use in PCI arm	1	0	0	100	0	82	0	97	98
IMA use in CABG arm	82	81	NR	96	39	95	74	93	93

*These trials, on average, enrolled relatively few patients with diabetes, congestive heart failure, and three-vessel disease, and internal mammary artery use in patients randomly assigned to CABG was less frequent than that of current clinical practice.

3VD, Three-vessel disease; ARTS, Arterial Revascularization Therapies Study; BARI, Bypass Angioplasty Revascularization Investigation; CABG, coronary artery bypass grafting; CABRI, Coronary Angioplasty versus Bypass Revascularisation Investigation; CHF, congestive heart failure; EAST, Emory Angioplasty versus Surgery Trial; ERACI, Argentine Randomised Trial of Coronary Angioplasty Versus Bypass Surgery in Multivessel Disease; GABI, German Angioplasty Bypass Surgery Investigation; IMA, internal mammary artery; LAD, left anterior descending artery; LV, left ventricular; MASS, Medicine, Angioplasty, or Surgery Study; NR, not reported; PCI, percutaneous coronary intervention; PVD, peripheral vascular disease; RITA, Randomised Intervention Treatment of Angina trial; SoS, Stent or Surgery trial.

Adapted from Hlatky MA, Boothroyd DB, Bravata DM, et al. Coronary artery bypass surgery compared with percutaneous coronary interventions for multivessel disease: a collaborative analysis of individual patient data from ten randomised trials. *Lancet* 2009;373:1190-1197.

(RR, 4.03; 95% CI, 2.70-6.01]) leading to a greater risk of 12-month MACCEs (RR, 1.74; 95% CI, 1.24-2.44]).[14] Although caution should be used when applying these data to clinical practice, these observational, nonrandomized data serve to provide equipoise regarding the comparative efficacy of PCI for the treatment of multivessel disease—in particular for the safety endpoint of death, myocardial infarction, and stroke—setting the foundation for more definitive, randomized clinical trials in patients who are suitable for either revascularization strategy.

Modern Randomized Clinical Trials of Stenting Versus Surgery

In the clinical trials and observational studies that compared outcomes after surgery with bare metal stents, the need for repeat revascularization was a major limitation of PCI. Randomized clinical trials involving relatively simple target lesions have demonstrated that DES significantly reduces the incidence of angiographic restenosis and clinically driven target revascularization.[12,15] Therefore, this raised the possibility that PCI with DES could provide better outcomes for the treatment of multivessel disease. Several randomized clinical trials of DES versus cardiac surgery have been performed or are planned (Table 13-2), although to date the duration of follow-up is limited given the relatively recent introduction of DES.

MULTICENTER REGISTRIES WITH HISTORICAL CORONARY ARTERY BYPASS GRAFTING CONTROLS FROM EARLIER RANDOMIZED TRIALS

ARTS II

The second Arterial Revascularisation Therapy Study (ARTS) evaluated the safety and efficacy of PCI with sirolimus-eluting stents (SES) in patients with multivessel coronary artery disease and used the bare metal stent and CABG arms of the first, randomized ARTS trial as historical controls.[16] In the original ARTS trial, bare metal stents were inferior to CABG in reducing the incidence of MACCEs, driven

entirely by the need for repeat revascularization.[9,17] ARTS II followed similar inclusion criteria as ARTS I, although the enrolled population was older, had a larger percentage of diabetic patients, and had more complex coronary anatomy that resulted in a greater number of stents implanted per patient. Patients who received SES had a significantly lower risk of MACCEs at 1 year compared with patients randomly assigned to bare metal stents in ARTS I (10.4% vs. 26.4%; RR, 0.39; 95% CI, 0.30-0.51), whereas MACCE rates in the SES patients were similar to those of the historical CABG controls (10.5% vs. 11.7%; RR, 0.89; 95% CI, 0.65-1.23), with fewer events in the combined death, stroke, or myocardial infarction endpoint (3.0% vs. 8.0%, RR, 0.37; 95% CI, 0.22-0.63) balanced by a significantly higher need for repeat revascularization (8.5% vs. 4.2%; RR, 2.03; 95% CI, 1.23-3.34). At 5-year follow-up, however, the MACCE rate in the SES patients was significantly higher than that of the historical CABG controls (27.5% vs. 21.1%; P = .02), entirely because of repeat revascularization, with no differences in the rates of death or of the composite of death, myocardial infarction, or stroke (Figure 13-1).[18] The differences in repeat revascularization were heightened among diabetic patients, and MACCE-free survival was worse with increasing Synergy Between PCI with Taxus and Cardiac Surgery (SYNTAX) score (Figure 13-2).[18]

ERACI III

The Argentine Randomized Study: Coronary Angioplasty with Stenting Versus Coronary Bypass Surgery in Multi-Vessel Disease (ERACI) III trial compared the safety and efficacy of PCI with DES (paclitaxel-eluting or SES) in 225 patients with multivessel disease with historical controls from the bare metal stent and CABG arms of the randomized ERACI II trial.[20] The inclusion and exclusion criteria of the two studies were identical, and the same sites were used. At 1 year, MACCE rates were superior in the patients treated with DES compared with CABG (12.0% vs. 19.6%; P = .038), but this difference was attenuated at 3-year follow-up (22.7% vs. 22.7%; P = 1.0) because of repeat revascularization in the DES arm. The ERACI III trial results highlight the phenomenon of late catch-up with first-generation DES and, in turn, the importance of long-term follow-up in studies that compare PCI with CABG.

TABLE 13-2	Clinical Trials of Percutaneous Versus Surgical Revascularization for Multivessel Disease in the Modern Era								
						Event Rate (%)		
Trial	*Total No. of Patients**	*Stent Type*	*Study Design*	*Follow-up (yr)*	*Primary Endpoint*	DES	CABG	*P value*
ARTS II	1212	SES	Superiority, historical CABG control[†]	5	MACCEs	27.5	21.1	.02
ERACI III	433	SES and PES	Superiority, historical CABG control[‡]	3	MACCEs	22.7	22.7	NS
SYNTAX (3VD)	1095	PES	Noninferiority	3	MACCEs	28.8	18.8	<.001[§]
CARDia	432	SES	Noninferiority	1	Death, MI, stroke	13.0	10	.93[§]
FREEDOM	1900	DES	Superiority	5	Death, MI, stroke	26.6	18.7	0.03

3VD, Three-vessel disease; *ARTS*, Arterial Revascularisation Therapy Study II; *CABG*, coronary artery bypass grafting; *CARDia*, Coronary Artery Revascularization in Diabetes; *DES*, drug-eluting stent; *ERACI*, Argentine Randomized Study: Coronary Angioplasty with Stenting Versus Coronary Bypass Surgery in Multi-Vessel Disease; *FREEDOM*, Future Revascularization Evaluation in patients with Diabetes mellitus: Optimal management of Multivessel disease; *MI*, myocardial infarction; *MACCEs*, major adverse cardiovascular and cerebrovascular events; *PES*, paclitaxel eluting stent; *SES*, sirolimus-eluting stent; *SYNTAX*, Synergy Between PCI with Taxus and Cardiac Surgery.
*Total patients is the sum of the patients in the CABG arms and the arm receiving DES.
[†]CABG arm from ARTS I served as the historical control group.
[‡]CABG arm from ERACI II served as the control group.
[§]PCI failed to meet criteria for noninferiority.
Adapted from AM, Al Badarin FJ, Cha SS, Rihal CS. Percutaneous coronary intervention with drug-eluting stents versus coronary artery bypass surgery for multivessel coronary artery disease: a meta-analysis of data from the ARTS II, CARDIA, ERACI III, and SYNTAX studies and systematic review of observational data. *EuroIntervention* 2010;6:269-276.

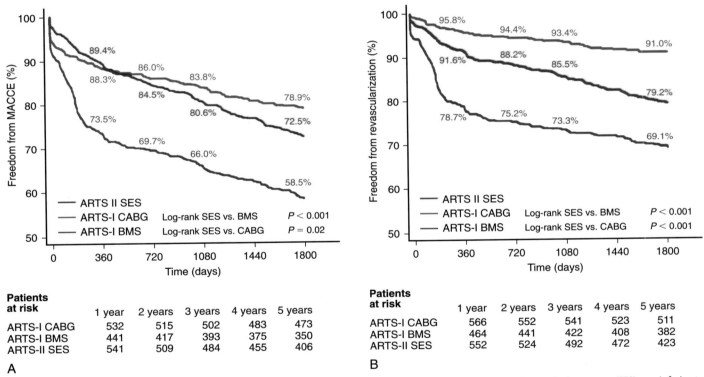

Figure 13-1   Results of the ARTS II trial at 5-year follow-up. Percutaneous coronary intervention *(PCI)* with sirolimus-eluting stents *(SES)* was inferior to coronary artery bypass grafting *(CABG)* for major adverse cardiovascular and cerebrovascular events *(MACCE)*, driven entirely by the need for repeat revascularization. Shown are freedom from MACCEs **(A)** and freedom from revascularization **(B)** in ARTS II, the CABG arm of ARTS I, and the bare metal stent *(BMS)* arm of ARTS I. (Adapted from Serruys PW, Onuma Y, Garg S, et al. 5-year clinical outcomes of the ARTS II [Arterial Revascularization Therapies Study II] of the sirolimus-eluting stent in the treatment of patients with multivessel de novo coronary artery lesions. *J Am Coll Cardiol* 2010;55:1093-1101.)

PROSPECTIVE, RANDOMIZED CLINICAL TRIALS

SYNTAX Trial

Design and Patient Characteristics

The Synergy Between PCI with Taxus and Cardiac Surgery (SYNTAX) trial was a prospective, randomized, multicenter noninferiority trial of PCI with paclitaxel-eluting stents compared with cardiac surgery for the treatment of three-vessel disease or left main obstruction in patients deemed by a heart team to be candidates for either treatment strategy.[21] The primary endpoint of the trial was MACCEs, defined as a composite of all-cause death, stroke, myocardial infarction, or repeat revascularization. The definitions of myocardial infarction after PCI and after CABG were identical. An absolute difference of 6.6% between treatments was selected as the noninferiority margin; if the

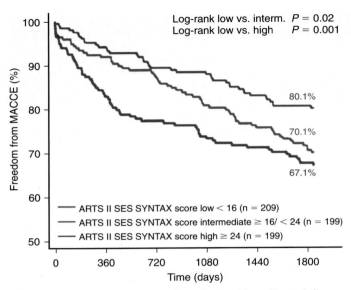

Figure 13-2 **Outcomes at 5 years in patients with multivessel disease treated with sirolimus-eluting stents** *(SES)* **in the ARTS II trial, stratified by SYNTAX score.** Patients in the lowest tercile of SYNTAX scores (i.e., least anatomic complexity) had the highest freedom from major adverse cardiovascular and cerebrovascular events *(MACCE)*. (Adapted from Serruys PW, Onuma Y, Garg S, et al. 5-year clinical outcomes of the arts ARTS II [Arterial Revascularization Therapies Study II] of the sirolimus-eluting stent in the treatment of patients with multivessel de novo coronary artery lesions. *J Am Coll Cardiol* 2010;55:1093-1101.)

upper bound of the one-sided 95% CI of the difference in the primary endpoint between treatments was less than this margin, then PCI would be considered noninferior. A total of 1800 patients were enrolled, of whom 1095 had three-vessel disease. Of these patients, 25% had a EuroSCORE higher than 6, indicative of high surgical risk. In the PCI arm, a mean of 4.6 ± 2.3 stents were implanted per patient, whereas in the CABG arm, patients received an average of 2.8 ± 0.7 grafts and 27.6% received bilateral internal mammary grafts. CABG provided complete revascularization more frequently than PCI (63.2% vs. 56.7%; $P = .005$).

Clinical Outcomes

At 1-year follow-up, PCI was not noninferior to CABG in the overall study (MACCE rates, 17.8% for PCI vs. 12.4% for CABG; $P = 0.002$; upper bound of the 95% CI for the difference = 8.3%).[21] Subgroup analysis of the cohort with three-vessel disease must be considered exploratory and hypothesis-generating because noninferiority in the overall population was not proven. In the patients with three-vessel disease in the absence of left main obstruction, MACCE rates were significantly higher with PCI compared with CABG (19.2% vs. 11.5%; $P < .001$). In contradistinction, MACCE rates were similar in the subgroup of patients with left main disease (13.7% vs. 15.8%; $P = .44$). Although speculative, this difference could in part be explained by the observation that patients with three-vessel disease but no left main obstruction had higher rates of comorbidities compared with those with left main obstruction, including worse left ventricular function and more diabetes, prior myocardial infarction, and lesions with adverse anatomic characteristics. Both PCI and CABG resulted in significant relief from angina and improvements in overall health status over the first year of follow-up. At both 6 and 12 months, there was a small but significant reduction in angina frequency with CABG as compared with PCI in the overall population.[22]

At 3-year follow-up, CABG provided superior outcomes in the overall cohort with respect to MACCEs (20.2% vs. 28.0%; $P = 0.001$).[23] The 3-year rates of the key secondary endpoints in the overall cohort according to treatment assignment are shown in Figure 13-3. Among patients with multivessel disease, MACCEs occurred in 18.8% of the CABG group compared with 28.8% of the PCI group ($P < .001$); CABG was also superior with respect to the individual endpoints of all-cause death (5.7% vs. 9.5%; $P = .02$), myocardial infarction (3.3% vs. 7.1%; $P = .005$), and repeat revascularization (10.0% vs. 19.4%; $P < 0.01$), whereas there was no difference in the two treatments in the incidence of stroke (2.9% vs. 2.6%, $P = .64$). The safety endpoint of all-cause death, myocardial infarction, or stroke also favored CABG (10.6% vs. 14.8%; $P = .04$).

Further post hoc analysis has demonstrated a consistent relationship between anatomic risk according to SYNTAX score and the comparative safety and efficacy of PCI in the group of patients with three-vessel disease, with CABG providing greater benefit in patients with increasing anatomic complexity (Figure 13-4).[23] Similar MACCE rates were observed in patients with the least complex anatomy (SYNTAX scores in the lowest tercile ≤ 22), whereas the safety endpoint of myocardial infarction was significantly increased with PCI in the intermediate tercile (SYNTAX score = 23 to 32) and both myocardial infarction and mortality were increased with PCI in the highest tercile (SYNTAX score > 32; 1.9% vs. 7.2%; $P = .02$; 4.5% vs. 11.1% for myocardial infarction and mortality, respectively).

SPECIAL POPULATIONS: DIABETES

According to a meta-analysis of randomized trials that compared bare metal stents or angioplasty with cardiac surgery, mortality was lower in diabetics treated with CABG[10] and, in subgroup analysis of the relatively large ART trial that used bare metal stents, diabetics had significantly increased repeat revascularization rates with PCI at 1 year and a trend toward a higher rate of the composite of death, myocardial infarction, or stroke at late follow-up.[19] Despite the antiproliferative effect of DES, restenosis rates are significantly higher after DES implantation in diabetics compared with nondiabetics, which may worsen the efficacy of DES compared with cardiac surgery. In the 367 diabetic patients enrolled in ARTS I and II, there were no significant differences in the rates of mortality or myocardial infarction between DES and CABG at 5-year follow-up, but continued accrual of repeat revascularization in the DES arm led to marked differences in MACCE rates (diabetics, 40.5% vs. 23.4%; $P < .001$ for DES and CABG respectively; nondiabetics, 22.9% vs. 20.7%; $P = .57$), although the interaction between diabetic status and treatment type was not significant.[19] Similarly, MACCE rates were higher in diabetics compared with nondiabetics in ERACI III, with a nonsignificant trend toward more death and nonfatal myocardial infarction among diabetics.[20] In SYNTAX, there was no statistically significant interaction between diabetic status and the treatment effect of PCI compared with CABG, although diabetes was associated with increased MACCEs in the PCI arm, driven by increased rates of repeat revascularization (Figure 13-5).[23,24] Similar to the overall trial, diabetics with low anatomic risk (SYNTAX score < 22) had similar MACCE rates with PCI or CABG (29.8% vs. 30.5%; $P = .98$), but those with high anatomic risk (SYNTAX score > 32) randomly assigned to PCI did significantly worse compared with CABG with respect to MACCE (45.9% vs. 18.5%; $P = .001$), as well as the composite of death, myocardial infarction, or stroke (22.9% vs. 8.9%; $P = .03$). Although limited, these subgroup analyses suggest that diabetics with complex disease do better with CABG, including with respect to mortality and myocardial infarction. Two randomized clinical trials, CARDia and FREEDOM, have specifically assessed the comparative efficacy of CABG or PCI in patients with diabetes and multivessel coronary artery disease.

CARDia Trial

Design and Patient Characteristics

The Coronary Artery Revascularization in Diabetes (CARDia) trial was a prospective, multicenter noninferiority trial that randomly assigned symptomatic diabetic patients with multivessel or complex

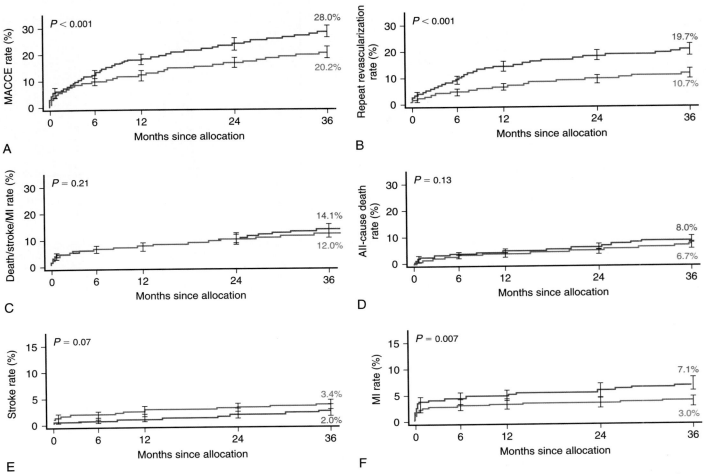

Figure 13-3 The 3-year outcomes in the overall cohort of the SYNTAX trial according to treatment assignment. **A,** Primary endpoint of major adverse cardiovascular and cerebrovascular events *(MACCE)*. **B,** Repeat revascularization. **C,** Composite of all-cause death, myocardial infarction *(MI)*, and stroke. **D,** All-cause death. **E,** Stroke. **F,** MI. (Adapted from Kappetein AP, Feldman TE, Mack MJ, et al. Comparison of coronary bypass surgery with drug-eluting stenting for the treatment of left main and/or three-vessel disease: 3-year follow-up of the SYNTAX trial. *Eur Heart J* 2011;32:2125-2134.)

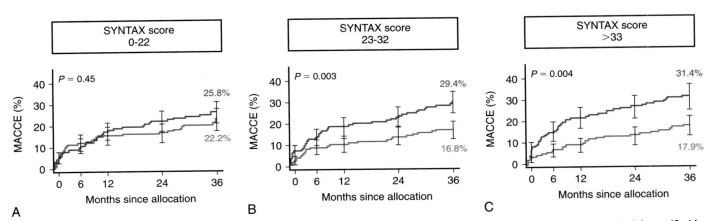

Figure 13-4 Major adverse cardiovascular and cerebrovascular events *(MACCE)* in the three-vessel disease cohort of the SYNTAX trial, stratified by anatomic complexity. The rate of the primary endpoint was similar between percutaneous coronary intervention and coronary artery bypass grafting in patients with low complexity but favored coronary artery bypass grafting in patients with intermediate or high complexity. **A,** Low complexity (SYNTAX score < 23). **B,** Intermediate complexity (SYNTAX score = 23-32). **C,** High complexity (SYNTAX score > 33). (Adapted from Kappetein AP, Feldman TE, Mack MJ, et al. Comparison of coronary bypass surgery with drug-eluting stenting for the treatment of left main and/or three-vessel disease: 3-year follow-up of the SYNTAX trial. *Eur Heart J* 2011;32:2125-2134.)

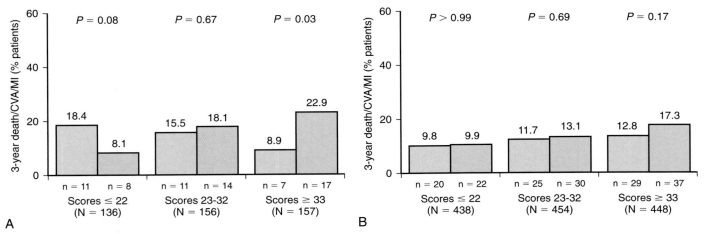

Figure 13-5 **Safety outcomes in the SYNTAX trial at 3 years according to diabetic status.** Consistent with the overall trial, patients in the highest tercile of SYNTAX score had the worst outcomes with percutaneous coronary intervention compared with coronary artery bypass grafting. The blue-green columns represent coronary artery bypass grafting, and the purple columns represent the paclitaxel-eluting stent. **A,** Rate of the composite endpoint of death, cerebrovascular accident *(CVA)*, or myocardial infarction *(MI)* in patients with diabetes. **B,** Rate of the composite endpoint of death, CVA, or MI in patients without diabetes. (Adapted from Mack MJ, Banning AP, Serruys PW, et al. Bypass versus drug-eluting stents at three years in syntax patients with diabetes mellitus or metabolic syndrome. *Ann Thorac Surg* 2011;92:2140-2146.)

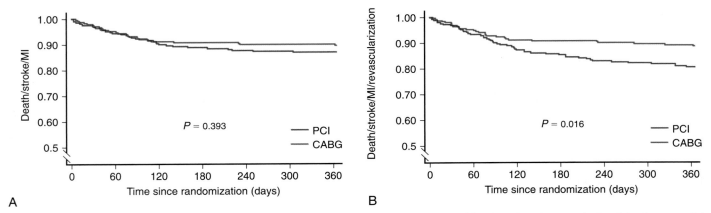

Figure 13-6 **Results of the Coronary Artery Revascularization in Diabetes (CARDia) trial. A,** Survival free from the primary endpoint of death, myocardial infarction *(MI)*, or stroke for patients randomly assigned to percutaneous coronary intervention *(PCI)* or coronary artery bypass grafting *(CABG)*. **B,** Survival free from major adverse cardiovascular and cerebrovascular events (death, MI, stroke, or repeat revascularization). PCI was not noninferior to CABG for the primary endpoint. (Adapted from Kapur A, Hall RJ, Malik IS, et al. Randomized comparison of percutaneous coronary intervention with coronary artery bypass grafting in diabetic patients. 1-year results of the CARDia [Coronary Artery Revascularization in Diabetes] trial. *J Am Coll Cardiol* 2010;55:432-440.)

single vessel disease to cardiac surgery or PCI with bare metal stents or DES.[25] The primary endpoint was a composite of all-cause death, myocardial infarction, and stroke at 1 year, and the study was powered such that noninferiority for PCI could be declared if the hazard ratio (HR) for the primary endpoint was 0.69 in favor of PCI (with an upper 95% CI boundary of 1.3). Among the 510 enrolled patients (only 85% of the anticipated sample size), 38% had insulin-treated diabetes and 62% had three-vessel disease. Patients in the PCI arm were treated with an average of 3.6 stents, with SES used in 69% of cases and bare metal stents in the remainder; an average of 2.9 grafts were used in the CABG arm, with 17% of patients receiving bilateral internal mammary artery grafts. The rate of complete revascularization was similar between the PCI and CABG arms in the patients with three-vessel disease.

Clinical Outcomes

At 1-year follow-up, the rate of the primary endpoint of all-cause death, myocardial infarction, or stroke was 13.0% in the PCI arm versus 10.5% in the CABG arm (HR, 1.25; 95% CI, 0.75-2.09), and therefore PCI did not meet the criteria for noninferiority because the

upper bound of the 95% CI of the HR was greater than 1.3 (Figure 13-6).[25] The individual endpoint of all-cause mortality was similar between groups (3.2% vs. 3.2%; HR, 0.98; 95% CI, 0.37-2.61; *P* = .97). In the patients randomly assigned to PCI, the rate of nonfatal myocardial infarction tended to be higher (9.8% vs. 5.7%; HR, 1.77; 95% CI, 0.92-3.40; *P* = .09) and the need for repeat revascularization was significantly greater (11.8% vs. 2.0%; HR, 6.18; 95% CI, 2.40-15.94; *P* < .001), whereas the risk of stroke tended to be lower (0.4% vs. 2.8%; HR, 0.14; 95% CI, 0.02-1.14; *P* = .07). More applicable are the results in the DES subgroup, although such an analysis is underpowered and hypothesis-generating. In the 178 patients randomly assigned to PCI who received DES, the incidence of the primary endpoint was similar compared with CABG in the patients enrolled during the same time period (11.6% vs. 12.4% for PCI and CABG, respectively; HR, 0.93; 95% CI, 0.51-1.71). Therefore, with the caveats that the trial was underpowered and had a relatively short duration of follow-up, the results of the CARDia trial support the contention that in diabetic patients with multivessel disease, PCI is not noninferior to CABG for death, myocardial infarction, or stroke and is associated with a greater risk of myocardial infarction and of

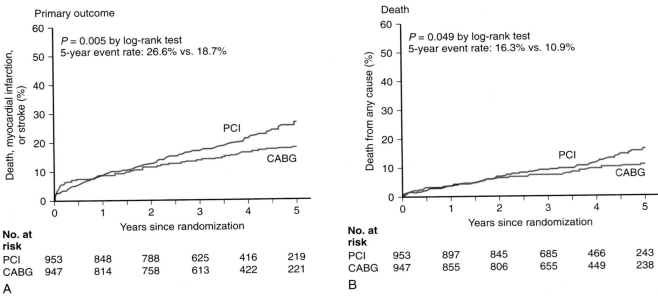

Figure 13-7   Results of the FREEDOM trial—coronary artery bypass grafting *(CABG)* versus percutaneous coronary intervention *(PCI)* in diabetic patients treated with optimal medical therapy. Kaplan-Meier estimates of the primary outcome of death, nonfatal myocardial infarction, or stroke **(A)** and death at 5 years after randomization **(B)**. Compared with PCI using paclitaxel- or sirolimus-eluting stents, CABG significantly reduced the incidence of death and myocardial infarction compared with PCI at the cost of more strokes in diabetic patients with predominantly three-vessel disease. (Adapted from Farkouh ME, Domanski M, Sleeper LA, et al; FREEDOM Trial Investigators. Strategies for multivessel revascularization in patients with diabetes. *N Engl J Med* 2012;367: 2375-2384.)

repeat revascularization but less stroke. Moreover, the results are generally consistent with SYNTAX[21,23] in that patients receiving DES appear to have similar rates of the composite of death, myocardial infarction, or stroke as CABG but still exhibit inferior repeat revascularization rates.

In a meta-analysis of the 782 diabetic patients enrolled in the ARTS II, CARDia, ERACI III, and SYNTAX trials, PCI with DES had a similar risk of the combined endpoint of death, myocardial infarction, or stroke (8.0% vs. 8.1%, respectively; RR, 0.99; 95% CI, 0.71-1.39; $P = 0.96$), but was associated with higher MACCE rates compared with CABG (18.8% vs. 10.4%, respectively; RR, 1.69; 95% CI, 1.23-2.31; $P = .001$) because of a significantly higher rate of repeat revascularization (14.1% vs. 4.1%, respectively; RR, 2.99; 95% CI, 1.87-4.77; $P < .001$).[26] However, this meta-analysis included only the 1-year follow-up of the SYNTAX trial.[21] Thus, it appears from these studies that diabetic patients fare worse overall with DES compared with CABG, with clearly higher rates of repeat revascularization, and possibly differences in death and myocardial infarction, particularly in those patients with very complex coronary anatomy.

FREEDOM Trial

The results of DES in the diabetic cohorts in the SYNTAX and CARDia trials are both from subgroup analyses of negative trials and are underpowered, exploratory, and hypothesis-generating. The Future Revascularization Evaluation in Patients with Diabetes Mellitus: Optimal Management of Multivessel Disease (FREEDOM) trial was a prospective, randomized, multicenter superiority trial sponsored by the National Heart, Lung, and Blood Institute that compared the safety and efficacy of multivessel PCI with first-generation DES compared with CABG in at least 1900 diabetic patients.[27,28] The primary endpoint was a composite of all-cause death, nonfatal myocardial infarction, and stroke. Three-vessel disease was present in 83% of the randomized patients, and the median SYNTAX score was 26, consistent with an anatomically complex population. Almost one third of randomized patients were treated with insulin. PCI was performed with sirolimus-eluting or paclitaxel-eluting stents, and 94.4% of patients randomly assigned to CABG received a left internal mammary

artery graft. At 5-year follow-up, the primary composite endpoint occurred in 26.6% of patients randomly assigned to PCI compared with 18.7% of patients randomly assigned to CABG ($P = .005$), driven by differences in mortality (16.3% vs. 10.9%; $P = .049$) and myocardial infarction (13.6% vs. 6.0%; $P < .001$). However, as observed in earlier trials, CABG was associated with an increased risk of stroke (2.4% vs. 5.2%; $P = .03$). According to survival curves, the mortality benefit with CABG appeared to occur at more than 2 years after randomization (Figure 13-7).

Risk Prediction Models for Percutaneous Coronary Intervention and Coronary Artery Bypass Grafting

Clinical outcomes in registry and randomized studies can be used to identify comorbidities associated with adverse events, which in turn can be used to build models to predict patient risk for a particular treatment strategy. Optimally, in the setting of the clinical decision of CABG versus PCI, a risk score (or scores) could help the practitioner and patient select the treatment strategy that would most likely provide the best clinical outcome. Several risk models have been developed and validated in the PCI or CABG population, but only a few have been validated for both treatment strategies (Table 13-3). In general, for CABG, risk models have incorporated clinical characteristics (i.e., outcomes appear to be independent of coronary anatomy), whereas risk models for PCI incorporate anatomic and/or clinical variables.

RISK SCORES INCORPORATING CLINICAL VARIABLES ALONE

Age, Creatinine, and Ejection Fraction Score

The Age, Creatinine, and Ejection Fraction (ACEF) score is a simple risk score that has been validated to predict mortality in elective CABG[29] (Figure 13-8). It is calculated as follows:

TABLE 13-3	Summary of Risk Stratification Models for Revascularization of Obstructive Coronary Artery Disease			
	No. of Variables Used to Calculate Scores		**Validated in PCI and CABG**	
Risk Model	*Clinical*	*Angiographic*	**PCI**	**CABG**
ACEF	3	0	Yes	Yes
Mayo Clinic Risk Score	7	0	Yes	Yes
NCDR-Cath PCI score	9	0	Yes	No
SYNTAX score	0	11 (per lesion)	Yes	No
Clinical SYNTAX score	3	11 (per lesion)	Yes	Yes
Functional SYNTAX score	0	11 (per lesion)	Yes	No
EuroSCORE	17	0	Yes	Yes
Society of Thoracic Surgery score	40	2	No	Yes
Global Risk Classification (GRC)	17	11 (per lesion)	Yes	Yes
New Risk Stratification (NRS)	17	33 (per lesion)	Yes	No

PCI, Percutaneous coronary intervention; *CABG*, coronary artery bypass grafting; *ACEF*, age, creatinine, ejection fraction; *NCDR*, National Cardiovascular Data Registry; *SYNTAX*, Synergy Between PCI with Taxus and Cardiac Surgery.
Adapted from Garg S, Stone GW, Kappetein AP, et al. Clinical and angiographic risk assessment in patients with left main stem lesions. *JACC Cardiovasc Interv* 2010;3:891-901.

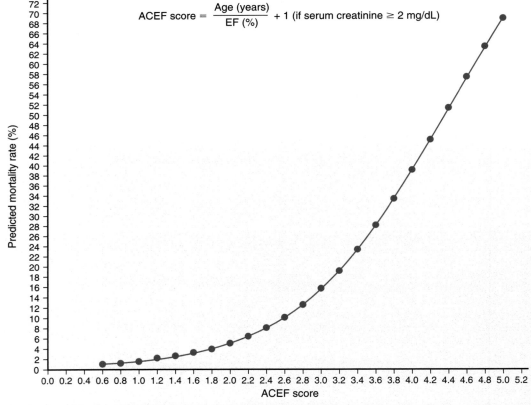

Figure 13-8   **Age, Creatinine, Ejection Fraction *(ACEF)* score and mortality in elective coronary artery bypass surgery.** The score is calculated using the formula [age/ejection fraction *(EF)* (%)] + 1 (if serum creatinine value is ≥2 mg/dL). This score was derived from a cohort of 4557 patients undergoing elective cardiac surgery. (Adapted from Ranucci M, Castelvecchio S, Menicanti L, et al. Risk of assessing mortality risk in elective cardiac operations: age, creatinine, ejection fraction, and the law of parsimony. *Circulation* 2009;119:3053-3061.)

$$ACEF = \frac{Age}{Ejection\ fraction\ (\%)} + 1 \quad \begin{array}{l} \text{(if the serum creatinine level is} \\ \ge 2\ mg/dL) \end{array}$$

In a study of 29,659 consecutive patients who underwent elective cardiac surgeries, the ACEF score provided an accuracy level comparable to the EuroSCORE, with superior clinical performance.[30] A modified ACEF score has been proposed, incorporating creatinine clearance rather than an absolute threshold of a creatinine level of 2 mg/dL or higher, but this has not been validated in a surgical population.[31]

The prognostic usefulness of the ACEF score has also been explored in the PCI population. The ACEF score had significant discriminatory ability for the endpoints of mortality as well as myocardial infarction in the Limus Eluted From A Durable Versus ERodable Stent Coating (LEADERS) all-comers trial, in ARTS II, and in the Randomized,

Two-arm, Noninferiority Study Comparing Endeavor-Resolute Stent With Abbot Xience-V Stent (RESOLUTE) All Comers trial (c-statistics for mortality, 0.73, 0.65, and 0.78, respectively), but not for the endpoint of repeat revascularization.[32-34]

EuroSCORE

The European System for Cardiac Operative Risk Evaluation (EuroS-CORE) was developed between 1995 and 1999 from data obtained from over 19,000 consecutive patients undergoing open heart surgery in 128 centers in eight European countries.[35] Weights were allocated to each risk factor found to be independently associated with operative mortality on the basis of the odds ratios so that in the case of the additive EuroSCORE, the percentage predicted mortality for a patient can be calculated by adding the weighted values of risk factors present. The score includes 17 clinical variables (see Table 13-3), and an online calculator is available at www.euroscore.org. The risk model was subsequently validated in a large cohort of patients undergoing coronary or valve surgery in North America.[36] Subsequent iterations of the EuroSCORE include the logistic model and, most recently, the EuroSCORE II, which provides better calibration than the original model.[20]

A high EuroSCORE is also an independent predictor of adverse outcomes after PCI.[37-39] The baseline EuroSCORE significantly predicted MACCEs in patients randomly assigned to PCI or CABG in the left main cohort of the SYNTAX trial[40] and also had significant predictive ability for all-cause death and MACCE in the CABG and PCI arms of the cohort with three-vessel disease.[41] Among this three-vessel disease cohort, adding the EuroSCORE to the SYNTAX score improved risk prediction for patients treated with PCI whereas, in contradistinction, the SYNTAX score provided little extra value to the EuroSCORE in patients treated with CABG.[41] A combination of the EuroSCORE and SYNTAX score (a so-called global risk score) may be useful in determining the optimal treatment strategy for patients with multivessel disease (see later, "Global Risk Classification").[41]

Mayo Clinic Risk Score

The Mayo Clinic Risk Score for PCI incorporates seven preprocedural clinical variables and provides excellent discrimination for the endpoints of procedural death and major adverse cardiovascular events.[42] The score is also predictive of in-hospital mortality after CABG.[43] Its role in selecting the optimal revascularization strategy in patients with multivessel disease has not been examined.

RISK SCORES INCORPORATING ANATOMIC VARIABLES ALONE

SYNTAX Score

The SYNTAX score is a lesion-based scoring system derived from a host of anatomic variables, incorporating the number of lesions, lesion location, lesion length, presence of chronic total occlusions, bifurcations or trifurcations, aorto-ostial stenoses, vessel tortuosity, calcification, thrombus, and diffuse disease. A higher score reflects more complex anatomy. An online calculator is available at www.syntaxscore.com. In the overall and three-vessel disease cohorts of the SYNTAX trial, increasing terciles of SYNTAX score were significantly associated with MACCEs in patients randomly assigned to PCI, but were not associated with clinical outcomes in patients randomly assigned to CABG.[21,23] The ability of the SYNTAX score to predict major adverse cardiovascular events has been confirmed in several other studies of PCI with DES for all-comer populations.[33,44] In a pooled, patient-level analysis of six randomized clinical trials of DES, the SYNTAX score was significantly associated with the independent endpoints of death, myocardial infarction, repeat revascularization, and stent thrombosis.[45] As noted later, current guidelines recommend the use of the SYNTAX score to select treatment strategies in patients who are good candidates for CABG.[46] The addition of the EuroSCORE to the SYNTAX score may enhance the

identification of low-risk patients who could be treated with CABG or PCI safely and efficaciously.[41]

Functional SYNTAX score

The Functional SYNTAX score is calculated by separately adding the individual scores of lesions with a fractional flow reserve (FFR) value of 0.80 or lower and ignoring lesions with an FFR higher than 0.80. The functional SYNTAX score resulted in a significant downward classification compared with the standard SYNTAX score in the Fractional Flow Reserve Versus Angiography in Multivessel Evaluation (FAME) study and provided better classification of death or myocardial infarction, repeat revascularization, and major adverse cardiovascular events.[47] Therefore, the functional SYNTAX score increases the proportion of patients with multivessel disease who fall into lower risk categories for adverse events after PCI. The usefulness of the functional SYNTAX score to determine an optimal revascularization strategy must be confirmed in a prospective fashion.

RISK SCORES INCORPORATING ANATOMIC AND CLINICAL VARIABLES

Global Risk Classification

Because the SYNTAX score incorporates only anatomic variables to select the appropriate revascularization strategy, its prognostic usefulness may be diminished because it does not include important clinical factors that have prognostic value. The EuroSCORE uses only clinical variables; a high score is predictive of mortality for both PCI and CABG, and therefore it cannot be used alone to guide revascularization strategy. The global risk classification combines the SYNTAX score and additive EuroSCORE so that patients are classified as low global risk if the SYNTAX score is low to intermediate (<33) and the EuroSCORE is low (<6); intermediate if the SYNTAX score is high and the EuroSCORE is low, or vice versa; and high if both the SYNTAX score and EuroSCORE are high.[41] Patients in the overall SYNTAX trial with low global risk had similar outcomes with PCI or CABG at 3 years; among the cohort of patients in the three-vessel disease, those with low SYNTAX score but high EuroSCORE obtained a mortality benefit with CABG compared with PCI.[41] This would argue that patients with significant comorbidities and three-vessel disease are best served by surgical revascularization if the surgical risk is not prohibitive. A treatment algorithm has been proposed that incorporates clinical and anatomic variables to determine the appropriate revascularization strategy for patients with three-vessel disease (Figure 13-9). Because the global risk classification and proposed algorithm are based on post hoc and subgroup analyses, this score must be validated by further studies.

Clinical SYNTAX Score

The clinical SYNTAX score combines the anatomically based SYNTAX score with the clinically based modified ACEF score. It is calculated by multiplying the SYNTAX score by ([age/ejection fraction] + 1 for each 10 mL the creatinine clearance is less than 60 mL/min/1.73 m^2). When applied to patients undergoing PCI in the ARTS II study, the clinical SYNTAX score improved the ability to predict mortality and MACCEs at 5 years. In a cohort of patients undergoing CABG or PCI for unprotected left main disease, the clinical SYNTAX score, unlike the SYNTAX score alone, did not serve to identify patients with differential outcomes with one treatment strategy or the other.[31]

Society of Thoracic Surgery Score

The Society of Thoracic Surgery (STS) score incorporates 40 clinical variables and two angiographic variables (presence of left main disease and number of diseased vessels). An online calculator is available at http://riskcalc.sts.org/STSWebRiskCalc273. It can be used to predict the risk of operative morbidity and mortality after cardiac surgery. Data are lacking to support a role for the STS score to predict outcomes after PCI.

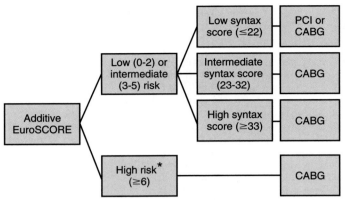

Figure 13-9 Proposed algorithm that incorporates anatomic and clinical variables to determine revascularization strategy for three-vessel disease, derived from the SYNTAX trial. Percutaneous coronary intervention *(PCI)* may be the preferred strategy in low-risk patients because outcomes appear comparable. *CABG,* Coronary artery bypass grafting. *In patients at high-risk according to EuroSCORE, PCI should be considered if an acceptable threshold for operative risk is exceeded. (Adapted from Serruys PW, Farooq V, Vranckx P, et al. A global risk approach to identify patients with left main or three-vessel disease who could safely and efficaciously be treated with percutaneous coronary intervention: the SYNTAX trial at 3 years. *JACC Cardiovasc Interv* 2012;5: 606-617.)

SUMMARY OF USING RISK STRATIFICATION SCORES TO SELECT APPROPRIATE REVASCULARIZATION STRATEGY

Although several models can stratify risk in patients undergoing CABG or PCI, few are able to provide information regarding differential outcomes with one strategy over the over. For example, a high EuroSCORE or ACEF score is predictive of mortality after both PCI and CABG. On the other hand, the SYNTAX score, which is associated with outcomes after PCI, has no predictive accuracy for CABG and therefore can be used to identify patients who would do poorly with percutaneous revascularization. Exploratory analyses of the SYNTAX trial have supported the use of combined clinical and anatomic variables to identify low-risk patients in whom outcomes with PCI and CABG are comparable and therefore in whom PCI could be a preferred strategy. Further work is needed to validate these models to individualize the decision tree in patients with three-vessel coronary disease who require revascularization.

🔹 Society Guidelines

The American College of Cardiology Foundation (ACC)/American Heart Association (AHA)/Society of Cardiovascular Angiography and Intervention (SCAI) 2011 Guideline for Percutaneous Coronary Intervention incorporates the study design features and analyses of the SYNTAX trial into its recommendations (Table 13-4).[46] These guidelines recommend that patients with complex coronary artery disease be evaluated by a heart team (class I, level of evidence C). The heart team is composed of an interventional cardiologist, cardiac surgeon, and often the patient's general cardiologist. The team reviews the patient's medical condition and coronary anatomy, determines that PCI and/or CABG are technically feasible and reasonable, and discusses revascularization options with the patient before a treatment strategy is selected. The guidelines further state the following: (1) calculations of SYNTAX and STS scores are reasonable to help determine patient risk for each treatment strategy (class IIa, level of evidence B); (2) CABG is preferred in patients with three-vessel disease who are good candidates for surgery and have SYNTAX scores higher than 22 (class IIa, level of evidence B); and (3) CABG is

	Recommendations for Revascularization Strategy in Patients with Complex Coronary Artery Disease (CAD) *		
TABLE 13-4			
Classification	*Level of Evidence*	*Recommendation*[†]	
I	C	A heart team approach to revascularization is recommended in patients with unprotected left main or complex CAD.	
IIa	B	Calculation of the STS and SYNTAX scores is reasonable in patients with unprotected left main and complex CAD.	
IIa	B	It is reasonable to choose CABG over PCI to improve survival in patients with complex three-vessel CAD (e.g., SYNTAX score > 22), with or without involvement of the proximal LAD artery, who are good candidates for CABG.	
IIa	B	It is reasonable to choose CABG over PCI to improve symptoms in patients with complex three-vessel CAD (e.g., SYNTAX score > 22), with or without involvement of the proximal LAD artery, who are good candidates for CABG.	
IIa	B	CABG is probably recommended in preference to PCI to improve survival in patients with multivessel CAD and diabetes mellitus, particularly if a LIMA graft can be anastomosed to the LAD artery.	

CABG, Coronary artery bypass grafting; *LAD,* left anterior descending; *LIMA,* left internal mammary artery; *PCI,* percutaneous coronary intervention; *STS,* Society of Thoracic Surgeons; *SYNTAX,* Synergy Between Percutaneous Coronary Intervention with Taxus and Cardiac Surgery.
*Without involvement of the left main coronary artery.
[†]Adapted from Levine GN, Bates ER, Blankenship JC, et al. 2011 ACCF/AHA/SCAI Guideline for Percutaneous Coronary Intervention: a report of the American College of Cardiology Foundation/American Heart Association Task Force on Practice Guidelines and the Society for Cardiovascular Angiography and Interventions. *Circulation* 2011;124:e574-e651.

recommended over PCI in diabetics with multivessel disease (class IIa, level of evidence B).

The European Society of Cardiology (ESC) and European Association for Cardio-Thoracic Surgery (EACTS) 2010 Guidelines for Myocardial Revascularization incorporate data from the SYNTAX trial as well as data regarding the benefit of complete revascularization.[48] In patients at low risk for surgery, these guidelines provide a class IIa (level of evidence B) recommendation for PCI in (1) the setting of one- or two-vessel disease involving the proximal left anterior descending (LAD) artery and (2) patients with three-vessel disease, SYNTAX score of 22 or lower, in whom full revascularization can be achieved. PCI is not recommended for patients with three-vessel disease and SYNTAX scores higher than 22 and in whom full revascularization cannot be achieved. CABG is favored in all these scenarios (class I recommendation). CABG rather than PCI should be considered in diabetic patients when the extent of coronary artery disease justifies a surgical approach (especially multivessel disease) and the patient's risk profile is acceptable (class IIa, level of evidence B).

🔹 Future Directions

Late and very late stent thrombosis was a significant issue with early-generation DES, particularly in patients who underwent complex stenting procedures.[49] Stent thrombosis occurred in 3.9% of patients randomly assigned to paclitaxel-eluting stents in the SYNTAX trial.[23] Catch-up, or late restenosis, has also been observed with early-generation sirolimus-eluting and paclitaxel-eluting stents,[19,20,50] but does not appear to occur with newer generation stents, possibly because of differences in drug, polymer type, and/or drug load.[51-53] In the setting of acute coronary syndrome, the newer oral P2Y$_{12}$ antagonists are superior to clopidogrel in reducing recurrent major adverse cardiovascular events,[54] including cardiac mortality in the case of ticagrelor.[55] These advances will likely continue to reduce major adverse cardiovascular events, including death or myocardial infarction, in patients treated with PCI for multivessel disease.[18] With respect to CABG, optimal secondary prevention therapy postsurgery, which was achieved less frequently among surgical patients in SYNTAX,[21] and increased use of bilateral internal mammary artery grafts, which are relatively underused in the United States, may further improve long-term surgical outcomes.[56]

Conclusion

The early trials of CABG versus PCI with stand-alone angioplasty or bare metal stents are difficult to apply to current practice. In the DES era, synthesis of observational nonrandomized studies with various lengths of follow-up appears to show that PCI with DES provides similar rates of death and myocardial infarction than CABG, with less stroke but more repeat revascularization. In randomized trials, PCI for DES was noninferior to CABG, with increased rates of revascularization, particularly in diabetics, and possibly increased mortality and myocardial infarction in patients with highly complex disease. The SYNTAX score is an angiographic risk model predictive of outcomes in patients with unprotected left main or three-vessel disease undergoing PCI and can be used to identify patients with three-vessel disease in whom PCI or CABG may provide comparable outcomes. In the FREEDOM trial, diabetic patients with predominantly three-vessel disease had better outcomes with CABG, driven by reductions in all-cause mortality and nonfatal myocardial infarction, but at the cost of more strokes. Outcomes after PCI are a moving target because of constant technologic and operator innovation,[57] and newer DES, functional assessment, and other advances will continue to have an impact on the comparative efficacy of PCI and CABG in patients with multivessel disease.

REFERENCES

1. BARI Investigators. The final 10-year follow-up results from the BARI randomized trial. *J Am Coll Cardiol* 2007;49:1600-1606.
2. CABRI Trial Participants. First-year results of CABRI (Coronary Angioplasty versus Bypass Revascularisation Investigation). *Lancet* 1995;346:1179-1184.
3. King 3rd SB, Kosinski AS, Guyton RA, et al. Eight-year mortality in the Emory Angioplasty versus Surgery Trial (EAST). *J Am Coll Cardiol* 2000;35:1116-1121.
4. Rodriguez AE, Baldi J, Fernandez Pereira C, et al. Five-year follow-up of the Argentine randomized trial of coronary angioplasty with stenting versus coronary bypass surgery in patients with multiple vessel disease (ERACI II). *J Am Coll Cardiol* 2005;46:582-588.
5. Kaehler J, Koester R, Billmann W, et al. 13-year follow-up of the German angioplasty bypass surgery investigation. *Eur Heart J* 2005;26:2148-2153.
6. Hueb W, Lopes N, Gersh BJ, et al. Ten-year follow-up survival of the Medicine, Angioplasty, or Surgery Study (MASS II): a randomized controlled clinical trial of 3 therapeutic strategies for multivessel coronary artery disease. *Circulation* 2010;122:949-957.
7. Henderson RA, Pocock SJ, Sharp SJ, et al. Long-term results of RITA-1 trial: clinical and cost comparisons of coronary angioplasty and coronary-artery bypass grafting. Randomised Intervention Treatment of Angina. *Lancet* 1998;352:1419-1425.
8. Booth J, Clayton T, Pepper J, et al. Randomized, controlled trial of coronary artery bypass surgery versus percutaneous coronary intervention in patients with multivessel coronary artery disease: six-year follow-up from the Stent or Surgery trial (SoS). *Circulation* 2008;118:381-388.
9. Serruys PW, Ong AT, van Herwerden LA, et al. Five-year outcomes after coronary stenting versus bypass surgery for the treatment of multivessel disease: the final analysis of the arterial revascularization therapies study (arts) randomized trial. *J Am Coll Cardiol* 2005;46:575-581.
10. Hlatky MA, Boothroyd DB, Bravata DM, et al. Coronary artery bypass surgery compared with percutaneous coronary interventions for multivessel disease: a collaborative analysis of individual patient data from ten randomised trials. *Lancet* 2009;373:1190-1197.
11. Stone GW, Ellis SG, Cox DA, et al; TAXUS-IV Investigators. A polymer-based, paclitaxel-eluting stent in patients with coronary artery disease. *N Engl J Med* 2004;350:221-231.
12. Moses JW, Leon MB, Popma JJ, et al. Sirolimus-eluting stents versus standard stents in patients with stenosis in a native coronary artery. *N Engl J Med* 2003;349:1315-1323.
13. Kastrati A, Mehilli J, Pache J, et al. Analysis of 14 trials comparing sirolimus-eluting stents with bare metal stents. *N Engl J Med* 2007;356:1030-1039.
14. Yan TD, Padang R, Poh C, et al. Drug-eluting stents versus coronary artery bypass grafting for the treatment of coronary artery disease: a meta-analysis of randomized and nonrandomized studies. *J Thor Cardiovasc Surg* 2011;141:1134-1144.
15. Stone GW, Ellis SG, Cannon L, et al. Comparison of a polymer-based paclitaxel-eluting stent with a bare metal stent in patients with complex coronary artery disease: a randomized controlled trial. *Jama* 2005;294:1215-1223.
16. Serruys PW, Ong AT, Morice MC, et al. Arterial revascularisation therapies study. Part II. Sirolimus-eluting stents for the treatment of patients with multivessel de novo coronary artery lesions. *EuroIntervention* 2005;1:147-156.
17. Serruys PW, Unger F, Sousa JE, et al. Comparison of coronary-artery bypass surgery and stenting for the treatment of multivessel disease. *N Engl J Med* 2001;344:1117-1124.

18. Serruys PW, Onuma Y, Garg S, et al. 5-year clinical outcomes of the ARTS II (Arterial Revascularization Therapies Study II) of the sirolimus-eluting stent in the treatment of patients with multivessel de novo coronary artery lesions. *J Am Coll Cardiol* 2010;55:1093-1101.
19. Onuma Y, Wykrzykowska JJ, Garg S, et al. 5-year follow-up of coronary revascularization in diabetic patients with multivessel coronary artery disease: insights from ARTS (Arterial Revascularization Therapy Study)-II and ARTS-I trials. *JACC Cardiovasc Interv* 2011;4:317-323.
20. Rodriguez AE, Maree AO, Mieres J, et al. Late loss of early benefit from drug-eluting stents when compared with bare metal stents and coronary artery bypass surgery: 3 years follow-up of the eraci iii registry. *Eur Heart J* 2007;28:2118-2125.
21. Serruys PW, Morice MC, Kappetein AP, et al. Percutaneous coronary intervention versus coronary-artery bypass grafting for severe coronary artery disease. *N Engl J Med* 2009;360:961-972.
22. Cohen DJ, Van Hout B, Serruys PW, et al. Quality of life after PCI with drug-eluting stents or coronary-artery bypass surgery. *N Engl J Med* 2011;364:1016-1026.
23. Kappetein AP, Feldman TE, Mack MJ, et al. Comparison of coronary bypass surgery with drug-eluting stenting for the treatment of left main and/or three-vessel disease: 3-year follow-up of the SYNTAX trial. *Eur Heart J* 2011;32:2125-2134.
24. Mack MJ, Banning AP, Serruys PW, et al. Bypass versus drug-eluting stents at three years in syntax patients with diabetes mellitus or metabolic syndrome. *Ann Thorac Surg* 2011;92:2140-2146.
25. Kapur A, Hall RJ, Malik IS, et al. Randomized comparison of percutaneous coronary intervention with coronary artery bypass grafting in diabetic patients. 1-year results of the CARDIA (Coronary Artery Revascularization in Diabetes) trial. *J Am Coll Cardiol* 2010;55:432-440.
26. From AM, Al Badarin FJ, Cha SS, Rihal CS. Percutaneous coronary intervention with drug-eluting stents versus coronary artery bypass surgery for multivessel coronary artery disease: a meta-analysis of data from the ARTS II, CARDIA, ERACI III, and SYNTAX studies and systematic review of observational data. *EuroIntervention* 2010;6:269-276.
27. Farkouh ME, Dangas G, Leon MB, et al. Design of the future revascularization evaluation in patients with diabetes mellitus: optimal management of multivessel disease (freedom) trial. *Am Heart J* 2008;155:215-223.
28. Farkouh ME, Domanski M, Sleeper LA, et al. Strategies for multivessel revascularization in patients with diabetes. *N Engl J Med* 2012.
29. Ranucci M, Castelvecchio S, Menicanti L, et al. Risk of assessing mortality risk in elective cardiac operations: age, creatinine, ejection fraction, and the law of parsimony. *Circulation* 2009;119:3053-3061.
30. Ranucci M, Castelvecchio S, Conte M, et al. The easier, the better: age, creatinine, ejection fraction score for operative mortality risk stratification in a series of 29,659 patients undergoing elective cardiac surgery. *J Thor Cardiovasc Surg* 2011;142:581-586.
31. Capodanno D, Caggegi A, Miano M, et al. Global risk classification and clinical SYNTAX (Synergy Between Percutaneous Coronary Intervention with Taxus and Cardiac Surgery) score in patients undergoing percutaneous or surgical left main revascularization. *JACC Cardiovasc Interv* 2011;4:287-297.
32. Wykrzykowska JJ, Garg S, Onuma Y, et al. Value of age, creatinine, and ejection fraction (ACEF score) in assessing risk in patients undergoing percutaneous coronary interventions in the "all-comers" leaders trial. *Circ Cardiovasc Interv* 2011;4:47-56.

33. Garg S, Serruys PW, Silber S, et al. The prognostic utility of the syntax score on 1-year outcomes after revascularization with zotarolimus- and everolimus-eluting stents: a substudy of the resolute all comers trial. *JACC Cardiovasc Interv* 2011;4:432-441.
34. Garg S, Sarno G, Garcia-Garcia HM, et al. A new tool for the risk stratification of patients with complex coronary artery disease: the clinical syntax score. *Circ Cardiovasc Interv* 2010;3:317-326.
35. Nashef SA, Roques F, Michel P, et al. European system for cardiac operative risk evaluation (euroscore). *Eur J Cardiothorac Surg* 1999;16:9-13.
36. Nashef SA, Roques F, Hammill BG, et al. Validation of European System for Cardiac Operative Risk Evaluation (EuroSCORE) in North American cardiac surgery. *Eur J Cardiothorac Surg* 2002;22:101-105.
37. Romagnoli E, Burzotta F, Trani C, et al. EuroSCORE as predictor of in-hospital mortality after percutaneous coronary intervention. *Heart* 2009;95:43-48.
38. Morice MC, Serruys PW, Sousa JE, et al. A randomized comparison of a sirolimus-eluting stent with a standard stent for coronary revascularization. *N Engl J Med* 2002;346:1773-1780.
39. Min SY, Park DW, Yun SC, et al. Major predictors of long-term clinical outcomes after coronary revascularization in patients with unprotected left main coronary disease: analysis from the MAIN-COMPARE study. *Circ Cardiovasc Interv* 2010;3:127-133.
40. Morice MC, Serruys PW, Kappetein AP, et al. Outcomes in patients with de novo left main disease treated with either percutaneous coronary intervention using paclitaxel-eluting stents or coronary artery bypass graft treatment in the Synergy Between Percutaneous Coronary Intervention with TAXUS and Cardiac Surgery (SYNTAX) trial. *Circulation* 2010;121:2645-2653.
41. Serruys PW, Farooq V, Vranckx P, et al. A global risk approach to identify patients with left main or three-vessel disease who could safely and efficaciously be treated with percutaneous coronary intervention: the SYNTAX trial at 3 years. *JACC Cardiovasc Interv* 2012;5:606-617.
42. Singh M, Rihal CS, Lennon RJ, et al. Bedside estimation of risk from percutaneous coronary intervention: the new Mayo Clinic risk scores. *Mayo Clin Proc* 2007;82:701-708.
43. Singh M, Gersh BJ, Li S, et al. Mayo Clinic risk score for percutaneous coronary intervention predicts in-hospital mortality in patients undergoing coronary artery bypass graft surgery. *Circulation* 2008;117:356-362.
44. Girasis C, Garg S, Raber L, et al. SYNTAX score and Clinical SYNTAX score as predictors of very long-term clinical outcomes in patients undergoing percutaneous coronary interventions: a substudy of SIRolimus-eluting stent compared with pacliTAXel-eluting stent for coronary revascularization (SIRTAX) trial. *Eur Heart J* 2011;32:3115-3127.
45. Garg S, Sarno G, Girasis C, et al. A patient-level pooled analysis assessing the impact of the SYNTAX (synergy between percutaneous coronary intervention with taxus and cardiac surgery) score on 1-year clinical outcomes in 6,508 patients enrolled in contemporary coronary stent trials. *JACC Cardiovasc Interv* 2011;4:645-653.
46. Levine GN, Bates ER, Blankenship JC, et al. 2011 ACCF/AHA/SCAI guideline for percutaneous coronary intervention: a report of the American College of Cardiology Foundation/American Heart Association Task Force on Practice Guidelines and the Society for Cardiovascular Angiography and Interventions. *Circulation* 2011;124:e574-e651.
47. Nam CW, Mangiacapra F, Entjes R, et al. Functional syntax score for risk assessment in multivessel coronary artery disease. *J Am Coll Cardiol* 2011;58:1211-1218.

48. Task Force on Myocardial Revascularization of the European Society of Cardiology (ESC) and the European Association for Cardio-Thoracic Surgery (EACTS); European Association for Percutaneous Cardiovascular Interventions (EAPCI); Wijns W, Kolh P, Danchin N, et al. Guidelines on myocardial revascularization. *Eur Heart J* 2010;31:2501-2555.

49. Daemen J, Wenaweser P, Tsuchida K, et al. Early and late coronary stent thrombosis of sirolimus-eluting and paclitaxel-eluting stents in routine clinical practice: data from a large two-institutional cohort study. *Lancet* 2007;369:667-678.

50. Nakagawa Y, Kimura T, Morimoto T, et al. Incidence and risk factors of late target lesion revascularization after sirolimus-eluting stent implantation (3-year follow-up of the j-Cypher Registry). *Am J Cardiol* 2010;106:329-336.

51. Palmerini T, Biondi-Zoccai G, Della Riva D, et al. Stent thrombosis with drug-eluting and bare metal stents: evidence from a comprehensive network meta-analysis. *Lancet* 2012;379: 1393-1402.

52. Stone GW, Rizvi A, Newman W, et al. Everolimus-eluting versus paclitaxel-eluting stents in coronary artery disease. *N Engl J Med* 2010;362:1663-1674.

53. Raber L, Magro M, Stefanini GG, et al. Very late coronary stent thrombosis of a newer-generation everolimus-eluting stent compared with early-generation drug-eluting stents: a prospective cohort study. *Circulation* 2012;125:1110-1121.

54. Wiviott SD, Braunwald E, McCabe CH, et al. Prasugrel versus clopidogrel in patients with acute coronary syndromes. *N Engl J Med* 2007;357:2001-2015.

55. Wallentin L, Becker RC, Budaj A, et al. Ticagrelor versus clopidogrel in patients with acute coronary syndromes. *N Engl J Med* 2009;361:1045-1057.

56. Grau JB, Ferrari G, Mak AW, et al. Propensity matched analysis of bilateral internal mammary artery versus single left internal mammary artery grafting at 17-year follow-up: validation of a contemporary surgical experience. *Eur J Cardiothorac Surg* 2012;41:770-775.

57. Price MJ, Kandzari DE, Teirstein PS. Change we can believe in: the hyper-evolution of percutaneous coronary intervention for unprotected left main disease with drug-eluting stents. *Circ Cardiovasc Interv* 2008;1:164-166.

CHAPTER 14

Left Main Coronary Artery Stenting

GILL LOUISE BUCHANAN | **ALAIDE CHIEFFO**

KEY POINTS

- Significant unprotected left main coronary artery (ULMCA) disease remains a class I indication for coronary artery bypass grafting (CABG).

- Registries and randomized studies have shown a higher rate of repeat revascularization after percutaneous coronary intervention (PCI) compared with CABG, but a lower incidence of cerebrovascular events; no differences were reported in overall major adverse cardiovascular events.

- It is important to use adjunctive techniques to evaluate the significance of ULMCA lesions (e.g., intravascular ultrasound and fractional flow reserve).

- The location of the ULMCA lesion affects the optimal stent technique; factors that also need to be considered include plaque distribution, side branch size, severity and distribution of the side branch lesion, and bifurcation angle.

- Drug-eluting stents (DES) should be the stent of choice, unless there are contraindications to or anticipated poor compliance with prolonged dual antiplatelet therapy.

- Hemodynamic support should be considered when there is evidence of severe left ventricular systolic dysfunction or hemodynamic instability or patients with acute presentations.

- Future randomized studies are awaited to definitively assess the long-term outcomes of patients undergoing PCI of the ULMCA compared with CABG.

Unprotected left main coronary artery (ULMCA) disease is a class I indication for coronary artery bypass grafting (CABG).[1,2] First, the location of the disease means that a substantial amount of myocardium can potentially be jeopardized; second, it commonly affects the distal bifurcation, which is known to be at higher risk for restenosis. Furthermore, a large proportion of patients with ULMCA disease have triple-vessel coronary artery disease.

In more recent years, with the advent of drug-eluting stents (DES), a significant reduction in restenosis and target lesion revascularization (TLR) has been shown after the percutaneous treatment of ULMCA (Table 14-1). This is in comparison to the bare metal stent (BMS) era, which was limited by restenosis and, in some series, sudden death.[3-17] In addition, operators have increased experience, better equipment, and more effective antiplatelet agents at their disposal. These factors have led to an increasing enthusiasm among interventional cardiologists to undertake treatment of these lesions, with favorable results. This chapter will discuss the issues surrounding percutaneous coronary intervention (PCI) of the ULMCA—the available data, case selection, and methods and technology available.

Current Guidelines

Current practice guidelines still recommend CABG as standard therapy for patients with significant ULMCA disease.[2,18] The most recent European Society of Cardiology guidelines for PCI of the ULMCA state a class IIa indication (level of evidence B) for isolated or one-vessel disease if the ULMCA lesion is located in the ostium or body (Table 14-2). When the distal bifurcation is involved, this becomes a class IIb indication. If there is associated two- or three-vessel coronary artery disease with a Synergy between Percutaneous

Coronary Intervention with TAXUS and Cardiac Surgery (SYNTAX) score of 32 or lower, the indication is class IIb (level of evidence B); however, when the SYNTAX score is 33 or higher, this becomes class IIIb.[2]

The American Heart Association (AHA)/American College of Cardiology (ACC)/Society for Cardiovascular and Angiographic Interventions (SCAI) recently modified their recommendation for PCI of the ULMCA (see Table 14-2) from a class IIb to a class IIa (level of evidence B) indication in those with favorable anatomy for PCI (SYNTAX ≤ 22) and clinical conditions that confer an increased risk of adverse events with CABG. Furthermore, the guidelines state that in the setting of acute coronary syndrome, ULMCA PCI is a class IIa (level of evidence B) indication, and in ST elevation myocardial infarction when PCI can be performed more promptly than CABG, a class IIa (level of evidence C) indication.[1]

Risk Stratification

Most risk stratification methods used for the patient with ULMCA disease are derived from traditional surgical scoring systems, such as the EuroSCORE.[19] The SYNTAX score is a prospective angiographic tool devised to grade the anatomic complexity of coronary artery disease (an online calculator can be found at www.syntaxscore.com). In the prespecified subgroup of patients enrolled in the SYNTAX trial with ULMCA obstruction, there were no differences in the occurrence of major adverse cardiovascular and cerebrovascular events (MACCE) up to 3 years in patients with low and intermediate SYNTAX scores treated with PCI or CABG. Conversely, in those with high SYNTAX scores, PCI was associated with higher MACCE up to 3 years.[20] Moreover, it was demonstrated that the single independent anatomic factor predicting 1-year MACCE was the increasing number of vessels requiring interventional treatment.[21,22]

Since the SYNTAX score is based purely on anatomic features, other scoring methods have subsequently been tested to incorporate additional clinical parameters in an attempt to achieve a superior system of risk stratification and thereby deliver full informed consent and advise patients regarding the most appropriate treatment modality. One such risk model using anatomic and clinical features is the recently described Global Risk Classification, which combines the SYNTAX score with the EuroSCORE.[23] This has been shown to be a better predictor of cardiac mortality in patients undergoing ULMCA PCI. A further novel score using clinical and anatomic parameters, in addition to procedural factors, is the New Risk Stratification score. This has been demonstrated to show superior sensitivity and sensitivity compared with the SYNTAX score in predicting MACCE in high-risk patients undergoing PCI for ULMCA,[24] with a New Risk Stratification score of 25 or higher being the sole predictor of MACCE and stent thrombosis.

Percutaneous Coronary Intervention Versus Coronary Artery Bypass Grafting

Several nonrandomized, observational registry studies have shown no significant differences in MACCE between CABG and PCI in patients with ULMCA obstruction up to a follow-up period of 5 years (Table 14-3).[7,25-40] The Revascularization for Unprotected Left Main Coronary Artery Stenosis: Comparison of Percutaneous Coronary

TABLE 14-1	Observational Registries Evaluating the Drug-Eluting Stent in the Treatment of Unprotected Left Main Coronary Artery Disease									
	Study									
Parameter	De Lezo et al[3]	Chieffo et al[4]	Park et al[5]	Valgimigli et al[6]	Chieffo et al[9]	Sheiban et al[10]	Palmerini et al[54]	Kim et al[13]	Meliga et al[17]	Vaquerizo et al[63]
Year	2004	2005	2005	2005	2007	2007	2008	2008	2008	2009
No. of patients	52	85	102	95	147	85	1111	63	358	291
Type of DES	SES	SES and PES	SES	SES and PES	SES and PES	SES	SES and PES	SES and PES	SES and PES	PES
Distal lesion location (%)	42	88	71	65	0*	61	70	73	73.7	78.4
TLR/TVR (%)	6/2	14.1/18.8	7/2	6 (TVR)	0.7/0.7	10.8 (TLR)	11.8 (TLR)	16 (TLR)	3.9/10	7.9 (TVR)
Cardiac death (%)	0	3.5	14	14	2.7	2.4	7.8	5	9.2	5.2

DES, Drug-eluting stent; *PES,* paclitaxel-eluting stent; *SES,* sirolimus-eluting stent; *TLR,* target lesion revascularization; *TVR,* target vessel revascularization; *ULMCA,* unprotected left main coronary artery.
*All ostial and/or body lesions.

TABLE 14-2	Current Recommendations for Revascularization in Patients with Significant Unprotected Left Main Coronary Artery Disease	
	Therapy	
Guidelines	**PCI**	**CABG**
ACC/AHA/SCAI Guidelines*		
ULMCA	—	IB
ULMCA (anatomically favorable for PCI and significant risk with CABG)	Class IIa, level of evidence B	—
ESC/EACTS Guidelines†		
ULMCA (isolated or one-VD, ostium or body)	Class IIa, level of evidence B	IA
ULMCA (isolated or one-VD, bifurcation)	Class IIb, level of evidence B	IA
ULMCA + two- or three-VD and SYNTAX score < 32	Class IIb, level of evidence B	IA
ULMCA + two- or three-VD and SYNTAX score ≥ 33	Class III, level of evidence B	IA

CABG, Coronary artery bypass grafting; *PCI,* percutaneous coronary intervention; *ULMCA,* unprotected left main coronary artery; *VD,* vessel disease.
*American College of Cardiology Foundation/American Heart Association/Society of Cardiovasular Angiographic Interventions 2011 Guidelines for Percutaneous Coronary Intervention.[1]
†European Society of Cardiology/European Association for Cardiothoracic Surgery Guidelines on Myocardial Revascularization.[2]

Angioplasty Versus Surgical Revascularization (MAIN-COMPARE) trial was the first large, multicenter, nonrandomized study comparing these two treatment groups in the treatment of ULMCA. It incorporated a total of 2240 patients who underwent PCI (BMS, n = 318; DES, n = 784) or CABG (n = 1138). After propensity matching, no significant differences were observed in death (hazard ratio [HR] in the PCI group, 1.18; 95% confidence interval [CI], 0.77-1.80) or the composite of death, myocardial infarction, and cerebrovascular events (HR, 1.10; 95% CI, 0.75-1.62). Conversely, target vessel revascularization (TVR) was higher in the PCI cohort (HR, 4.76; 95% CI, 2.80-8.11).[29] Extended follow-up to 5 years has subsequently been reported, confirming no significant differences in death (HR, 1.13; 95% CI, 0.88-1.44; P = .35) or the combined endpoint of death, myocardial infarction, or cerebrovascular events (HR, 1.07; 95% CI, 0.84-1.3; P = .59).[38]

These findings were consistent with that of a single-center registry that reported no differences between CABG (n = 142) and first-generation DES (n = 107) in cardiac death (adjusted odds ratio [OR], 0.502; 95% CI, 0.162-1.461; P = .24). As in MAIN-COMPARE, patients undergoing CABG experienced a lower rate of TVR (adjusted

OR for PCI, 4.411; 95% CI, 1.825-.371; P = .0004); in contrast, those treated with PCI had a trend toward a lower rate of the composite endpoint of cardiac death and myocardial infarction (adjusted OR, 0.408; 95% CI, 0.146-1.061; P = .06).[25,37]

The number of randomized trials evaluating DES compared with CABG for ULMCA disease are limited.[40a] The Study of Unprotected Left Main Stenting Versus Bypass Surgery (LE MANS) enrolled 105 patients with >50% left main narrowing, with or without multivessel coronary artery disease, who were equally suitable for PCI or CABG. The primary endpoint was the change in left ventricular ejection fraction by echocardiography at 12 months; clinical outcomes were key secondary endpoints. At 1-year follow-up, the mean ejection fraction increased with PCI compared with CABG (3.3 ± 6.7% vs. 0.5 ± 0.8%, p = 0.047), resulting in a greater ejection fraction in the PCI group (58.0 ± 6.8% vs. 54.1 ± 8.9%, P = 0.01). The risk of MACCE at 30 days was lower with PCI (2% vs. 13%; RR 0.88, 95% CI 0.79 to 0.99; p = 0.03), whereas the risk of MACCE at 1 year was similar (31% vs. 25%, RR 1.09, 95% CI 0.85 to 1.38), primarily because of the need for repeat revascularization in the PCI group. Left main restenosis occurred in 5 patients (9.6%), of whom 4 had received BMS. At longer-term follow-up of 28.0 ± 9.9 months, there was a trend toward better survival after PCI (p = 0.08).[40b]

The major landmark trial comparing the outcomes of CABG versus PCI with DES has been the SYNTAX study, which had a prespecified ULMCA subgroup (CABG, n = 348; PCI, n = 357). Noninferiority in MACCE at 12 months was achieved in the ULMCA subgroup (13.7% vs. 15.8%; P = .44), although noninferiority was not achieved in the overall trial. Therefore, these observations in the left main cohort must be considered exploratory hypothesis-generating. Despite the higher rates of repeat revascularization among the PCI patients (11.8% vs. 6.5%; P = .02), there was a significantly higher rate of cerebrovascular events in those undergoing CABG (2.7% vs. 0.3%; P = .01).[41] At 5-year follow up, MACCE rates did not significantly differ according to treatment strategy (CABG 31.0% vs. PCI 36.9%; p = 0.12). The results were similar in those with a low SYNTAX scores (0 to 22; 31.5% vs. 30.4%; p = 0.74) and intermediate SYNTAX scores (23 to 32; 32.3% vs. 32.7%; p = 0.88). However, in the high SYNTAX score group (≥33), non-inferiority in MACCE was not achieved, and CABG appeared to be a superior treatment strategy (29.7% vs. 46.5%; p = 0.003).[41a]

The SYNTAX results are encouraging for the use of PCI in ULMCA, particularly in those with low anatomic risk (SYNTAX score < 33). However, as noted previously, this subgroup analysis was hypothesis-generating and further, more definitive trials are awaited that are adequately powered.

The Premier of Randomized Comparison of Bypass Surgery Versus Angioplasty Using Sirolimus-Eluting Stent in Patients with Left Main Coronary Artery Disease (PRECOMBAT) randomly assigned 300 patients to CABG and 300 patients to PCI with sirolimus-eluting

TABLE 14-3	Studies Comparing Percutaneous Coronary Intervention Versus Coronary Artery Bypass Grafting for the Treatment of Unprotected Left Main Coronary Artery Disease							
	Study							
Parameter	Palmerini et al[26]	Lee et al[7]	Sanmartin et al[32]	Buszman et al[28]	Chieffo et al[37]	Park et al[38]	Kappetein et al[20]	Park et al[40]
Year	2006	2006	2007	2008	2010	2010	2011	2011
No. of patients	311	173	335	106	249	2240	695	600
Study design	Registry	Registry	Registry	Randomized	Registry	Registry	Randomized	Randomized
EuroSCORE (%)	6 vs. 5	NA	27 vs. 25.3*	3.3 vs. 3.5	4.4 vs. 4.3	NA	3.9 vs. 3.9	2.6 vs. 2.8
SYNTAX score	NA	NA	NA	25 vs. 24	28 vs. 29	NA	29.6 vs. 30.2	NA
Follow-up (yr)	1	1	1	1	5	5	3	2
Cardiac death (%)	NA	2 vs. 1.6	NA	NA	7.5 vs. 11.9	9.9†	7.3 vs. 8.4	2.4 vs. 3.4
MI (%)	8 vs. 5	NA	0 vs. 1.3	1.9 vs. 5.6	0.9 vs. 7.7	1†	6.9 vs. 4.1	1.7 vs. 1.0
TLR (%)	25.5 vs. 2.6‡	NA	NA	NA	18.7 vs. 8.4	NA	20.0 vs. 11.7	NA
TVR (%)	NA	7 vs. 1	5.2 vs. 0.8§	28.8 vs. 9.4‖	28 vs. 8.4	9.7†	NA	6.1 vs. 3.4
CVA (%)	NA	NA	0 vs. 0.8	0 vs. 3.7	0.9 vs. 4.2	1.8†	1.2 vs. 4.0	0.7 vs. 0.4
MACCE (%)	NA	17 vs. 25	10.4 vs. 11.4	30.7 vs. 24.5	32.4 vs. 38.3	NA	26.8 vs. 22.3	12.2 vs. 8.1

CVA, Cerebrovascular accident; DES, drug-eluting stent; MACCE, major adverse cardiac and cerebrovascular event; MI, myocardial infarction; NA, not available. TLR, target lesion revascularization; TVR, target vessel revascularization.
*Logistic EuroSCORE.
†Cumulative for overall.
‡$P = .0001$.
§$P = .02$.
‖$P = .01$.

stents (SES). This was a noninferiority study with a primary composite endpoint of MACCE at 1-year follow-up. PCI was non-inferior to CABG (cumulative event rate, 8.7% vs. 6.7%; absolute risk difference, 2.0 percentage points; 95% confidence interval [CI], −1.6 to 5.6; $P = .01$ for non-inferiority). Of note, the margin allowed to achieve non-inferiority was rather wide, particularly given the lower-than-expected event rate in the CABG arm. At 2 years, the cumulative event rate was 12.2% versus 8.1% (HR, 1.50; 95% CI 0.90-2.52; $P = .12$). The two groups had similar rates of the individual components of death (CABG, 3.4%, vs. PCI, 2.4%; $P = .45$), myocardial infarction (1.0% vs. 1.7%; $P = .49$), and cerebrovascular events (0.7% vs. 0.4%; $P = .56$). However, as with prior studies, the rate of ischemia-driven TVR was higher in the PCI group (4.2% vs. 9.0%; $P = .02$).[42]

The results of larger ongoing multicenter randomized trials, such as the Evaluation of Xience Prime Versus Coronary Artery Bypass Surgery for Effectiveness of Left Main Revascularization trial (EXCEL, clinicaltrials.gov identifier NCT01205776), are awaited to clarify outcomes with currently available second-generation DES versus CABG. In this study, 2634 patients with ULMCA and a SYNTAX score of 32 or lower will be randomized to CABG or second-generation DES (Xience Prime, Abbott Vascular, Redwood City, Calif). The primary endpoint is the composite incidence of death, myocardial infarction, or cerebrovascular events at a median follow-up duration of 3 years. The trial is powered for sequential noninferiority and superiority testing.

Lesion Assessment and Imaging

Conventional coronary angiography is widely used in the evaluation of ULMCA lesions. It is a useful tool to evaluate lesion length, morphology, plaque burden, and the anatomic relationship of the ostium and distal bifurcation. However, angiography does not allow assessment of the true luminal size of the ULMCA because of factors such as positive remodeling. Additionally, the ULMCA segment is the least reproducible part of the coronary tree because it is often short and lacks a normal segment for comparison, rendering the assessment subject to large intraobserver and interobserver variability.[43,44] Therefore, invasive diagnostic methods, such as intravascular ultrasound

(IVUS) or fractional flow reserve (FFR), are often necessary to allow full evaluation of the lesion. IVUS is an important adjunctive imaging modality in this complex subset of patients, first to determine plaque composition and distribution and also to allow adequate sizing of the vessel diameter and lesion length before stent selection. Also, IVUS is essential after stent implantation to enable the assessment of stent expansion and apposition (Figure 14-1). After IVUS, approximately 25% of lesions require additional inflation because of underexpansion. IVUS guidance was shown to confer a mortality benefit at 3 years over angiography guidance alone in a subgroup analysis of patients treated with DES from the MAIN-COMPARE registry (IVUS, 4.7%, vs. no IVUS, 16.0%; $P = .049$).[45]

Another tool that may be useful in assessing the severity of angiographically intermediate lesions is the FFR, with a value of 0.75 or lower considered a reliable indicator of significant stenosis. In patients with an equivocal ULMCA stenosis, a strategy of revascularization versus medical therapy based on the FFR measurement was associated with excellent survival and freedom from adverse events at up to 3 years follow-up.[46]

More recently, optical coherence tomography has been demonstrated to be safe and feasible in the assessment of vascular response after DES implantation.[47] In view of the ability of this tool to define stent struts and arterial tissue clearly, there may be a future role for this imaging technique to identify predisposing features of stent thrombosis, which is catastrophic after ULMCA PCI, including delayed or incomplete stent endothelialization and stent malapposition.

Lesion Subsets and Stenting Techniques

The left main coronary artery is comprised of three distinct segments—the ostium, body, and distal bifurcation. The latter is associated with an increased incidence of disease as a result of low shear stresses causing flow disturbance, which is associated with the formation of atherosclerotic plaques.[48] In contradistinction, the carina typically remains free of disease. This distal location poses additional complexity to the PCI procedure, with clinical outcomes after ULMCA bifurcation PCI less favorable compared with those for lesions elsewhere in the ULMCA.[9] Disease in this location has been identified as the most significant

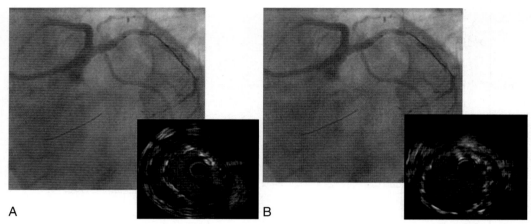

A   B

Figure 14-1   Importance of intravascular ultrasound (IVUS) in the treatment of the unprotected left main coronary artery. A, Angiographic and intra-vascular ultrasound (IVUS) images of a left main after implantation of a drug-eluting stent, demonstrating a good angiographic result but evident underex-pansion at IVUS. **B,** Images after post-dilation, with properly sized balloons and a clear improvement in the IVUS results.

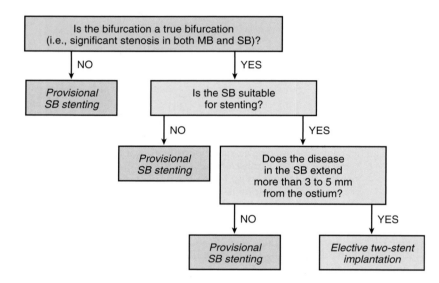

Figure 14-2   Recommended approach to the percutaneous treatment of bifurcation lesions. This includes the unpro-tected left main coronary artery. *MB,* Main branch; *SB,* side branch.

predictor of overall MACCE and the need for repeat revascularization in a meta-analysis of 17 trials of PCI for ULMCA disease.[11]

The treatment of the ostial ULMCA is similar to that for any aorto-ostial lesion, with the exception that it is often much larger in diameter. It is important to predilate the lesion adequately to ensure that the stent can be adequately deployed. The stent length should aim not to cover the distal bifurcation and should be allowed to protrude back into the aorta by 1 to 2 mm. Multiple cine projections should be used to ensure adequate positioning of the stent. In addi-tion, as noted, IVUS guidance is advisable for optimum stent sizing and deployment. Similarly, ULMCA lesions in the body should be treated in this fashion with the possible goal of avoiding the distal bifurcation. Low event rates have been observed in patients treated percutaneously for ostial and body ULMCA stenoses.[4-6,49] In a multi-center study of 147 patients undergoing DES implantation for lesions of the ULMCA not affecting the bifurcation, there was a TLR rate of 0.7%, a cardiac death rate of 2.7%, and a MACE rate of 7.4% at long-term clinical follow-up (886 ± 308 days).[9]

ULMCA disease involves the distal bifurcation in 60% to 90% of those requiring intervention.[50] Because of the heterogeneity of distal bifurcation lesions, no single stent strategy for PCI of the ULMCA bifurcation can be applied (Figure 14-2). The most important factors to consider when deciding on an appropriate technique include the plaque distribution, size of the side branch, severity and length of the

side branch lesion, and bifurcation angulation (Figure 14-3). In a ULMCA bifurcation lesion, the main branch is generally regarded to be the left anterior descending coronary artery, with the side branch the circumflex or intermediate artery. However, this latter vessel may be as important in terms of size and territory of distribution. When the bifurcation has plaque involving the main branch alone (Medina classification 1,1,0 or 1,0,0) a stent should be implanted using a pro-visional one-stent strategy from the ULMCA into the main branch. After stent implantation, the decision for a second stent should be made only after adequate post-dilation and final kissing balloon infla-tion if there is evidence of dissection associated with reduced Throm-bolysis In Myocardial Infarction (TIMI) flow or a significant residual stenosis. If feasible, PCI of the ULMCA distal bifurcation with a single-stent approach has been shown to have better outcomes[51,52] with a TLR rate almost equivalent to that for PCI of the ostium or body when DES are used.[4,53] Elective use of two stents should be considered at the outset of the procedure if there is significant disease affecting both branches, if the side branch is of significant size with a large area of distribution and if the side branch disease extends 3 to 5 mm beyond the ostium. It is important to note that studies have shown the TLR rate to be up to 25% when a two-stent strategy has been used, with restenosis confined mainly to the circumflex ostium.[52,54] Final kissing balloon inflation is critical for effective PCI of the ULMCA, regardless of the technique used. Figure 14-4

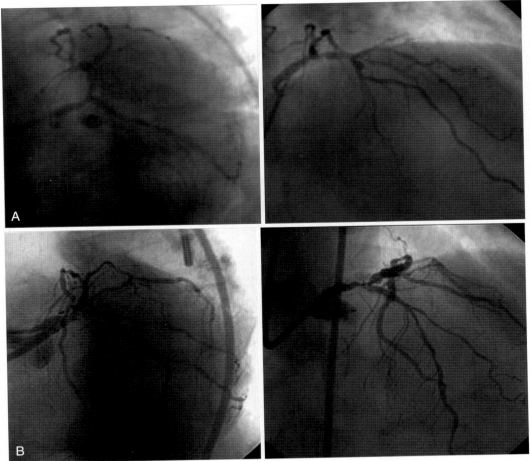

Figure 14-3 Examples of left main disease requiring a one-stent versus a two-stent strategy. **A,** Left main disease not significantly affecting the side-branch, favoring a one-stent strategy. **B,** Disease requiring a two-stent strategy from the outset.

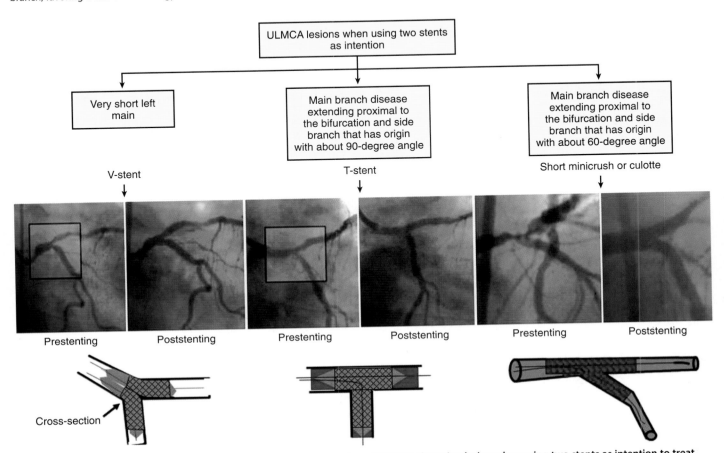

Figure 14-4 Approach to the distal unprotected left main coronary artery *(ULMCA)* bifurcation lesion when using two stents as intention to treat.

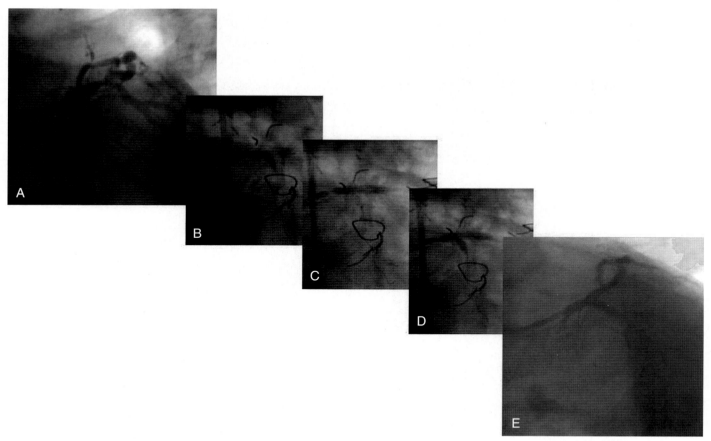

Figure 14-5 **Culotte technique in treatment of the left main coronary artery. A,** Angiogram before intervention. **B,** Angiogram of stent deployment in the side branch. **C,** Angiogram of stent deployment in the main branch. **D,** Angiogram of final kissing balloon inflation with noncompliant balloons. **E,** Final angiographic result.

illustrates our approach to treatment of the distal ULMCA lesion when using two stents as an intention to treat. Figures 14-5 and 14-6 demonstrate case examples of the results with the culotte and mini-crush techniques for the treatment of the ULMCA.

Type of Stent

Clinical outcomes after ULMCA PCI have improved greatly with the advent of DES. At midterm follow-up in observational registries of elective DES implantation for ULMCA disease, the 1-year mortality was up to 5%, the need for TLR varied from 0% to 14%, and TVR ranged from 0% to 19%.* Therefore, unless there are significant concerns regarding prolonged treatment with dual antiplatelet therapy, the use of DES should be considered in all cases.

Several observational registry studies have compared outcomes among the first-generation DES.[8,57] In addition, the Intracoronary Stenting and Angiographic Results: Drug-eluting Stents for Unprotected Left Main Lesions (ISAR-LEFT MAIN) study randomly assigned 607 patients undergoing PCI for ULMCA disease to SES or paclitaxel-eluting stents (PES). At 12 months, there were no significant differences in outcomes, including the composite outcome of death, myocardial infarction, and TLR (SES 15.8% vs. PES 13.6%; relative risk [RR], 0.85; 95% CI, 0.56-1.29) or in-stent restenosis (SES 19.4% vs. PES 16.0%; $P = .30$). At 2 years, no significant differences in ULMCA-specific revascularization (10.7% SES vs. 9.2% PES; $P = .47$) or definite stent thrombosis (0.3% SES vs. 0.7% PES) were identified.[54]

*References 3-6, 13, 17, 51, and 53-64.

There remains limited evidence regarding the use of second-generation DES in the treatment of ULMCA lesions. The LEft MAin Xience V (LEMAX) observational registry compared 173 patients treated with everolimus-eluting stents (EES) with a historical control group of 291 patients who had received PES for ULMCA disease. Follow-up at 12 months showed a lower incidence of TLR and stent thrombosis with EES.[65] ISAR-LEFT MAIN 2, a randomized, non-inferiority trial, (clinicaltrials.gov identifier NCT00598637) assessed the safety and efficacy of EES versus Resolute zotarolimus-eluting stents (ZES) (Abbott Vascular, Redwood City, California) in ULMCA lesions, with a primary endpoint of MACE at 1-year follow-up. A preliminary report stated that there was no difference in the incidence of the primary endpoint between groups (14.3% vs. 17.5% for EES and ZES, respectively; p = 0.25). The upper bound of the 95% CI of the difference between treatments was 8.0%, less than the 9.0% non-inferiority margin, and ergo the Resolute ZES achieved the criteria for non-inferiority. Therefore it appears that these DES may provide similar outcomes between groups in this high-risk patient population, although the non-inferiority margin was wide and thus cannot exclude differences that may be clinically significant.

Further Considerations

HEMODYNAMIC SUPPORT

There is no generalized consensus as to when hemodynamic support should be used for patients undergoing PCI for ULMCA disease. There is an 8% risk of acute hemodynamic instability that usually necessitates intra-aortic balloon pump support.[66] Those with preserved left ventricular function can generally tolerate the ischemia

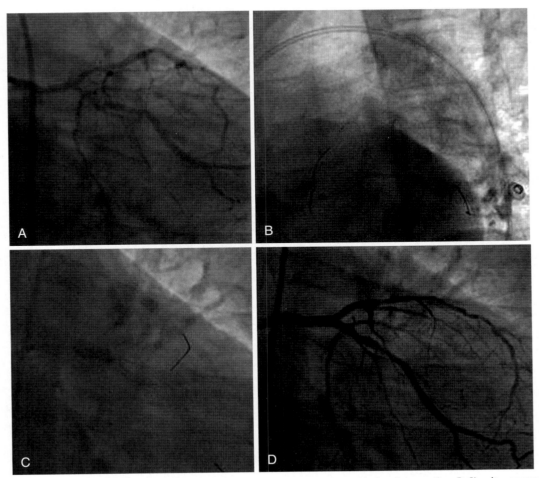

Figure 14-6   **Minicrush technique in treatment of the left main coronary artery. A,** Angiogram before intervention. **B,** Simultaneous positioning of drug-eluting stent in the left anterior descending and circumflex arteries. **C,** Two-step final kissing balloon inflation (first post-dilation of the side branch with a noncompliant balloon and then kissing balloon inflation). **D,** Final angiographic result.

that occurs during balloon inflation, and insertion of an intra-aortic balloon pump is usually not required. However, there are certain situations in which intra-aortic balloon pump placement should be considered before PCI, including severe left ventricular dysfunction, a systolic blood pressure of 90 mm Hg or lower, or acute coronary syndrome. In addition, certain anatomic features may be an indication for intra-aortic balloon pump insertion, such as an occluded right coronary artery, dominant circumflex artery, or heavy calcium burden that requires rotational atherectomy. An alternative option for hemodynamic support in those patients deemed to be high risk is the Impella system (Abiomed, Danvers, Mass), a minimally invasive left ventricular assist device.[67]

DUAL ANTIPLATELET THERAPY

After elective DES implantation, current European guidelines support the use of 6 to 12 months and American guidelines support the use of at least 12 months of dual antiplatelet therapy (DAPT), with aspirin therapy continued indefinitely thereafter.[1,2] This guidance, however, is not specific for ULMCA PCI, and many interventionalists have advocated extended DAPT in this subset of patients as a result of the potentially fatal consequences if stent thrombosis occurs. A study of 215 patients undergoing ULMCA PCI with DES assessed platelet reactivity before PCI by light transmittance aggregometry after a loading dose of clopidogrel 600 mg. High residual platelet reactivity was observed in 18.6% of patients, and the 3-year cardiac

mortality rate was 28.3% ± 10.4% in this group compared with 8.0% ± 3.1% in those with low residual platelet reactivity ($P = .005$). There was also a significant difference in stent thrombosis at 3 years, favoring better outcomes in those with low residual platelet activity (16.0% ± 7.3% vs. 4.2% ± 1.8%; $P = .021$). Moreover, high residual platelet reactivity was the only predictor of cardiac death (HR, 3.82; 95% CI, 1.38-10.54; $P = .010$) and stent thrombosis (HR, 3.69; 95% CI, 1.12-12.09; $P = .31$).[22] Further studies are necessary to clarify the optimal regimen and duration of DAPT after the treatment of ULMCA with DES.

SURVEILLANCE

Previously, it was standard practice to perform routine coronary angiography after ULMCA PCI in view of concerns regarding the serious consequences if restenosis were to occur. However, this recommendation was removed from guidelines published by the ACC/AHA/SCAI in 2009 because it was thought to be difficult to predict angiographically whether patients will suffer a stent thrombosis, in addition to the unnecessary risks posed to the patient undergoing angiography after an LM stent.[68] Therefore, surveillance with coronary angiography is currently not recommended unless specific procedural features may cause concern regarding durability of the stent. However, it has been suggested that coronary multislice computed tomography with optimal heart rate control may enable a noninvasive evaluation of selected patients after ULMCA stenting.[69]

Conclusion

Treatment of the ULMCA with PCI remains a complex procedure because of the location of the lesion and other concomitant anatomic features. However, recent technologic advances, including newer generation DES, imaging techniques, and antiplatelet agents, have led to improved outcomes. Individual risk stratification through modalities such as the SYNTAX score enables the assessment of the optimal treatment strategy for a particular patient. Despite encouraging results for ULMCA PCI, further studies using the newer technologies are essential to assess long-term outcomes in these patients.

REFERENCES

1. Levine GN, Bates ER, Blankenship JC, et al. 2011 ACCF/AHA/SCAI guideline for percutaneous coronary intervention: a report of the American College of Cardiology Foundation/American Heart Association Task Force on Practice Guidelines and the Society for Cardiovascular Angiography and Interventions. *Circulation* 2011;124:e574-e651.
2. Wijns W, Kolh P, Danchin N, et al. Guidelines on myocardial revascularization: the task force on myocardial revascularization of the European Society of Cardiology (ESC) and the European Association for Cardio-Thoracic Surgery (EACTS). *Eur Heart J* 2010;31(20):2501-2555.
3. de Lezo JS, Medina A, Pan M, et al. Rapamycin-eluting stents for the treatment of unprotected left main coronary disease. *Am Heart J* 2004;148:481-485.
4. Chieffo A, Stankovic G, Bonizzoni E, et al. Early and mid-term results of drug-eluting stent implantation in unprotected left main. *Circulation* 2005;111:791-795.
5. Park SJ, Kim YH, Lee BK, et al. Sirolimus-eluting stent implantation for unprotected left main coronary artery stenosis: comparison with bare metal stent implantation. *J Am Coll Cardiol* 2005;45:351-356.
6. Valgimigli M, van Mieghem CA, Ong AT, et al. Short- and long-term clinical outcome after drug-eluting stent implantation for the percutaneous treatment of left main coronary artery disease: insights from the Rapamycin-Eluting and Taxus Stent Evaluated At Rotterdam Cardiology Hospital registries (RESEARCH and T-SEARCH). *Circulation* 2005;111:1383-1389.
7. Lee MS, Kapoor N, Jamal F, et al. Comparison of coronary artery bypass surgery with percutaneous coronary intervention with drug-eluting stents for unprotected left main coronary artery disease. *J Am Coll Cardiol* 2006;47:864-870.
8. Valgimigli M, Malagutti P, Aoki J, et al. Sirolimus-eluting vs. paclitaxel-eluting stent implantation for the percutaneous treatment of left main coronary artery disease: a combined RESEARCH and T-SEARCH long-term analysis. *J Am Coll Cardiol* 2006;47:507-514.
9. Chieffo A, Park SJ, Valgimigli M, et al. Favorable long-term outcome after drug-eluting stent implantation in nonbifurcation lesions that involve unprotected left main coronary artery: a multicenter registry. *Circulation* 2007;116:158-162.
10. Sheiban I, Meliga E, Moretti C, et al. Long-term clinical and angiographic outcomes of treatment of unprotected left main coronary artery stenosis with sirolimus-eluting stents. *Am J Cardiol* 2007;100:431-435.
11. Biondi-Zoccai GG, Lotrionte M, et al. A collaborative systematic review and meta-analysis on 1278 patients undergoing percutaneous drug-eluting stenting for unprotected left main coronary artery disease. *Am Heart J* 2008;155:274-283.
12. Chieffo A, Park SJ, Meliga E, et al. Late and very late stent thrombosis following drug-eluting stent implantation in unprotected left main coronary artery: a multicentre registry. *Eur Heart J* 2008;29:2108-2115.
13. Kim YH, Dangas GD, Solinas E, et al. Effectiveness of drug-eluting stent implantation for patients with unprotected left main coronary artery stenosis. *Am J Cardiol* 2008;101:801-806.
14. Tamburino C, Di Salvo ME, Capodanno D, et al. Are drug-eluting stents superior to bare-metal stents in patients with unprotected non-bifurcational left main disease? Insights from a multicentre registry. *Eur Heart J* 2009;30:1171-1179.
15. Tamburino C, Di Salvo ME, Capodanno D, et al. Comparison of drug-eluting stents and bare-metal stents for the treatment of unprotected left main coronary artery disease in acute coronary syndromes. *Am J Cardiol* 2009;103:187-193.
16. Kim YH, Park DW, Lee SW, et al. Long-term safety and effectiveness of unprotected left main coronary stenting with drug-eluting stents compared with bare-metal stents. *Circulation* 2009;120:400-407.
17. Meliga E, Garcia-Garcia HM, Valgimigli M, et al. Longest available clinical outcomes after drug-eluting stent implantation for unprotected left main coronary artery disease: the DELFT (Drug-Eluting Stent For Left Main) registry. *J Am Coll Cardiol* 2008;51:2212-2219.
18. Patel MR, Dehmer GJ, Hirshfeld JW, et al; American College of Cardiology Foundation Appropriateness Criteria Task Force; Society for Cardiovascular Angiography and Interventions; Society of Thoracic Surgeons; American Association for Thoracic Surgery; American Heart Association, and the American Society of Nuclear Cardiology Endorsed by the American Society of Echocardiography; Heart Failure Society of America; Society of Cardiovascular Computed Tomography. ACCF/SCAI/STS/AATS/AHA/ASNC 2009 Appropriateness Criteria for Coronary Revascularization: a report by the American College of Cardiology Foundation Appropriateness Criteria Task Force, Society for Cardiovascular Angiography and Interventions, Society of Thoracic Surgeons, American Association for Thoracic Surgery, American Heart Association, and the American Society of Nuclear Cardiology Endorsed by the American Society of Echocardiography, the Heart Failure Society of America, and the Society of Cardiovascular Computed Tomography. *J Am Coll Cardiol* 2009;53:530-553.
19. Nashef SA, Roques F, Michel P, et al. European system for cardiac operative risk evaluation (EuroSCORE). *Eur J Cardiothorac Surg* 1999;16:9-13.
20. Kappetein AP, Feldman TE, Mack MJ, et al. Comparison of coronary bypass surgery with drug-eluting stenting for the treatment of left main and/or three-vessel disease: 3-year follow-up of the Syntax trial. *Eur Heart J* 2011;32:2125-2134.
21. Morice MC, Serruys PW, Kappetein AP, et al. Outcomes in patients with de novo left main disease treated with either percutaneous coronary intervention using paclitaxel-eluting stents or coronary artery bypass graft treatment in the Synergy Between Percutaneous Coronary Intervention with TAXUS and Cardiac Surgery (SYNTAX) trial. *Circulation* 2010;121:2645-2653.
22. Migliorini A, Valenti R, Marcucci R, et al. High residual platelet reactivity after clopidogrel loading and long-term clinical outcome after drug-eluting stenting for unprotected left main coronary disease. *Circulation* 2009;120:2214-2221.
23. Capodanno D, Miano M, Cincotta G, et al. EuroSCORE refines the predictive ability of SYNTAX score in patients undergoing left main percutaneous coronary intervention. *Am Heart J* 2010;159:103-109.
24. Chen SL, Chen JP, Mintz G, et al. Comparison between the NERS (New Risk Stratification) score and the SYNTAX (Synergy between Percutaneous Coronary Intervention with Taxus and Cardiac Surgery) score in outcome prediction for unprotected left main stenting. *JACC Cardiovasc Interv* 2010;3(6):632-641.
25. Chieffo A, Morici N, Maisano F, et al. Percutaneous treatment with drug-eluting stent implantation vs. bypass surgery for unprotected left main stenosis: a single-center experience. *Circulation* 2006;113:2542-2547.
26. Palmerini T, Marzocchi A, Marrozzini C, et al. Comparison between coronary angioplasty and coronary artery bypass surgery for the treatment of unprotected left main coronary artery stenosis (the Bologna Registry). *Am J Cardiol* 2006;98:54-59.
27. Palmerini T, Barlocco F, Santarelli A, et al. A comparison between coronary artery bypass grafting surgery and drug eluting stent for the treatment of unprotected left main coronary artery disease in elderly patients (aged > or = 75 years). *Eur Heart J* 2007;28:2714-2719.
28. Buszman PE, Kiesz SR, Bochenek A, et al. Acute and late outcomes of unprotected left main stenting in comparison with surgical revascularization. *J Am Coll Cardiol* 2008;51:538-545.
29. Seung KB, Park DW, Kim YH, et al. Stents vs. coronary-artery bypass grafting for left main coronary artery disease. *N Engl J Med* 2008;358:1781-1792.
30. Park DW, Kim YH, Yun SC, et al. Long-term outcomes after stenting vs. coronary artery bypass grafting for unprotected left main coronary artery disease: 10-year results of bare-metal stents and 5-year results of drug-eluting stents from the ASAN-MAIN (ASAN Medical Center-Left MAIN Revascularization) Registry. *J Am Coll Cardiol* 2010;56(17):1366-1375.
31. Brener SJ, Galla JM, Bryant R 3rd, et al. Comparison of percutaneous vs. surgical revascularization of severe unprotected left main coronary stenosis in matched patients. *Am J Cardiol* 2008;101:169-172.
32. Sanmartin M, Baz JA, Claro R, et al. Comparison of drug-eluting stents vs. surgery for unprotected left main coronary artery disease. *Am J Cardiol* 2007;100:970-973.
33. Hsu JT, Chu CM, Chang ST, et al. Percutaneous coronary intervention vs. coronary artery bypass graft surgery for the treatment of unprotected left main coronary artery stenosis: in-hospital and 1-year outcome after emergent and elective treatments. *Int Heart J* 2008;49:355-370.
34. Makikallio TH, Niemela M, Kervinen K, et al. Coronary angioplasty in drug-eluting stent era for the treatment of unprotected left main stenosis compared to coronary artery bypass grafting. *Ann Med* 2008;40:437-443.
35. Rodes-Cabau J, Deblois J, Bertrand OF, et al. Nonrandomized comparison of coronary artery bypass surgery and percutaneous coronary intervention for the treatment of unprotected left main coronary artery disease in octogenarians. *Circulation* 2008;118:2374-2381.
36. Wu C, Hannan EL, Walford G, Faxon DP. Utilization and outcomes of unprotected left main coronary artery stenting and coronary artery bypass graft surgery. *Ann Thorac Surg* 2008;86:1153-1159.
37. Chieffo A, Magni V, Latib A, et al. 5-year outcomes following percutaneous coronary intervention with drug-eluting stent implantation vs. coronary artery bypass graft for unprotected left main coronary artery lesions: the Milan experience. *JACC Cardiovasc Interv* 2010;3(6):595-601.
38. Park DW, Seung KB, Kim YH, et al. Long-term safety and efficacy of stenting vs. coronary artery bypass grafting for unprotected left main coronary artery disease: 5-year results from the main-compare (revascularization for unprotected left main coronary artery stenosis: comparison of percutaneous coronary angioplasty vs. surgical revascularization) registry. *J Am Coll Cardiol* 2010;56(2):117-124.
39. Park IS, Cho AH, Lee SJ, et al. Life-threatening anaphylactoid reaction in an acute ischemic stroke patient with intravenous rt-PA thrombolysis, followed by successful intra-arterial thrombolysis. *J Clin Neurol* 2008;4:29-32.
40. Cho S, Park TS, Yoon DH, et al. Identification of genetic polymorphisms in FABP3 and FABP4 and putative association with back fat thickness in Korean native cattle. *BMB Rep* 2008;41:29-34.

40a. Teirstein PS, Price MJ. Left main percutaneous coronary intervention. *J Am Coll Cardiol* 2012;60:1605-1613.

40b. Buszman PE, Buszman PP, Kiesz RS, et al. Early and long-term results of unprotected left main coronary artery stenting: the LE MANS (Left Main Coronary Artery Stenting) registry. *J Am Coll Cardiol* 2009;54:1500-1511.

41. Serruys PW, Morice MC, Kappetein AP, et al. Percutaneous coronary intervention vs. coronary-artery bypass grafting for severe coronary artery disease. *N Engl J Med* 2009;360:961-972.

41a. Mohr FW, Morice MC, Kappetein AP, et al. Coronary artery bypass graft surgery versus percutaneous coronary intervention in patients with three-vessel disease and left main coronary disease: 5 year follow-up of the randomized clinical SYNTAX trial. *Lancet* 2013;381:629-638.

42. Park SJ, Kim YH, Park DW, et al. Randomized trial of stents vs. bypass surgery for left main coronary artery disease. *N Engl J Med* 2011;364:1718-1727.
43. Fisher LD, Judkins MP, Lesperance J, et al. Reproducibility of coronary arteriographic reading in the coronary artery surgery study (CASS). *Cathet Cardiovasc Diagn* 1982;8:565-575.
44. Isner JM, Kishel J, Kent KM, et al. Accuracy of angiographic determination of left main coronary arterial narrowing: angiographic-histologic correlative analysis in 28 patients. *Circulation* 1981;63:1056-1064.

45. Park SJ, Kim YH, Park DW, et al. Impact of intravascular ultrasound guidance on long-term mortality in stenting for unprotected left main coronary artery stenosis. *Circ Cardiovasc Interv* 2009;2:167-177.

46. Jasti V, Ivan E, Yalamanchili V, et al. Correlations between fractional flow reserve and intravascular ultrasound in patients with an ambiguous left main coronary artery stenosis. *Circulation* 2004;110:2831-2836.

47. Parodi G, Maehara A, Giuliani G, et al. Optical coherence tomography in unprotected left main coronary artery stenting. *EuroIntervention* 2010;6:94-99.

48. Prosi M, Perktold K, Ding Z, Friedman MH. Influence of curvature dynamics on pulsatile coronary artery flow in a realistic bifurcation model. *J Biomech* 2004;37:1767-1775.

49. Valgimigli M, Malagutti P, Rodriguez-Granillo GA, et al. Distal left main coronary disease is a major predictor of outcome in patients undergoing percutaneous intervention in the drug-eluting stent era: an integrated clinical and angiographic analysis based on the Rapamycin-Eluting Stent Evaluated At Rotterdam Cardiology Hospital (RESEARCH) and Taxus-Stent Evaluated At Rotterdam Cardiology Hospital (T-SEARCH) registries. *J Am Coll Cardiol* 2006;47:1530-1537.

50. Park SJ, Park DW. Percutaneous coronary intervention with stent implantation vs. coronary artery bypass surgery for treatment of left main coronary artery disease: is it time to change guidelines? *Circ Cardiovasc Interv* 2009;2:59-68.

51. Kim YH, Park SW, Hong MK, et al. Comparison of simple and complex stenting techniques in the treatment of unprotected left main coronary artery bifurcation stenosis. *Am J Cardiol* 2006;97:1597-1601.

52. Palmerini T, Marzocchi A, Tamburino C, et al. Impact of bifurcation technique on 2-year clinical outcomes in 773 patients with distal unprotected left main coronary artery stenosis treated with drug-eluting stents. *Circ Cardiovasc Interv* 2008;1:185-192.

53. Agostoni P, Valgimigli M, Van Mieghem CA, et al. Comparison of early outcome of percutaneous coronary intervention for unprotected left main coronary artery disease in the drug-eluting stent era with vs. without intravascular ultrasonic guidance. *Am J Cardiol* 2005;95:644-647.

54. Mehilli J, Kastrati A, Byrne RA, et al. Paclitaxel- vs. sirolimus-eluting stents for unprotected left main coronary artery disease. *J Am Coll Cardiol* 2009;53:1760-1768.

55. Price MJ, Cristea E, Sawhney N, et al. Serial angiographic follow-up of sirolimus-eluting stents for unprotected left main coronary artery revascularization. *J Am Coll Cardiol* 2006;47:871-877.

56. Palmerini T, Marzocchi A, Tamburino C, et al. Two-year clinical outcome with drug-eluting stents vs. bare-metal stents in a real-world registry of unprotected left main coronary artery stenosis from the Italian Society of Invasive Cardiology. *Am J Cardiol* 2008;102:1463-1468.

57. Lee SH, Ko YG, Jang Y, et al. Sirolimus- vs. paclitaxel-eluting stent implantation for unprotected left main coronary artery stenosis. *Cardiology* 2005;104:181-185.

58. Carrie D, Lhermusier T, Hmem M, et al. Clinical and angiographic outcome of paclitaxel-eluting stent implantation for unprotected left main coronary artery bifurcation narrowing. *EuroIntervention* 2006;1:396-402.

59. Christiansen EH, Lassen JF, Andersen HR, et al. Outcome of unprotected left main percutaneous coronary intervention in surgical low-risk, surgical high-risk, and acute myocardial infarction patients. *EuroIntervention* 2006;1:403-408.

60. Migliorini A, Moschi G, Giurlani L, et al. Drug-eluting stent supported percutaneous coronary intervention for unprotected left main disease. *Catheter Cardiovasc Interv* 2006;68:225-230.

61. Sheiban I, Meliga E, Moretti C, et al. Sirolimus-eluting stents vs bare metal stents for the treatment of unprotected left main coronary artery stenosis. *EuroIntervention* 2006;2:356-362.

62. Gao RL, Xu B, Chen JL, et al. Immediate and long-term outcomes of drug-eluting stent implantation for unprotected left main coronary artery disease: comparison with bare-metal stent implantation. *Am Heart J* 2008;155:553-561.

63. Carrie D, Eltchaninoff H, Lefevre T, et al. Twelve-month clinical and angiographic outcome after stenting of unprotected left main coronary artery stenosis with paclitaxel-eluting stents—results of the Multicentre Friend Registry. *EuroIntervention* 2009;4:449-456.

64. Vaquerizo B, Lefevre T, Darremont O, et al. Unprotected left main stenting in the real world: two-year outcomes of the French Left Main Taxus Registry. *Circulation* 2009;119:2349-2356.

65. Salvatella N, Morice MC, Darremont O, et al. Unprotected left main stenting with a second-generation drug-eluting stent: one-year outcomes of the LEMAX Pilot study. *EuroIntervention* 2011;7:689-696.

66. Briguori C, Airoldi F, Chieffo A, et al. Elective vs. provisional intraaortic balloon pumping in unprotected left main stenting. *Am Heart J* 2006;152:565-572.

67. Dixon SR, Henriques JP, Mauri L, et al. A prospective feasibility trial investigating the use of the Impella 2.5 system in patients undergoing high-risk percutaneous coronary intervention (the PROTECT I Trial): initial U.S. experience. *JACC Cardiovasc Interv* 2009;2:91-96.

68. Kushner FG, Hand M, Smith Jr SC, et al. 2009 focused updates: ACC/AHA guidelines for the management of patients with ST-elevation myocardial infarction (updating the 2004 guideline and 2007 focused update) and ACC/AHA/SCAI guidelines on percutaneous coronary intervention (updating the 2005 guideline and 2007 focused update): a report of the American College of Cardiology Foundation/American Heart Association Task Force on Practice Guidelines. *J Am Coll Cardiol* 2009;54:2205-2241.

69. Van Mieghem CA, Cademartiri F, Mollet NR, et al. Multislice spiral computed tomography for the evaluation of stent patency after left main coronary artery stenting: a comparison with conventional coronary angiography and intravascular ultrasound. *Circulation* 2006;114:645-653.

CHAPTER 15

Stenting Approaches to the Bifurcation Lesion

ANDREJS ĒRGLIS | MATTHEW J. PRICE

KEY POINTS

- Percutaneous coronary intervention (PCI) and stent implantation in bifurcation lesions are a particular challenge because they are associated with lower procedural success, increased complication rates, and worse late clinical outcomes compared with nonbifurcation lesion interventions.

- Low endothelial shear stress promotes atherosclerotic plaque formation, and the anatomic distribution of atherosclerosis at the coronary bifurcation is consistent with the spatial variation in shear stress at that site—low stress along the lateral walls of the main vessel and side branches and high stress along the carina.

- The Medina classification is a simple and validated method of systematically describing bifurcation lesions. The presence or absence of a greater than 50% stenosis is denoted by the numeral 1 or 0, respectively, in each of the three arterial segments in the following order: proximal main vessel, distal main vessel, and proximal side branch.

- A two-stent approach to bifurcation lesion PCI does not provide benefit compared with a simple treatment strategy (stenting of the main vessel with provisional stenting of the side branch).

- A simple, provisional stenting approach is associated with less fluoroscopy time, lower incidence of periprocedural myocardial infarction, and similar rates of target vessel revascularization compared with a routine two-stent strategy.

- Stenting of the main vessel and provisional stenting of the side branch should be the preferred approach in bifurcation lesions involving a side branch of intermediate size, with stent deployment in the side branch only in the setting of suboptimal angiographic results, such as flow-limiting dissection, significant residual stenosis, or reduced thrombolysis in myocardial infarction (TIMI) flow.

- A planned two-stent approach might be more appropriate when both the parent vessel and side branch are large, particularly when there is significant disease distal to the ostium of a side branch that arises from the main vessel at a shallow angle.

Introduction and Historical Perspective

Approximately 15% to 20% of all coronary interventions are performed to treat coronary bifurcations.[1,2] Long before the nomenclature of lesion complexity matured, side branch (SB) involvement was recognized as an unfavorable determinant of angioplasty success. Meier and associates[3] were among the first to define the risks of side branch occlusion associated with parent vessel angioplasty, emphasizing the importance of plaque extension into the SB as a predictor of postpercutaneous coronary intervention (PCI) occlusion. Optimal treatment of bifurcation lesions is still a major challenge for coronary intervention and has a lower procedural success, increased complication rates, and worse late clinical outcomes compared with nonbifurcation lesion interventions. Several important factors, such as anatomic variation, angulation between branches, downstream territory, and extent of plaque burden, should be taken into consideration when addressing the bifurcation lesion to choose the most appropriate approach and achieve an optimal result.

Plaque and endothelial characteristics of ostial lesions appear to lead to increased recoil and increased risk of dissection, with compromise of SBs and/or the main vessel; further complexity arises from dynamic changes in anatomy during intervention in either branch of the bifurcation lesion, which in turn risks SB occlusion because of plaque redistribution—so-called plaque shift—across the carina of the bifurcation. The kissing balloon technique was developed to lower the risk of such a plaque shift.[4] However, the results after balloon dilation of bifurcation lesions were frequently suboptimal, with a high incidence of complications and restenosis.[4,5] Treatment of bifurcations with directional atherectomy was shown to improve the immediate procedural outcome compared with balloon dilation alone, but the incidence of restenosis remained high.[6] Debulking with directional atherectomy or rotational atherectomy and adjunctive balloon angioplasty not only improved acute angiographic results but also decreased target vessel revascularization compared with balloon angioplasty alone.[7]

The use of coronary stents has improved the treatment of bifurcation lesions; however, the incidence of side branch compromise persisted.[8-10] Bare metal stent (BMS) implantation was associated with a major adverse cardiac event (MACE) rate of 30% at 1 year.[11] The introduction of drug-eluting stents (DES) has been promising and resulted in a reduction in MACE and target lesion revascularization (TLR) rates for bifurcation lesions compared with historical BMS controls.[2,12] Several two-stent techniques were developed, and many of them are currently used in selected cases. Nevertheless because of bifurcation lesion complexity, adverse event rates are relatively high and SB ostial restenosis remains an area in which further improvement is needed. Optimal treatment of bifurcation lesions is therefore still a major challenge for coronary intervention and has a lower procedural success, increased complication rates, and worse late clinical outcomes compared with nonbifurcation lesion interventions. Given their heterogeneity, a variety of different strategies and stenting techniques have been proposed to treat bifurcation stenoses, but an optimal strategy for every anatomic subset has not yet been established.[13] Because of these concerns, such lesions are often treated less aggressively, leading to greater residual stenosis and therefore greater restenosis.[14]

Atherosclerosis in Coronary Bifurcations

DISTRIBUTION

Coronary flow is complex because of pulsatile conditions, curvature of the artery, contraction and relaxation of the myocardium, and extensive branching that leads to large variations in wall shear stress levels. Since systemic factors are for the most part identical along the arterial bed, the differential distribution of atherosclerosis has been attributed to the local effect of flow-related hemodynamic forces and endothelial shear stress; that is, flow disturbances influence the localization and progression of atheroma.[15-17]

Autopsy and intravascular ultrasound studies have demonstrated that atherosclerosis within coronary bifurcations most frequently occurs in the lateral walls of both the main vessel and SBs, with a substantially lower incidence and reduced extent of atherosclerosis in the region of the carina.[18-24] Histopathology has shown that the degree of intimal thickening and necrotic core formation in the carina is considerably less than that of the lateral walls.[25] A study using multislice computed tomography documented plaque in the carina region in only 31% of cases and, in those cases in which the carina was affected, plaque was invariably in other areas of the bifurcation.[26]

Endothelial Shear Stress

Endothelial shear stress is the tangential force exerted on the endothelial surface that results from the friction of the flowing blood. It is calculated as the product of the blood viscosity (μ) and the radial gradient of axial blood velocity (dv/dy) at the endothelial surface (i.e., $\mu \times$ dv/dy) and is expressed in units of force per area, N/m^2 or pascal, or dyne/cm^2 (1 N/m^2 = 1 pascal = 10 dyne/cm^2).[27]

Endothelial shear stress = Blood viscosity (μ) $\times$ Radial gradient of axial blood velocity (dv/dy) at the endothelial surface

Blood Flow Patterns

The pulsatile nature of the arterial blood flow in combination with the complex geometric configuration of the coronary arteries determine the pattern of endothelial shear stress, which is characterized by direction and magnitude.[15,28,29] In relatively straight arterial segments, endothelial shear stress is pulsatile and unidirectional, with a magnitude that varies within a range of 15 to 70 dyne/cm^2 over the cardiac cycle and yields a positive time average (Figure 15-1). In contrast, in geometrically irregular regions in which laminar flow is disturbed, pulsatile flow generates low and/or oscillatory endothelial shear stress.[30-32] Low endothelial shear stress typically occurs at the inner areas of curvatures as well as upstream of stenoses.[33] Oscillatory endothelial shear stress is characterized by significant changes in direction (is bidirectional) and in magnitude between systole and diastole, resulting in a very low time average that is usually close to zero (see Figure 15-1).[30-32] Oscillatory endothelial shear stress occurs primarily downstream of stenoses, at the lateral walls of bifurcations, and in the vicinity of branch points.[15,17,32,33] In addition to these temporal oscillations, significant spatial oscillations in endothelial shear stress can occur over short distances, especially in geometrically irregular regions, resulting in high spatial gradients, which are also involved in the development and progression atherosclerosis.[17,34-36]

An arterial bifurcation or branching point imposes an anatomic substrate for the development of disturbed flow. This is because a proportion of blood flow is subject to an abrupt change in direction, from purely axial to the direction of the branches. As a result, flow separation occurs and secondary flow patterns develop, often manifesting as vortices. These events lead to low and oscillatory endothelial shear stress, as well as low-pressure gradients along the lateral walls of the main vessel and SB (Figure 15-2; also see Figure 15-1).[25,37-40] In contradistinction, high endothelial shear stress develops in the carina region.[26] This spatial variation in shear stress is generally consistent with the anatomic distribution of atherosclerosis in coronary bifurcations.

Endothelial Shear Stress and Arterial Plaque Formation

In arterial regions with disturbed flow, low endothelial shear stress reduces the bioavailability of nitric oxide by decreasing eNOS messenger ribonucleic acid and protein expression, thereby exposing the endothelium to the atherogenic effect of local and systemic risk factors (Figure 15-3).[41-44] In addition, low shear stress downregulates prostacyclin, an endothelial vasodilator,[18,30] while upregulating endothelin-1,[30,43,44] thus precipitating atherosclerosis. Low endothelial shear stress furthermore promotes permeability and the uptake of

Figure 15-1 Pulsatile, low, and oscillatory endothelial shear stress *(ESS)*. (Adapted from Chatzizisis YS, Coskun AU, Jonas M, et al. Role of endothelial shear stress in the natural history of coronary atherosclerosis and vascular remodeling: molecular, cellular, and vascular behavior. *J Am Coll Cardiol* 2007; 49:2379-2393.)

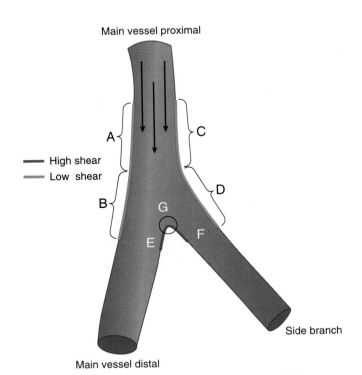

Figure 15-2 Distribution of endothelial shear stress within coronary artery bifurcations. *A,* Proximal main vessel on the lateral wall. *B,* Distal main vessel on the lateral wall. *C,* Proximal main vessel on the branch side. *D,* Distal side branch on the lateral wall. *E,* Distal main vessel on the flow divider side. *F,* Distal side branch on the flow divider side. *G,* Carina. (Adapted from Nakazawa G, Yazdani SK, Finn AV, et al. Pathologic findings at bifurcation lesions: the impact of flow distribution on atherosclerosis and arterial healing after stent implantation. *J Am Coll Cardiol* 2010;55:1679-1687.)

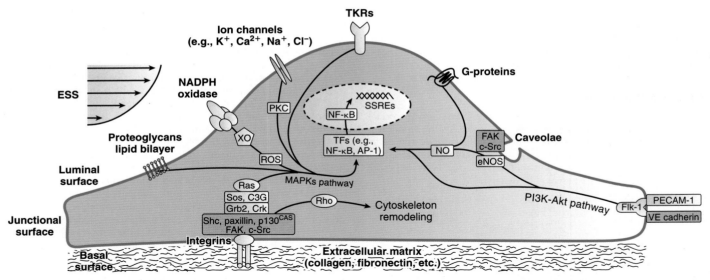

Figure 15-3 **Role of endothelial shear stress in atherosclerosis development.** In arterial regions with disturbed laminar flow, low endothelial shear stress shifts the endothelial function and structure toward a phenotype that promotes atherogenesis, atherosclerotic plaque formation and progression, and vascular remodeling. Local endothelial shear stress *(ESS)* is sensed by luminal endothelial mechanoreceptors, such as ion channels (K+, Ca2+, Na+, Cl−), G-proteins, caveolae, tyrosine kinase receptors *(TKRs)*, nicotinamide adenine dinucleotide phosphate *(NADPH)* oxidase and xanthine oxidase *(XO)*, plasma membrane lipid bilayer, and heparan sulfate proteoglycans. Also, ESS signals are transmitted through the cytoskeleton to the basal or junctional endothelial surface, where certain integrins or a mechanosensory complex consisting of platelet endothelial cell adhesion molecule-1 *(PECAM-1)* and Flk-1 are activated, respectively, and initiate a downstream signaling cascade. Activated integrins phosphorylate and activate a multiple complex of nonreceptor tyrosine kinases (FAK, c-Src, Shc, paxillin, and p130CAS), adaptor proteins (Grb2, Crk), and guanine nucleotide exchange factors (Sos, C3G), thereby activating Ras family GTPase. Active Ras plays a pivotal role in the intracellular transduction of ESS signals as it triggers various parallel downstream cascades of serine kinases; each of these kinases phosphorylates and hence activates the next one downstream, ultimately activating mitogen-activated protein kinases *(MAPKs)*. Besides integrin-mediated mechanotransduction, ESS activates a number of other downstream signaling pathways initiated by luminal or junctional mechanoreceptors. These pathways include the production of reactive oxygen species *(ROS)* from NADPH oxidase and XO, activation of protein kinase C *(PKC)*, activation of Rho family small GTPases (which mediate the remodeling cytoskeleton, resulting in temporary or permanent structural changes of ECs), release of endothelial nitric oxide *(NO)* synthase *(eNOS)* and other signaling molecules from caveolae, and activation of the phosphoinositide-3 kinase *(PI3K)*–Akt cascade. Ultimately, all of these signaling pathways lead to phosphorylation of several transcription factors *(TFs)*, such as nuclear factor-kappa β *(NF-κB)* and activator protein-1 *(AP-1)*. These TF proteins bind positive or negative shear stress–responsive elements *(SSREs)* at promoters of mechanosensitive genes, inducing or suppressing their expression, thereby modulating cellular function and morphology. *VE cadherin,* Vascular endothelial–cadherin. (Adapted from Chatzizisis YS, Coskun AU, Jonas M, et al. Role of endothelial shear stress in the natural history of coronary atherosclerosis and vascular remodeling: molecular, cellular, and vascular behavior. *J Am Coll Cardiol* 2007;49:2379-2393.)

low-density lipoprotein cholesterol, enhancing oxidative stress, which further promotes inflammation. Low endothelial shear stress also promotes vascular smooth muscle cell migration, differentiation, and proliferation and extracellular matrix degradation in the vascular wall and plaque fibrous cap.[40]

Serial intravascular ultrasound and immunohistochemical analyses in a diabetic atherosclerotic pig model have demonstrated that low endothelial shear stress is an independent predictor of plaque location and development and the progression of high-risk features, such as intensive lipid accumulation, inflammation, thin fibrous cap, internal elastic lamina fragmentation, medial thinning, and excessive expansive remodeling.[40] Furthermore, the magnitude of low shear stress at baseline was significantly associated with the severity of high-risk plaque characteristics at follow-up. In areas of low endothelial shear stress in which high-risk plaque developed, excessive expansive remodeling also occurred and was associated with the persistence of a low endothelial shear stress environment, despite continued plaque growth, thereby fostering a vicious cycle of low shear stress, excessive expansive remodeling, and high-risk plaque characteristics.[40] The proximal wall opposite to the carina represents the area with the lowest shear stress and a higher risk of developing vulnerable plaque and rupture. Importantly, this area represents the landing zone of multiple layers of stent struts in cases of two-stent techniques, in which incomplete stent apposition, nonuniform strut deployment, and disturbances in drug distribution may occur. This may in part explain the worse outcomes of bifurcational lesion stenting irrespective of technique used.[45]

Vascular Profiling

The most comprehensive technique for investigating the relationship between endothelial shear stress and vascular pathobiology is a methodology termed *vascular profiling,* which uses intravascular ultrasound and coronary angiography to create an accurate three-dimensional representation of the coronary artery that forms the basis of identifying local shear stress and vascular remodeling behavior.[31,46] Vascular profiling is accurate and highly reproducible and can be used to track changes in lumen, wall thickness, and endothelial shear stress over periods as short as 6 to 9 months in animals and humans.[40,46-51] Future technologies may be able to assess local endothelial shear stress and remodeling behavior noninvasively with multislice computed tomography, magnetic resonance imaging, or other imaging modalities.[52]

🔲 Bifurcation Lesion Definition, Geometry, and Classification

DEFINITION

In general, the term *coronary artery bifurcation* is used for the following: (1) when a coronary artery divides into two equally important branches or (2) when the main branch has an SB, which is large enough to be of hemodynamic significance.[53] The European Bifurcation Club defines a bifurcation lesion as a coronary artery narrowing occurring adjacent to and/or involving the origin of a significant SB, for which acute closure or loss would be substantially detrimental within the global context of a particular patient (e.g., symptoms, location of ischemia, viability, collateralization, vessel, left ventricular function).[54]

BIFURCATION GEOMETRY AND REFERENCE VESSEL SIZE PREDICTION

Coronary bifurcations are transitional junctions that allow the divergence of the system that nourishes the myocardium. The coronary tree consists of a self-similar pattern of branching, based on energetic efficiency (the principle of minimum work for blood transport). Interventional management of bifurcations should aim to restore optimal flow and minimize further hemodynamic disturbances by obeying the rules of geometry and hence function.[55]

There are many theories of vascular tree design based on the concept of minimum work.[56,57] Murray[56] has proposed a cost function that is the sum of friction power loss and metabolic power dissipation proportional to blood volume. The consequence of this minimum energy hypothesis is Murray's law, also known as the *cube law*, which states that the sum of the cubes of the daughter-vessel diameters is equal to the cube of the mother-vessel diameter as $D^3 = Dd1^3 + Dd2^3$, where D is the diameter of the mother vessel and $Dd1$ and $Dd2$ are the diameters of the daughter vessels. Zhou, Kassab, and others[57-59] have shown that Murray's law does not hold in the entire tree because Murray's analysis considered each bifurcation in isolation rather than as an integrated whole; they proposed the HK model, $D^{7/3} = Dd1^{7/3} + Dd2^{7/3}$, which has been rigorously validated.[57-60] Finet and colleagues[61] have observed a linear relation ($D = 0.678 \times [Dd1+Dd2]$) based on regression analysis of Y-type bifurcation. The HK model gives rise to a ratio of 0.673 for the case of the Y-type bifurcation, in which the daughter vessels are of equal diameter. Hence, the HK model is not only consistent with the Finet rule for Y bifurcations but also holds for T bifurcations, which were not considered by Finet and associates.[61]

This systematic differential between mother and daughter vessel diameters may lead to challenges in stent diameter selection and result in acute proximal stent malapposition that should be taken into account in the interventional management of bifurcations.[61] A stent that is sized to the diameter of the major daughter vessel will systematically show proximal malapposition in the mother vessel.[62] The degree of this malapposition (ΔD) can easily be calculated in advance of implantation:

$$\Delta D = D_{\text{mother vessel}} - D_{\text{major daughter vessel}}$$

Post-dilation of the proximal segment by a balloon having the diameter of the mother vessel is a well-accepted practice for fixing this phenomenon. A final kissing balloon inflation can also mechanically correct the malapposition at the cost of asymmetric deformation of the mother vessel induced by the proximal juxtaposition of the two balloons.

In summary, the prediction rules for bifurcation vessel sizing are as follows:

Murray's Law:

$$D^3 = Dd1^3 + Dd2^3$$

HK model:

$$D^{7/3} = Dd1^{7/3} + Dd2^{7/3}$$

Finet rule (for Y-type bifurcations):

$$D = 0.678 \times (Dd1 + Dd2)$$

where D is the diameter of the mother vessel and $Dd1$ and $Dd2$ are the diameters of the daughter vessels.

LESION CLASSIFICATION

Bifurcations vary in the degree of plaque burden, plaque location, angle between branches, diameter of the branches, and bifurcation site. No two bifurcations are identical, and no single interventional strategy can be applied to every bifurcation. Bifurcation lesion classification schemes involve several anatomic characteristics that vary according to the position of the lesion(s) in one or more of the three segments of the bifurcation: proximal main vessel, distal main vessel, or SB. The angle between the main branch and SB is prognostically important. With Y angulation (i.e., <70 degrees), SB access is usually straightforward, but plaque shifting is more pronounced and precise stent placement at the SB ostium is difficult, whereas with T angulation (i.e., >70 degrees), SB access is usually more difficult, but plaque shifting is often minimal and precise stent placement in the ostium is straightforward. Thus, the critical issue in bifurcation PCI is the selection of the most appropriate strategy for an individual bifurcation. There are six major bifurcation lesion classifications published in the literature that are currently used (Figure 15-4). Older bifurcation classification schemes, such as the Lefevre classification (Figure 15-5), require significant memorization.[63]

Medina Classification

The Medina classification (see Figure 15-4) is a simplified and universal classification of bifurcation lesions validated by the European Bifurcation Club, is straightforward, and does not require memorization.[64] It consists of recording any narrowing in excess of 50% in each of the three arterial segments of the bifurcation in the following order: proximal main vessel, distal branch, and SB; 1 is used to indicate the presence of a significant stenosis, and 0 represents the absence of stenosis. Commas separate the three numerals. Simple bifurcations are those that have SB origins without significant stenoses ([1,1,0], [1,0,0], and [0,1,0]). Their treatment is straightforward because it is often sufficient simply to implant a stent in the main vessel as long as it covers the SB origin. Intervention on the SB should be performed only if its ostium is compromised. Treatment with two stents could be effective in complex bifurcations, in which the proximal [1,0,1], distal [0,1,1], or both [1,1,1] components of the main vessel and the SB origin are involved. The results of some studies have suggested that the Medina classification could be reduced to two lesion types, either [1,1,1] or non–[1,1,1].[65,66] Given limitations associated with angiographic assessment, a Medina IVUS index has been proposed, based on the localization of plaque rather than those of significant lesions, although IVUS findings may not automatically influence treatment outcome. A Medina FFR index has also been considered.

Movahed Classification

Movahed[67-69] has proposed a clinically relevant, simple, and complete classification system that allows a relationship to be built intuitively among several characteristics of a lesion and a potential treatment strategy (Figure 15-6). It is based on a system composed of a single prefix to which up to four different suffixes can be added. The description begins with the prefix B (for bifurcation lesion). Each suffix describes a technically important feature of a bifurcation lesion in the context of technical decision making. This classification is complete and includes two other important technical features of bifurcation lesions not described in any other major classifications, the proximal healthy segment and angle of bifurcation branches.[67,70] However, this classification is difficult to memorize and its use has not been supported by any randomized study.

Classification of the Left Main Bifurcation

Intervention on distal left main bifurcation lesions is more complex because of its potential impact on important clinical outcomes, such as mortality. Compared with non–left main bifurcation lesions, the left main commonly displays a relatively larger bifurcation angle. The loss of an SB, the left anterior descending (LAD) or left circumflex (LCX) artery, could result in fatal complications. Compared with bifurcation lesions in other sites, high residual stenosis at the ostium of the LAD or LCX artery results in higher incidences of TLR or MACE. A novel classification that differentiates distal left main bifurcation lesions has been proposed (Figure 15-7).

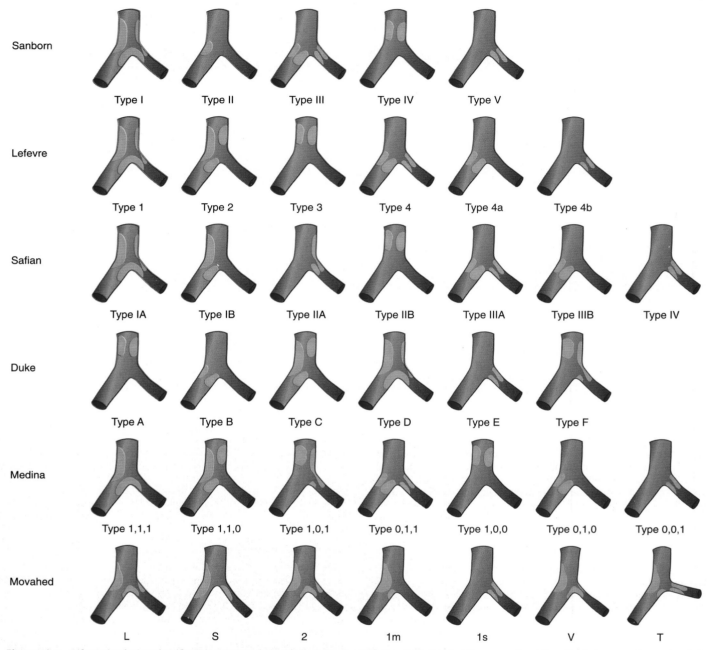

Figure 15-4 **Bifurcation lesion classification systems.** (Adapted from Movahed MR, Kern K, Thai H, et al. Coronary artery bifurcation lesions: a review and update on classification and interventional techniques. *Cardiovasc Revasc Med* 2008;9:263-268.)

Bifurcation Stenting Techniques

TECHNIQUE CLASSIFICATION

Many techniques have been described and used successfully in the treatment of bifurcation lesions. Classification of treatments has been complicated and has caused confusion in the past.[71] The European Bifurcation Club has suggested a MADS (*m*ain, *a*cross, *d*istal, *s*ide) classification, taking into account initial stent deployment, which often corresponds to a technical strategy related to the importance of the vessel that is treated first.[54] MADS is a family classification system that facilitates the description of techniques by listing only the variants of each individual technique, allowing comparisons between techniques in various anatomic and clinical settings (Figure 15-8).

The first family of techniques (M) starts by stent implantation in the proximal main vessel relatively close to the carina. This initial step may be followed by the opening of the stent toward both branches, with subsequent successive or simultaneous stent placement in one or both distal branches. The second family (A) starts with the stenting of the proximal main vessel to the distal main branch across the SB. This may be the first and last step of the procedure but may also be followed by the opening of the stent struts, delivery of a second stent in the SB, and with or without kissing balloon inflation. The third family (D) involves the distal branches and historically starts with simultaneous stent placement at the ostium of both distal branches (V stenting). A recent variant consists of creating a new carina by stent implantation in the proximal segments (i.e., simultaneous kissing stent [SKS]). The fourth family (S) involves strategies in which the SB is stented first, either at the ostium level or with relatively pronounced protrusion into the proximal main vessel. The SB stent may be crushed with a balloon inflated in the main vessel, or a second stent may be deployed in the main vessel across the SB.[54]

The MADS classification does not exhaustively describe all technical aspects of interventional techniques, which include the use of wires, lesion preparation, single balloon inflation, kissing balloon inflations, or using one or two stents. Therefore, Movahed and Stinis[67] have suggested classifying the most common bifurcation techniques with regard to stenting into six categories: one-stent technique (OST), stent with balloon technique (SBT), kissing stent technique (KST), T stent technique (TST), crush stent technique (CRT), and culotte stent technique (CUT) (Figure 15-9).

INITIAL STRATEGY AND DECISION MAKING

The most important issue in bifurcation intervention is selecting the most appropriate strategy for an individual bifurcation and optimizing the performance of this technique.[37] An appropriate and timely decision affects the results, saves time, lowers costs, and lowers the risk of complications. Latib and Colombo[72] have suggested that there are three questions an operator needs to answer to decide the appropriate primary strategy (Figure 15-10). An individualized strategy for treating true bifurcation lesions is mostly dictated by the SB. These questions determine the likelihood of success with a provisional approach

and determine whether the operator is willing to accept a suboptimal result in the SB with balloon angioplasty only. If the answers to all these questions are in the affirmative, the bifurcation may still be treated with one stent, but the operator should strongly consider a two-stent approach as intention to treat.[72] The provisional approach of implanting one stent in the main branch is now considered to be the default approach for most bifurcations lesions. This approach is used mainly because the routine implantation of two stents does not give superior results compared with selective usage.[73] Thus, the approach to bifurcation PCI can be divided into three strategies set forth as follows: (1) main branch stenting only; (2) provisional SB stenting; and (3) a two-stent strategy.

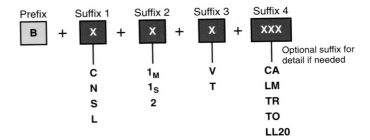

Suffix 1: C = Close to bifurcation
N = Nonsignificant sidebranch
S = Small proximal segment
L = Large proximal segment

Suffix 2: 1_M = Only main branch ostium diseased
1_S = Only sidebranch ostium diseased
2 = Both main and sidebranch ostia diseased

Suffix 3: V = Angle between branch vessels less than 70 degrees
T = Angle between branch vessels more than 70 degrees

Suffix 4: CA = Calcified
LM = Left main involved in bifurcation
TR = Thrombus-containing lesion
TO = Total occlusion
LL20 = Lesion length of the main branch less than 20

Figure 15-6 **Detailed description of the Movahed coronary bifurcation classification.** (Adapted from Movahed MR, Kern K, Thai H, et al. Coronary artery bifurcation lesions: a review and update on classification and interventional techniques. *Cardiovasc Revasc Med* 2008;9:263-268.)

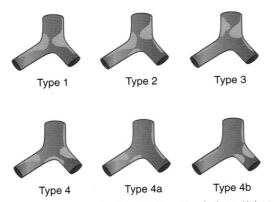

Figure 15-5 **Lefevre classification of bifurcation lesions.** (Adapted from Lefevre T, Louvard Y, Morice MC, et al. Stenting of bifurcation lesions: classification, treatments, and results. *Catheter Cardiovasc Interv* 2000;49:274-283.)

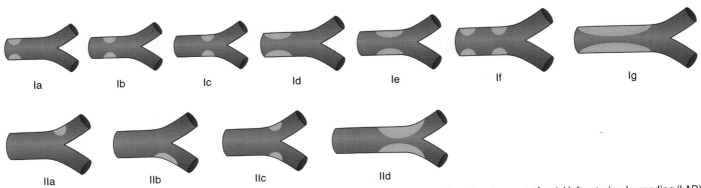

Figure 15-7 **Classification scheme for left main disease.** Type I, Lesion in entire left main stem without involvement of ostial left anterior descending (LAD) artery or circumflex. Type Ia, Ostial left main stenosis. Type Ib, Stenosis in left main shaft. Type Ic, Distal nonbifurcated stenosis. Type Id, Proximal stenosis in both first and second areas (type Ia + type Ib). Type Ie, Distal stenosis in both second and third areas (type Ib + type Ic). Type If, Ostial and distal nonbifurcated stenosis (type Ia + type Ic). Type Ig, Lesion in entire main stem without involvement of ostial LAD artery or circumflex. Type II, Distal bifurcated stenosis involving both ostium of LAD artery and circumflex artery. Type IIa, Ostial LAD stenosis. Type IIb, Continuous stenosis from ostial LAD artery or circumflex to third area of left main. Type IIc, Both ostial left anterior and circumflex stenosis without stenosis in third area of left main. (Adapted from Chen SL, Louvard Y, Runlin G. Perspective on bifurcation PCI. *J Interv Cardiol* 2009;22:99-109.)

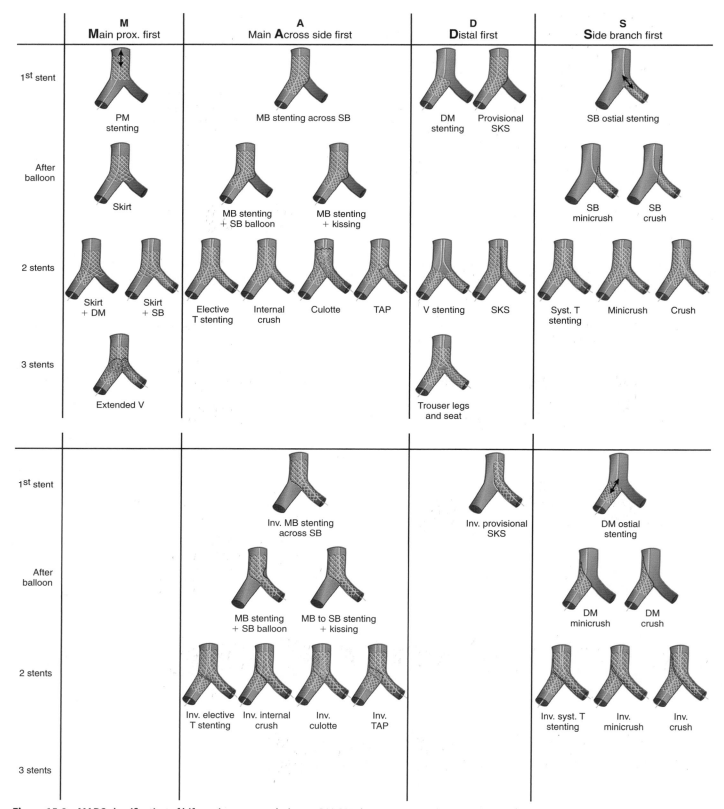

Figure 15-8   **MADS classification of bifurcation stent techniques.** *DM,* Distal main; *MB,* main branch; *Inv,* inverted; *PM,* proximal main; *SB,* side branch; *SKS,* simultaneous kissing stents; *TAP,* T stenting and protrusion. (Adapted from Louvard Y, Thomas M, Dzavik V, et al. Classification of coronary artery bifurcation lesions and treatments: time for a consensus! *Catheter Cardiovasc Interv* 2008;71:175-183.)

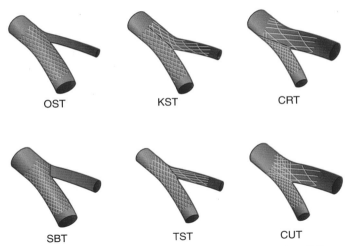

Figure 15-9 Mohaved and Stinis classifications of interventional bifurcation techniques. *CRT,* Crush stent technique; *CUT,* culotte stent technique; *KST,* kissing stent technique; *OST,* one-stent technique; *SBT,* stent with balloon technique; *TST,* T stent technique.

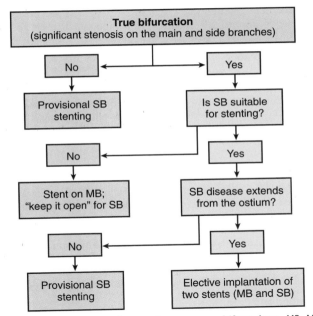

Figure 15-10 Algorithm for treating coronary bifurcations. *MB,* Main branch; *SB,* side branch. (Adapted from Latib A, Colombo A. Bifurcation disease: what do we know, what should we do? *JACC Cardiovasc Interv* 2008;1: 218-226.)

Main Branch Stenting Only

This strategy is used when the SB has ostial or diffuse disease and is not suitable (too small) for stenting or is clinically irrelevant.[72] Two guidewires should be placed in most bifurcations, and the SB guidewire should be jailed in most of them after deployment of the stent in the main branch. This approach of "just keep it open" for the SB was the strategy used in the provisional stenting group of the Nordic study. It is important in protecting the SB from closure because of plaque shift and/or obstructing stent struts after main branch stenting. The guidewire jailed in the SB by the main branch stent facilitates rewiring of the SB if SB post-dilation, stenting, or final kissing balloon inflation is needed or if the SB occludes. The jailed guidewire also acts as a marker for the SB ostium and changes the angle of the SB take off to ease re-access. In the French multicenter TULIPE study,

the absence of this jailed wire was associated with a greater rate of reinterventions during follow-up.[74] There is usually no need to remove this guidewire during high-pressure stent dilation in the main branch; however, it is preferable to avoid jailing hydrophilic guidewires because there is a risk of stripping the polymer coating on wire removal.[75] Careful handling of the guiding catheter to prevent deep migration into the ostium of the coronary vessel is important to allow for the safe removal of the jailed guidewire.

Provisional Side Branch Stenting

This strategy is quick, safe, and easy to perform and is associated with results comparable to a more complex approach if the SB is suitable for stenting and has minimal disease or disease at the ostium only.[72] Wiring of both branches should be done routinely. The main advantages are that wire protection may help prevent SB occlusion and has been shown to be a predictor of PCI success in the SB.[74]

The branch with the most unfavorable anatomy (typically the SB) should be wired first. Predilation of the main and SBs should be performed if necessary, preferably with atherotomy by cutting balloon or noncompliant balloon.[75] SBs without significant disease usually do not require predilation; in most cases, predilation of the SB should be avoided because it does not seem to prevent the risk of SB occlusion during main branch stenting. After stenting of the main branch, the SB wire should be left in place. Current opinion favors DES placement in the main branch. If the angiographic results in the main branches and SBs are satisfactory, the procedure is complete and the SB wire that is jailed behind the main branch stent struts can be removed gently. In situations with a suboptimal result, the SB is rewired before the removal of the confined wire. If recrossing into the SB through the main branch stent struts is difficult, a hydrophilic wire is an excellent option. The jailed wire in the SB should always be left in place as a marker until recrossing has been completed.

The next step is SB balloon dilation and final kissing inflation, if necessary. A final kissing inflation is mandatory if the SB is dilated through the main branch stent struts to correct main branch stent distortion and optimize expansion.[74,76] There is uncertainty as to whether final kissing inflation is mandatory when a provisional approach is used. Benchtop studies have demonstrated that final kissing inflation has the advantage of opening stent struts that can scaffold the SB ostium and thus deliver drug appropriately and facilitate future SB access. There is also concern that stenting across a bifurcation without opening the stent struts into the SB results in malapposed struts across the SB ostium that will not endothelialize. The use of final kissing inflation should be performed only in bifurcations in which the SB is suitable for stenting in case dissection occurs.[72]

Assessment of the procedural outcome after final kissing inflation is the key moment of the provisional SB stenting strategy. If the result remains unsatisfactory (e.g., suboptimal result, plaque shift with >75% residual stenosis or thrombolysis in myocardial infarction [TIMI] flow grade < 3 in an SB ≥ 2.5 mm) or SB balloon dilation is complicated by a flow-limiting dissection, then SB stenting should be performed. A second stent in the SB may be required in 20% to 30% of cases. Even with a 50% to 70% residual angiographic SB obstruction (but without dissection), the stenting procedure could be considered complete. If the SB result is suboptimal, stenting can be performed in a reverse T approach, advancing the stent through the main branch stent struts and with final kissing balloon inflation.[37]

Two-Stent Strategy

Correct patient selection for elective two-stent techniques requires accurate assessment of lesion severity, distribution, extension, and presence of concomitant disease.[77] The decision to perform double stenting depends predominantly on SB characteristics and as intention to treat should generally be reserved for true bifurcations with SBs that are relatively large in diameter (>2.5 mm), that subtend a substantial amount of myocardium, have severe disease that extends well beyond the ostium (i.e., >10 mm or more), and/or have an unfavorable angle for recrossing after main branch stent implantation.

These variables should not be considered in isolation, but usually a combination of these factors dictates the decision to perform double stenting electively. The decision to implant a second stent may also be made at an intermediate time, such as after wire insertion that may favorably modify the bifurcation angle or after predilation of the main branches and/or SBs.[78] A variety of two-stent techniques can be performed based on the operator's choice and skills. A detailed description of those techniques is provided later in this chapter. After the two-stent implantation, final kissing balloon inflation should be performed using moderate pressure.[75]

PROCEDURAL CONSIDERATIONS

Arterial Access and Guiding Catheter

The guide catheter selection for coronary bifurcation intervention should be based on the same general criteria as for nonbifurcation PCI. The catheter shape should provide good support at the ostium using coaxial catheterization or active support by deep-seated intubation. Nevertheless, guide catheter diameter is primarily determined by chosen treatment technique, because many techniques frequently require the simultaneous insertion of two balloons or two stents. It is possible to insert simultaneously two low-profile balloon catheters inside a 6-Fr guide with an internal lumen diameter of more than 0.070 inch (1.75 mm). A 6-Fr guide can be used if provisional stenting requires implantation of a second stent in the SB, whereas if implantation of two stents is needed, the stent delivery systems can be inserted only one after the other. Techniques such as T stenting, reverse crush, and step crush (see later) can all be accomplished with a 6-Fr guide. However, the standard crush, V stenting, and simultaneous kissing stents techniques cannot be performed unless a larger guide is used, because these techniques require the simultaneous advancement of two stent delivery systems through the guide.

Arterial Approach

Radial access has the advantage over the conventional femoral approach with respect to access site complications, but in some cases backup support and necessary guide catheter diameter can be an issue. Although use of a 7-Fr and larger guide catheter for the radial approach can be feasible in selected patients,[79] it is not a routine practice because of anatomic considerations in some individuals, arterial spasm, and operator experience.

Choice of Coronary Guidewires and Wiring Techniques

For most bifurcation lesions, the placement of two wires (one in the main branch and one in the SB) should be considered as a default approach. In most cases, wire placement in the SB should be performed before wire placement in the main branch. However, the vessel in which wire placement is expected to be most complicated because of unfavorable anatomy, calcification, tortuosity, or severe stenosis should be wired first. With one wire already in place, the maneuverability of a second wire is limited, which may jeopardize the successful wiring of the least accessible branch. Even after successful wire placement, wrapping of the wires can occur, preventing the sequential advancement of balloons and stents. Wire wrapping can be avoided by limiting the rotation of the second wire to less than 180 degrees during advancement and keeping the wires separately on the table in the same position throughout the procedure, even after rewiring and wire exchange. One must also anticipate the jailing of the SB wire between a stent and the main branch; in general, it is wise to avoid jailing hydrophilic jacketed or hybrid guidewires because there is a potential risk of peeling off the hydrophilic coating or losing the distal part in the SB during wire removal.

There are some situations in which, because of the location of the plaque in the main branch and/or the angulation of the SB, wiring of the SB cannot be achieved, even after attempting different types of wires with various tip curves and techniques. In this situation, the following options are available: (1) stop the procedure because the risk of losing the SB will be too high, considering the size and distribution of the branch (typically an angulated circumflex artery when stenting the distal bifurcation of an unprotected left main); (2) use the Venture wire control catheter (St. Jude Medical, Minnetonka, Minn) to direct guidewire entry in the SB; or (3) attempt to modify the plaque at the bifurcation to facilitate access into the SB by dilating the main vessel with a balloon and then redirecting the second wire into the SB ostium. In the past, plaque removal by directional coronary atherectomy has been suggested to facilitate the wire passage into the SB ostium.[37]

DEDICATED TWO-STENT TECHNIQUES

T Stenting

Classic T Stenting

Both branches are wired and dilated. Positioning a stent first at the ostium of the SB is done carefully to avoid stent protrusion into the main branch (MB) while at the same time trying to minimize any possible gap. After deployment of the stent, the balloon from the SB is removed with the wire in place. The next step is to advance and deploy the stent in the main branch. Rewiring of the SB and removal of the jailed wire are done before SB balloon dilation and final kissing inflation (FKI). This description of T stenting describes the situation in which the operator decides to stent the SB first. However, in most cases, the T stenting technique is performed after MB and provisional SB stenting for a suboptimal result or flow-limiting dissection in the SB.

Modified T Stenting

Modified T stenting (Figure 15-11) is a variation performed by simultaneously positioning stents at the SB and MB, with the SB stent minimally protruding into the MB, when the angle between the branches is close to 90 degrees.[80,81] The SB stent is deployed first and then after wire and balloon removal from the SB, the MB stent is deployed. The procedure is completed with a final kissing balloon inflation.

Reverse T Stenting

Reverse T stenting is a widely used provisional stenting strategy and is the best suitable bail-out technique after initial MB branch stenting and SB balloon angioplasty if the SB result remains suboptimal or major dissection of the SB requires additional stenting. However, this technique requires rewiring the SB through the MB stent struts after first stent deployment in the MB, followed by ballooning and stenting of the SB, with the risk that advancement of the SB stent could be difficult. Final kissing balloon inflations are recommended.

T Stenting and Protrusion

The T stenting and protrusion (TAP) technique is used to enhance SB ostial coverage. It is an intentional protrusion of the SB stent within the MB that ensures SB ostial coverage and facilitates final kissing balloon inflation.[82] Therefore, this technique is advantageous compared with conventional T stenting, which is associated with a risk of incomplete SB ostial coverage, especially when the angle between the MB and SB is acute. The first steps of TAP and provisional T stenting are identical—stenting of the MB, rewiring of the SB, and kissing balloon inflation. If the operator is not satisfied with the obtained result, an uninflated balloon catheter to be used for final kissing inflation is advanced into the MB, and a stent of the appropriate length and size is advanced into the SB. The position of the SB stent is adjusted to cover the proximal (or upper) part of the SB ostium fully. Bench testing demonstrates that this location results in the protrusion of stent struts within the MB only in the distal part of the SB ostium. The SB stent is then deployed while the MB balloon is kept uninflated. Finally, the stent balloon is withdrawn slightly and final kissing balloon inflation is performed by simultaneously inflating the SB stent balloon and MB balloon. The kissing balloon inflation reorients the protruding SB stent struts, resulting in a small neocarina.[82]

1. Wire both branches and
predilate if needed.

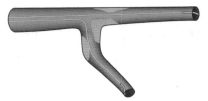

2. Advance the two stents. SB stent is
positioned with minimal protrusion into MB.

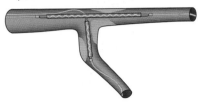

3. SB stent is deployed at
nominal pressure.

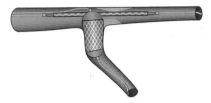

4. Check for optimal result in the SB and
then remove balloon and wire from SB.
Deploy the MB stent at high pressure.

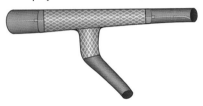

5. Rewire the SB and perform
high-pressure dilation.

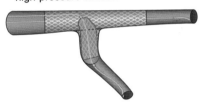

6. Perform final kissing inflation after
advancement of a balloon into the MB.

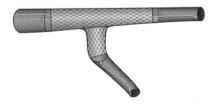

Figure 15-11   Modified T stenting technique.
MB, Main branch; *SB,* side branch. (Adapted from
Latib A, Colombo A, Moussa I, Sheiban I. When are
two stents needed? Which technique is the best?
How to perform? *EuroIntervention* 2010;6[Suppl]:
J81-J87.)

Culotte Technique

Although the culotte technique, sometimes also referred as Y stenting or trouser legs, was associated with high restenosis rates in the past, it has regained popularity in the DES era.[83-85] This technique provides near-perfect coverage of the carina and SB ostium at the expense of an excess of metal covering the proximal end.[85] It provides the best immediate angiographic result and may guarantee a more homogeneous drug distribution at the site of the bifurcation. The culotte technique can be used in almost all true bifurcation lesions, irrespective of the bifurcation angle. The only anatomic limitation is when there is a large mismatch between the proximal MB and SB diameters, which may lead to malapposition of the SB stent within the proximal part of the MB.[78] Stents with open cell designs are preferred when the SB diameter is more than 3 mm because with some closed cell stents, the intrastrut opening may reach a maximum diameter of only 3 mm. The main disadvantage of this technique is that rewiring of both branches through the stent struts is required, which can be difficult, technically demanding, and time-consuming.

The procedure can be performed using a 6-Fr guiding catheter (Figure 15-12). Both branches are wired and predilated. First, a stent is deployed across the smaller, more angulated branch, usually the SB. The nonstented branch is then rewired through the stent struts, and dilation is performed to facilitate passage of the second stent. This is advanced and expanded into the nonstented branch, usually the main branch. Finally, kissing balloon inflation is performed. For the final kissing balloon inflation, noncompliant balloons are preferred, and each limb of the culotte should be dilated at high pressure individually before simultaneously inflating both balloons to nominal pressure.

Although the culotte technique may be technically more challenging than other procedures, a number of factors can facilitate success. When rewiring the other branch after stent placement, it is reasonable always to first place the guidewire distal into the stented branch to ensure that the wire has not passed under the stent struts before recrossing into the branch. The branch with the sharpest angle should be stented first, because wire recrossing and advancement of the second stent through the first stent struts will be more easily accomplished. However, this conventional practice has recently been challenged in the Nordic Stent Technique Study, in which the authors recommended stenting of the main branch first to avoid acute closure.[86] It is preferable not to perform the culotte technique if there is a dissection in both branches after predilation.[78]

Crush Technique

The crush technique is described schematically in Figure 15-13. Its main advantage is that patency of both branches is ensured; therefore, this approach should be applied in conditions of clinical instability or complex anatomy.[87] As such, the crush technique is very useful when the SB is functionally relevant or difficult to wire. In addition, this technique provides excellent coverage of the ostium of the SB. It can be used in almost all true bifurcation lesions but should be avoided in bifurcations with a wide angle; an angle of 50 degrees or more between the two branches has been suggested to be an independent predictor of major adverse cardiac events after crush stenting.[88]

The standard crush and minicrush technique require use of a 7- or an 8-Fr guiding catheter. Both branches are wired and fully dilated. Stents are positioned in the MB and SB. The SB stent is positioned so that about 1 to 2 mm of the proximal end (minicrush) is within the main branch; this position is verified in at least two projections. The SB stent is deployed. An angiogram is taken to verify that the SB has an appropriate lumen, normal flow, and no distal dissection or residual lesions are present. If an additional stent is needed in the SB, this is the time to implant it; otherwise, the wire from SB is removed. The main branch stent is then deployed at high pressure, flattening the protruding cells of the SB stent—hence the name *crush.*

1. Wire both branches and predilate if needed.

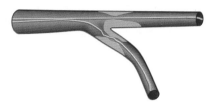

2. Leave the wire in the straighter branch (MB) and deploy a stent in the more angulated branch (SB).

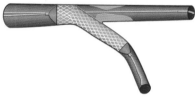

3. Rewire the unstented branch and dilate the stent struts to unjail the branch (MB).

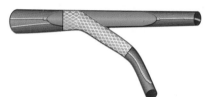

4. Place a second stent into the unstented branch (MB) and expand the stent, leaving some proximal overlap.

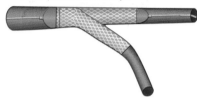

5. Re-cross the second stent's (MB) struts into the first stent (SB) with a wire and perform kissing balloon inflation.

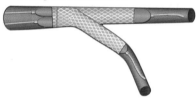

Figure 15-12 Culotte technique. *MB,* Main branch; *SB,* side branch. (Adapted from Latib A, Colombo A, Moussa I, Sheiban I. When are two stents needed? Which technique is the best? How to perform? *EuroIntervention* 2010;6[Suppl]:J81-J87.)

After rewiring of the SB, it is important to perform a two-step postdilation. Dilation of the SB with a high-pressure balloon inflation of a diameter at least equal to that of the stent is necessary,[76] and then final kissing balloon inflation is recommended.[89,90] This allows better strut contact against the ostium of the SB and therefore better drug delivery. The main disadvantage is that to perform final kissing inflation, one must recross multiple struts with a wire and a balloon.[80,91] The minicrush (i.e., minimizing the length of SB stent crushed by the MB) may be associated with more complete endothelialization and, in turn, theoretically less stent thrombosis, as well as easier recrossing of the crushed stent.[78]

Step Crush Technique

The step crush or modified balloon crush techniques can be used when a crush technique is required through a 6-Fr guiding catheter (e.g., the radial approach).[78] The result is identical to that obtained with the standard crush technique, except that each stent is advanced and deployed separately. Similar to the standard crush, both branches are wired and fully dilated. A stent is advanced into the SB protruding a few millimeters into the main branch; a balloon—rather than a second stent—is advanced into the MB spanning the bifurcation, the stent in the SB is deployed, and the stent balloon is removed. Angiography is performed and if the SB result is adequate, the wire is also removed. The MB balloon is then inflated to crush the protruding SB stent and is removed, and a second stent is advanced in the main branch and deployed. The next steps are identical to those of the classic crush technique and involve recrossing into the SB, SB stent dilation, and final kissing balloon inflation.[78,92]

Reverse Crush Technique

The reverse, or internal, crush is an option in the setting of provisional SB stenting when using a 6-Fr guide catheter.[37] Both branches are wired routinely, a stent is deployed in the main branch, and balloon dilation with final kissing inflation toward the SB is performed. If the result at the ostium or the proximal segment of the SB is suboptimal, a second stent is advanced into the SB and left in position without being deployed. Then, a balloon sized according to the diameter of the MB is positioned at the level of the bifurcation, making sure to stay inside the stent previously deployed in the MB. The stent in the SB is retracted about 2 to 3 mm into the MB and deployed, the stent balloon is removed, and an angiogram is obtained to verify that a good result is present at the SB (i.e., no further distal stent in the side branch is needed). If this is the case, the wire from the SB is removed, and the balloon in the MB is inflated to high pressure. The other steps are similar to those of the crush technique and involve recrossing into the SB, SB dilation, and final kissing balloon inflation. This technique shares the same disadvantages as the standard crush technique.

Double Kissing Crush Technique

This double kissing (DK) crush technique is a modification of the step crush procedure, in which a balloon kissing inflation is performed twice, first after a main branch balloon crushes the SB stent and then the standard final kissing inflation at the end of the procedure. The DK crush technique therefore consists of five steps: SB stenting, balloon crush, first kissing, MB stenting and crushing, and final kissing.[93] The specific steps are as follows:

1. A balloon is advanced into the MB, and a stent is positioned in the SB.
2. The SB stent is deployed; the balloon in the main branch is inflated after removing the guidewire and the SB stent balloon, thereby crushing the protruding SB stent against the MB wall.
3. The first kissing balloon inflation is performed after successfully rewiring the SB.

1. Wire both branches and predilate
   if needed.

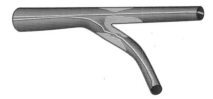

2. Advance the two stents. MB stent is
   positioned proximally. SB stent will
   protrude only minimally into MB.

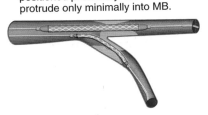

3. Deploy the SB stent.

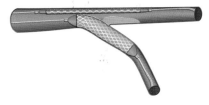

4. Check for optimal result in the SB and then
   remove balloon and wire from SB. Deploy the
   MB stent, crushing the MB stent.

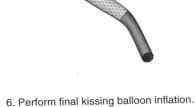

5. Rewire the SB and perform
   high-pressure dilation.

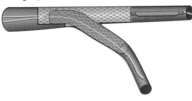

6. Perform final kissing balloon inflation.

Figure 15-13 Minicrush technique. *MB,* Main branch; *SB,* side branch. (Adapted from Latib A, Colombo A, Moussa I, Sheiban I. When are two stents needed? Which technique is the best? How to perform? *EuroIntervention* 2010; 6[Suppl]:J81-J87.)

4. The SB balloon and wire are removed, and another stent in the MB is positioned and deployed to crush the SB stent further.
5. Final kissing balloon inflations are performed after successfully rewiring the SB.

DK crush may result in less stent distortion, improved stent apposition, and facilitate final kissing inflation. The DK crush may be superior to the classic crush technique with respect to acute procedural results and clinical outcomes by facilitating successful final kissing inflation in all patients.[93] The Double Kissing Crush II study randomly assigned 370 patients with true bifurcations lesions to treatment with the DK crush or provisional stenting[94] and found that the DK crush approach was associated with a lower rate of restenosis and repeat revascularization. This was the only randomized trial to suggest that double stenting may be superior to provisional stenting. However, stent thrombosis was numerically higher in the DK crush arm (2.2% vs. 0.5%; $P = .37$). In the Double Kissing Crush III randomized trial of 419 patients with unprotected left main bifurcation lesions, the DK crush technique was associated with significantly less 1-year major adverse cardiovascular events compared with the culotte technique (16.3% versus 6.2%, $p < 0.05$), driven by a reduced rate of target vessel revascularization.[94a]

V-Stent, Simultaneous Kissing Stent, and Trouser Simultaneous Kissing Stent Techniques

The V and SKS techniques share some technical similarities. Both are performed by delivering and simultaneously implanting two stents.[95,96] One stent is advanced into the SB and the other into the MB. The V technique consists of the delivery and implantation of two stents together, forming a small proximal stent carina (<2 mm). V stenting is ideal for Medina [0,1,1] bifurcations with a large proximal MB that is relatively free from disease and a less than 90-degree angle between both branches (Figure 15-14).[37] When the two stents

protrude into the MB with the creation of a double barrel and a new stent carina that extends a considerable length (≥3 mm) into the MB, the technique is called SKS. SKS is best suited to easily accessible bifurcations with a large proximal vessel containing plaque and when both branches are of similar diameter. The proximal part of the MB should be able to accommodate the two stents, approximately two thirds of the aggregate diameter of the two size stents.[37] Case reports have described the development of a thin, diaphragmatic, membranous structure at the new carina (at the level of the kissing struts), resulting in an angiographic filling defect. Other than producing a very distressing angiographic appearance, the exact long-term significance and relation to adverse advents of this membrane are not known.[77] The subacute stent thrombosis rate for this technique has been low in the DES era, according to two studies.[104,105]

A modified approach, termed the *trouser* SKS, is used for the treatment of long proximal lesions to avoid formation of very long new carina.[103,104] A large-diameter stent is first deployed proximally in the MB over a single guidewire. Then, the SB is wired through the lumen of the proximal stent and two stents are advanced and deployed in the more distal main and SBs.

The main advantage of the V and SKS techniques is that access to both branches is always preserved during the procedure, with no need for branch rewiring. The main disadvantage is that simultaneous double-stenting techniques also require the use of larger guiding catheters as well as aggressive predilation of both branches.

There are several limitations of the V and the SKS techniques. Balloon barotrauma to the proximal main branch during stent deployment or post-dilation can lead to dissection, progression of disease, or proximal edge restenosis. If a proximal stent becomes necessary to treat a proximal dissection, there is the risk of leaving a small gap. If restenosis occurs in the neocarina or at the proximal stent edge, percutaneous treatment would require converting to the crush

1. Wire both branches and predilate if needed.

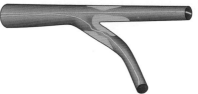

2. Position two parallel stents covering both branches and extending into the MB.
V: minimal protrusion into MB. SKS: double barrel into the MB

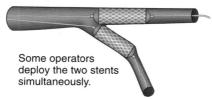

3. Deploy one stent.

4. Deploy the second stent.

Some operators deploy the two stents simultaneously.

5. Perform high-pressure single-stent post-dilation and medium-pressure kissing inflation with short and noncompliant balloons.

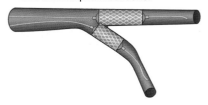

Figure 15-14 **V stenting technique.** *MB,* Main branch; *SKS,* simultaneous kissing stent. (Adapted from Latib A, Colombo A, Moussa I, Sheiban I. When are two stents needed? Which technique is the best? How to perform? *EuroIntervention* 2010; 6[Suppl]:J81-J87.)

technique, which would make recrossing into the branch covered by the crushed stent potentially challenging because four layers of stent struts would need to be traversed. If disease distal to the V stenting or SKS site needs to be treated at follow-up, rewiring the stented vessels may be complicated by wire passage behind stent struts.[78]

🔵 Clinical Outcomes of Bifurcation Stenting

Outcomes of different stent techniques and stenting strategies have been examined in several randomized trials, analyses of nonrandomized studies, and observational registries (Tables 15-1 and 15-2).[89,97-103] The interpretation of these studies is challenging, because operators use different treatment strategies based on plaque burden and bifurcation anatomy.

PROVISIONAL STENTING VERSUS DOUBLE STENTING

In the Nordic study, 413 patients were randomized to a simple treatment strategy (stenting of the main vessel with optional stenting of the SB) or to a complex stenting strategy involving stenting of both the main vessel and SB. In this study, only sirolimus-eluting stents were used. The simple stenting strategy used in the main vessel was associated with lower rates of procedure-related biomarker elevation. After 14 months of follow-up, the rates of stent thrombosis and MACE were low and not significantly different between the simple and complex strategy groups (9.5% and 8.2%). The mortality rate was 2.4% versus 1.0%, and the rate of non–PCI-related myocardial infarction was 2.0% versus 1.0% in the single- and double-stent strategies, respectively.[10,127]

The British Bifurcation Coronary (BBC) ONE randomized trial examined the safety and efficacy of simple compared with complex stenting strategies for bifurcation lesions using DES. In the simple strategy, the main vessel was stented, followed by optional kissing

balloon dilation–T stent placement. In the complex strategy, both vessels were systematically stented (culotte or crush techniques), with mandatory final kissing balloon dilation. This study enrolled a total of 500 patients, of which 82% had true bifurcation lesions according to Medina classification. In the simple group, 66 patients (26%) received kissing balloon inflation in addition to main vessel stenting, and 7 (3%) underwent T stenting. In the complex group, 89% of culotte (n = 75) and 72% of crush (n = 169) cases were completed successfully with final kissing balloon inflations. MACEs occurred in 8.0% of those in the simple group versus 15.2% of the complex group (hazard ratio [HR], 2.02; 95% confidence interval [CI], 1.17-3.47; P = .009), myocardial infarction occurred in 3.6% versus 11.2% (P = .001), and in-hospital MACEs occurred in 2.0% versus 8.0% (P = .002).[104]

Gao and associates[103] have prospectively compared single- versus double-stent techniques using DES in 566 consecutive patients. In the one-stent strategy, kissing balloon inflation was mandatory; the two-stent strategy included crush, culotte, Y, V, and kissing stent techniques. MACE rates were higher in the two-DES group than in the one-DES group (5.5% vs. 2.0%; P = .032), which were mainly driven by myocardial infarction (4.5% vs. 1.4%; P = .032) rather than death or TLR (0% vs. 0.5%, P = .389; 1.4% vs. 2.7%, P = .352). Stent thrombosis rates were higher in the two-DES group than in the one-DES group (2.7% vs. 0.6%; P = .042). At 7-month angiographic follow-up, there was no difference in the rate of restenosis in the one-DES group compared with the two-DES group in the MB (9.8 vs. 11.9%; P = .652), but in the SB, the restenosis rate was higher in the one-DES group (33.6% vs. 15.5%; P = .004).

The Coronary Bifurcations: Application of the Crushing Technique Using Sirolimus Eluting Stents (CACTUS) trial[87] was a prospective, randomized, multicenter study comparing two different stenting techniques using sirolimus-eluting stents and mandatory final kissing balloon inflation in 350 patients with true bifurcation lesions. One group was randomly assigned to crush stenting, and the other was randomly assigned to stenting of only the MB with provisional

TABLE 15-1	Randomized Trials of Different Techniques for Percutaneous Treatment of Bifurcation Lesions						
Study (Year)	No. of Patients in Study	Technique	Stents	FU (mo)	Endpoint	Result (%)	P Value
Pan et al (2004)[107]	91	OST with SBT vs. mandatory TST	RES	6	TLR	5.0 vs. 2.0	ns
Colombo et al (2004)[106]	85	OST with provisional SBST vs. complex; no culotte allowed	SES	6	MACE	13.6 vs. 19.0	ns
DKCRUSH I Trial (2008)[93]	312	Classic CRT vs. DK CRT	PES, SES	8	MACE	24.4 vs. 11.4	.02
					TLR	18.9 vs. 9.0	.03
					ST	3.2 vs. 1.3	ns
Ferenc et al (2008)[105]	202	OST with provisional TST and mandatory FKBD vs. mandatory TST and mandatory FKBD	SES	12	MACE	12.9 vs. 11.9	ns
					Definite ST	1.0 vs. 1.0	ns
Nordic Bifurcation Study (2008)[2,174]	413	OST with provisional SBST vs. complex CRT 50%, CUT 21%, TST 29%	SES	14	MACE	9.5 vs. 8.2	ns
					MI	2.0 vs. 1.0	ns
					Definite ST	1.0 vs. 0.5	ns
CACTUS Trial (2009)[87]	350	OST with provisional TST 31% and mandatory FKBD vs. CRT with mandatory FKBD	SES	6	MACE	15.0 vs. 15.8	ns
					MI	0.5 vs. 0.5	ns
					ST	1.1 vs. 1.7	ns
British Bifurcation Coronary Study (2010)[104]	500	OST with provisional SBST/FKBD vs. complex CRT, CUT with mandatory FKBD	PES	9	MACE	8.0 vs. 15.2	.009
					MI	3.6 vs. 11.2	.001
Nordic Stent Technique Study (2009)[86]	424	CRT with mandatory FKBD vs. CUT with mandatory FKBD	SES	6	MACE	4.3 vs. 3.7	ns
					MI	1.9 vs. 1.4	ns
					ST	1.4 vs. 1.9	ns
Nordic-Baltic Bifurcation Study III (2011)[130]	477	OST with provisional SBST and FKBD vs. OST with provisional SBST without FKBD	DES	6	MACE	2.1 vs. 2.5	ns
DKCRUSH II Trial (2011)[94]	370	OST with provisional TST with FKBD vs. DK CRT	DES	12	MACE	17.3 vs. 10.3	ns
					MI	2.2 vs. 3.2	ns
					Definite ST	0.5 vs. 2.2	ns
					TLR	13.0 vs. 4.3	.005

CRT, Crush technique; CUT, culotte technique; DES, drug-eluting stent; DK CRT, double kissing crush technique; FKBD, final kissing balloon dilation; FU, follow-up; MACE, major adverse cardiac event; MI, myocardial infarction; ns, nonsignificant; OST, one-stent technique; PES, paclitaxel-eluting stent; RES, rapamycin-eluting stent; SBST, side branch stenting technique; SBT, side-branch balloon technique; SES, sirolimus-eluting stent; ST, stent thrombosis; TLR, target lesion revascularization; TST, T stent technique.

TABLE 15-2	Nonrandomized Studies of Different Techniques for Percutaneous Treatment of Bifurcation Lesions						
Study	No. of Patients in Study	Technique	Stents	FU (mo)	Endpoint	Result (%)	P Value
Yamashita et al (2000)[100]	92	OST with SBT vs. complex	BMS	6	MACE	38.0 vs. 51.0	ns
					TLR	36.0 vs. 38.0	ns
Al Suwaidi et al (2000)[102]	131	OST with SBT vs. complex (TST, YST)	BMS	12	Death	0.0 vs. 2.4	ns
					MI	2.1 vs. 8.8	ns
					TLR	20.5 vs. 19.4	ns
Anzuini et al (2001)[101]	90	OST with SBT vs. complex (TST)	BMS	12	Death	0.0 vs. 0.0	ns
					MI	0.0 vs. 0.0	ns
					TLR	15.6 vs. 35.6	ns
Gao et al (2008)[103]	566	OST with mandatory FKBD vs. complex (CRT, CUT, YST, VST, KST)	DES	7	MACE	2.0 vs. 5.5	.032
					MI	3.6 vs. 11.2	.032
					ST	0.6 vs. 2.7	.042

BMS, Bare metal stent; CRT, crush technique; CUT, culotte technique; DES, drug-eluting stent; FKBD, final kissing balloon dilation; FU, follow-up; KST, kissing stent technique; MACE, major adverse cardiac event; MI, myocardial infarction; OST, one-stent technique; SBT, side branch balloon technique; ST, stent thrombosis; TLR, target lesion revascularization; ns, nonsignificant; TST, T stent technique; VST, V stent technique; YST, Y stent technique.

SB T stenting. Additional stenting of the SB in the provisional stenting group was required in 31% of cases. At 6 months, MACE rates were similar in the two groups (15.8% in the crush group vs. 15% in the provisional stenting group). The rates of restenosis were similar for the main branch (4.0% vs. 8.7%; $P = .09$) and the SB (14.6% vs. 12.5%; $P = .61$) for the double-stenting and MB-only stenting groups, respectively.

Ferenc and coworkers[105] randomly assigned 202 patients with a coronary bifurcation lesion to routine T stenting with a sirolimus-eluting stent in both branches or to provisional T stenting with sirolimus-eluting stent placement in the MB followed by kissing-balloon angioplasty. Angiographic follow-up demonstrated an SB restenosis rate of 23.0% ± 20.2% after provisional T stenting and 27.7% ± 24.8% after routine T stenting ($P = .15$). The 1-year rates of target lesion revascularization were 10.9% after provisional and 8.9% after routine T stenting ($P = .64$).

Colombo and colleagues[106] randomly assigned patients to undergo stenting of both branches or stenting of the MB with provisional stenting of the SB. In total, 85 patients were enrolled and only a sirolimus-eluting stent (SES) was used. The restenosis rate at 6 months was not significantly different between the double-stenting (28.0%) and provisional SB stenting (18.7%) groups.

Pan and associates[107] compared single stenting versus double stenting for coronary bifurcations in a randomized study of 91 patients with true coronary bifurcation lesions. All patients received SES in the main vessel, covering the SB. A total of 44 patients were randomized to receive a second stent at the SB origin (T stent and modified T stent techniques were used). At 6-month angiographic reevaluation, restenosis of the main vessel was observed in 1 patient (2%) from the single-stent group and in 4 patients (10%) from the double-stent group, and restenosis of the SB appeared in 2 (5%) and 6 (15%) patients, respectively.

Yamashita and coworkers[100] treated 92 patients with bifurcation lesions with a two-stent strategy versus a one-stent strategy in the MB and balloon angioplasty of the SB. In this study, BMS were used. At 6-month follow-up, the angiographic restenosis rate in the two-stent group was 62% compared with 48% in the one-stent group; target lesion revascularization rates were similar in the two groups (38% vs. 36%, respectively), as were the MACE rates (51% vs. 38%).

Meta-analyses of randomized trials that compared a simple versus a complex strategy using DES found that a provisional strategy was associated with a significantly lower rate of myocardial infarction and a numerically lower rate of stent thrombosis.[108,109] Brar and colleagues[109] published a meta-analysis of six randomized controlled trials involving 1641 patients that compared a provisional with a two-stent strategy. There were no differences in efficacy, measured by target vessel revascularization or percentage diameter stenosis, between provisional T stenting and a routine two-stent strategy. Although death and stent thrombosis occurred at similar rates in both treatment groups, myocardial infarction was more common with the two-stent strategy. The relative and absolute reductions in myocardial infarction with provisional stenting were 43% and 3.0%, respectively ($P = .01$). A patient-level, pooled meta-analysis of the British Bifurcation Coronary Study (BBC ONE) and Nordic Bifurcation Study has confirmed the findings of the individual studies and further demonstrated that a two-stent strategy was not superior to a provisional approach even in more complex patient groups (e.g., those with large-diameter SBs and those with disease involving >5 mm of the SB ostium).[110]

These data suggest that no additional benefit is associated with a mandatory two-stent strategy. Provisional stenting should be performed in bifurcation lesions with an intermediate-size SB (diameter ≥ 2 to 2.75 mm), with stent deployment in the SB only for suboptimal angiographic results, including flow-limiting dissection, residual stenosis more than 70%, or TIMI flow less than 2.[2,87,104] An elective two-stent approach might be more appropriate when both the parent vessel and SB are large, (>2.5 to 2.75 mm), especially with significant disease distal to the ostium and when the SB arises at a shallow angle.[111]

FINAL KISSING BALLOON INFLATION AND OUTCOMES

Final kissing balloon inflation has been reported to have a protective effect against stent thrombosis.[97] In addition, after the crush technique, final kissing balloon inflation significantly reduced SB late lumen loss (0.24 ± 0.50 mm vs. 0.58 ± 0.77 mm; $P < .001$) at 9-month angiographic follow-up.[112] In all modern bifurcation trials (e.g., BBC ONE and CACTUS), kissing balloon inflation after the use of complex two-stent techniques has been mandatory.

PLAQUE MODIFICATION

Plaque debulking with directional coronary atherectomy or modification with a scoring device before stent deployment could minimize arterial injury and subsequent neointimal proliferation and could prevent restenosis formation. In addition, it minimizes plaque shifting between the MB and SB and thus could help avoid SB stenting and provide better stent apposition with reduced inflation pressure, even if very long stents are deployed. Tsuchikane and colleagues[113] have reported registry data of 99 patients with bifurcation lesions who

received directional coronary atherectomy before stenting. Simple stenting was performed in 97 patients. The 9-month binary restenosis rates in the MB and SB were 1.1% and 3.4%, respectively; target lesion revascularization was performed only in 2 patients. The safety and efficacy of plaque modification with a scoring device before main vessel stenting and/or SB treatment in bifurcation lesions was examined in 556 patients undergoing intervention with a cutting balloon ($n = 209$) or without ($n = 347$).[114] Target lesion revascularization was lower in the cutting balloon group compared with the noncutting balloon group (5.3% vs. 11.0%, $P = .021$). These outcomes are promising and support the hypothesis that plaque debulking before stenting, especially in complex bifurcated lesions, may help the operator avoid the need for complex stenting and may provide a good long-term outcome in patients within the first year postprocedure.[113,114]

TREATMENT OF UNPROTECTED LEFT MAIN CORONARY ARTERY BIFURCATION

Up to 80% of left main disease involves the bifurcation. The introduction of DES has significantly improved the outcome of patients with unprotected left main coronary artery stenosis treated with PCI.[115-120] In an observational study, the adjusted HR of the risk of 2-year MACEs in patients treated for unprotected left main bifurcations compared with patients without bifurcations was 1.50 ($P = .024$). There was a significant difference between patients with bifurcations treated with two stents and those without bifurcations ($P = .001$) but not between patients with bifurcations treated with one stent and those without bifurcations ($P = .38$).[121] The results of this study suggest that not all unprotected left main coronary artery (ULMCA) bifurcations should be considered in the same way and that those patients who can be treated with one stent, irrespective of lesion location, have more favorable outcomes.

BARE METAL STENTS

No large prospective randomized trials have addressed long-term clinical outcomes after the placement of BMS compared with stand-alone balloon dilation or surgery, or with different stenting techniques. Most evidence has been obtained from registries and retrospective studies.*

High rates of restenosis are the major limitation in the treatment of bifurcation stenoses with BMS, in particular with the two-stent strategy, with restenosis rates reportedly as high as 48% with single-stent strategy and 62% with a two-stent strategy. In the bare metal era, the provisional T stent approach was the method of choice, and studies do not suggest a benefit in stenting both vessels rather than one.

BARE METAL STENTS VERSUS DRUG-ELUTING STENTS

DES reduces the risk of restenosis compared with BMS for the treatment of nonbifurcation lesions. Analysis of the 126 patients with bifurcation lesions treated in the Stenting Coronary Arteries in Non-Stress/Benestent Disease (SCANDSTENT) trial has shown that sirolimus-eluting stent implantation improves angiographic and clinical outcomes considerably compared with BMS. SES were associated with significant reduction in restenosis rates at the MB (4.9% vs. 28.3%; $P < .001$) and SB (14.8% vs. 43.4%; $P < .001$) and were associated with a significant decrease in MACE rates at 7-month follow-up (9% vs. 28%; $P = .01$).[12] Similarly, registry studies have shown reductions in MACE rates and target lesion revascularization rates compared with historical BMS controls. These reductions occurred irrespective of whether a one-stent (MACE, 5.4% vs. 38%; TLR, 5.4% vs. 38%) or two-stent (MACE, 13.3% vs. 51%; TLR, 8.9% vs. 38%) strategy was used.[98,107]

---

*References 74, 85, 101, 102, 122, and 123.

Complications of Bifurcation Stenting

PCI for coronary bifurcations is associated with more procedural complications and higher restenosis and adverse event rates than for nonbifurcation lesions.[11,124-127] The introduction of DES for the treatment of bifurcation lesions has dramatically decreased restenosis rates from, in some subsets, up to 60%[100,128] to 5% to 10%, and in the latest trials,[106,107,129,130] even to 2.5% in the MB, especially for patients suffering from diabetes.[131] However, abrupt SB closure and SB ostial restenosis remain areas for which further improvement is needed. A higher risk of subacute and late stent thrombosis is a major concern as well.[76,106,127,132-134]

SIDE BRANCH CLOSURE

Acute SB closure may be defined as TIMI flow grade 0 or 1. The incidence of SB compromise after coronary stent implantation is greater than after balloon angioplasty.[8,9,135] Initial studies have reported an incidence of SB closure ranging from 4.5% to 26% of cases using a one-stent technique, attributable to plaque shifting, SB ostial recoil, and/or propagation of dissection.[9,63,136] Studies using everolimus-eluting stents have reported an SB occlusion rate ranging from 6.1% to 9.9%.[137] Anatomic features associated with an increased risk of SB closure include smaller SB reference vessel diameter,[9] angulation of the SB take off,[8] involvement of the ostium of the SB, and SB ostial composition. Acute coronary syndrome has also been reported as a predictor of abrupt SB closure.[84] The rates of myocardial infarction, both during the periprocedural period and during follow-up, are higher in patients with SB occlusion compared with those without occlusion.[137]

When the SB ostium is not diseased, the likelihood of its narrowing after the main vessel is stented is low, and the SB can be rescued by kissing balloon inflation of the main vessel stent and SB if it is compromised. A challenging situation is a significant true bifurcation lesion with atherosclerotic involvement of both the main vessel and SB ostia. In these situations, the risk of SB occlusion is increased.[63]

SB occlusion should be anticipated whenever a stent is placed across a bifurcation. A large SB or a smaller diameter SB with a diseased ostium should be protected with a second guidewire before PCI. Of note, revascularization of an SB vessel with a diameter less than 1.5 mm is unlikely to yield any clinical benefit; therefore, vessels of this size are routinely excluded from studies comparing bifurcation stenting strategies.[2,87] Wiring of the SB usually preserves patency if occlusion occurs and serves as a locator for the SB origin.

SIDE BRANCH RESTENOSIS

Despite the adoption of drug-eluting stents, restenosis at the ostium of the SB remains a stubborn problem and cause for repeated revascularizations.[92] Potential mechanisms include focal stent underexpansion at the ostium, inadequate ostial scaffolding, and uneven drug distribution.[138-140] The less favorable outcomes associated with PCI of bifurcation compared with nonbifurcation lesions may in part result from the inability of current devices and techniques to scaffold adequately and preserve the SB ostium.[106,107] Dedicated bifurcation stents could be advantageous by achieving complete lesion coverage and scaffolding.[141]

FRACTURE OF A JAILED WIRE

Hydrophilic guidewires should be used cautiously for wire jailing and when recrossing into the SB because of the risk of stripping the polymer coating when withdrawing and the risk of wire-induced dissection or perforation, respectively. When the jailed wire technique is used, the stent in the main vessel should be implanted with low pressure; rewiring should then be performed, and only then should post-dilation of the main vessel stent at a higher atmosphere be undertaken.[142] Jailing a long segment of wire in the parent vessel should be

avoided. Fracture of the jailed wire is a rarely reported complication.[11] Removal of a broken wire is very difficult or even impossible because of the force needed to withdraw the wire, especially if high pressures were used for stent implantation. Use of a snare could be the method of choice when a jailed wire is broken and the free proximal filament is located in the guiding catheter or proximally in the MB. Before pulling the system out, a second guidewire should be introduced under the stent struts into the SB and a small balloon used to dilate the space between the vessel wall and stent struts. Another method in the case of a jailed broken wire is high-pressure balloon inflation of a balloon within the guiding catheter to trap the free part of the filament, allowing removal of the whole system together with the guiding catheter from the coronary artery. However, this method carries some risks, may be ineffective, and is applicable in cases in which a free proximal filament of the jailed wire is in the guiding catheter. If the interventions described are not possible or successful, or if a free filament of broken wire is located in the coronary artery and the wire is broken proximally to the floppy part, surgery may be required.[143]

STENT EMBOLIZATION

Stent embolization refers to the loss of the stent from the delivery system and is a rare complication. Risk factors for stent embolization include heavy vessel calcification, pronounced vessel tortuosity, diffuse disease, and attempts to deliver a stent to a distal lesion through a previously implanted proximal stent, such as bifurcation stenting when manipulating one stent through the struts of another. If the guidewire is still across the stent and has been maintained in the distal coronary artery, a low-profile balloon may be placed back through the stent, allowing it to be repositioned across the target lesion and expanded or implanted at a safe location within the coronary vessel. If the stent cannot be repositioned, the balloon can be placed distal to the stent and inflated to trap the stent between the balloon and guiding catheter, withdrawing all components together into the femoral sheath. If the guidewire position has been lost and the unexpanded stent is located in a proximal portion of the coronary artery, or has embolized into a peripheral artery, it may be removed using a variety of forceps or snare devices. If displaced from the wire or more distal, a series of wires can be wrapped around it to ensnare it. Alternatively, a second stent may be expanded adjacent to the dislodged stent to trap it against the vessel wall, effectively excluding it from the lumen.

STENT THROMBOSIS

Pathologic studies have suggested that arterial branch points are the foci of low shear stress and low flow velocity and are sites predisposed to the development of atherosclerotic plaque, thrombus, and inflammation. The two or three layers of stent struts apposed to the vessel wall with some bifurcation techniques (e.g., crush stenting) initially raised concerns about possible increased thrombogenicity, especially with DES.[144] Several studies have found a higher risk of stent thrombosis in bifurcation lesions compared with lesions in the body of the vessel.[76,106,127,132-134,145] Stent thrombosis occurred in as many as 4.4% of patients after PCI with paclitaxel-eluting stents of bifurcation lesions compared with approximately 1% in nonbifurcation lesions[126]; treatment of bifurcations has been identified as an independent predictor of late stent thrombosis.[146] The risk of subacute stent thrombosis has been higher using two-stent techniques in most trials.[89,97,106] Moreover, stent thrombosis rates appear to be approximately doubled when two DES rather than one are implanted in a bifurcation.[106,134] However, the data are inconsistent. In randomized trials of bifurcation PCI, only one reported a statistically significant difference in stent thrombosis with two-stent techniques compared with a provisional one-stent technique,[103] whereas in the other trials, the differences in stent thrombosis rates did not meet statistical significance.[10,77,78,101,127]

Although in-stent restenosis has been dramatically reduced by the advent of DES, the inhibition of stent endothelialization has been shown in autopsy studies to correlate with the occurrence of in-stent thrombosis.[126,149,150] Data have futher suggested that late or very late thrombosis after placing DES is related to the percentage of stent strut endothelialization.[147-149] This is important in the context of bifurcation stenting, especially with two-stent techniques, in which uncovered struts sometimes may persist indefinitely. In one study, neointimal coverage was observed in 100% of bare metal bifurcation struts compared with 70% in DES at 8 months after implantation; this could potentially be reduced by newer generation DES that show better apposition and strut coverage over the longer-term.[150,151]

Dedicated Bifurcation Stents

The conventional one-stent technique with provisional SB stenting is the prevailing approach to bifurcation stenting. Despite the apparent advantages of this technique, there are situations in which two stents are needed, such as a large SB or SB with extensive disease and substantial myocardial territory at risk. For these situations, there are still a number of limitations, such as (1) maintenance of access to the SB throughout the procedure; (2) MB stent struts jailing the SB ostium, resulting in difficulty in rewiring or passing balloon and/or stent into the SB through the stent struts in the MB; (3) distortion of the MB stent by SB dilation; (4) inability to cover and scaffold the SB ostium fully; and (5) dependence on operator skills and technical experience.[152] Various dedicated bifurcation stents have been designed to address these limitations.

CLASSIFICATION OF DEDICATED BIFURCATION STENT DEVICES

Numerous dedicated bifurcation stents have been developed and are already available outside the United States or under clinical investigation. These devices can be broadly divided into four groups:
1. Stents for treating the MB with some degree of SB scaffolding. These stents maintain direct access to the SB after MB stenting and facilitate provisional SB stenting if necessary. Such dedicated stents include the Multi-Link Frontier (Abbott Vascular, Abbott Park, Ill),[170] Petal (Boston Scientific, Natick, Mass), Antares (TriReme Medical, Pleasanton, Calif), Invatec Twinrail (Invatec [Medtronic], Minneapolis), Nile Croco (Minvasys, Gennevilliers, France), SLK-view (Advanced Stent Technologies [Boston Scientific]), StenTys (StenTys, Princeton, NJ), and Y-Med Side-Kick (Y-Med, San Diego, Calif).
2. Stents for treating the SB first. These stents are intended to treat the SB with significant ostial and proximal disease. A second stent implantation is needed for the MB. Examples are the Sideguard (Cappella Medical Devices, Galway, Ireland) and Tryton (Tryton Medical, Durham, NC) stents.
3. Proximal main branch bifurcation stents. The conically shaped stent design maintains the geometry of the ostium after implantation. It must be precisely placed at the carina of the bifurcation to be effective. In most cases, another stent—for MB, SB, or both—is required to treat the bifurcation lesion fully. The Devax AXXESS PLUS (Devax, Lake Forest, Calif) is such a stent.
4. Bifurcated stents. An example is the Medtronic Bifurcation Stent System (Medtronic, Minneapolis).

Intravascular Imaging and Functional Assessment

Selection of the appropriate stenting strategy of a coronary bifurcation is crucial for achieving optimal results. However, currently available classification schemes are based on angiography and are therefore limited by the inherent inability of this imaging modality to determine atheroma distribution and volume at the level of the bifurcation. In addition, angiography cannot identify several characteristics that may complicate the procedure and adversely affect outcome. Important parameters that can guide treatment decisions include the

accurate determination of stenosis severity, diameter of the vessels involved, lesion length and location in the MB and SBs, and morphologic and compositional characteristics of the plaque, such as calcification, lipid content, and thickness of the fibrous cap.

INTRAVASCULAR ULTRASOUND

IVUS should be considered for the assessment of patients with coronary bifurcation lesions, particularly in those with angiographically ambiguous left main coronary artery disease. Better insight into plaque configuration with IVUS can diminish the unnecessary use of the two-stent procedure by distinguishing true stenosis from pseudostenosis caused by artifacts, including coronary spasm or calcification at the SB. SBs that on IVUS display diffuse plaque around the ostium with more then 50% stenosis have been demonstrated to be at higher risk for occlusion.[153] IVUS visualization of coronary bifurcation anatomy may allow better selection of the most appropriate stenting technique, reduce the need for a two-stent strategy, and improve outcomes.

Left Main Bifurcation Percutaneous Coronary Intervention

IVUS may reduce the long-term mortality rate of PCI, especially when DES are used for unprotected left main stenosis.[154,155] Use of IVUS may also provide a criterion that can be useful in defining a critical left main stenosis. IVUS-determined minimal lumen diameter and minimal lumen area cutoff values of 2.8 mm and 5.9 mm², respectively, provide the best sensitivity and specificity to predict the physiologic significance of a left main stenosis and are well correlated with a fractional flow reserve cut off point of 0.75.[156] The long-term assessment of the effect of IVUS guidance in 758 patients with de novo non–left main bifurcation lesions who were assigned to IVUS or angiographic guidance has shown that IVUS-guided stenting significantly reduces all-cause mortality in patients receiving DES at 4-year follow-up. The long-term survival benefit of IVUS guidance in patients receiving DES was driven primarily by a reduction in very late stent thrombosis.[155] In the Revascularisation for unprotected left MAIN coronary artery stenosis: COMparison of Percutaneous coronary Angioplasty vs. surgical Revascularization (MAIN-COMPARE) multicenter registry, there was a strong trend toward a lower mortality risk with IVUS guidance (6% vs. 13.6%; log rank P = .063; HR, 0.54; 95% CI, 0.28-1.03; Cox-model P = .061) at 3-year follow-up.[157]

Non–Left Main Bifurcation Percutaneous Coronary Intervention

IVUS studies have in general specifically excluded bifurcation segments from the assessment of incomplete stent apposition.[158,159] Little evidence is currently available on bifurcation lesion treatment with IVUS guidance. Costa and associates[160] have analyzed 40 patients with bifurcation lesions who underwent crush stenting with sirolimus-eluting stents under IVUS guidance. Incomplete crushing, defined as incomplete apposition of the SB or main vessel stent struts against the main vessel wall proximal to the carina, was observed in more than 60% of non–left main lesions. The authors concluded that in most bifurcation lesions treated with the crush technique, the smallest minimum stent area appeared at the SB ostium, which contributed to a higher restenosis rate at this location.

Virtual Histology

An IVUS virtual histology (VH) study designed to evaluate the compositional characteristics of atherosclerotic plaque in coronary bifurcations demonstrated that left main–left anterior descending artery bifurcation sites have a greater necrotic core and dense calcium at the bifurcation and distal segments of the bifurcation sites compared with proximal segments. In contrast, bifurcation sites of non–left main coronary arteries showed a greater necrotic core in the proximal segments. Among the non–left main bifurcation sites, the percentage of necrotic core of proximal segments at the left anterior descending artery–diagonal, left circumflex artery–obtuse marginal artery, and right coronary artery–acute marginal artery bifurcation sites were significantly greater than those at the bifurcation or distal segments. However, dense calcium was only greater in the proximal segments at the right coronary artery–acute marginal artery bifurcation sites than in those at the bifurcation and distal segments. These results might be attributed to different anatomic locations and other factors, such as shear stress and the vessel structure of the bifurcation sites. The data suggest a heterogeneous, nonuniform distribution of atherosclerotic plaques between left main–left anterior descending artery and non–left main bifurcation sites.[161]

In a study of 103 bifurcations from 30 patients imaged with both IVUS-VH and optical coherence tomography (OCT), the amount of necrotic core was higher at the proximal rim of the ostium of the SB; a thin fibrous cap was also identified more often in the proximal rim. The percentage of necrotic core decreased from the proximal to distal rim (16.8% vs. 13.5%, respectively; $P = .01$), whereas the cap thickness showed an inverse tendency (130 ± 105 μm vs. 151 ± 68 μm for the proximal and distal rims, respectively; $P = .05$). The thin caps were more often located in the proximal rim (15 of 34; 44.1%), followed by the in-bifurcation segment (14 of 34; 41.2%), and were less frequent in the distal rim (5 of 34; 14.7%).[45]

OPTICAL COHERENCE TOMOGRAPHY

OCT has emerged as a technologic breakthrough in the field of intracoronary imaging by providing high-resolution in vivo images with almost histologic detail. Coronary OCT consists of a fiberoptic wire that emits light in the near-infrared spectrum (1.250 to 1.350 nm); it records reflected light signals while rotating and being simultaneously pulled back along the long axis of a coronary vessel.[162] In a substudy of Optical Coherence Tomography for Drug-Eluting Stent Safety (ODESSA), a prospective randomized trial designed to evaluate the healing of overlapped DES versus BMSs, bifurcation segments with SB diameters more than 1.5 mm by angiography were analyzed and demonstrated a variable pattern of strut coverage among the different types of stents used.[163] In total, there were 12,656 struts in 61 bifurcation segments from 46 patients obtained at 6 months. Paclitaxel-eluting stents had the highest rate of uncovered struts in the SB ostium (paclitaxel-eluting stents, 60.1%; sirolimus-eluting stents, 17.0%; zotarolimus-eluting stents, 13.2%; BMS, 12.3%; $P < .0001$), whereas sirolimus-eluting stents demonstrated the highest rate of uncovered struts opposite to the ostium (paclitaxel-eluting stents, 3.8%; sirolimus-eluting stents, 14.0%; zotarolimus-eluting stents, 1.5%; BMS, 0.0%; $P = .0025$).

In another study, 31 patients underwent T stenting for bifurcation lesions. Of these, 17 patients underwent simple crossover stent implantation (main vessel stenting followed by kissing balloon dilation), whereas 14 underwent more complex reconstruction of the bifurcation using the culotte or T stenting technique. Strut malapposition occurred most frequently at the SB ostium and the use of complex stenting did not significantly increase the prevalence of strut malapposition compared with a simple technique, perhaps because of the use of the kissing balloon technique to ensure improved strut apposition in the latter group.[164]

In summary, OCT studies have demonstrated that malapposed stent struts are found frequently in the region of coronary bifurcations. However, these findings must be analyzed in relation to clinical events, which have not been assessed. If better strut apposition could be achieved with OCT guidance in bifurcation PCI, with a contribution to a decreased incidence of clinical events, then this approach could be recommended for routine use in this setting.

FRACTIONAL FLOW RESERVE

During a provisional strategy in coronary bifurcation stenting, the operator has to decide whether the SB needs further treatment after main vessel stent implantation. The significance of an ostial SB stenosis can be evaluated by visual estimation of angiographic stenosis severity, quantitative coronary analysis, TIMI flow evaluation,

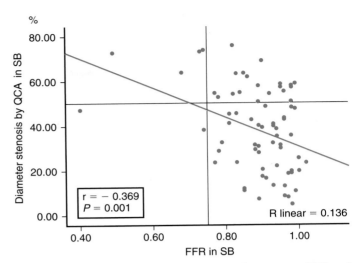

Figure 15-15 Comparison between fractional flow reserve *(FFR)* and angiographic percentage diameter stenosis in jailed side branches *(SB)*. For the most part, SB with angiographically severe narrowings were not physiologically significant according to FFR. *QCA,* Quantitative coronary angiography. (Adapted from Kumsars I, Narbute I, Thuesen L, et al. Side-branch fractional flow reserve measurements after main vessel stenting: a Nordic-Baltic Bifurcation Study III substudy. *EuroIntervention* 2012;7:1155-1161.)

intravascular imaging (IVUS, OCT), and/or FFR. FFR is a stenosis-specific physiologic parameter reflecting the degree of functional significance and the downstream myocardial territory.[165-167] Angiographic stenosis severity of a jailed SB after main vessel stenting is weakly correlated to functional severity as assessed by FFR,[168-171] whereas TIMI flow evaluation has been shown to be effective in identifying SBs with a need for treatment after main vessel stenting.[2,130] Accurate lesion assessment with two-dimensional quantitiative coronary angiography is limited by vessel overlap, foreshortening, and out-of-plane magnification.[172] The SB FFR substudy of Nordic Baltic Bifurcation III trial has suggested that in 75% of cases, angiography overestimates the functional severity of SB lesions after main vessel stenting when applying the more than 50% stenosis limit, and that the functional severity of jailed SB lesions after DES implantation in the main vessel does not change significantly during 8-month follow-up. Figure 15-15 shows the comparison between FFR and angiographic percentage diameter stenosis within the jailed SB of this trial.[173] The discordance between angiographic and functional assessment in part results from difficulties in visualizing ostial lesions in multiple orthogonal views, as well as the fact that such lesions are often very short, reducing the likelihood that they affect blood flow significantly.

A study that tested a strategy of DES placement in the MB, with required kissing balloon angioplasty and provisional treatment of the diseased SB only if the FFR was lower than 0.75, has shown that patients whose treatment has been guided by FFR have excellent outcomes at a median follow-up of 6 months, similar to patients whose SB treatment was guided by angiography. Interestingly, not one patient in the FFR group required a stent in the SB after balloon angioplasty.[168]

The FFR pressure wire is stiffer compared with a floppy wire, and therefore the use of this wire may be difficult to advance into a jailed SB. SB FFR evaluation prolongs the procedure, additional devices such as microcatheters could be needed, and the procedure may lead to complications such as dissections and the need for additional stenting. The data appear to support a strategy to keep the SB open with TIMI 3 flow; FFR-guided treatment of the SB is recommended only in selected cases with an unsatisfactory result even after final kissing balloon treatment. In these patients, FFR may identify the lesions that require reintervention and therefore possibly avoid the use of unnecessarily complex strategies.

Conclusion

Results from randomized trials as well as observational registry data support the contention that stenting of the main vessel and provisional SB stenting should be first-line treatment for most bifurcation lesions. Selective use of IVUS, with or without tissue characterization and/or OCT, may play a role in the selection of optimal techniques and final balloon size. However, the mechanisms of SB restenosis and clinical outcomes of the different two-stent bifurcation stent techniques require further evaluation.

REFERENCES

1. Myler RK, Shaw RE, Stertzer SH, et al. Lesion morphology and coronary angioplasty: current experience and analysis. *J Am Coll Cardiol* 1992;19:1641-1652.
2. Steigen TK, Maeng M, Wiseth R, et al. Randomized study on simple versus complex stenting of coronary artery bifurcation lesions: the Nordic bifurcation study. *Circulation* 2006;114:1955-1961.
3. Meier B, Gruentzig AR, King 3rd SB, et al. Risk of side branch occlusion during coronary angioplasty. *Am J Cardiol* 1984;53:10-14.
4. Oesterle SN. Coronary interventions at a crossroads: the bifurcation stenosis. *J Am Coll Cardiol* 1998;32:1853-1854.
5. Mathias DW, Mooney JF, Lange HW, et al. Frequency of success and complications of coronary angioplasty of a stenosis at the ostium of a branch vessel. *Am J Cardiol* 1991;67:491-495.
6. Brener SJ, Leya FS, Apperson-Hansen C, et al. A comparison of debulking versus dilation of bifurcation coronary arterial narrowings (from the CAVEAT I Trial). Coronary Angioplasty Versus Excisional Atherectomy Trial-I. *Am J Cardiol* 1996;78:1039-1041.
7. Dauerman HL, Higgins PJ, Sparano AM, et al. Mechanical debulking versus balloon angioplasty for the treatment of true bifurcation lesions. *J Am Coll Cardiol* 1998;32:1845-1852.
8. Aliabadi D, Tilli FV, Bowers TR, et al. Incidence and angiographic predictors of side branch occlusion following high-pressure intracoronary stenting. *Am J Cardiol* 1997;80:994-997.
9. Fischman DL, Savage MP, Leon MB, et al. Fate of lesion-related side branches after coronary artery stenting. *J Am Coll Cardiol* 1993;22:1641-1646.
10. Pan M, Medina A, Suarez de Lezo J, et al. Follow-up patency of side branches covered by intracoronary Palmaz-Schatz stent. *Am Heart J* 1995;129:436-440.
11. Al Suwaidi J, Yeh W, Cohen HA, et al. Immediate and one-year outcome in patients with coronary bifurcation lesions in the modern era (NHLBI dynamic registry). *Am J Cardiol* 2001;87:1139-1144.
12. Thuesen L, Kelbaek H, Klovgaard L, et al. Comparison of sirolimus-eluting and bare metal stents in coronary bifurcation lesions: subgroup analysis of the Stenting Coronary Arteries in Non-Stress/Benestent Disease Trial (SCANDSTENT). *Am Heart J* 2006;152:1140-1145.
13. Wijns W, Kolh P, Danchin N, et al. Guidelines on myocardial revascularization: the Task Force on Myocardial Revascularization of the European Society of Cardiology (ESC) and the European Association for Cardio-Thoracic Surgery (EACTS). *Eur Heart J* 2010;31:2501-2555.
14. Nguyen T. *Practical Handbook of Advanced Interventional Cardiology: Tips and Tricks*. Malden, Mass: Blackwell; 2008.
15. Ku DN, Giddens DP, Zarins CK, et al. Pulsatile flow and atherosclerosis in the human carotid bifurcation: positive correlation between plaque location and low oscillating shear stress. *Arteriosclerosis* 1985;5:293-302.
16. Friedman MH, Bargeron CB, Deters OJ, et al. Correlation between wall shear and intimal thickness at a coronary artery branch. *Atherosclerosis* 1987;68:27-33.
17. Soulis JV, Giannoglou GD, Chatzizisis YS, et al. Spatial and phasic oscillation of non-Newtonian wall shear stress in human left coronary artery bifurcation: an insight to atherogenesis. *Coron Artery Dis* 2006;17:351-358.
18. Toggweiler S, Urbanek N, Schoenenberger AW, et al. Analysis of coronary bifurcations by intravascular ultrasound and virtual histology. *Atherosclerosis* 2010;212:524-527.
19. Svindland A. The localization of sudanophilic and fibrous plaques in the main left coronary bifurcation. *Atherosclerosis* 1983;48:139-145.
20. Grottum P, Svindland A, Walloe L. Localization of atherosclerotic lesions in the bifurcation of the main left coronary artery. *Atherosclerosis* 1983;47:55-62.
21. Fox B, James K, Morgan B, et al. Distribution of fatty and fibrous plaques in young human coronary arteries. *Atherosclerosis* 1982;41:337-347.
22. Oviedo C, Maehara A, Mintz GS, et al. Intravascular ultrasound classification of plaque distribution in left main coronary artery bifurcations: where is the plaque really located? *Circ Cardiovasc Interv* 2010;3:105-112.
23. Colombo A, Al-Lamee R. Bifurcation lesions: an inside view. *Circ Cardiovasc Interv* 2010;3:94-96.
24. Medina A, Martin P, Suarez de Lezo J, et al. Vulnerable carina anatomy and ostial lesions in the left anterior descending coronary artery after floating-stent treatment. *Rev Esp Cardiol* 2009;62:1240-1249.
25. Nakazawa G, Yazdani SK, Finn AV, et al. Pathological findings at bifurcation lesions: the impact of flow distribution on atherosclerosis and arterial healing after stent implantation. *J Am Coll Cardiol* 2010;55:1679-1687.
26. van der Giessen AG, Wentzel JJ, Meijboom WB, et al. Plaque and shear stress distribution in human coronary bifurcations: a multislice computed tomography study. *EuroIntervention* 2009;4:654-661.
27. Giannoglou GD, Antoniadis AP, Koskinas KC, et al. Flow and atherosclerosis in coronary bifurcations. *EuroIntervention* 2010;6(Suppl):J16-J23.
28. Feldman CL, Stone PH. Intravascular hemodynamic factors responsible for progression of coronary atherosclerosis and development of vulnerable plaque. *Curr Opin Cardiol* 2000;15:430-440.
29. Papaioannou TG, Karatzis EN, Vavuranakis M, et al. Assessment of vascular wall shear stress and implications for atherosclerotic disease. *Int J Cardiol* 2006;113:12-18.
30. Malek AM, Alper SL, Izumo S. Hemodynamic shear stress and its role in atherosclerosis. *Jama* 1999;282:2035-2042.
31. Stone PH, Coskun AU, Yeghiazarians Y, et al. Prediction of sites of coronary atherosclerosis progression: in vivo profiling of endothelial shear stress, lumen, and outer vessel wall characteristics to predict vascular behavior. *Curr Opin Cardiol* 2003;18:458-470.
32. Gimbrone Jr MA, Topper JN, Nagel T, et al. Endothelial dysfunction, hemodynamic forces, and atherogenesis. *Ann N Y Acad Sci* 2000;902:230-239.
33. Ku DN. Blood flow in arteries. *Annu Rev Fluid Mech* 1997;29:399-434.
34. Nagel T, Resnick N, Dewey Jr CF, et al. Vascular endothelial cells respond to spatial gradients in fluid shear stress by enhanced activation of transcription factors. *Arterioscler Thromb Vasc Biol* 1999;19:1825-1834.
35. Giannoglou GD, Soulis JV, Farmakis TM, et al. Haemodynamic factors and the important role of local low static pressure in coronary wall thickening. *Int J Cardiol* 2002;86:27-40.
36. Buchanan JR Jr, Kleinstreuer C, Truskey GA, et al. Relation between non-uniform hemodynamics and sites of altered permeability and lesion growth at the rabbit aorto-celiac junction. *Atherosclerosis* 1999;143:27-40.
37. Sharma SK, Sweeny J, Kini AS. Coronary bifurcation lesions: a current update. *Cardiol Clin* 2010;28:55-70.
38. Richter Y, Groothuis A, Seifert P, et al. Dynamic flow alterations dictate leukocyte adhesion and response to endovascular interventions. *J Clin Invest* 2004;113:1607-1614.
39. Moses JW, Leon MB, Popma JJ, et al. Sirolimus-eluting stents versus standard stents in patients with stenosis in a native coronary artery. *N Engl J Med* 2003;349:1315-1323.
40. Chatzizisis YS, Coskun AU, Jonas M, et al. Role of endothelial shear stress in the natural history of coronary atherosclerosis and vascular remodeling: molecular, cellular, and vascular behavior. *J Am Coll Cardiol* 2007;49:2379-2393.
41. Gambillara V, Chambaz C, Montorzi G, et al. Plaque-prone hemodynamics impair endothelial function in pig carotid arteries. *Am J Physiol Heart Circ Physiol* 2006;290:H2320-H2328.
42. Cheng C, van Haperen R, de Waard M, et al. Shear stress affects the intracellular distribution of eNOS: direct demonstration by a novel in vivo technique. *Blood* 2005;106:3691-3698.
43. Ziegler T, Bouzourene K, Harrison VJ, et al. Influence of oscillatory and unidirectional flow environments on the expression of endothelin and nitric oxide synthase in cultured endothelial cells. *Arterioscler Thromb Vasc Biol* 1998;18:686-692.
44. Qiu Y, Tarbell JM. Interaction between wall shear stress and circumferential strain affects endothelial cell biochemical production. *J Vasc Res* 2000;37:147-157.
45. Gonzalo N, Garcia-Garcia HM, Regar E, et al. In vivo assessment of high-risk coronary plaques at bifurcations with combined intravascular ultrasound and optical coherence tomography. *JACC Cardiovasc Imaging* 2009;2:473-482.
46. Stone PH, Coskun AU, Kinlay S, et al. Effect of endothelial shear stress on the progression of coronary artery disease, vascular remodeling, and in-stent restenosis in humans: in vivo 6-month follow-up study. *Circulation* 2003;108:438-444.
47. Slager CJ, Wentzel JJ, Schuurbiers JC, et al. True 3-dimensional reconstruction of coronary arteries in patients by fusion of angiography and IVUS (ANGUS) and its quantitative validation. *Circulation* 2000;102:511-516.
48. Giannoglou GD, Chatzizisis YS, Sianos G, et al. In-vivo validation of spatially correct three-dimensional reconstruction of human coronary arteries by integrating intravascular ultrasound and biplane angiography. *Coron Artery Dis* 2006;17:533-543.
49. Chatzizisis YS, Giannoglou GD, Matakos A, et al. In-vivo accuracy of geometrically correct three-dimensional reconstruction of human coronary arteries: is it influenced by certain parameters? *Coron Artery Dis* 2006;17:545-551.
50. Coskun AU, Yeghiazarians Y, Kinlay S, et al. Reproducibility of coronary lumen, plaque, and vessel wall reconstruction and of endothelial shear stress measurements in vivo in humans. *Catheter Cardiovasc Interv* 2003;60:67-78.
51. Stone PH, Coskun AU, Kinlay S, et al. Regions of low endothelial shear stress are the sites where coronary plaque progresses and vascular remodeling occurs in humans: an in vivo serial study. *Eur Heart J* 2007;28:705-710.
52. Wentzel JJ, Corti R, Fayad ZA, et al. Does shear stress modulate both plaque progression and regression in the thoracic aorta? Human study using serial magnetic resonance imaging. *J Am Coll Cardiol* 2005;45:846-854.
53. Jorgensen E, Helqvist S. Stent treatment of coronary artery bifurcation lesions. *Eur Heart J* 2007;28:383-385.
54. Louvard Y, Thomas M, Dzavik V, et al. Classification of coronary artery bifurcation lesions and treatments: time for a consensus! *Catheter Cardiovasc Interv* 2008;71:175-183.
55. Finet G, Huo Y, Rioufol G, et al. Structure-function relation in the coronary artery tree: from fluid dynamics to arterial bifurcations. *EuroIntervention* 2010;6(Suppl):J10-J15.
56. Murray CD. The physiological principle of minimum work: I. The vascular system and the cost of blood volume. *Proc Natl Acad Sci U S A* 1926;12:207-214.
57. Zhou Y, Kassab GS, Molloi S. On the design of the coronary arterial tree: a generalization of Murray's law. *Phys Med Biol* 1999;44:2929-2945.
58. Zhou Y, Kassab GS, Molloi S. In vivo validation of the design rules of the coronary arteries and their application in the assessment of diffuse disease. *Phys Med Biol* 2002;47:977-993.
59. Kassab GS. Design of coronary circulation: a minimum energy hypothesis. *Comput Methods Appl Mech Engrg* 2007;196:3033-3042.
60. Huo Y, Kassab GS. A scaling law of vascular volume. *Biophys J* 2009;96:347-353.
61. Finet G, Gilard M, Perrenot B, et al. Fractal geometry of arterial coronary bifurcations: a quantitative coronary angiography and intravascular ultrasound analysis. *EuroIntervention* 2008;3:490-498.
62. Guerin P, Pilet P, Finet G, et al. Drug-eluting stents in bifurcations: bench study of strut deformation and coating lesions. *Circ Cardiovasc Interv* 2010;3:120-126.
63. Lefevre T, Louvard Y, Morice MC, et al. Stenting of bifurcation lesions: classification, treatments, and results. *Catheter Cardiovasc Interv* 2000;49:274-283.
64. Medina A, Suarez de Lezo J, Pan M. [A new classification of coronary bifurcation lesions.] *Rev Esp Cardiol* 2006;59:183.
65. Todaro D, Burzotta F, Trani C, et al. Evaluation of a strategy for treating bifurcated lesions by single or double stenting based on the Medina classification. *Rev Esp Cardiol* 2009;62:606-614.
66. Medina A, Suarez de Lezo J. Percutaneous coronary intervention in bifurcation lesions: does classification aid treatment selection? *Rev Esp Cardiol* 2009;62:595-598.
67. Movahed MR, Stinis CT. A new proposed simplified classification of coronary artery bifurcation lesions and bifurcation interventional techniques. *J Invasive Cardiol* 2006;18:199-204.
68. Sanborn TA. Bifurcation classification schemes: impact of lesion morphology on development of a treatment strategy. *Rev Cardiovasc Med* 2010;11(Suppl 1):S11-S16.
69. Movahed MR. B2 lesions are true bifurcation lesions simply categorized as one group according to the Movahed bifurcation classification. *J Invasive Cardiol* 2010;22:252.
70. Movahed MR, Kern K, Thai H, et al. Coronary artery bifurcation lesions: a review and update on classification and interventional techniques. *Cardiovasc Revasc Med* 2008;9:263-268.
71. Movahed MR. Coronary artery bifurcation lesion classifications, interventional techniques and clinical outcome. *Expert Rev Cardiovasc Ther* 2008;6:261-274.
72. Latib A, Colombo A. Bifurcation disease: what do we know, what should we do? *JACC Cardiovasc Interv* 2008;1:218-226.
73. Latib A, Colombo A, Sangiorgi GM. Bifurcation stenting: current strategies and new devices. *Heart* 2009;95:495-504.
74. Brunel P, Lefevre T, Darremont O, et al. Provisional T-stenting and kissing balloon in the treatment of coronary bifurcation lesions: results of the French multicenter "TULIPE" study. *Catheter Cardiovasc Interv* 2006;68:67-73.
75. Colombo A, Stankovic G, eds. *Problem-oriented approaches in interventional cardiology*. London: Informa Healthcare; 2007.

76. Ormiston JA, Currie E, Webster MW, et al. Drug-eluting stents for coronary bifurcations: insights into the crush technique. *Catheter Cardiovasc Interv* 2004;63:332-336.
77. Moussa ID, Colombo A. *Tips and Tricks in Interventional Therapy of Coronary Bifurcation Lesions*. New York: Informa Healthcare; 2010.
78. Latib A, Colombo A, Moussa I, et al. When are two stents needed? Which technique is the best? How to perform? *EuroIntervention* 2010;6(Suppl. J):J81-J87.
79. Saito S, Ikei H, Hosokawa G, et al. Influence of the ratio between radial artery inner diameter and sheath outer diameter on radial artery flow after transradial coronary intervention. *Catheter Cardiovasc Interv* 1999;46:173-178.
80. Colombo A, Stankovic G, Orlic D, et al. Modified T-stenting technique with crushing for bifurcation lesions: immediate results and 30-day outcome. *Catheter Cardiovasc Interv* 2003; 60:145-151.
81. Kobayashi Y, Colombo A, Akiyama T, et al. Modified "T" stenting: a technique for kissing stents in bifurcational coronary lesion. *Catheterization and Cardiovascular Diagnosis* 1998;43: 323-326.
82. Burzotta F, Gwon H-C, Hahn J-Y, et al. Modified T-stenting with intentional protrusion of the side-branch stent within the main vessel stent to ensure ostial coverage and facilitate final kissing balloon: the T-stenting and small protrusion technique (TAP-stenting). Report of bench testing and first clinical Italian-Korean two-centre experience. *Catheter Cardiovasc Interv* 2007;70:75-82.
83. Melikian N, Mario CD. Treatment of bifurcation coronary lesions: a review of current techniques and outcome. *J Interv Cardiol* 2003;16:507-513.
84. Louvard Y, Lefevre T, Morice MC. Percutaneous coronary intervention for bifurcation coronary disease. *Heart* 2004;90: 713-722.
85. Chevalier B, Glatt B, Royer T, et al. Placement of coronary stents in bifurcation lesions by the "culotte" technique. *Am J Cardiol* 1998;82:943-949.
86. Ērglis A, Kumsars I, Niemela M, et al. Randomized comparison of coronary bifurcation stenting with the crush versus the culotte technique using sirolimus eluting stents: the Nordic Stent Technique Study. *Circ Cardiovasc Interv* 2009;2:27-34.
87. Colombo A, Bramucci E, Sacca S, et al. Randomized study of the crush technique versus provisional side-branch stenting in true coronary bifurcations: the CACTUS (Coronary Bifurcations: Application of the Crushing Technique Using Sirolimus-Eluting Stents) study. *Circulation* 2009;119:71-78.
88. Dzavik V, Kharbanda R, Ivanov J, et al. Predictors of long-term outcome after crush stenting of coronary bifurcation lesions: importance of the bifurcation angle. *Am Heart J* 2006;152: 762-769.
89. Ge L, Airoldi F, Iakovou I, et al. Clinical and angiographic outcome after implantation of drug-eluting stents in bifurcation lesions with the crush stent technique: importance of final kissing balloon post-dilation. *J Am Coll Cardiol* 2005;46: 613-620.
90. Ge L, Tsagalou E, Iakovou I, et al. In-hospital and nine-month outcome of treatment of coronary bifurcational lesions with sirolimus-eluting stent. *Am J Cardiol* 2005;95:757-760.
91. Galassi AR, Colombo A, Buchbinder M, et al. Long-term outcomes of bifurcation lesions after implantation of drug-eluting stents with the mini-crush technique. *Catheter Cardiovasc Interv* 2007;69:976-983.
92. Iakovou I, Ge L, Colombo A. Contemporary stent treatment of coronary bifurcations. *J Am Coll Cardiol* 2005;46: 1446-1455.
93. Chen SL, Zhang JJ, Ye F, et al. Study comparing the double kissing (DK) crush with classical crush for the treatment of coronary bifurcation lesions: the DKCRUSH-1 Bifurcation Study with drug-eluting stents. *Eur J Clin Invest* 2008;38:361-371.
94. Chen SL, Santoso T, Zhang JJ, et al. A randomized clinical study comparing double kissing crush with provisional stenting for treatment of coronary bifurcation lesions: results from the DKCRUSH-II (Double Kissing Crush versus Provisional Stenting Technique for Treatment of Coronary Bifurcation Lesions) trial. *J Am Coll Cardiol* 2011;57:914-920.
94a. Chen SL, Xu B, Han YL, et al. Comparison of double kissing crush versus culotte stenting for unprotected distal left main bifurcation lesions. *J Am Col Cardiol* 2013; doi:10.1016/j.jacc. 2013.01.023.
95. Schampaert E, Fort S, Adelman AG, et al. The V-stent: a novel technique for coronary bifurcation stenting. *Catheterization and Cardiovascular Diagnosis* 1996;39:320-326.
96. Sharma SK. Simultaneous kissing drug-eluting stent technique for percutaneous treatment of bifurcation lesions in large-size vessels. *Catheter Cardiovasc Interv* 2005;65:10-16.
97. Hoye A, Iakovou I, Ge L, et al. Long-term outcomes after stenting of bifurcation lesions with the "crush" technique: predictors of an adverse outcome. *J Am Coll Cardiol* 2006;47: 1949-1958.
98. Ge L, Iakovou I, Cosgrave J, et al. Treatment of bifurcation lesions with two stents: one year angiographic and clinical follow up of crush versus T-stenting. *Heart* 2006;92:371-376.
99. Tsuchida K, Colombo A, Lefevre T, et al. The clinical outcome of percutaneous treatment of bifurcation lesions in multivessel coronary artery disease with the sirolimus-eluting stent: insights from the Arterial Revascularization Therapies Study part II (ARTS II). *Eur Heart J* 2007;28:433-442.
100. Yamashita T, Nishida T, Adamian MG, et al. Bifurcation lesions: two stents versus one stent–immediate and follow-up results. *J Am Coll Cardiol* 2000;35:1145-1151.
101. Anzuini A, Briguori C, Rosanio S, et al. Immediate and long-term clinical and angiographic results from Wiktor stent treatment for true bifurcation narrowings. *Am J Cardiol* 2001;88:1246-1250.
102. Al Suwaidi J, Berger PB, Rihal CS, et al. Immediate and long-term outcome of intracoronary stent implantation for true bifurcation lesions. *J Am Coll Cardiol* 2000;35:929-936.
103. Gao Z, Yang YJ, Gao RL. Comparative study of simple versus complex stenting of coronary artery bifurcation lesions in daily practice in Chinese patients. *Clin Cardiol* 2008;31:317-322.
104. Hildick-Smith D, de Belder AJ, Cooter N, et al. Randomized trial of simple versus complex drug-eluting stenting for bifurcation lesions: the British Bifurcation Coronary Study: old, new, and evolving strategies. *Circulation* 2010;121:1235-1243.
105. Ferenc M, Gick M, Kienzle RP, et al. Randomized trial on routine vs. provisional T-stenting in the treatment of de novo coronary bifurcation lesions. *Eur Heart J* 2008;29:2859-2867.
106. Colombo A, Moses JW, Morice MC, et al. Randomized study to evaluate sirolimus-eluting stents implanted at coronary bifurcation lesions. *Circulation* 2004;109:1244-1249.
107. Pan M, de Lezo JS, Medina A, et al. Rapamycin-eluting stents for the treatment of bifurcated coronary lesions: a randomized comparison of a simple versus complex strategy. *Am Heart J* 2004;148:857-864.
108. Zhang F, Dong L, Ge J. Simple versus complex stenting strategy for coronary artery bifurcation lesions in the drug-eluting stent era: a meta-analysis of randomised trials. *Heart* 2009;95: 1676-1681.
109. Brar SS, Gray WA, Dangas G, et al. Bifurcation stenting with drug-eluting stents: a systematic review and meta-analysis of randomised trials. *EuroIntervention* 2009;5:475-484.
110. Behan MW, Holm NR, Curzen NP, et al. Simple or complex stenting for bifurcation coronary lesions: a patient-level pooled-analysis of the Nordic Bifurcation Study and the British Bifurcation Coronary Study. *Circ Cardiovasc Interv* 2011;4: 57-64.
111. Baber U, Kini AS, Sharma SK. Stenting of complex lesions: an overview. *Nat Rev Cardiol* 2010;7:485-496.
112. Adriaenssens T, Byrne RA, Dibra A, et al. Culotte stenting technique in coronary bifurcation disease: angiographic follow-up using dedicated quantitative coronary angiographic analysis and 12-month clinical outcomes. *Eur Heart J* 2008; 29:2868-2876.
113. Tsuchikane E, Aizawa T, Tamai H, et al. Pre-drug-eluting stent debulking of bifurcated coronary lesions. *J Am Coll Cardiol* 2007;50:1941-1945.
114. Ērglis A. *Arterial scoring: cosmetic or curative. Presented at the meeting of Transcatheter Cardiovascular Therapeutics*. San Francisco, September 21-25, 2009.
115. Chieffo A, Stankovic G, Bonizzoni E, et al. Early and mid-term results of drug-eluting stent implantation in unprotected left main. *Circulation* 2005;111:791-795.
116. Kim YH, Dangas GD, Solinas E, et al. Effectiveness of drug-eluting stent implantation for patients with unprotected left main coronary artery stenosis. *Am J Cardiol* 2008;101: 801-806.
117. Meliga E, Garcia-Garcia HM, Valgimigli M, et al. Longest available clinical outcomes after drug-eluting stent implantation for unprotected left main coronary artery disease: the DELFT (Drug Eluting stent for LeFT main) Registry. *J Am Coll Cardiol* 2008;51:2212-2219.
118. Palmerini T, Marzocchi A, Marrozzini C, et al. Preprocedural levels of C-reactive protein and leukocyte counts predict 9-month mortality after coronary angioplasty for the treatment of unprotected left main coronary artery stenosis. *Circulation* 2005;112:2332-2338.
119. Park SJ, Kim YH, Lee BK, et al. Sirolimus-eluting stent implantation for unprotected left main coronary artery stenosis: comparison with bare metal stent implantation. *J Am Coll Cardiol* 2005;45:351-356.
120. Seung KB, Park DW, Kim YH, et al. Stents versus coronary-artery bypass grafting for left main coronary artery disease. *N Engl J Med* 2008;358:1781-1792.
121. Palmerini T, Marzocchi A, Tamburino C, et al. Impact of bifurcation technique on 2-year clinical outcomes in 773 patients with distal unprotected left main coronary artery stenosis treated with drug-eluting stents. *Circ Cardiovasc Interv* 2008;1: 185-192.
122. Pan M, Suarez de Lezo J, Medina A, et al. Simple and complex stent strategies for bifurcated coronary arterial stenosis involving the side branch origin. *Am J Cardiol* 1999;83: 1320-1325.
123. Rux S, Sonntag S, Schulze R, et al. Acute and long-term results of bifurcation stenting (from the Coroflex Registry). *Am J Cardiol* 2006;98:1214-1217.
124. Garot P, Lefevre T, Savage M, et al. Nine-month outcome of patients treated by percutaneous coronary interventions for bifurcation lesions in the recent era: a report from the Prevention of Restenosis with Tranilast and its Outcomes (PRESTO) trial. *J Am Coll Cardiol* 2005;46:606-612.
125. Wilensky RL, Selzer F, Johnston J, et al. Relation of percutaneous coronary intervention of complex lesions to clinical outcomes (from the NHLBI Dynamic Registry). *Am J Cardiol* 2002;90:216-221.
126. Brilakis ES, Lasala JM, Cox DA, et al. Two-year outcomes after utilization of the TAXUS paclitaxel-eluting stent in bifurcations and multivessel stenting in the ARRIVE registries. *J Interv Cardiol* 2011;24:342-350.
127. Yeo KK, Mahmud E, Armstrong EJ, et al. Contemporary clinical characteristics, treatment, and outcomes of angiographically confirmed coronary stent thrombosis: results from a multicenter California registry. *Catheter Cardiovasc Interv* 2012;79:550-556.
128. Sheiban I, Albiero R, Marsico F, et al. Immediate and long-term results of "T" stenting for bifurcation coronary lesions. *Am J Cardiol* 2000;85:1141-1144.
129. Tanabe K, Hoye A, Lemos PA, et al. Restenosis rates following bifurcation stenting with sirolimus-eluting stents for de novo narrowings. *Am J Cardiol* 2004;94:115-118.
130. Niemela M, Kervinen K, Ērglis A, et al. Randomized comparison of final kissing balloon dilation versus no final kissing balloon dilation in patients with coronary bifurcation lesions treated with main vessel stenting: the Nordic-Baltic Bifurcation Study III. *Circulation* 2011;123:79-86.
131. Capodanno D, Tamburino C, Sangiorgi GM, et al. Impact of drug-eluting stents and diabetes mellitus in patients with coronary bifurcation lesions: a survey from the Italian Society of Invasive Cardiology. *Circ Cardiovasc Interv* 2011;4:72-79.
132. Vigna C, Biondi-Zoccai G, Amico CM, et al. Provisional T-drug-eluting stenting technique for the treatment of bifurcation lesions: clinical, myocardial scintigraphy and (late) coronary angiographic results. *J Invasive Cardiol* 2007;19: 92-97.
133. Jim MH, Ho HH, Chan AO, et al. Stenting of coronary bifurcation lesions by using modified crush technique with double kissing balloon inflation (sleeve technique): immediate procedure result and short-term clinical outcomes. *Catheter Cardiovasc Interv* 2007;69:969-975.
134. Iakovou I, Schmidt T, Bonizzoni E, et al. Incidence, predictors, and outcome of thrombosis after successful implantation of drug-eluting stents. *JAMA* 2005;293:2126-2130.
135. Poerner TC, Kralev S, Voelker W, et al. Natural history of small and medium-sized side branches after coronary stent implantation. *Am Heart J* 2002;143:627-635.
136. Mazur W, Grinstead WC, Hakim AH, et al. Fate of side branches after intracoronary implantation of the Gianturco-Roubin flex-stent for acute or threatened closure after percutaneous transluminal coronary angioplasty. *Am J Cardiol* 1994; 74:1207-1210.
137. Lansky AJ, Yaqub M, Smith Jr RS, et al. Side branch occlusion with everolimus-eluting and paclitaxel-eluting stents: three-year results from the SPIRIT III randomised trial. *EuroIntervention* 2010;6(Suppl):J44-J52.
138. Colombo A, Latib A. The artisan approach for stenting bifurcation lesions. *JACC Cardiovasc Interv* 2010;3:66-67.
139. Sonoda S, Morino Y, Ako J, et al. Impact of final stent dimensions on long-term results following sirolimus-eluting stent implantation: serial intravascular ultrasound analysis from the sirius trial. *J Am Coll Cardiol* 2004;43:1959-1963.
140. Fujii K, Mintz GS, Kobayashi Y, et al. Contribution of stent underexpansion to recurrence after sirolimus-eluting stent implantation for in-stent restenosis. *Circulation* 2004;109: 1085-1088.
141. Stankovic G, Darremont O, Ferenc M, et al. Percutaneous coronary intervention for bifurcation lesions: 2008 consensus document from the fourth meeting of the European Bifurcation Club. *EuroIntervention* 2009;5:39-49.
142. Hermiller JB. Bifurcation intervention: keep it simple. *J Invasive Cardiol* 2006;18:43-44.
143. Balbi M, Bezante GP, Brunelli C, et al. Guide wire fracture during percutaneous transluminal coronary angioplasty: possible causes and management. *Interact Cardiovasc Thorac Surg* 2010;10:992-994.
144. Virmani R, Guagliumi G, Farb A, et al. Localized hypersensitivity and late coronary thrombosis secondary to a sirolimus-eluting stent: should we be cautious? *Circulation* 2004;109: 701-705.
145. de la Torre Hernandez JM, Alfonso F, Gimeno F, et al. Thrombosis of second-generation drug-eluting stents in real practice results from the multicenter Spanish registry ESTROFA-2 (Estudio Espanol Sobre Trombosis de Stents Farmacoactivos de Segunda Generacion-2). *JACC Cardiovasc Interv* 2010;3: 911-919.
146. Baran KW, Lasala JM, Cox DA, et al. A clinical risk score for the prediction of very late stent thrombosis in drug eluting stent patients. *EuroIntervention* 2011;6:949-954.
147. Finn AV, Joner M, Nakazawa G, et al. Pathological correlates of late drug-eluting stent thrombosis: strut coverage as a marker of endothelialization. *Circulation* 2007;115:2435-2441.
148. Joner M, Finn AV, Farb A, et al. Pathology of drug-eluting stents in humans: delayed healing and late thrombotic risk. *J Am Coll Cardiol* 2006;48:193-202.
149. Kim JS, Hong MK, Fan C, et al. Intracoronary thrombus formation after drug-eluting stents implantation: optical coherence tomographic study. *Am Heart J* 2010;159:278-283.
150. Li S, Wang Y, Gai L, et al. Evaluation of neointimal coverage and apposition with various drug-eluting stents over 12 months after implantation by optical coherence tomography. *Int J Cardiol* 2013;162:166-171.

151. Kim JS, Kim JS, Shin DH, et al. Optical coherence tomographic comparison of neointimal coverage between sirolimus- and resolute zotarolimus-eluting stents at 9 months after stent implantation. *Int J Cardiovasc Imaging* 2012;28:1281-1287.

152. Abizaid A, de Ribamar Costa Jr J, et al. Bifurcated stents: giving to Caesar what is Caesar's. *EuroIntervention* 2007;2:518-525.

153. Furukawa E, Hibi K, Kosuge M, et al. Intravascular ultrasound predictors of side branch occlusion in bifurcation lesions after percutaneous coronary intervention. *Circ J* 2005;69:325-330.

154. Hahn JY, Song YB, Lee SY, et al. Serial intravascular ultrasound analysis of the main and side branches in bifurcation lesions treated with the T-stenting technique. *J Am Coll Cardiol* 2009;54:110-117.

155. Kim SH, Kim YH, Kang SJ, et al. Long-term outcomes of intravascular ultrasound-guided stenting in coronary bifurcation lesions. *Am J Cardiol* 2010;106:612-618.

156. Jasti V, Ivan E, Yalamanchili V, et al. Correlations between fractional flow reserve and intravascular ultrasound in patients with an ambiguous left main coronary artery stenosis. *Circulation* 2004;110:2831-2836.

157. Park SJ, Kim YH, Park DW, et al. Impact of intravascular ultrasound guidance on long-term mortality in stenting for unprotected left main coronary artery stenosis. *Circ Cardiovasc Interv* 2009;2:167-177.

158. Cook S, Wenaweser P, Togni M, et al. Incomplete stent apposition and very late stent thrombosis after drug-eluting stent implantation. *Circulation* 2007;115:2426-2434.

159. Kimura M, Mintz GS, Carlier S, et al. Outcome after acute incomplete sirolimus-eluting stent apposition as assessed by serial intravascular ultrasound. *Am J Cardiol* 2006;98:436-442.

160. Costa RA, Mintz GS, Carlier SG, et al. Bifurcation coronary lesions treated with the "crush" technique: an intravascular ultrasound analysis. *J Am Coll Cardiol* 2005;46:599-605.

161. Han SH, Puma J, Garcia-Garcia HM, et al. Tissue characterisation of atherosclerotic plaque in coronary artery bifurcations: an intravascular ultrasound radiofrequency data analysis in humans. *EuroIntervention* 2010;6:313-320.

162. Bezerra HG, Costa MA, Guagliumi G, et al. Intracoronary optical coherence tomography: a comprehensive review clinical and research applications. *JACC Cardiovasc Interv* 2009;2:1035-1046.

163. Kyono H, Guagliumi G, Sirbu V, et al. Optical coherence tomography (OCT) strut-level analysis of drug-eluting stents (DES) in human coronary bifurcations. *EuroIntervention* 2010;6:69-77.

164. Tyczynski P, Ferrante G, Moreno-Ambroj C, et al. Simple versus complex approaches to treating coronary bifurcation lesions: direct assessment of stent strut apposition by optical coherence tomography. *Rev Esp Cardiol* 2010;63:904-914.

165. Pijls NH, van Son JA, Kirkeeide RL, et al. Experimental basis of determining maximum coronary, myocardial, and collateral blood flow by pressure measurements for assessing functional stenosis severity before and after percutaneous transluminal coronary angioplasty. *Circulation* 1993;87:1354-1367.

166. Pijls NH, De Bruyne B, Peels K, et al. Measurement of fractional flow reserve to assess the functional severity of coronary-artery stenoses. *N Engl J Med* 1996;334:1703-1708.

167. De Bruyne B, Bartunek J, Sys SU, et al. Relation between myocardial fractional flow reserve calculated from coronary pressure measurements and exercise-induced myocardial ischemia. *Circulation* 1995;92:39-46.

168. Koo BK, Park KW, Kang HJ, et al. Physiological evaluation of the provisional side-branch intervention strategy for bifurcation lesions using fractional flow reserve. *Eur Heart J* 2008;29:726-732.

169. Ziaee A, Parham WA, Herrmann SC, et al. Lack of relation between imaging and physiology in ostial coronary artery narrowings. *Am J Cardiol* 2004;93:1404-1407.

170. Koo BK, Kang HJ, Youn TJ, et al. Physiologic assessment of jailed side branch lesions using fractional flow reserve. *J Am Coll Cardiol* 2005;46:633-637.

171. Koo BK, Waseda K, Kang HJ, et al. Anatomic and functional evaluation of bifurcation lesions undergoing percutaneous coronary intervention. *Circ Cardiovasc Interv* 2010;3:113-119.

172. Green NE, Chen SY, Hansgen AR, et al. Angiographic views used for percutaneous coronary interventions: a three-dimensional analysis of physician-determined vs. computer-generated views. *Catheter Cardiovasc Interv* 2005;64:451-459.

173. Kumsars I, Narbute I, Thuesen L, et al. Side branch fractional flow reserve measurements after main vessel stenting: a Nordic-Baltic Bifurcation Study III substudy. *EuroIntervention* 2012;7:1155-11561.

174. Chen SL, Louvard Y, Runlin G. Perspective on bifurcation PCI. *J Interv Cardiol* 2009;22:99-109.

CHAPTER 16

Chronic Total Occlusions

J. AARON GRANTHAM | **WILLIAM L. LOMBARDI** | **DAVID DANIELS**

KEY POINTS

- Chronic total occlusions (CTOs) are identified in as many as 18% of coronary angiograms, but CTOs account for only 5% of percutaneous coronary interventions (PCIS) in the United States.

- Key barriers to PCI of CTOs include lower success rates, longer procedure time, and lack of clarity regarding clinical benefit.

- Potential mechanisms of clinical benefit from CTO revascularization include improvement in angina, relief of significant ischemia burden, prevention of ventricular arrhythmias, and complete revascularization.

- Procedural planning, including fastidious diagnostic angiography, proper vascular access and guide selection, and appropriate procedural anticoagulation, are key elements of successful CTO-PCI.

- An approach to crossing the CTO segment successfully with a hybrid strategy to PCI-CTO—identification of a primary anterograde or retrograde approach from the outset and rapid switching from one approach to the other as needed—requires a specific set of coronary wires and microcatheters and knowledge of specific techniques that are not used during, and are at times antithetical to, traditional PCI.

- The skill set for the hybrid approach can be acquired through mentoring relationships and educational resources (e.g., www.CTOFundamentals.org).

Coronary chronic total occlusions (CTOs) are commonly encountered complex lesions that are most frequently treated with medical therapy or surgical revascularization rather than with percutaneous coronary intervention (PCI).[1] A renewed interest in CTO-PCI has emerged from the development of novel techniques and technologic advances that have improved procedural success and procedural efficiency, in combination with a growing evidence base supporting its potential clinical benefit. In this chapter, we review the barriers to, indications for, and benefits of CTO-PCI and provide an overview of the advances responsible for the reemergence of PCI as a viable strategy for revascularization in this patient subset.

Background

A coronary CTO is defined as a 100% occlusion with thrombolysis in myocardial infarction (TIMI) grade 0 flow for at least 3 months. These complex lesions are found in 18% of patients with significant coronary artery disease at angiography; evidence of myocardial infarction in the territory subtended by the CTO is present in only 25% of cases.[2] Despite this frequent finding, only 13.7% of eligible CTOs are treated with PCI,[3] and CTOs account for only 5% of interventions in the United States.[4] The disparity in treatment selection observed among patients with a CTO as compared with those without a CTO in the Bypass Angioplasty Revascularization Investigation (BARI) Registry suggests that CTOs are preferentially treated with medical therapy or surgical revascularization rather than with PCI.[1] However, the benefits of CTO-PCI appear comparable to those of surgical revascularization and medical therapy. Successful durable revascularization may be more likely with CTO-PCI than coronary artery bypass grafting (CABG), in which 1-year saphenous vein graft patency rates have been reported to be as low as 23%.[5] Nonetheless, substantial barriers to CTO-PCI adoption persist.

BARRIERS TO CTO-PCI

Barriers to the adoption of CTO-PCI include lack of clarity regarding long-term clinical benefit, concerns over increased complication rates, low success rates, and long procedure times. Over the past decade, there has been substantial growth in the evidence base regarding the quality and quantity of life after CTO-PCI, procedural safety compared with non–CTO-PCI, success rates, and procedural efficiency.

Quality of Life

PCI was shown to be superior to medical therapy in reducing patient reported angina frequency and quality of life, even in a population of patients with a high prevalence of only mild ischemia.[6] No prospective randomized trial has compared patient-reported health status after PCI or optimal medical therapy for the treatment of CTO. Several observational studies have demonstrated that angina-free survival after successful CTO-PCI is superior to that after failed CTO-PCI. In a meta-analysis of 13 observational studies encompassing 7288 patients over an average of 6 years of follow-up, successful recanalization was associated with a significant reduction in residual or recurrent angina (odds ratio [OR], 0.45; 95% confidence interval [CI], 0.30-0.67; $P < .01$.)[7] Grantham and colleagues[8] have reported that among symptomatic patients in the FlowCardia Approach to CTO Recanalization (FACTOR) trial, the mean improvement in all three health status domains of the Seattle Angina Questionnaire (angina frequency, physical limitation, and quality of life) were significantly better with successful compared with unsuccessful CTO-PCI. Furthermore, Borgia and associates[9] have reported that at 1 year, angina frequency scores deteriorated by 9 points with a failed CTO-PCI but improved by 30 points with successful CTO-PCI.

During the acquisition of a medical history in patients with CTO, special attention should be paid to the presence or absence of angina-type symptoms. Many patients with chronic obstructive coronary artery disease may accommodate their lifestyle or, because of the chronicity of disease, be less aware of symptoms and are thereby inappropriately considered to be asymptomatic. Patients with CTOs should be informed that fatigue and dyspnea are common angina equivalents, and operators should carefully query spouses and relatives about atypical symptoms that may reflect functional limitations related to the presence of a CTO.

Quantity of Life

A considerable body of evidence suggests that ischemia is associated with adverse cardiovascular events and that reductions in ischemic burden are associated with reductions in mortality.[10-12] In large study of 10,627 patients undergoing adenosine myocardial perfusion stress imaging, revascularization compared with medical therapy had greater survival benefit (absolute and relative) in patients with inducible ischemia involving more than 10% of the total myocardium.[10] In the Clinical Outcomes Utilizing Revascularization and Aggressive Drug Evaluation (COURAGE) nuclear substudy,[11] patients who achieved a more than 5% reduction in ischemic burden with PCI and optimal medical therapy or optimal medical therapy alone had a lower unadjusted risk of death or myocardial infarction, particularly if they displayed moderate or severe ischemia before treatment. PCI and optimal medical therapy provided significantly greater reductions in ischemic burden compared with optimal medical therapy alone. In the Fractional flow reserve versus Angiography for Multivessel Evaluation (FAME) trial, ischemia-driven complete revascularization was associated with superior outcomes compared with angiographically driven complete revascularization.[13]

Ischemia is frequently present among patients with CTO who do not have infarction in the territory subtended by the obstruction, even in the presence of substantial collaterals on angiography.[14] Among patients with a CTO and no Q waves in the territory subtended by the obstruction, the fractional flow reserve (FFR) was less than 0.80 in 107 of 107 cases.[14] As noted in the COURAGE trial, PCI is more effective than medical therapy at reducing ischemia, particularly in those patients with a moderate to large ischemic burden.[11] The International Study of Comparative Health Effectiveness with Medical and Invasive Approaches (ISCHEMIA) trial (clinicaltrials.gov identifier NCT01471522) will examine whether a routine invasive strategy with catheterization followed by revascularization, plus optimal medical therapy, in patients with moderate or severe ischemia on stress imaging is superior to a conservative strategy of optimal medical therapy alone.

In a meta-analysis of observational CTO studies, the hazard for death was significantly lower after successful CTO recanalization compared with failed CTO recanalization (OR, 0.56; 95% CI, 0.43-0.72), thereby suggesting a survival advantage for CTO recanalization.[7] The importance of complete revascularization after PCI with regard to survival has been highlighted by several prospective studies. In an analysis of the New York State's Percutaneous Coronary Interventions Reporting System, incomplete revascularization was a significant predictor of mortality after adjustment for differences in preprocedural risk[15]; patients with two-vessel incomplete revascularization with at least one CTO were the cohort at greatest risk. In patients with ischemic heart disease and implantable cardioverter-defibrillators (ICDs), the presence of a CTO is associated with higher rates of ventricular arrhythmia and mortality and is independently and strongly associated with appropriate ICD intervention.[16] Although speculative, this observation supports the contention that one mechanism of mortality benefit in patients undergoing successful CTO-PCI could be the avoidance of sudden death. CTO-PCI also improves parameters of left ventricular performance,[17] known to be a predictor of mortality.

The 2011 American College of Cardiology Foundation/American Heart Association/Society of Cardiovascular Angiography and Interventions Guideline for PCI stated that PCI of a CTO in patients with appropriate clinical indications and suitable anatomy is reasonable when performed by operators with appropriate expertise (class IIa, level of evidence B).[18] Among patients with CTOs and myocardial viability or ischemia and no symptoms, we believe CTO-PCI can be justified for the potential benefit of a survival advantage as long as the ischemic burden is high (e.g., >10%). This is based on observational data of the benefit of revascularization on short-term mortality rates in this subgroup.[19] The nuances of this recommendation should be clearly communicated to the patient during a detailed informed consent process that should take place in an office environment, not the catheterization laboratory.

Complications of Chronic Total Occlusion Intervention

CTO-PCI is associated with complication rates equal to non–CTO-PCI among highly experienced operators.[3,20,21] Although the risk of perforation with CTO-PCI is higher than with non–CTO-PCI, the rates of tamponade, need for covered stents, and coiling are low. This level of safety can be maintained only if operators are properly trained in CTO-PCI techniques, with an emphasis on knowing when to abort a case and a deep understanding of avoidance maneuvers for complications.

Fundamentals of Percutaneous Coronary Intervention for Chronic Total Occlusions

Techniques and technology have been rapidly evolving over the last decade, with a growing movement of CTO specialists worldwide and in North America. A paradigm shift from the traditional teaching of true lumen PCI to a "by any means necessary" approach began with the introduction of anterograde dissection and reentry by Colombo and colleagues.[22] A major breakthrough in further increasing success rates came with the evolution of retrograde PCI through collateral channels.[23] Current success rates for CTO intervention have reached 90% with the addition of retrograde techniques and dedicated CTO training.[24]

PROCEDURAL PLANNING

Although CTO-PCI can be performed ad hoc after diagnostic angiography, this approach is generally not recommended. The potential risks specific to CTO-PCI should be discussed with the patient so that true informed consent can be obtained. In addition, procedural planning requires careful scrutiny of the diagnostic angiogram to formulate the PCI strategy. An in-depth familiarity with all major collateral routes can help improve procedural efficiency and success. Also, because CTO-PCI procedures are longer than traditional PCI, setting up a CTO day can appropriately set the expectations of the operator, staff, and patient without interrupting the flow of the cardiac catheterization laboratory with a prolonged ad hoc procedure.

Diagnostic Angiography

Well-performed diagnostic coronary angiography is critical to proper CTO-PCI planning. Specific measures should be taken to elucidate the important characteristics of the anatomy fully as soon as the CTO is recognized from the initial injections. Acquisitions should be long enough to allow for full collateral filling of the distal CTO vessel. Two orthogonal views of the proximal CTO cap should be obtained. Injections of the donor artery should be set up to encompass the donor artery, collateral origins, and destination, as well as complete retrograde filling of the occluded vessel, to define the distal cap. The image intensifier and table should be set up to minimize panning, which can degrade the visualization of small communicating collateral channels; often, this may require a lower magnification to increase the field of view. Suggested fluoroscopic angles helpful in demonstrating collateral origin, course, and distal targets are listed in Table 16-1.

Vascular Access and Guide Catheters

Although recanalization of a CTO with a 5-Fr single-access radial approach can be performed, the average success rate for most operators will be lower under those conditions, and extra equipment will be needed for support. Chances for success can be maximized through bilateral access with 8-Fr, 45-cm femoral sheaths, when feasible, to provide extra passive support. The use of 8-Fr guiding catheters that offer back wall support are advantageous because of the available

TABLE 16-1	Suggested Angulations for Common Collateral Angiography			
Artery	Artery	Collateral	Primary Angulation	Secondary Angulation
LAD	PDA	Septal-septal	RAO cranial	RAO caudal
LAD	PDA	Apical epicardial	LAO caudal	LAO/AP cranial
LCX	RCA	AV groove epicardial	LAO cranial	RAO caudal
OM	Diagonal	Epicardial	RAO caudal	LAO cranial

AP, Anteroposterior; *AV,* atrioventricular; *LAD,* left anterior descending; *LAO,* left anterior oblique; *LCX,* left circumflex; *OM,* obtuse marginal; *PDA,* posterior descending artery; *RAO,* right anterior oblique; *RCA,* right coronary artery.

BOX 16-1   KEY POINTS FOR VASCULAR ACCESS AND GUIDING CATHETER SELECTION IN PCI FOR CHRONIC TOTAL OCCLUSIONS

- Strong consideration for 8-Fr guide catheters
- Bilateral 8-Fr, 45-cm sheaths to improve support
- Side holes for the anterograde guide
- Short (90-cm) length for retrograde guide (donor vessel)
- No side holes for retrograde guide
- Access, guide consistency: anterograde from right femoral, retrograde from left femoral
- Use of a plunger-type hemostatic valve
- Avoid power injectors
- Unfractionated heparin for procedural anticoagulation
- Goal: activated clotting time of >300 seconds

TABLE 16-2   Japanese Chronic Total Occlusion Scoring System* for Probability of Anterograde Guidewire Success

CTO Score	Success in <30 min (%)
0	92.3
1	58.3
2	34.8
>3	22.2

*The Japanese chronic total occlusion score is calculated by the sum of the number of the following characteristics: (1) previously failed lesion; (2) blunt stump; (3) tortuosity (>45 degrees); (4) calcification; and (5) lesion length (>20mm). CTO, Chronic total occlusion.
Adapted from Morino Y, Abe M, Morimoto T, et al. Predicting successful guidewire crossing through chronic total occlusion of native coronary lesions within 30 minutes. JACC Cardiovasc Interv 2011;4:213-221.

options they provide for different strategic approaches, as well as their backup support for device delivery. When contralateral coronary or bypass graft collaterals exist, simultaneous injection from the donor and recipient arteries enables the definition of CTO length and improves procedural success rates. Double-guide injections should be used, even when anterograde collaterals exist, because ipsilateral visualization is often impaired during attempted anterograde PCI. Without a retrograde catheter to opacify the target vessel, the operator is blind to the actual distal wire location, which often leads to loss of procedural momentum and ultimately failure. Retrograde injections are also critical when using anterograde dissection techniques in which forceful anterograde injections can cause hydraulic dissections, compressing the distal lumen and decreasing the probability of successful reentry. Visualization of the target vessel via the retrograde catheter is therefore required when any contralateral collaterals exist. Using a guide, rather than a diagnostic catheter, to opacify the retrograde circulation will not only improve visualization, but also enable rapid switching from anterograde to retrograde during the hybrid strategy to CTO revascularization (Box 16-1).

If the option for retrograde PCI is being considered, a 90-cm guiding catheter should be used for the collateral donor vessel to allow for the adequate delivery of retrograde gear all the way to the anterograde guide, if required. An 8-Fr, 90-cm guide catheter should also be used when collaterals are ipsilateral (e.g., left dominant system with occluded left anterior descending artery and collaterals provided by the left posterior descending artery). Radial access can be used for one or both catheters with high success rates, but this access should be restricted to experienced radial operators.[25,26] Side holes should be avoided for the retrograde guiding catheter, because this can prevent the recognition of deep guide seating while manipulating retrograde gear, which can lead to dissections of the donor vessel or donor vessel ischemia, with disastrous consequences. Y connectors with a nonrotating hemostatic valve, such as the Co-Pilot (Abbott Vascular, Abbott Park, Ill) or Guardian II (Vascular Solutions, Vascular Solutions, Minneapolis, Minn), allow free rotation of CTO-specific over the wire devices, such as the Tornus (Abbot Vascular), Corsair (Abbott Vascular), and CrossBoss (Bridgepoint Medical [Boston Scientific], Natick, Mass), with minimal blood loss and the ability to monitor guide catheter pressure constantly. Power injectors, although useful for improving efficiency and possibly contrast utilization, can be dangerous when injecting into the anterograde guide and can result in hydraulic dissections. Therefore, we think that hand injections, at least for the anterograde guide, should be used when performing CTO procedures.

Procedural Anticoagulation

Patients should be pretreated with aspirin plus a $P2Y_{12}$ receptor antagonist, usually clopidogrel, ideally more than 6 hours before the procedure.[27] We prefer unfractionated heparin for procedural anticoagulation while maintaining the activated clotting time between 300 and 350 seconds. A systematic approach of checking activated clotting time every 30 minutes can help avoid thrombotic complications.

Glycoprotein (GP) IIb/IIIa inhibitors should be avoided, given the inability to reverse them rapidly if a significant coronary perforation occurs. A recent retrospective study of clinical outcomes after coronary perforation has observed that the composite endpoint of in-hospital death, cardiac tamponade, or emergency cardiac surgery after perforation is no higher with bivalirudin than heparin,[28] suggesting that the choice of anticoagulant does not influence outcome when cardiac perforation occurs. Data supporting the use of bivalirudin during CTO intervention, however, are limited.

Strategic Approach to the Chronic Total Occlusion

Contemporary CTO-PCI is constantly evolving, but traditionally, an anterograde wiring approach is attempted first, regardless of lesion characteristics. Although an anterograde approach is the most time-efficient strategy, if successful, a long lesion, blunt stump, calcification, bridging collaterals, and poor distal vessel visualization are predictors of anterograde failure.[21,29-32] A CTO score was derived from the Japanese CTO Registry and has been validated to predict guidewire crossing in less than 30 minutes, primarily during anterograde procedures. This score includes the following variables (1 point each): previously failed lesion, a blunt stump, significant tortuosity, calcification, and lesion length more than 20 mm (Table 16-2).[32]

Mounting evidence has suggested that the addition of anterograde dissection and reentry techniques and the retrograde approach can facilitate efficient procedural success in these challenging lesion subsets.[24,33,34] The next step in this evolution is an algorithmic methodology to procedural planning and execution, termed the *hybrid approach*. In the hybrid approach, anterograde wiring, anterograde dissection and reentry, and retrograde techniques are all used interchangeably as needed to achieve rapid success on the first attempt (Figure 16-1).[35] The key element of the hybrid approach is to establish a base of operations where these multiple techniques can be used to increase success rates and efficiency. Although an initial approach should be selected based on lesion characteristics and operator experience, the ability to implement this algorithm fully can have powerful effects on procedural success and provides a framework for rapid, bailout decision making. Recently, we applied this algorithm to 17 consecutive cases performed over 3 days by five experienced North American CTO operators. Procedural success was 100%, with a mean procedure time of 95 ± 10 minutes. The first strategy was successful in approximately two thirds of cases, whereas one or two bailout strategies were required in the remaining third.[36]

Coronary Wires

Simplifying the inventory to five classes of wires will provide operators with all the tools needed to navigate a CTO successfully, improve operator familiarity with a limited amount of equipment, and is more judicious from an inventory and capital expenditure perspective. The five classes of wires required include the following (Tables 16-3 and 16-4):

1. Soft-tipped, tapered, polymer-jacketed wire (e.g., Fielder XT, Asahi-Intecc, Japan)
2. Soft-tipped, nontapered, polymer-jacketed wire (e.g., Fielder FC, Asahi-Intecc)
3. Stiff-tipped, nontapered, polymer-jacketed wire (e.g., Pilot 200, Abbott Vascular)
4. Stiff-tipped, tapered, unjacketed wire (e.g., Confianza Pro 12, Asahi-Intecc)
5. Externalization wire (e.g., Viperwire Advance, Cardiovascular Systems, St. Paul, Minn; RG3 [Asahi-Intecc] for non-U.S. operators; or R350, Vascular Solutions)

TABLE 16-3	Wires for Successful Percutaneous Coronary Intervention for Chronic Total Occlusion Using Hybrid Approach	
Type of Wire	**Use**	
Polymer-jacketed, soft-tipped, tapered	Probing microchannels, knuckling for subintimal tracking	
Polymer-jacketed, soft-tipped, nontapered	Crossing retrograde collaterals	
Polymer-jacketed, stiff-tipped, nontapered	Tortuous anatomy, knuckling for subintimal tracking	
Unjacketed, stiff-tipped, tapered	Directed puncture, wire-based reentry	
Externalization wire	Retrograde approach	

The Fielder XT can be used to probe for microchannels within the CTO, or it can be used as a knuckle wire to facilitate subintimal tracking. Wires specific to retrograde collateral crossing are nontapered, polymer-jacketed wires, such as the Fielder FC, Whisper, or Pilot 50 and now the Sion (Asahi-Intecc), which is the preferred epicardial collateral crossing wire. The Pilot 200 is useful for crossing the tortuous CTO, and if it enters the subintimal space, it can also be knuckled to allow for subintimal tracking. The Confianza Pro 12 should be used for directed puncture when anatomic ambiguity is minimal or during a wire-based reentry technique.

Anterograde Wiring

Anterograde wiring should be attempted as a first approach when the lesion contains favorable characteristics per the algorithm in Figure 16-1. These are good starter lesions for operators early in their experience with CTO-PCI. A workhorse, spring-coiled wire with a standard working bend is loaded in an over-the-wire balloon catheter or microcatheter. This wire is manipulated to the proximal cap and advanced as far into the occlusion as possible. Occasionally, the workhorse wire will find a microchannel and partly or completely cross the occlusion. These lesions often will be more recent occlusions and morphologically closer to an acute lesion rather than a CTO. Most of the time, the wire will buckle and not advance beyond the proximal cap or shortly within the occlusion segment. At this point, the over-the-wire catheter should be advanced as far as it will go and the workhorse wire removed. The next wire to use is a soft-tipped, polymer-jacketed, tapered wire such as the Fielder XT (Asahi-Intecc). This should be

TABLE 16-4	Specific Characteristics of Wires Suitable for Percutaneous Coronary Intervention for Chronic Total Occlusion						
Wire	**Surface**	**Company**	**Tip Load (gauge)**	**Tip Diameter (inch)**	**Construction**	**Use**	
Fielder XT	Full jacket	Asahi-Intecc	1.2	0.009	Core to tip	Microchannel, knuckle wire	
Fielder FC	Full jacket	Asahi-Intecc	1.6	0.014	Core to tip	Collateral crossing	
Sion	Hydrophilic	Asahi-Intecc	0.7	0.014	Composite double coil core to tip	Epicardial collateral crossing	
Pilot 200	Full jacket	Abbott	4.1	0.014	Core to tip	Tortuous CTO crossing	
Confianza Pro 12	Hybrid	Asahi-Intecc	12	0.009	Core to tip	Unambiguous CTO crossing	
Viper Wire Advance	Hydrophobic	Cardiovascular Systems		0.014	Core to tip	Externalization (335 cm)	

CTO, Chronic total occlusion.

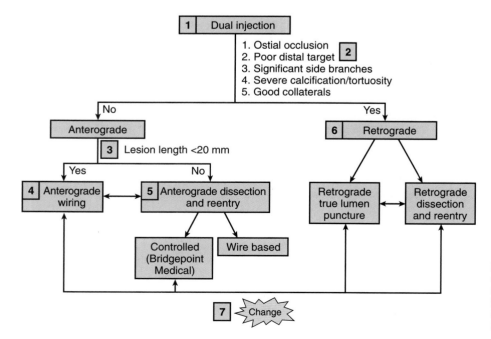

Figure 16-1 Hybrid approach to percutaneous coronary intervention for coronary chronic total occlusions. (Adapted from Brilakis ES, Grantham A, Rinfret S, et al. Percutaneous treatment algorithm for crossing coronary chronic total occlusions. *J Am Coll Cardiol Interv* 2012;5:367-379.)

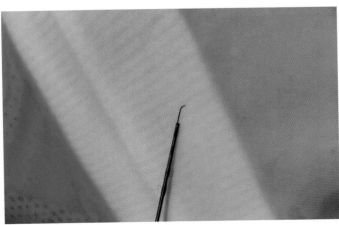

Figure 16-2   Typical wire bend for anterograde wiring approach, 30 to 45 degrees 1 mm from the tip. A secondary bend, 30 degrees 3 to 4 mm from the tip can be added if additional maneuverability is required within the chronic total occlusions.

shaped with a 30- to 45-degree, 1-mm tip by advancing the wire through the introducer needle and compressing it over the end (Figure 16-2). This wire should be manipulated in an attempt to dissect through the occlusion or cross a microchannel into the distal true lumen. As long as steady progress is made toward the distal cap, this wire is used. Advancing the microcatheter or balloon facilitates progress by stiffening the tip of the wire.

If at any time progress stops, the wire is exchanged for one with significantly different characteristics. The choice of the next wire depends on the operator's understanding of the anatomy of the CTO segment. If the occlusion is relatively short and seemingly straight, a heavyweight, high puncture force, CTO-specific crossing wire such as the Confianza Pro 12 (Asahi-Intecc) should be used. Although one could incrementally advance through the Miracle series of wires, starting with the 3- to 12-gauge tip, this approach does not afford any significant safety or efficacy advantage over going directly to the Confianza. In addition, the tapered hydrophobic tip of the Confianza Pro 12 can facilitate entry into a tough proximal cap by catching the cap, especially when the occlusion is at a major side branch.

If the occlusion segment anatomy is unclear or appears tortuous, a jacketed, stiff-tipped wire such as the Pilot 200 (Abbott Vascular) is used. The blunt and jacketed tip is less likely to penetrate the external elastic membrane. If at any time an anterograde wire enters the subintimal space beyond the distal cap, the strategy should be immediately changed to dissection and reentry (see later). Once the wire appears to cross the distal cap, careful confirmation of intraluminal position is critical before continuing. Angiography with filling from the collateral donor vessel should be performed in at least two orthogonal views before the anterograde wire is advanced more than a few millimeters beyond the distal cap. Easy advancement is not a guarantee of an intraluminal position. If distal visualization is poor, a true intraluminal position is more likely if the anterograde wire can make definite engagement of side branches as it is advanced. The over-the-wire catheter should be carefully advanced across the occlusion, with careful attention made to guide support. If a microcatheter was used and will not advance, it should be exchanged for a small-diameter, over-the-wire balloon catheter.[37] Careful, active guide manipulation can improve support to facilitate crossing, but care should be taken as the catheter is advanced to prevent sudden wire advancement or uncrossing of the lesion, causing distal perforation or loss of distal access, respectively. A guide extension (Guideliner, Vascular Solutions) or a side branch–anchoring balloon can enhance support and facilitate crossing. The guide extension can be advanced over a balloon catheter to provide better tracking of the extension through the proximal vessel.[38] Small side branches proximal to the CTO, such as right

ventricular marginal branches, can be wired and an appropriately sized balloon can be inflated within the branch to serve as an anchor. This provides strong support by holding the guiding catheter fixed in place while an over the wire balloon is advanced across the CTO.[38]

If one is still unable to cross, dottering devices such as the Tornus or Corsair catheters (Asahi-Intecc) can be used. The Tornus is available in 2.1 and 2.6 Fr, with the larger device providing the most support. Tornus is often successful when all other combinations of support and balloon catheters have failed.[39] The Tornus is advanced with a counterclockwise rotation and gentle forward pressure. Once the CTO is crossed with an over-the-wire catheter, it is critical to exchange the crossing wire for a spring-coiled, workhorse-type wire. This will prevent distal wire perforation or dissection during subsequent equipment delivery. We recommend using balloon trapping for all over the wire exchanges (see later) to prevent inadvertent wire movement and improve procedural efficiency (Figure 16-3). Balloon angioplasty and stenting can then be performed per usual practice.

Anterograde Dissection and Reentry

If the subintimal space is entered during anterograde wiring and wire redirection is unsuccessful, reentry should then be performed. This technique is safe and effective in recanalizing CTOs but requires a departure from traditional PCI teaching. The subcutaneous tracking and reentry technique consists of forming a J or knuckle with a hydrophilic jacketed wire and pushing this down an intentionally created dissection plane.[22,40] The adventitia serves as an elastic inner tube to contain interventional equipment within this plane without leading to a perforation outside the vessel architecture. The knuckle wire helps prevent perforation by bluntly propagating the dissection plane. The advantage of this technique is that very long occlusions can be traversed quickly, and the subintimal space usually offers less resistance to wire advancement than the occluded lumen. The rapid advancement of a knuckled wire is contradictory to the traditional approach of anterograde, true lumen wiring. With anterograde wiring, the focus is on trying to stay within the imaginary border of the lumen (a challenge especially in long occlusion segments), whereas with dissection techniques, the occlusion is usually quickly crossed and the challenge is reentry. Unfortunately, the original and modified subcutaneous tracking and reentry techniques are limited by a high incidence of side branch loss, subsequent myocardial infarction, and restenosis because of poorly controlled distal reentry localization. The technique is most suitable for the lesions within the right coronary and left circumflex arteries.

Bridgepoint

The Bridgepoint CTO crossing device (Boston Scientific) is a U.S. Food and Drug Administration (FDA) approved device that consists of three components—a blunt dissection catheter called the CrossBoss, the Stingray reentry balloon, and wire (Figure 16-4). In the FAST-CTO study, the system demonstrated a more than 80% success rate after initial failure with anterograde wiring.[41] In a recent allcomers study, the Bridgepoint system achieved significantly higher anterograde CTO-PCI success compared with a wires-only approach (86% vs. 64%, $P = .02$).[42]

CrossBoss Catheter.   The CrossBoss is an over-the-wire catheter with an atraumatic 3-Fr tip that can be advanced with or without a wire. A working wire is usually loaded in the device advanced to the proximal cap, especially if there are significant side branches in the proximal vessel. The torquing device on the catheter should be kept close to the hemostatic valve to prevent excessive advancement of the catheter. The CrossBoss is then advanced without a wire with a rapid spinning motion. Gentle forward pressure should be applied, but the key is rapid spinning, which takes some momentum to build. Once the device starts advancing, it often does so rapidly. The torque device has a tension relief mechanism that clicks if the torque exceeds design specification limits. If this occurs, the spin direction can be reversed and slightly less pressure applied. If the CrossBoss appears to deviate

Trapping technique

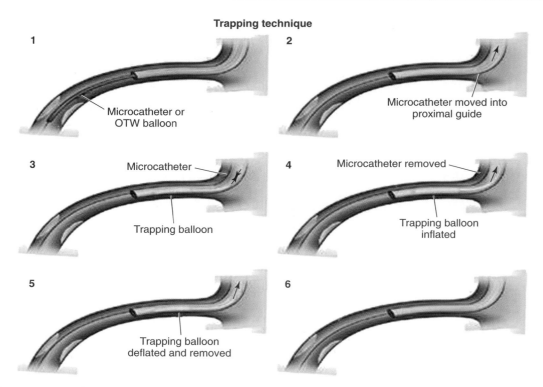

Figure 16-3 **Using a trapping balloon to decrease the risk of guidewire migration or movement.** A trapping balloon, 2.5 mm for a 7-Fr and 3.0 mm for an 8-Fr guide, decreases the risk of guidewire displacement during exchanges of over the wire (OTW) equipment while allowing the use of short guidewires and minimizing time and radiation expenditures. It is important to back-bleed air out of the system aggressively when the trapping balloon is removed.

from the expected vessel course, an angiogram should be performed before further advancement. Although perforation of the vessel is extraordinarily unlikely with the blunt-tipped design, tracking down side branches can occur and should be assiduously avoided.

Once the CrossBoss appears to have traveled beyond the distal cap, an angiogram should be obtained in at least two projections. At this point, the catheter will be either in the true lumen (≈30% of the time) or in the subintimal space adjacent to the distal target vessel. In the former case, a workhorse wire can be advanced through the over-the-wire lumen and the catheter exchanged for a balloon. If the CrossBoss is in the subintimal space, the next task is to select a reentry position. Ideally, this is on a relatively straight part of the vessel and before any major side branches. If reentry occurs distal to an important side branch, it will be cut off from anterograde flow after recanalization. The catheter should be advanced just beyond the intended site of reentry to create a path for the Stingray balloon. A workhouse wire is then advanced to the end of the dissection pouch and the CrossBoss is carefully withdrawn. We highly recommend using a trapping technique to remove all over-the-wire equipment such as the CrossBoss to prevent the loss of wire position. In a 7-Fr or larger guiding catheter, a 2.5- to 3.0-mm rapid exchange balloon catheter is advanced without a wire alongside the over-the-wire equipment to the distal end of the guide and is inflated to trap the wire in place. Over-the-wire catheters can then be pulled and withdrawn from the guide without losing wire position. This decreases radiation exposure and enables the use of short rather than exchange length coronary wires (Figure 16-3).

Stingray Balloon. The Stingray balloon is a flat balloon with two exit holes; when the balloon is inflated in the dissection plane, it facilitates reentry. There are two radiopaque markers on the Stingray balloon and an exit hole just proximal to each marker on opposite faces of the flat balloon. One exit port will lead the wire to the adventitial side of the vessel and the other to the luminal side of the vessel.

The Stingray balloon must be carefully prepared using a so-called double-prep technique. A three-way stopcock is attached to the balloon port and a 10-mL empty syringe is used to aspirate air. The stopcock is then turned off to the balloon and the sequence repeated. Then, 2 to 3 mL of 100% contrast is drawn up in the syringe and the sequence repeated twice with contrast to prepare the balloon. This meticulous preparation is critical to visualizing the small balloon to find the optimal reentry visualization angle. At this point, the Stingray balloon is advanced within the dissection plane beyond the distal cap so that it is overlying the distal vessel as visualized by injections, ideally from the contralateral artery, because forceful ipsilateral injections can lead to hydraulic dissections that will compress the distal lumen and obscure visualization by staining, making reentry more challenging. The image intensifier angle should then be adjusted to identify the projection that shows the balloon edge as a single radiopaque line. If two lines are seen, the balloon is being visualized en face, and the detector should be rotated until a single line is visualized. An angiogram should then clearly show the artery target on one side of the balloon.

Stingray Wire. The Stingray wire is a stiff wire platform with a preshaped, 28-degree tip and a barb on the end designed to facilitate reentry. The wire is carefully advanced within the Stingray balloon toward the tip. One never knows which port will be directed toward the lumen. Although we advocate a high field of view for CTO-PCI procedures because it decreases radiation exposure, a lower field of view may be necessary for this portion of the procedure to visualize the balloon orientation properly. Once the wire exits the balloon, it is advanced toward the true lumen until a pop is felt or the wire appears to have advanced into the artery. At this point, we generally favor using a so-called stick and swap maneuver. Once the fenestration is made with the Stingray wire, we remove it and replace it with a Pilot 200 wire. The advantage of wiring the distal vessel with a jacketed wire is that the Stingray barb, although very useful for

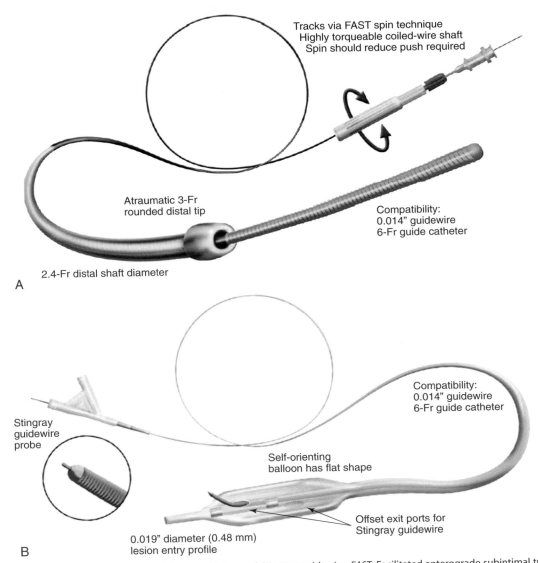

Tracks via FAST spin technique
Highly torqueable coiled-wire shaft
Spin should reduce push required

Atraumatic 3-Fr
rounded distal tip

Compatibility:
0.014" guidewire
6-Fr guide catheter

2.4-Fr distal shaft diameter

A

Stingray
guidewire
probe

Compatibility:
0.014" guidewire
6-Fr guide catheter

Self-orienting
balloon has flat shape

Offset exit ports for
Stingray guidewire

0.019" diameter (0.48 mm)
lesion entry profile

B

Figure 16-4. **A,** CrossBoss catheter. **B,** Stingray catheter and Stingray guidewire. *FAST,* Facilitated anterograde subintimal tracking.

catching the tissue to puncture into the true lumen, has a tendency to exit the opposite side of the artery or lift up plaque on the back wall of the artery and cause distal dissection. Once a wire is in the distal vessel, an angiogram should again be obtained in two views to confirm an intraluminal position. The Stingray balloon is then carefully removed; the balloon will have more than usual resistance on the wire because of the wire exiting a side port and being compressed in the vessel. Trapping is particularly useful at this stage. The lesion is then predilated. It is important to take a very gentle injection after adequate large balloon predilation and before stenting. The full extent of the subintimal dissection should be stented. Our usual practice is not to stent distal lesions beyond the CTO unless absolutely critical to outflow.

Retrograde Approach

The advent of retrograde techniques to facilitate CTO-PCI has improved overall success rates from 50% to 70% with anterograde-only approaches improved to more than 90% in contemporary series, with very low complication rates.[7,24,43] Kahn and Hartzler[44] first described the concept of retrograde PCI in 1990 using saphenous vein grafts as the retrograde conduit. Since then, the technique has evolved

using septal or epicardial collaterals for CTO access.[45,46] Retrograde PCI can be broadly defined as any technique using a donor collateral artery for the delivery of interventional equipment that ultimately facilitates successful CTO recanalization. Barriers to the widespread adoption of CTO-PCI include excessive procedural time, translating to higher radiation exposure, contrast use, and institutional costs when compared with those of routine PCI; this is coupled with relatively low success rates when restricted to anterograde-only techniques. We have demonstrated that with the addition of a retrograde option, dramatically higher success rates are achievable with lower procedural time and contrast use when retrograde operators are compared with nonretrograde operators.[24]

Indications for a Retrograde Approach and Appropriate Case Selection

Retrograde CTO techniques can be used as a bailout strategy for a failed anterograde attempt or, in the right circumstances, as a primary approach.[47] In patients with a failed anterograde attempt, retrograde success rates are significantly higher than another anterograde-only procedure. The presence of a suitable collateral and predictors of low anterograde success could be considered as an indication for primary retrograde approach and is associated with a high success rate.[34] Predictors of anterograde failure include long lesions (>20 mm), apparent small distal target, and a side branch at a flush proximal cap. Predictors of retrograde success include visible collateral connections, less than 90-degree collateral body tortuosity, and a less than 90-degree angle between the distal collateral anastomoses and CTO vessel.[48] Figure 16-1 illustrates a proposed algorithm for an approach to CTO-PCI incorporating the retrograde option in selected cases. To maximize the safety, efficiency, and potential benefits of the retrograde approach, we suggest the following guidelines:

1. An operator should have performed at least 100 anterograde CTO procedures before a retrograde attempt.
2. Initially, only septal collaterals should be traversed, and operators should avoid epicardial collaterals until they are sufficiently comfortable with retrograde wire and equipment handling.
3. On-site proctoring with an experienced retrograde operator is strongly recommended during initial cases.
4. An array of retrograde-specific equipment should be stocked, including devices for managing specific complications (see later, "Retrograde Approach Equipment").

Setting Up For Success

Review of the Diagnostic Angiogram. A careful review of the diagnostic angiogram is critical. One should focus initially on anterograde and retrograde ostial diameters and orientations for selecting the proper guiding catheters. The length of the CTO is often overestimated based on single-catheter injections, but one should attempt to get a sense of length to formulate a strategy ahead of time. Collateral sources—epicardial and septal—should be carefully assessed as potential retrograde conduits, paying particular attention to tortuosity, location, and entrance and exit angles. Both collateral size and distal vessel filling are often more prominent with injections through large-caliber guiding catheters, so one should be aware that all usable options may not be fully delineated until dual-injection, guiding catheter angiography is performed.

Guiding Catheter Selection and Setup. Support-type guides, including extra backup shapes for the left coronary and Amplatz shape for the right coronary, are useful, but guide selection should not be dogmatic, and careful scrutiny of the diagnostic angiogram is important in this respect. For example, Judkins Right guides may be more appropriate for a very proximal right coronary artery (RCA) occlusion, in which a more aggressive guide has a higher risk of proximal dissection. We recommend at least 7-Fr, and if allowable by ostial size, 8-Fr guiding catheters, both for improved support and equipment delivery. If review of the diagnostic angiogram suggests a small ostium, the use of side holes should be considered for the anterograde guide. Although damping during the procedure is not likely to be clinically relevant because the vessel is chronically occluded, hydraulic coronary dissection from injections can occur with a damped guide. This becomes increasingly more likely once an anterograde subintimal dissection has been created when performing reverse controlled anterograde and retrograde tracking (CART; see later, "Controlled Anterograde and Retrograde Tracking"). Side holes should never be used with the retrograde guide. Any damping should be recognized promptly, because donor vessel ischemia puts a large territory of myocardium at risk, including the collateralized territory, and hemodynamic compromise may ensue. The need for active retrograde guide management during delivery of devices, as well as the tendency for it to become deep-seated during removal of equipment, makes quick recognition of donor vessel ischemia important. If bilateral guides are engaged into the two native coronary ostia, it is advisable to place the left coronary guide first and then the right to avoid displacing the RCA catheter. Access guide consistency, such as always putting the anterograde guide in the right femoral and retrograde guide in the left femoral artery, can help avoid accidentally injecting via the anterograde guide at the wrong time (e.g., after anterograde subintimal ballooning but before distal recanalization) and creating a

TABLE 16-5	Rentrop Classification of Coronary Collaterals
Grade	**Classification**
0	No visible filling of any collateral channel
1	Filling of the side branch of the occluded artery
2	Partial filling of the occluded vessel
3	Complete collateral filling of the occluded vessel up to its occlusion

Adapted from Rentrop KP, Cohen M, Blanke H, et al. Changes in collateral channel filling immediately after controlled coronary artery occlusion by an angioplasty balloon in human subjects. *J Am Coll Cardiol* 1985;5:587-592.

TABLE 16-6	Werner Classification of Collateral Connections
Class	**Definition**
CC0	Collateral with no visible connection to the recipient artery
CC1	Tiny or faint connections
CC2	Small, vessel-like connections

Adapted from Werner GS, Ferrari M, Heinke S, et al. Angiographic assessment of collateral connections in comparison with invasively determined collateral function in chronic coronary occlusions. *Circulation* 2003;107:1972-1977. CC, Collateral connection.

hydraulic dissection. Acquiring short guides or the ability to shorten a guide is important for retrograde procedures, especially when planning to externalize a guidewire (see later, "Retrograde Approach Equipment").

Collateral Angiography. A careful evaluation of collaterals is critical to the planning and success of the retrograde approach. Ideally, good collateral angiography should be performed at the time of diagnostic angiography in all patients with CTOs. This will allow the operator the time to review a candidate's collaterals offline carefully. Collaterals can be classified according to the Rentrop or Werner classifications[49,50] (Tables 16-5 and 16-6).

Cineangiograms should be acquired in angulations intended to maximize the exposure of the collateral origin from the donor vessel and associated side branches, course of the collateral, and distal anastomosis with the CTO vessel (see Table 16-1). During acquisition, high field of view (low magnification) and avoidance of panning improves the resolution of very faint collaterals.

Retrograde Approach Equipment. Short (90-cm) guides are a necessity for these procedures, because standard length guides will often not allow the Corsair or other support catheters to reach the anterograde guide via collaterals. Full reach of the support catheter from retrograde guide to anterograde guide is required if one desires to externalize the guidewire to facilitate recanalization. The 90-cm guides are available for most curves, or a standard guide can be shortened. For wire externalization techniques, a long stiff wire such as the Viperwire Advance (330 cm) is the wire of choice. Although a Rotafloppy wire (Boston Scientific; 325 cm) is long enough and can be used for this purpose, it is more prone to kinking and therefore should be used only if a more suitable wire is not available. In addition to an externalization wire, a snare may be needed. We suggest the Merit 18-30 mm En Snare (Merit Medical Systems, South Jordan, Utah), which consists of three large nitinol snare loops; the Merit 18-30 mm En Snare is efficient for retrieving the retrograde wire from the aorta should this be necessary. To assist with collateral wire manipulation and allow for subsequent wire exchange, an over-the-wire support catheter or dedicated exchange catheter should be used. For the retrograde approach, the Corsair catheter, which is an over-the-wire, hydraulic support catheter and channel dilator specifically designed for retrograde PCI, has largely supplanted standard microcatheters. It consists of an array of eight thin wires wound together with two larger wires in a spiral structure allowing torque to be transmitted from shaft to tip; advancement is facilitated by rotation similar to that of the Tornus catheter. It has a hydrophilic polymer coating on the distal 60 cm to facilitate channel crossing. In a recent study, procedural retrograde CTO-PCI success in cases in which the retrograde channel was successfully crossed with a guidewire was significantly greater with the Corsair compared with standard techniques (99% vs. 92.5%; $P = 0.030$).[51] There was also a strong trend toward lower fluoroscopy and procedural time. Long, 1.2- and 1.5-mm over-the-wire balloon catheters should be available for septal dilation if needed for the advancement of retrograde equipment.

Wiring Coronary Collaterals. Septal collaterals should be attempted initially, because epicardial vessels have a higher risk of perforation and subsequent complications. Septal collaterals associated with a higher success rate are those with less than 90 degrees of tortuosity and good visibility of the collateral to recipient vessel connection.[48] For septal collaterals, a straight course is more important than size in achieving procedural success, whereas for epicardial collaterals, size is more important than tortuosity. Once a candidate collateral is identified, a nonjacketed workhorse wire with a standard curve is loaded into a Corsair catheter and maneuvered via the retrograde guide to the origin of the collateral identified for retrograde crossing. As noted, another type of microcatheter or a 1.20- to 1.5-mm over-the-wire balloon can be used for this purpose, but the Corsair has proven to be more efficient to support retrograde crossing. The tip of the catheter is advanced to the origin of the collateral, and then the working wire is exchanged for a nontapered, polymer-jacketed wire, such as the Fielder FC. The tip should be shaped with a very short bend (<1 mm) to facilitate collateral engagement and maneuvering. Once the collateral is engaged, the wire should be gently advanced, with close attention paid to ensuring free tip movement and preventing wire buckling, because collaterals are very susceptible to injury. A blind probing technique, so-called septal surfing, can often facilitate efficient crossing while minimizing contrast utilization. If little progress has been made after a few minutes, the support catheter can be advanced into the proximal collateral channel to obtain a selective angiogram as a road map.

After removal of the guidewire, a 3-mL syringe with contrast should be attached and air aspirated from the catheter before angiography. Before guidewire replacement, the catheter, particularly with the Corsair, should be flushed with saline to prevent guidewire sticking and problems with maneuverability. Different wire shapes may be needed to progress through the collateral, and the Corsair catheter may need to be advanced for support, depending on collateral tortuosity. The operator should rapidly progress through different wire shapes and paths through the collateral network and should not get stuck attempting to cross one particular collateral connection repeatedly. Forward progress that results in the appearance of the guidewire crossing the collateral can be the result of several phenomena, such as successful retrograde collateral crossing into the recipient artery true lumen, dissection and subintimal position in the collateral or recipient vessel, vessel exit into the pericardial space, or vessel exit into the ventricle, often heralded by ventricular ectopy.

Before advancement of the Corsair or the over-the-wire balloon catheter, the operator must be confident of the wire position in the distal true lumen. Other ipsilateral or contralateral collaterals can be confirmed with an angiogram from the appropriate guiding catheter, but contralateral injections are always preferable to avoid the risk of hydraulic dissection. At this point, the Corsair catheter should be advanced across the collateral into the distal portion of the occluded artery using gentle pressure and fast rotations, alternating four to five rotations counterclockwise and then clockwise. The key is momentum, and once the catheter is moving, it is important to continue alternating high-speed rotations while advancing. If an over-the-wire balloon is used, gentle low-pressure inflation (e.g., 4 to 5 atm) may be needed to dilate the septal vessel to allow for catheter

advancement. The catheter should then be advanced to the area of the distal cap to facilitate lesion crossing.

Lesion Crossing. Once a base of operations has been established at the distal cap, several techniques can be used to cross the CTO from the retrograde direction. The simplest technique is retrograde wiring; it has been observed that the distal cap is often softer and more penetrable than the proximal cap. Another advantage of crossing the CTO retrograde is the lower likelihood of engaging a side branch, so there is an increased chance of staying within the main vessel lumen or main vessel subintimal space.

An anterograde wire can be positioned as well to proceed with the simple landmark and kissing wire techniques, which are variations of the same approach. The landmark technique simply uses the retrograde wire as a landmark for the distal vessel. The retrograde wire is positioned at the distal cap of the occlusion to help navigate the anterograde wire in the proper direction. If the retrograde wire had initially advanced substantially within the occlusion, the technique is called kissing, because both wires are advanced toward each other. The meeting point can be within the lumen or in the subintimal space, because both wires are clearly within the true lumen distally and proximally.

The anterograde wire can initially serve as a marker for retrograde wiring attempts using the kissing wire approach and, if unsuccessful, subsequently as part of the setup for reverse CART. With the retrograde support catheter at the distal cap, the collateral crossing wire should be removed and replaced with a CTO crossing wire. If the path of the CTO segment is well defined, unambiguous, and short, we advocate using a Confianza Pro 12 because it combines steerability with maximal puncture force. If the path is ill defined, initially a Fielder XT, Pilot 200, or another hydrophilic-jacketed wire is more likely to stay within the vessel architecture. Advancing through the lesion should be expeditious but steady, and any significant progress should be checked with contrast injections from the appropriate guide; in general, we discourage injections through the microcatheter once out of the collaterals because if it is in the subintimal space, a large hydraulic dissection will be created, which can complicate further progress. If the retrograde wire passes into the proximal true lumen, as confirmed by two angiographic views, retrograde recanalization techniques can be used (see later). If the retrograde wire is difficult to advance and forms a loop or knuckle, this can be used to dissect up the subintimal space and is often easier to cross the lesion in this subintimal plane, as in the anterograde dissection techniques described earlier. Again, one should never attempt to knuckle a stiff hydrophobic wire such as a Confianza Pro 12 because doing so could result in a large perforation. Confianza and other stiff wires may be needed to enter the distal cap in a resistant lesion but can be exchanged for a softer wire once they have served their purpose. The Pilot 200 can be an effective knuckle wire but tends to make larger loops. The Fielder XT is an excellent wire for this technique because the tapered hydrophilic tip often enters the subintimal space easily and it tends to form a smaller controllable knuckle. Once the retrograde wire is knuckled and advanced into the midportion of the CTO in the subintimal space, we can then set up for reverse CART.

Controlled Anterograde and Retrograde Tracking. The CART technique was originally described by Surmely and associates in 2006; it consists of advancing the retrograde wire into the occlusion segment and inflating a retrograde balloon in the subintimal space to connect the subintimal retrograde wire with the anterograde wire in the true lumen.[52] This technique has an advantage over the subcutaneous tracking and reentry technique in which subintimal dissections can be extensive and side branches distal to the occlusion segment can be compromised. In CART, the dissection is limited to the CTO segment. Subintimal wire passage and reentry to the true lumen followed by true-false-true stenting can facilitate CTO recanalization by bypassing challenging intraluminal fibrocalcific plaque. Since its first description in the treatment of coronary CTOs, there has been some

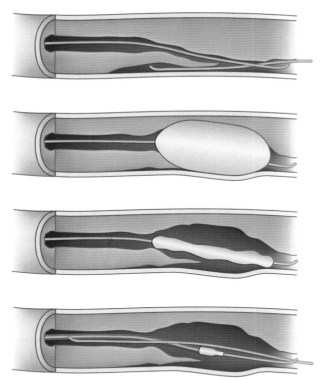

Figure 16-5 Reverse controlled anterograde and retrograde tracking. The anterograde wire is positioned in the occlusion segment within the subintimal space lying adjacent to the retrograde wire. A large balloon is inflated over the anterograde wire, enlarging this space, thereby connecting the subintimal and true lumen and allowing passage of the retrograde wire proximally into the true lumen. Once the retrograde wire is advanced to the coronary ostia, externalization and subsequent anterograde balloon dilation and stenting can be performed with excellent support.

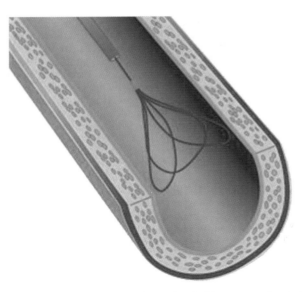

Figure 16-6   18-30 mm En Anare for retrieval of the retrograde wire from the aorta in case wiring the anterograde guide proves difficult. Snaring can be facilitated by pulling the anterograde guide into the aortic arch and snaring in the proximal arch.

controversy about its efficacy and safety.[53] However, a large series of CART stenting was presented, demonstrating reocclusion rates of only 6% and a 12-month target vessel revascularization (TVR) rate of 13%, which is comparable to that of traditional anterograde CTO outcomes with drug-eluting stents.[54-56]

Since the introduction of the Corsair septal dilator and support catheter, reverse CART has gained popularity (Figure 16-5). In this case, wires are advanced retrograde and anterograde and subintimal balloon inflations are carried out over the anterograde wire, which facilitates retrograde crossing into the true lumen. Before inflating a balloon, one must be certain that the catheter is within the vessel architecture. Confirmation of this is made easier with the retrograde technique because both wires can be seen lying adjacent to each other in multiple views. Once the anterograde subintimal balloon has been inflated, contrast injections via the anterograde guide should not be performed until recanalization has been achieved, because this can lead to a hydraulic dissection that can make the procedure more challenging. Large balloons (≥2.5 to 3.0 mm in diameter), sized appropriately to the reference vessel diameter, increase the chances of connecting the luminal and subintimal spaces. Recoil of the subintimal space can prevent retrograde wiring, and larger balloons may improve the chances of connecting the spaces. Reverse CART guided by intravascular ultrasound (IVUS) has had high success rates in the hands of very experienced operators.[57] IVUS can be used to size anterograde balloons to the reference vessel and evaluate the relative position of the retrograde and anterograde wires. The added complexity and cost of adding IVUS to routine retrograde procedures has not been evaluated.

Retrograde Recanalization Techniques. Once the retrograde wire appears proximal to the occlusion segment, the wire should advance easily to the aorta and appear to flop freely into the aortic root. Failure to observe this free motion suggests that the wire may still be subintimal, and withdrawal and readvancement should be attempted until the result is satisfactory. Special care should be taken when the retrograde wire is being advanced through the left main to the left coronary ostia. Subintimal wire position with subsequent advancement of the Corsair can impair flow to the uninvolved epicardial artery (left anterior descending or left circumflex), leading to ischemia or even acute vessel closure. IVUS may be performed at this point over the anterograde wire to confirm the intraluminal position of the retrograde wire if there is any concern. CTO recanalization may be performed via a number of techniques, including the following: (1) wire externalization and subsequent anterograde balloon and stent delivery[58]; (2) retrograde ballooning with or without retrograde wire trapping, followed by anterograde wiring and stent delivery; (3) retrograde ballooning and stenting with or without retrograde wire trapping; and (4) anterograde snaring of the retrograde wire with pull-through and subsequent anterograde ballooning and stenting (reverse wire trapping).[59]

Of these approaches, we advocate wire externalization as the primary technique that most effectively facilitates efficient recanalization and provides the most support for balloon and stent delivery in complex CTOs.[60] To accomplish wire externalization, one starts by advancing the retrograde wire into the lumen of the anterograde guide. If this cannot be easily achieved and the retrograde wire is in the aorta, a snare can be used via the anterograde guide to trap the wire (Figure 16-6). This is often easier to accomplish within the ascending aorta or the arch and may require withdrawing the anterograde guide to facilitate capture, followed by carefully reseating the guide once the retrograde wire is pulled inside. One must snare stiff wires distally because prolapsing the wire into the guide on the stiff portion may cause the wire to snap. Once the wire is established within the anterograde guide, the Corsair catheter is advanced over this wire until it is also within the anterograde guide, and then the retrograde wire is removed. At this point, if a short (90-cm) retrograde guide was not used, the Corsair catheter may not have the length to reach the anterograde guide. Once the wire is removed from the Corsair catheter that is within the anterograde wire, a dedicated externalization wire is then advanced through the Corsair.

Options for externalization wires in North America include the Viperwire Advance, which is a 330-cm stiff peripheral wire that can easily be advanced through the heart and has sufficient length to be easily externalized even through long collateral segments, or the Rotafloppy wire, which is a 325-cm wire. The Rotafloppy wire can be more challenging to use because the reverse taper to 0.008 inch can lead to kinking during advancement, and the lack of support can make advancing through the system painstakingly slow. The RG3 is a 0.010-inch dedicated externalization wire that is the wire of choice for this technique, but it is not currently approved for use within the United States. Once the retrograde externalization wire approaches the hemostatic valve of the anterograde guide, the valve should be removed and the retrograde wire advanced, with sufficient length protruding from the anterograde guide to reload the hemostatic valve over the wire. Retention of the introducer needle in the valve can make this step easier. From this point forward, great care should be exercised when pulling on the retrograde wire protruding from the anterograde guide's hemostatic valve or when backing out any retrograde gear because these maneuvers can cause deep seating of the retrograde guide and subsequent donor vessel ischemia and/or dissection.

For use of the retrograde wire for anterograde equipment delivery, the microcatheter (e.g., Corsair catheter) must be withdrawn to a position distal to the CTO. The microcatheter should remain across the collaterals to protect them from injury as balloons and stents are passed anterograde over the retrograde wire. The floppy tip of the wire can be cut off to facilitate easier loading of balloons and stents. An appropriately sized monorail balloon may be advanced anterograde over the externalized retrograde wire and angioplasty of the occlusion segment performed. Again, care must be taken when withdrawing any gear over the retrograde wire because this can cause deep seating of the retrograde guide. Fluoroscopic observation and attention to the degree of retrograde traction of a device is of paramount importance for preventing guide catheter dissection at this stage of the procedure. The likelihood of inadvertent guide displacement is higher in calcified or tortuous CTO segments, as with traditional PCI. Stenting and post-dilation can then be performed in the same fashion. At this point, a gentle angiogram should be obtained via the anterograde guide to document the result, and further stenting and post-dilation can be performed as indicated. In general, we favor restricting stenting

to the occlusion segment and any uncovered dissections and not stenting the distal vessel if it has a diffusely small diameter. The distal vessel size improves with blood flow, as is often documented in follow-up of these patients.

Retrieval of Retrograde Equipment. Once the PCI is complete, the retrograde equipment needs to be retrieved. The first step is to readvance the microcatheter to the anterograde guide to protect the vessel from the distal tip of the retrograde wire, especially if the tip was cut off to facilitate balloon and stent loading. The retrograde wire should then be pulled back through the collaterals, followed by the microcatheter, with attention to preventing deep seating of the retrograde guide. A final retrograde injection should be made to document that there is no dissection at the coronary ostium and to assess collaterals for damage. The collateral flow may be weak or reversed at this point, depending on the degree of anterograde flow in the CTO vessel.

Conclusion

CTOs are frequently encountered on coronary angiography but make up only a small fraction of target lesions for PCI. Revascularization of CTOs may provide benefit through several potential mechanisms, such as improvement in angina and quality of life, reduced ventricular arrhythmias, reduction in ischemic burden, particularly in those with significant ischemia at baseline and moderate to severe inducible ischemia on stress testing, and prevention of incomplete revascularization, which has been associated with decreased survival. There are several barriers to CTO-PCI, including lower rates of procedural success and longer procedure times compared with non-CTO intervention. The implementation of a hybrid approach, which incorporates both the anterograde and retrograde strategies to cross the CTO lesion quickly and efficiently, may improve procedural success rates and procedural speed and enable percutaneous revascularization to be offered to most patients with CTO. The most effective means of achieving successful implementation of the hybrid approach has been for operators to seek a mentoring relationship with an experienced CTO operator and work together intermittently over the course of a year. Continuous mentoring is now available though a new online resource at www.CTOFundamentals.org.

REFERENCES

1. Christofferson RD, Lehmann KG, Martin GV, et al. Effect of chronic total coronary occlusion on treatment strategy. Am J Cardiol 2005;95:1088-1091.
2. Fefer P, Knudtson ML, Cheema AN, et al. Current perspectives on coronary chronic total occlusions: the Canadian multicenter chronic total occlusions registry. J Am Coll Cardiol 2012;59:991-997.
3. Grantham JA, Marso SP, Spertus JA, et al. State of the art: chronic total occlusion angioplasty in the United States. JACC: Int 2009;2:479-486.
4. Abbott JD, Kip KE, Vlachos HA, et al. Recent trends in the percutaneous treatment of chronic total coronary occlusions. Am J Cardiol 2006;97:1691-1696.
5. Widimsky P, Straka Z, Stros P, et al. One-year coronary bypass graft patency: a randomized comparison between off-pump and on-pump surgery angiographic results of the PRAGUE-4 trial. Circulation 2004;110:3418-3423.
6. Weintraub WS, Spertus JA, Kolm P, et al. Effect of PCI on quality of life in patients with stable coronary disease. N Engl J Med 2008;359:677-687.
7. Joyal D, Afilalo J, Rinfret S. Effectiveness of recanalization of chronic total occlusions: a systematic review and meta-analysis. Am Heart J 2010;160:179-187.
8. Grantham JA, Jones PG, Cannon L, et al. Quantifying the early health status benefits of successful chronic total occlusion recanalization. Circulation 2010;3:284-290.
9. Borgia F, Viceconte N, Ali O, et al. Improved cardiac survival, freedom from mace and angina-related quality of life after successful percutaneous recanalization of coronary artery chronic total occlusions. Int J Cardiol 2012;161:31-38.
10. Hachamovitch R, Hayes SW, Friedman JD, et al. Comparison of the short-term survival benefit associated with revascularization compared with medical therapy in patients with no prior coronary artery disease undergoing stress myocardial perfusion single photon emission computed tomography. Circulation 2003;107:2900-2907.
11. Shaw LJ, Berman DS, Maron DJ, et al. Optimal medical therapy with or without percutaneous coronary intervention to reduce ischemic burden: results from the Clinical Outcomes Utilizing Revascularization and Aggressive Drug Evaluation (COURAGE) trial nuclear substudy. Circulation 2008;117:1283-1291.
12. Piccini JP, Starr AZ, Horton JR, et al. Single-photon emission computed tomography myocardial perfusion imaging and the risk of sudden cardiac death in patients with coronary disease and left ventricular ejection fraction >35%. J Am Coll Cardiol 2010;56:206-214.
13. Tonino PA, De Bruyne B, Pijls NH, et al. Fractional flow reserve versus angiography for guiding percutaneous coronary intervention. N Engl J Med 2009;360:213-224.
14. Werner GS, Surber R, Ferrari M, et al. The functional reserve of collaterals supplying long-term chronic total coronary occlusions in patients without prior myocardial infarction. Eur Heart J 2006;27:2406-2412.
15. Hannan EL, Racz M, Holmes DR, et al. Impact of completeness of percutaneous coronary intervention revascularization on long-term outcomes in the stent era. Circulation 2006;113:2406-2412.
16. Nombela-Franco L, Mitroi CD, Fernandez-Lozano I, et al. Ventricular arrhythmias among implantable cardioverter-defibrillator recipients for primary prevention: impact of chronic total coronary occlusion (VACTO Primary Study). Circ Arrhythm Electrophysiol 2012;5:147-154.
17. Cheng ASH, Selvanayagam JB, Jerosch-Herold M, et al. Percutaneous treatment of chronic total coronary occlusions improves regional hyperemic myocardial blood flow and contractility: insights from quantitative cardiovascular magnetic resonance imaging. J Am Coll Cardiol Interv 2008;1:44-53.
18. Levine GN, Bates ER, Blankenship JC, et al. 2011 ACCF/AHA/SCAI Guideline for Percutaneous Coronary Intervention: a report of the American College of Cardiology Foundation/American Heart Association Task Force on Practice Guidelines and the Society for Cardiovascular Angiography and Interventions. Circulation 2011;124:e574-e651.
19. Hachamovitch R, Hayes SW, Friedman JD, et al. Comparison of the short-term survival benefit associated with revascularization compared with medical therapy in patients with no prior coronary artery disease undergoing stress myocardial perfusion single photon emission computed tomography. Circulation 2003;107:2900-2907.
20. Suero JA, Marso SP, Jones PG, et al. Procedural outcomes and long-term survival among patients undergoing percutaneous coronary intervention of a chronic total occlusion in native coronary arteries: a 20-year experience. J Am Coll Cardiol 2001;38:409-414.
21. Morino Y, Kimura T, Hayashi Y, et al; J-CTO Registry Investigators. In-hospital outcomes of contemporary percutaneous coronary intervention in patients with chronic total occlusion: insights from the J-CTO Registry (Multicenter CTO Registry in Japan). JACC Cardiovasc Interv 2010;3:143-151.
22. Colombo A, Mikhail GW, Michev I, et al. Treating chronic total occlusions using subintimal tracking and reentry: the STAR technique. Catheter Cardiovasc Interv 2005;64:407-411.
23. Surmely JF, Katoh O, Tsuchikane E, et al. Coronary septal collaterals as an access for the retrograde approach in the percutaneous treatment of coronary chronic total occlusions. Catheter Cardiovasc Interv 2007;69:826-832.
24. Thompson CA, Jayne JE, Robb JF, et al. Retrograde techniques and the impact of operator volume on percutaneous intervention for coronary chronic total occlusions: an early U.S. experience. JACC Cardiovasc Interv 2009;2:834-842.
25. Rathore S, Hakeem A, Pauriah M, et al. A comparison of the transradial and the transfemoral approach in chronic total occlusion percutaneous coronary intervention. Catheter Cardiovasc Interv 2009;73:883-887.
26. Rinfret S, Joyal D, Nguyen CM, et al. Retrograde recanalization of chronic total occlusions from the transradial approach: early Canadian experience. Catheter Cardiovasc Interv 2011;78:366-374.

27. Kushner FG, Hand M, Smith SC, et al. 2009 focused updates: ACC/AHA guidelines for the management of patients with ST-elevation myocardial infarction (updating the 2004 guideline and 2007 focused update) and ACC/AHA/SCAI guidelines on percutaneous coronary intervention (updating the 2005 guideline and 2007 focused update): a report of the American College of Cardiology Foundation/American Heart Association Task Force on Practice Guidelines. *J Am Coll Cardiol* 2009;54: 2205-2241.

28. Romaguera R, Sardi G, Laynez-Carnicero A, et al. Outcomes of coronary arterial perforations during percutaneous coronary intervention with bivalirudin anticoagulation. *Am J Cardiol* 2011;108:932-935.

29. Dong S, Smorgick Y, Nahir M, et al. Predictors for successful angioplasty of chronic totally occluded coronary arteries. *J Interv Cardiol* 2005;18:1-7.

30. Stone GW, Rutherford BD, McConahay DR, et al. Procedural outcome of angioplasty for total coronary artery occlusion: an analysis of 971 lesions in 905 patients. *J Am Coll Cardiol* 1990;15:849-856.

31. Hsu JT, Kyo E, Chu CM, et al. Impact of calcification length ratio on the intervention for chronic total occlusions. *Int J Cardiol* 2011;150:135-141.

32. Morino Y, Abe M, Morimoto T, et al. Predicting successful guidewire crossing through chronic total occlusion of native coronary lesions within 30 minutes. *JACC Cardiovasc Interv* 2011;4:213-221.

33. Brilakis ES, Lombardi WB, Banerjee S. Use of the Stingray guidewire and the Venture catheter for crossing flush coronary chronic total occlusions due to in-stent restenosis. *Catheter Cardiovasc Interv* 2010;76:391-394.

34. Hsu JT, Tamai H, Kyo E, et al. Traditional anterograde approach versus combined anterograde and retrograde approach in the percutaneous treatment of coronary chronic total occlusions. *Catheter Cardiovasc Interv* 2009;74:555-563.

35. Brilakis ES, Grantham A, Rinfret S, et al. Percutaneous treatment algorithm for crossing coronary chronic total occlusions. *JACC Cardiovasc Interv* 2012;5:367-379.

36. Personal communication, William Lombardi.

37. Kandzari DE, Zankar AA, Teirstein PS, et al. Clinical outcomes following predilation with a novel 1.25-mm diameter angioplasty catheter. *Catheter Cardiovasc Interv* 2011;77:510-514.

38. Di Mario C, Ramasami N. Techniques to enhance guide catheter support. *Catheter Cardiovasc Interv* 2008;72:505-512.

39. Brilakis ES, Banerjee S. Crossing the balloon uncrossable chronic total occlusion: Tornus to the rescue. *Catheter Cardiovasc Interv* 2011;78:363-365.

40. Galassi AR, Tomasello SD, Costanzo L, et al. Mini-STAR as bail-out strategy for percutaneous coronary intervention of chronic total occlusion. *Catheter Cardiovasc Interv* 2012;79: 30-40.

41. Whitlow PL, Burke MN, Lombardi WL, et al. Use of a novel crossing and re-entry system in coronary chronic total occlusions that have failed standard crossing techniques: results of the FAST-CTOs (Facilitated Anterograde Steering Technique in Chronic Total Occlusions) Trial. *J Am Coll Cardiol Interv* 2012;5:393-401, doi:10.1016/j.jcin.2012.01.014.

42. Daniels D, Tremmel J, Yeung A, et al. CTO-PCI using device-based anterograde dissection and re-entry: improving success for all comers. *J Am Coll Cardiol Interv* 2012;59:E105.

43. Mehran R, Claessen BE, Godino C, et al. Multinational Chronic Total Occlusion Registry. Long-term outcome of percutaneous coronary intervention for chronic total occlusions. *JACC Cardiovasc Interv* 2011;4:952-961.

44. Kahn JK, Hartzler GO. Retrograde coronary angioplasty of isolated arterial segments through saphenous vein bypass grafts. *Catheter Cardiovasc Diagn* 1990;20:88-93.

45. Surmely J-F, Katoh O, Tsuchikane E, et al. Coronary septal collaterals as an access for the retrograde approach in the percutaneous treatment of coronary chronic total occlusions. *Catheter Cardiovasc Interv* 2007;69:826-832.

46. Zhang B, Liao H-T, Jin L-J, et al. [Retrograde percutaneous recanalization of chronic total occlusion of the coronary arteries via epicardial coronary collateral artery in 5 patients]. *Zhonghua Xin Xue Guan Bing Za Zhi* 2010;38:794-797.

47. Barlis P, Di Mario C. Retrograde approach to recanalising coronary chronic total occlusion immediately following a failed conventional attempt. *Int J Cardiol* 2009;133:e14-e17.

48. Rathore S, Katoh O, Matsuo H, et al. Retrograde percutaneous recanalization of chronic total occlusion of the coronary arteries: procedural outcomes and predictors of success in contemporary practice. *Circ Cardiovasc Interv* 2009;2:124-132.

49. Rentrop KP, Cohen M, Blanke H, et al. Changes in collateral channel filling immediately after controlled coronary artery occlusion by an angioplasty balloon in human subjects. *J Am Coll Cardiol* 1985;5:587-592.

50. Werner GS, Ferrari M, Heinke S, et al. Angiographic assessment of collateral connections in comparison with invasively determined collateral function in chronic coronary occlusions. *Circulation* 2003;107:1972-1977.

51. Tsuchikane E, Katoh O, Kimura M, et al. The first clinical experience with a novel catheter for collateral channel tracking in retrograde approach for chronic coronary total occlusions. *JACC Cardiovasc Interv* 2010;3:165-171.

52. Surmely JF, Tsuchikane E, Katoh O, et al. New concept for CTO recanalization using controlled anterograde and retrograde subintimal tracking: the CART technique. *J Invasive Cardiol* 2006;18:334-338.

53. Reimers B, Di Mario C, Colombo A. Subintimal stent implantation for the treatment of a chronic coronary occlusion. *G Ital Cardiol* 1997;27:1158-1163.

54. Kandzari DE, Rao SV, Moses JW, et al. Clinical and angiographic outcomes with sirolimus-eluting stents in total coronary occlusions. *JACC Cardiovasc Interv* 2009;2:97-106.

55. Kimura M, Tsuchikane E, Katoh O, et al. The safety and efficacy of a sub-intimal stenting after retrograde approach for chronic total occlusions: sub-analysis of the CARTTM registry. *J Am Coll Cardiol* 2011;57:E1627-E1627.

56. Rahel BM, Laarman GJ, Kelder JC, et al. Three-year clinical outcome after primary stenting of totally occluded native coronary arteries: a randomized comparison of bare-metal stent implantation with sirolimus-eluting stent implantation for the treatment of total coronary occlusions (Primary Stenting of Totally Occluded Native Coronary Arteries [PRISON] II study). *Am Heart J* 2009;157:149-155.

57. Rathore S, Katoh O, Tuschikane E, et al. A novel modification of the retrograde approach for the recanalization of chronic total occlusion of the coronary arteries intravascular ultrasound-guided reverse controlled anterograde and retrograde tracking. *JACC Cardiovasc Interv* 2010;3:155-164.

58. Nombela-Franco L, Werner GS. Retrograde recanalization of a chronic ostial occlusion of the left anterior descending artery: how to manage extreme takeoff angles. *J Invasive Cardiol* 2010;22:E7-E12.

59. Ge J, Zhang F. Retrograde recanalization of chronic total coronary artery occlusion using a novel reverse wire trapping technique. *Catheter Cardiovasc Interv* 2009;74:855-860.

60. Ge JB, Zhang F, Ge L, et al. Wire trapping technique combined with retrograde approach for recanalization of chronic total occlusion. *Chin Med J* 2008;121:1753-1756.

CHAPTER 17

Bypass Graft Intervention

LAWRENCE D. LAZAR | MICHAEL S. LEE

KEY POINTS

- Percutaneous interventions on vein grafts are more than twice as likely to be associated with major adverse cardiac events as compared with native vessel interventions.
- Embolic protection should be universal, with choice of proximal or distal occlusion systems or filter devices, depending on vessel anatomy and operator preference.
- Stents improve outcomes compared with balloon angioplasty alone, and drug-eluting stents appear to reduce target vessel revascularization.
- Impaired flow is a common complication that can be treated with vasodilators.
- Patients with prior bypass and acute coronary syndromes should be considered high risk and treated with an early invasive strategy.

Saphenous vein graft (SVG) disease ranks high among the most vexing lesions confronting interventional cardiologists. SVG intervention is associated with higher risk and lower long-term durability than native vessel intervention. Understanding the pathophysiology and natural history of SVG lesions allows one to approach them optimally, and knowing the history of tried techniques allows one to choose among therapies in which many devices may intuitively seem appropriate but few have been shown to improve outcomes. This chapter reviews the pathology of SVG disease and the evidence supporting the past and present armamentarium available for treatment of this difficult lesion subset.

Natural History and Pathology of Vein Graft Disease

Reviews of the surgical literature report that the attrition rate of vein grafts is approximately 10% early after surgery (typically within 4 weeks), an additional 5% to 10% close by the end of the first year, and thereafter the attrition rate is around 2%/year for the first 5 years.[1-3] After 5 years, the closure rate approximately doubles to around 4%/year so that by 10 years, approximately 50% of SVGs have occluded. Three processes are responsible for SVG closure. Thrombosis causes most failure within the first month. Fibrointimal hyperplasia causes most SVG failure after the first month and up to about 3 to 5 years after bypass grafting. Finally, atherosclerosis, which is accelerated in SVGs as compared with native arteries, is responsible for late closure.

SVG atherosclerosis differs from arterial atherosclerosis in ways important to the interventionalist. In contrast to the focal eccentric lesions with well-developed fibrous caps, which are commonly seen in arterial disease, venous lesions tend to be concentric and diffuse, with thin or absent fibrous caps.[2,4] Consequently, SVG lesions are friable and fragile and prone to cause distal vessel occlusion when disturbed during SVG intervention. SVG interventions are more than twice as likely to be associated with a major adverse cardiac event (MACE) compared with native vessel interventions.[5]

Approach to Ischemia Following Bypass Surgery

In clinical practice, a physician treats ischemia, not vein graft closure per se. Many SVGs that occlude have slow flow from small targets with poor runoff or from robust competitive flow from native coronaries. Given the higher potential morbidity from SVG intervention, one must take additional care to avoid the oculostenotic reflex, and treatment should be directed at symptomatic ischemia. Routine stress testing of asymptomatic patients after coronary artery bypass grafting (CABG) is not recommended.[6] In contrast, patients with prior CABG and acute coronary syndrome (ACS) should be stratified as high risk and treated with an early invasive strategy.

The decision to intervene on an SVG may be guided by symptoms, noninvasive imaging, angiography, or fractional flow reserve (FFR). Although FFR has not been prospectively studied in SVG disease, the standard cutoff values of 0.75 to 0.80 are typically used in clinical practice to determine hemodynamic significance. Disease progresses more rapidly in SVGs, however, and the safety of deferring intervention with an FFR greater than 0.80 has not been evaluated. Moderate nonobstructive stenoses are associated with low short-term event rates but are frequently the site of ischemic events over the long term, supporting a course of medical management with careful surveillance for these lesions.[7]

CABG patients undergoing percutaneous coronary intervention (PCI) have poorer long-term outcomes in terms of survival or event-free survival compared with patients with obstructive coronary artery disease without a previous CABG.[8] SVGs to the right coronary artery have the lowest patency, with progressively greater patency in SVGs to the left circumflex, diagonal branch, and left anterior descending (LAD) arteries.[9]

STAGES OF ISCHEMIA AFTER CORONARY ARTERY BYPASS GRAFTING

Very Early Ischemia

Ischemia within 30 days of CABG usually reflects SVG failure as a result of thrombosis.[2] Urgent coronary angiography and emergency PCI are indicated in the early postoperative period.[10] Balloon angioplasty across suture lines has been performed within days of surgery, although fatal avulsion of graft anastomoses has occurred and remains a concern until anastomotic healing occurs after about 2 months.[11]

Early Ischemia

Ischemia from 1 to 12 months after surgery is usually caused by perianastomotic graft stenosis. Stenoses occurring at the distal anastomosis may respond well to balloon dilation alone, with significantly lower rates of restenosis compared with midshaft or proximal SVG lesions.[12,13] Long-term outcomes throughout the SVG, including at the distal anastomosis, are generally improved with stent deployment.[14]

Late Ischemia

Ischemia presenting after the first postoperative year may result from SVG disease or progression of atherosclerotic disease. Up through 3 to 5 years after surgery, fibrointimal hyperplasia continues to be responsible for most SVG disease, whereas atherosclerotic disease predominates after that period. The distinction is important, because the former may be readily amenable to SVG intervention at a lower risk. In contrast, intervening on the fragile, friable atherosclerotic lesions that typically develop in SVGs is associated with distal embolization, slow flow, and periprocedural myocardial infarction (MI).[14] Diffuse SVG disease, large plaque volume, ulcerated lesion surface, and thrombus are predictors of distal coronary embolization.[15]

Not only do patients who undergo SVG intervention have more than twice the incidence of periprocedural complications compared with patients with native vessel PCI,[5] but they also continue to suffer a higher long-term rate of MI and need for repeat revascularization.[7,16] Within the first year following PCI, most events occur at the treated SVG sites, whereas later events occur more frequently from the progression of narrowing at previously untreated SVG sites.[7]

CHRONIC OCCLUSIONS

Balloon angioplasty[17] and stenting[7,16] of chronically occluded SVGs have produced acceptable short-term results, but complication rates were relatively high and long-term outcomes were poor. Prolonged infusions of fibrinolytics were associated with even higher complication rates and poor long-term patency (see later, "Fibrinolytics"). Consequently, intervention on chronically occluded SVGs is not recommended.[18]

Given the increased disease progression and higher risk of intervention in aged SVGs, patients with degenerative SVG disease should be evaluated for repeat surgical revascularization if they do not have a patent arterial conduit to the LAD artery. In contrast, because the main survival benefit from revascularization comes from the in situ arterial graft to the LAD, a percutaneous approach may be preferred (class IIa recommendation) in the presence of a patent arterial conduit to the LAD.[10]

⬤ Percutaneous Balloon Angioplasty and Stenting

BALLOON ANGIOPLASTY

Soon after the first coronary balloon angioplasty was performed in 1977, the first successful SVG angioplasty was reported in 1979.[19] Through the 1980s and 1990s, numerous case series of balloon angioplasty in SVGs documented short-term success but poor long-term outcomes. A review of 16 series from 1983 through 1991 found that short-term outcomes were favorable, with an average initial overall success rate of 88%.[13] The major complication rate was low, with a procedure-related death rate less than 1%, MI rate of approximately 4%, and the need for urgent CABG less than 2%. The risk of embolization into the native circulation was less than 3%, more commonly occurring in older, more diseased SVGs (see earlier).

Restenosis after balloon angioplasty, defined as more than 50% lumen diameter narrowing after initial successful intervention, occurred at an overall rate of 42%, with follow-up times ranging from 17 to 60 months.[13] The restenosis risk depended heavily on the site of dilation in the SVG. Proximal and midshaft lesions tended to have very high restenosis rates, averaging 58% and 52%, respectively. In contrast, the restenosis rate in the distal anastomosis was 28%. These results are likely overestimates because not all asymptomatic patients received follow-up angiography. Long-term adverse events, including death, MI, and recurrent angina, were almost twice as likely in older SVGs, occurring in 64% of SVGs more than 3 years old compared with 33% in SVGs less than 3 years old. The largest study included 454 patients followed for 5 years; it found that only 26% of patients remained alive and event-free.[20]

STENTING

Bare Metal Stents

Bare metal stents (BMS), approved by the U.S. Food and Drug Administration (FDA) in 1994, brought advancements in procedural

success along with some, albeit less pronounced, improvements in long-term outcomes. The SAVED (Stent Placement Compared With Balloon Angioplasty for Obstructed Coronary Bypass Grafts) randomized trial compared BMS with balloon angioplasty in SVG lesions and demonstrated superior procedural efficacy (defined as a reduction in stenosis to <50% without a major cardiac complication) in the stent group (92% vs. 69%; P < .001).[21] A larger acute gain in luminal diameter and a reduction in periprocedural major cardiac events were also noted. The 6-month freedom from MACE was significantly higher in the stent group (73% vs. 58%, P = 0.03). The primary outcome of the study was not significantly different between groups, although restenosis at 6 months occurred in 37% in the stent group compared with 46% in the angioplasty group (P = .24).

Although the use of a BMS in SVGs consistently improves short-term results compared with the use of balloon angioplasty, outcomes are more discouraging the longer the follow-up duration. Case series reported 6-month restenosis rates of approximately 20% with Palmaz-Schatz stents[22] and Wiktor I stents.[23] The 2-year repeat revascularization rate was almost 50% with longer follow-up, although most cases were caused by progressive disease at other sites.[22] At 5-year follow-up in a study that predominantly used the self-expanding Wallstent, event-free survival dropped to 30%, driven by a high incidence of MI and the need for repeat revascularization.[16] Aggressive vascular disease, rather than failure of target lesion treatment, primarily drives these grim long-term results. Synthesizing the available data, it seems clear that BMS implantation for focal SVG stenoses has an initial success rate more than 90%, with a 6-month restenosis rate of approximately 20%, but this population experiences progressive vascular disease and should expect recurrent cardiac events.

Drug-Eluting Stents

Drug-eluting stents (DES) have consistently shown superiority over BMS in reducing target vessel revascularization (TVR) after native vessel PCI. Evidence supports a similar conclusion in the setting of SVG intervention.

Over 20 studies comparing DES with BMS in SVG interventions have provided conflicting results, in part because of small sample sizes. The RRISC (Reduction of Restenosis in Saphenous Vein Grafts with Cypher Sirolimus-Eluting Stent) trial included 75 patients and found that sirolimus-eluting stents (Cypher, Cordis, Miami Lakes, FL) reduced late loss, binary restenosis, and TLR and TVR compared with BMS at 6-month follow-up.[24] However, the DELAYED RRISC (Death and Events at Long-Term Follow-Up Analysis: Extended Duration of the Reduction of Restenosis in Saphenous Vein Grafts With Cypher Stent) study, which was a 3-year post hoc analysis of RRISC, reported similar rates of TVR.[25] Although statistically underpowered for clinical outcomes, significantly higher all-cause mortality at 3 years was reported with sirolimus-eluting stents compared with BMS. The SOS (Stenting of Saphenous Vein Grafts) trial randomly assigned 80 patients to paclitaxel-eluting stents (Taxus, Boston Scientific, Natick, MA) or BMS and demonstrated a significant reduction in MACE driven by lower TLR rates with paclitaxel-eluting stents, without increased death or MI through almost 3 years of follow-up.[26,27] The primary endpoint of the RRISC and SOS trials was angiographic restenosis. The results showed similar angiographic restenosis rates between DES and BMS at 6-month (RRISC) and 12-month (SOS) follow-up, but higher mortality at long-term follow-up in the RRISC trial.

The ISAR-CABG (Is Drug-Eluting-Stenting Associated with Improved Results in Coronary Artery Bypass Grafts?) trial, the largest randomized controlled trial completed to date, randomly assigned 620 patients to DES or BMS and demonstrated a significant 6% absolute reduction in ischemia-driven target lesion revascularization (TLR) with DES compared with BMS (7% vs. 13%; P = .02), without a difference in risk of death, MI, or stent thrombosis.[28]

A number of meta-analyses that pooled the randomized controlled trials and observational studies observed a lower risk of TVR with DES.[29-31] MI also occurred less frequently, and there were trends toward lower risks of death and stent thrombosis in the DES group.[29] This potential reduction in mortality observed by meta-analysis, but not in ISAR-CABG, may result from selection bias or confounding, because a mortality reduction was seen only in the cohort studies.[30,31] Furthermore, the mortality difference is absent when the efficacy of DES is compared in a temporal fashion with the efficacy of BMS use before 2003, when DES were not commercially available, an analytical method that reduces the possibility of confounding or other biases.[30] One possibility is that the cohort studies may reflect the contemporary preference for BMS in patients with more comorbidities or other unmeasured confounders incorporated into physician decision making when selecting a particular stent type.

In ISAR-CABG, the 1-year event-free survival after DES implantation was 85%.[28] The overall incidences of all-cause mortality (5%), MI (4%), and TVR (7%) continue to be higher than those seen in native coronary disease. These findings are consistent with recent, "real world" registries with longer follow-up, which showed 3-year event-free survival rates of 73% to 78%.[30,32] Newer generations of DES hold the promise of improved outcomes. However, there are limited data to assist in the choice of the type of DES to be used for SVG lesions. In a multicenter study of 172 patients comparing first-generation DES for SVG intervention, there were no significant differences in mortality (hazard ratio [HR], 1.28; 95% confidence interval [CI], 0.39-4.25; $P = .69$) or TVR (HR, 2.54; 95% CI, 0.84-7.72; $P = .09$) with sirolimus- and paclitaxel-eluting stents.[33] There are no studies comparing second-generation stents in SVG interventions. SOS-Xience V (Study of the Xience V Everolimus-eluting Stent in Saphenous Vein Graft Lesions) was an observational cohort study of 40 patients with SVG lesions treated with Xience everolimus-eluting stents (Abbott Vascular, Abbott Park, Ill). This study demonstrated a 22% binary restenosis rate at 12-month follow-up angiography.[34] A total of 12 patients underwent optical coherence tomography evaluation at follow-up, which demonstrated high rates of stent strut coverage.[35]

Direct Stenting

Direct stenting has the theoretical benefit of decreasing distal embolization through trapping debris as well as by simply reducing the number of assaults on the friable vessel wall. In an observational registry of patients treated with SVG intervention, direct stenting was associated with significantly fewer periprocedural MIs (10.7% vs. 18.4%; $P = .24$) than conventional stenting on multivariate analysis.[36] The safety and efficacy of direct stenting have not been compared with predilation in a randomized trial.

◆ Adjunctive Devices

EMBOLIC PROTECTION

The use of embolic protection devices in SVG interventions carries a class I recommendation[18] based on multiple studies demonstrating a reduction in embolic complications (Table 17-1). Embolic protection devices can be divided into three categories—distal balloon occlusion aspiration, proximal balloon occlusion, and filter devices.[37]

Distal balloon occlusion aspiration systems include a balloon with as low as a 2.1F crossing profile mounted on a 0.014-inch hollow-core guidewire with a shapeable tip, as well as an aspiration catheter compatible with a 6F guide. The wire with occluding balloon crosses the lesion, and the angioplasty balloon or stent is positioned. The occluding balloon is inflated to a low pressure, and the angioplasty balloon or stent is deployed. The balloon or stent delivery system is removed; an aspiration catheter is advanced over the occluder wire and used to aspirate the column of blood with debris. Finally, the occluding balloon is deflated and angiography is repeated (Figure 17-1). In the SAFER (Saphenous Vein Graft Angioplasty Free of Emboli Randomized) trial, the use of the PercuSurge GuardWire system (Medtronic, Santa Rosa, CA; Figure 17-2) resulted in a significant, 6.9% absolute reduction in the 30-day primary endpoint of death, MI, emergency

TABLE 17-1	Comparison of Different Embolic Protection Devices		
		Balloon Occlusion	
Parameter	**Distal Filter**	**Distal**	**Proximal**
Complete occlusion	No	Yes	Yes
Allows perfusion	Yes	No	No
Ischemia	No	Yes	Yes
Allows visualization	Yes	No	No
Protects before crossing lesion	No	No	Yes
Crossing profile	High (3.2F)*	Low (2.7F)†	NA
Maneuverability	Reduced	Good	Good
Ease of use	Simple	Complex	Complex
Capture of smaller particles	No	Yes	Yes
Capture of neurohormonal substances	No	Yes	Yes

*FilterWire EZ.
†PercuSurge GuardWire.

bypass, or TLR by 30 days (9.6% for GuardWire vs. 16.5% for controls; $P = .001$) and a significant reduction in the incidence of no-reflow (3% vs. 9%; $P = .02$; Table 17-2).[38] A second-generation distal balloon occlusion device, the TriActiv system (Kensey Nash, Exton, PA), was subsequently shown to be noninferior to the GuardWire or FilterWire systems.[37]

Filter devices deploy a distal filter mounted on a 0.014-inch guidewire. The FilterWire EZ (Boston Scientific; Figure 17-3) uses a polyurethane filter, deployed from a 3.2F delivery sheath. The FIRE (FilterWire EX Randomized Evaluation) trial compared the first-generation FilterWire EX device with the GuardWire Plus system and demonstrated similar rates of procedural success and of MACE at 30 days and 6 months.[39] The second-generation FilterWire EZ has a lower crossing profile compared with the FilterWire EX (3.2 vs. 3.9F), an improved delivery system with a retooled nose cone, greater filter apposition of bends, and a smaller pore size (100 vs. 110 μm). The competing SpiderFX (eV3), which uses a nitinol mesh filter system with similar pore size (110 μm) and 3.2F crossing profile, has the advantage of being delivered via a monorail over a conventional 0.014-inch guidewire. In the SPIDER (Saphenous Vein Graft Protection in a Distal Embolic Protection Randomized) trial, the SpiderFX nitinol filter was noninferior to the FilterWire and the GuardWire (MACE, 9.1% vs. 8.4%; $P = .001$ for noninferiority).[40]

Anatomy frequently limits the use of distal embolic protection because of lesion proximity to the distal anastomosis or severe stenosis that prevents passing the 2.1 to 3.2F embolic protection device. Filtration systems have been observed not to be feasible for 42% of lesions, and distal balloon occlusion is not feasible for 57% of lesions.[41] For these interventions, proximal embolic protection can be used. Occlusive devices carry the major advantage of being able to capture smaller particulate matter because most fine particles produced during intervention are smaller than the pores in the distal filtration systems.[42] In addition, occlusive devices may remove soluble factors that may contribute to downstream vasospasm and no-reflow. The main disadvantage of occlusive devices is that they cause cessation of antegrade flow.[37] This may result in ischemia, which is poorly tolerated by some patients. Furthermore, angiography cannot be performed during distal occlusion. Finally, anatomy may dictate the choice between a proximal versus distal embolic protection system. The Proxis system (St. Jude Medical, Minneapolis; Figures 17-4 and 17-5) occludes flow proximal to the lesion and then allows for the aspiration of debris at the completion of the procedure. After balloon inflation, a small amount of contrast is injected and remains in the vessel, demonstrating adequate occlusion and patient tolerance as well as maintaining visibility during device placement. The PROXIMAL (Proximal

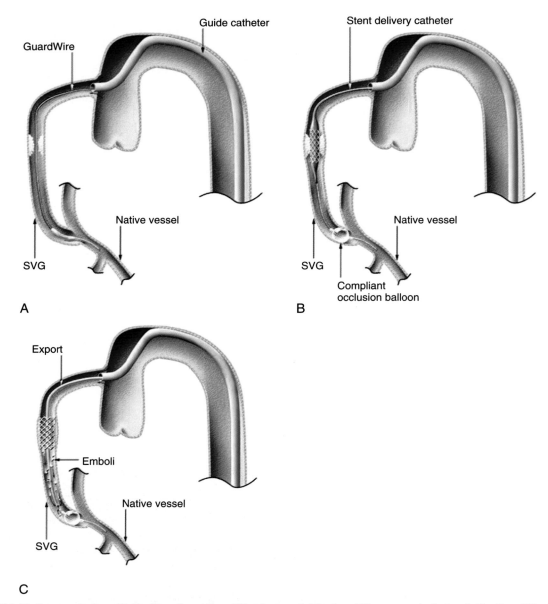

Figure 17-1   Distal balloon occlusion with the PercuSurge GuardWire System. A, The GuardWire crosses the lesion. **B,** The GuardWire balloon is inflated and PCI performed with distal embolic protection. **C,** An Export catheter removes embolic debris and soluble mediators before deflation of the GuardWire balloon. *SVG,* Saphenous vein graft.

Protection During Saphenous Vein Graft Intervention) trial showed Proxis to be noninferior to distal protection (FilterWire or Guard-Wire).[43] Subgroup analyses of lesions amenable to proximal or distal protection showed a trend toward superiority for the Proxis system (Figure 17-6), with 30-day MACE occurring in 6.2% with Proxis compared with 11.2% with FilterWire or GuardWire (*P* = .089 for superiority). Currently, the Proxis system is no longer commercially available.

OTHER DEVICES AND PROCEDURAL APPROACHES

Rheolytic Thrombectomy

Apart from embolic protection systems, rheolytic thrombectomy is one of the only devices with a specific FDA indication for SVG intervention. Patients receiving PCI to SVGs with thrombotic lesions were randomized to intervention with AngioJet (Possis Medical, Minneapolis) or prolonged urokinase infusion for a mean of 13 hours.[44]

The thrombectomy group had greater angiographic success, less frequent periprocedural MI, and a lower incidence of 30-day MACE, although there was no difference in the primary composite endpoint (death, Q-wave MI, stroke, TVR, or stent thrombosis).

Laser Angioplasty

Excimer laser coronary angioplasty with adjunctive balloon angioplasty was shown to open old, diseased SVGs successfully, although restenosis occurred in more than 50%.[45] More favorable results may be obtained with discrete lesions located at the ostia of grafts or in the body of smaller grafts.[46]

Atherectomy

Rotational atherectomy of SVGs is contraindicated by the manufacturer (Boston Scientific), although limited cases have reported successful use in resistant SVG stenoses. In a randomized comparison with balloon angioplasty, directional atherectomy was associated with

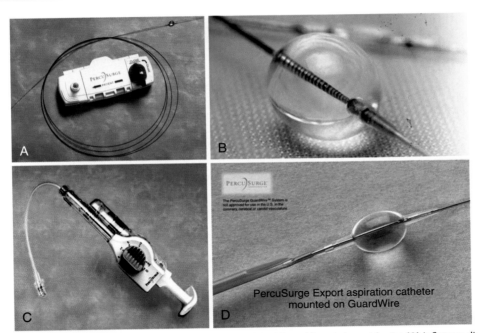

Figure 17-2 **PercuSurge GuardWire Distal Protection System.** A 0.014-inch nitinol-based hypotube guidewire **(A)** inflates a distal occlusion balloon **(B)**, which transiently stops perfusion to the distal microvasculature. A Microseal adapter controls a miniature valve within the hypotube to keep the occlusion balloon inflated while PCI is performed over the wire. The EZ-Flator **(C)** inflates the occlusion balloon to stop blood flow in the SVG. The Export aspiration catheter removes embolic debris while the occlusion balloon is inflated. The occlusion balloon **(D)** is deflated to permit restoration of blood flow.

TABLE 17-2	30-Day Outcomes of Selected Trials of Embolic Protection Devices			
	Outcome			
Trial	MACE (%)	Death (%)	MI (%)	No-Reflow (%)
SAFER				
GuardWire	9.6	1.0	8.6	3
Control	16.5	2.3	14.7	9
P value	0.004	0.17	0.008	0.001
FIRE				
FilterWire EX	9.9	0.9	9.0	NA
GuardWire	11.6	0.9	10.0	NA
P value	0.53	0.99	0.69	NA
BLAZE				
FilterWire EZ	6.7	0	6.7	NA
Pride				
TriActiv	11.2	1.3	9.9	NA
GuardWire, FilterWire EZ	10.1	0.6	8.8	NA
P value	0.65	0.45	0.64	NA
SPIDER				
Spider	9.1	0.3	7.7*	NA
GuardWire, FilterWire EZ	8.4	0.6	7.0*	NA
P value	.79	NS	NS	NA

BLAZE, Embolic Protection Transluminally with the FilterWire EZ Device in Saphenous Vein Grafts; *FIRE,* FilterWire EX Randomized Evaluation; *MACE,* major adverse cardiac event; *MI,* myocardial infarction; *NA,* not available; *NS,* nonsignificant; *SAFER,* Saphenous Vein Graft Angioplasty Free of Emboli Randomized trial; *SPIDER,* Saphenous Vein Graft Protection in a Distal Embolic Protection Randomized.
*Non–Q-wave MI.

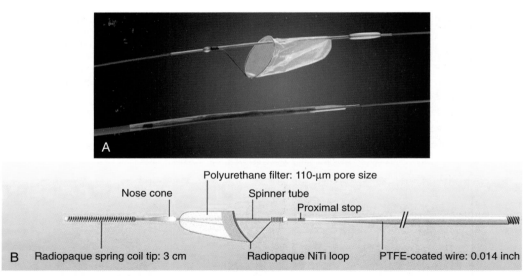

Figure 17-3 **FilterWire EZ. A,** The FilterWire is composed of a polyurethane filter basket (pore size, 110 μm) premounted on an 0.014-inch guidewire and preloaded on a delivery sheath. **B,** The FilterWire can be used with a 6F guiding catheter, protect saphenous vein grafts (SVGs) 3.5 to 5.5 mm in diameter, and is available in wire lengths of 190 and 300 cm. A landing zone more than 30 mm is needed. A retrieval sheath captures and removes the FilterWire from the SVG. A FilterWire for use in grafts with smaller reference diameters is also available. *PTFE,* Polytetrafluoroethylene.

improved initial angiographic success and luminal diameter but also with increased distal embolization and no difference in restenosis rates.[47] Another atherectomy device that is no longer in clinical use includes the Transluminal Extraction catheter, which had high primary success and low complication rates but was associated with restenosis rates of 60%. The X-SIZER (eV3, Plymouth, Minneapolis) reduced the size of procedural MIs but failed to reduce 30-day MACE.

Brachytherapy

Intracoronary brachytherapy successfully reduces the risk of recurrent in-stent restenosis in SVGs. Although effective, brachytherapy is laborious and expensive and requires coordination with a radiation oncologist. Brachytherapy is less frequently used than previously, given data demonstrating that DES are at least as effective and safe for the treatment of BMS restenosis.[48]

Covered Stents

Covered stents were studied to contain the friable atheroemboli, but randomized trials found no benefit compared with BMS.[49] One study actually found an increase in nonfatal MI.[50]

Adjunctive Pharmacotherapy

ANTITHROMBOTIC STRATEGY

Foundation antithrombotic strategy is essentially the same as for native vessel interventions with the same choices of anticoagulant and antiplatelet therapies.[51] Given the propensity for thrombus formation and impaired flow in SVG interventions, however, careful attention to thrombus prevention is doubly important. In addition to universal dual antiplatelet therapy, procedural anticoagulation choices include heparin alone, heparin plus glycoprotein (GP) IIb/IIIa inhibitor, and bivalirudin.

Although there have been no dedicated trials evaluating antithrombotic therapy in SVG intervention, the ACUITY (Acute Catheterization and Urgent Intervention Triage Strategy) trial included a postrandomization subset of 329 patients undergoing SVG intervention.[52] In this trial, patients with an ACS were randomly allocated to bivalirudin monotherapy, bivalirudin plus GP IIb/IIIa inhibitor, or heparin plus GP IIb/IIIa inhibitor. Within the group of patients undergoing SVG PCI, the primary composite endpoints, including 30-day MACE, major bleeding, and net adverse clinical events, were similar

among the three groups. Minor bleeding was significantly lower with bivalirudin alone compared with heparin plus a GP IIb/IIIa inhibitor (26% vs. 38%; *P* = .05). Thus, bivalirudin may be an equally effective anticoagulant with a better safety profile, although this has not been definitively demonstrated in an adequately powered randomized trial.

GLYCOPROTEIN IIB/IIIA INHIBITORS

Although initial studies with GP IIb/IIIa inhibitors showed promise in facilitating SVG PCI, overall results were not favorable. A meta-analysis pooling five trials of intravenous (IV) GP IIb/IIIa inhibitors found no improvement in outcomes after SVG PCI.[53] In the absence of embolic protection, SVG intervention with GP IIb/IIIa inhibitors was still associated with a high incidence of death and nonfatal MI. In current practice, GP IIb/IIIa inhibitors no longer have a role for routine upstream use in elective SVG intervention. The 2011 American College of Cardiology Foundation/American Heart Association/Society for Cardiovascular Angiography and Interventions Guideline for Percutaneous Coronary Intervention provide a class III recommendation for the use of GP IIb/IIIa inhibitors during SVG intervention (no benefit), stating that "platelet GP IIb/IIIa inhibitors are not beneficial as adjunctive therapy during SVG PCI."[18]

Delayed, selective use of GP IIb/IIIa inhibitors may be useful for treating slow flow or no-reflow.[54] Case reports have also shown success with prolonged IV infusions to stabilize or improve thrombus-laden SVGs. GP IIb/IIIa inhibitors also carry a class I recommendation as a possible component of adjunctive pharmacotherapy for ACSs.[55] Select patients with an acute presentation and a large thrombus burden may also benefit from use of a GP IIb/IIIa inhibitor.

VASODILATORS

SVG interventions are prone to complication by slow flow or no-reflow, defined as Thrombolysis in Myocardial Infarction (TIMI) 2 flow or TIMI 0 to 1 flow, respectively, not attributable to abrupt closure, high-grade stenosis, or spasm of the target lesion. Slow flow and no-reflow are clinically important, associated with tenfold higher incidence of in-hospital deaths and acute MI.[56] Numerous pharmacologic therapies have been tested to treat this complication. Acute microvascular spasm also contributes to impaired flow, as demonstrated by many studies showing improvement with the intragraft administration of vasodilators.

developed slow or no-reflow, high doses of intragraft adenosine (≥five boluses of 24 μg each) resulted in reversal of slow or no-reflow compared with low doses (more than five boluses; 91% vs. 33%; $P = .02$), and final TIMI flow grade was significantly improved (2.7 ± 0.6 vs. 2.0 ± 0.8; $P = .04$). High-velocity injections of intragraft adenosine to reverse slow or no-reflow resulted in TIMI 3 flow in 91% of cases.[58]

Nitroprusside

Nitroprusside is a direct donor of nitric oxide. In a study of 20 cases of slow flow or no-reflow, 9 (45%) of which were SVG interventions, intracoronary administration of nitroprusside (50 to 1000 μg; median dose = 200 μg) resulted in significant improvement in angiographic flow and blood flow velocity ($P = .01$ for each compared with pretreatment angiogram).[59] Nitroprusside was not associated with significant hypotension or other adverse clinical events in this study, but can cause profound hypotension in patients who are hypovolemic or hypotensive at baseline.

Verapamil

In 22 patients randomized to prophylactic intragraft administration of verapamil versus placebo, verapamil tended to reduce the occurrence of no-reflow (0% vs. 33.3%; $P = .10$), increase the TIMI frame count (53.3 ± 22.4% faster vs. 11.5 ± 38.9%; $P = .016$), and result in a trend toward improved TIMI myocardial perfusion grade.[60] In a prospective study of 32 episodes of no-reflow, intragraft verapamil (100 to 500 μg) improved the flow in all cases (TIMI flow grade 1.4 ± 0.8 preintragraft verapamil to 2.8 ± 0.5 postintragraft verapamil, $P = .001$) and reestablished TIMI flow grade 3 in 88% of cases.[61]

Nicardipine

The prophylactic intragraft administration of nicardipine, a potent arteriolar vasodilator, was followed by direct stenting for degenerated SVG without the use of a distal protection device in 83 patients and resulted in a creatine kinase–MB (CK-MB) level more than three times the upper limit of normal in 4.4% of patients.[62] Slow flow or no-reflow occurred transiently in 2.4% of patients. In-hospital MACE occurred in 4.4% (all CK-MB level elevation), and no additional MACE occurred from hospital discharge to 30 days.

FIBRINOLYTICS

Operators reported initial success opening chronically occluded SVGs with prolonged infusions of fibrinolytics. One series used prolonged administration (31-hour average) via infusion wire into the SVG.[63] Recanalization occurred in up to 80% of SVGs and 1-year angiographic patency was maintained in 65% of successfully treated SVGs. Prolonged infusions of fibrinolytics also successfully accomplished thrombus lysis in cases of nonocclusive intragraft thrombi.[64] A larger multicentered study presented a less optimistic picture, however.[65] Intragraft prolonged administration achieved initial patency in almost 70% of patients, but 6-month follow-up angiography of those with initial success demonstrated patency in only 40%. Treatment was complicated by MI (5%), enzyme level elevation (17%), emergency CABG (4%), stroke (3%), and death (6.5%). Prolonged infusion of fibrinolytics has also been associated with intracranial hemorrhage and intramyocardial hemorrhage, as well as vascular access site complications.

🔷 Treatment of Acutely Failed Grafts

Percutaneous intervention on an acutely occluded SVG follows the same principles discussed earlier. Whereas one should generally avoid intervening on a chronically, total occluded SVG, rapid reperfusion of an acutely occluded SVG is a priority. Patients with prior bypass who present with ACS should be stratified as high risk and treated with an early invasive strategy. For ST-elevation MIs, standard 90-minute, first medical contact to device times continue to apply. Redo CABG is reasonable for patients with multiple SVG stenoses,

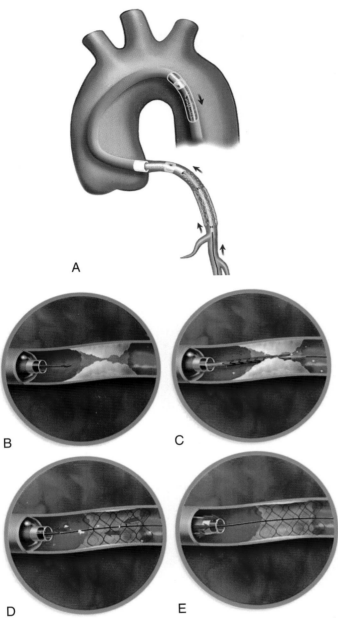

Figure 17-4   Proximal embolic protection. A, Proxis device. **B,** The Proxis is advanced over a guidewire into the saphenous vein graft (SVG) proximal to the lesion. **C,** After the occlusion balloon is inflated to stop SVG blood flow temporarily, SVG intervention can be performed. **D,** After stenting, embolic debris is aspirated from the SVG. **E,** Blood flow in the SVG is restored after the balloon is deflated.

Adenosine

Adenosine is an endogenous purine nucleoside, a vasodilator of arteries and arterioles, that inhibits platelet activation and aggregation. Although severe bradycardia may occur as a result of its effect on sinoatrial and atrioventricular nodal conduction, the half-life of adenosine is very short, so these effects rarely last more than a few seconds. Prophylactic administration of intragraft adenosine does not appear to decrease the risk of slow flow or no-reflow, but it can reverse slow or no-reflow with multiple boluses.[57] In a retrospective study of 143 patients, the incidence of slow or no-reflow was similar in patients who received preprocedural administration of intragraft adenosine and those who did not (14.2% vs. 13.6%; $P = 0.9$). In patients who

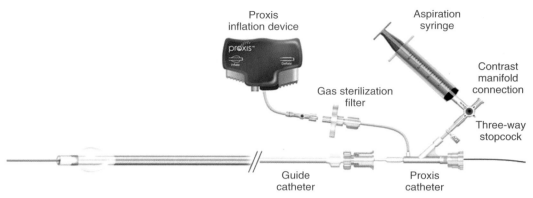

Figure 17-5   **Proxis proximal embolic protection device.** The carbon dioxide inflation device attached to the Proxis catheter inflates and deflates the Proxis sealing balloon. An aspiration syringe removes embolic debris and soluble mediators before balloon deflation.

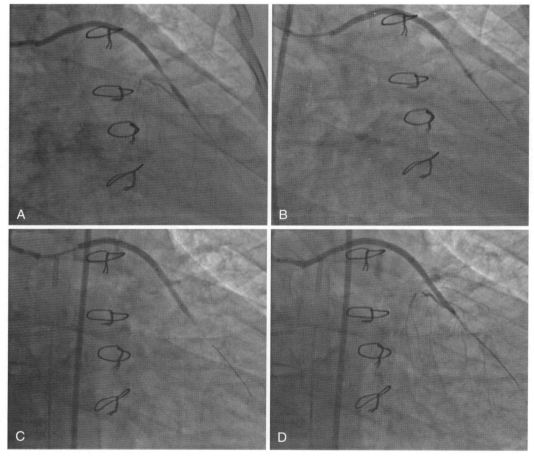

Figure 17-6   **Intervention with proximal occlusion embolic protection.** This was done in a 20-year-old aortocoronary saphenous vein graft (SVG) to the left anterior descending artery. **A,** SVG lesion with severe stenosis preintervention. **B,** Predilation, flow is occluded with the Proxis embolic protection system. The lumen is opacified to demonstrate adequate occlusion with patient tolerance and ease device placement. After dilation, the opacified column of blood with debris is aspirated and the proximal balloon deflated. **C,** Stent delivery with proximal occlusion. **D,** Final result, with good reflow. Patient had no postprocedure rise in troponin or creatine kinase–MB levels.

especially when there is significant stenosis of a graft that supplies the LAD artery. Routine antithrombotic strategies should be followed, with universal dual antiplatelet therapy and procedural anticoagulation with heparin alone, heparin plus a GP IIb/IIIa inhibitor, or bivalirudin. If not routinely used as part of an institution's ACS protocol, a GP IIb/IIIa inhibitor may be added to heparin or bivalirudin in cases of heavy thrombus burden. Aspiration thrombectomy

may be indicated, although judgment must be exercised to avoid traumatizing an older, diffusely friable graft. Rheolytic thrombectomy may be considered for patients with heavily thrombotic lesions. Embolic protection should be deployed when possible, although it is only an option after flow has been reestablished and an appropriate landing zone for the device can be clearly visualized. As in elective cases, stenting is preferred over balloon angioplasty alone, and DES may be preferred in appropriately selected patients. Acute SVG interventions are frequently complicated by slow flow or no-reflow and may be treated with vasodilators and GPIIb/IIIa inhibitors. Finally, the adage "better is the enemy of good" holds especially true in SVG interventions, in which the simplest possible intervention carries the least potential for complications.

Conclusions

Even in contemporary practice, long-term event-free survival remains less than 50% in patients treated with SVG intervention. Symptomatic SVG stenosis is treated with stenting, with the possible exception of distal anastomosis lesions in which balloon angioplasty alone may be sufficient. DES appear to decrease restenosis and the need for TVR, but results from large trials are needed for confirmation. Some form of embolic protection should be used whenever feasible. Thrombus may be treated with rheolytic thrombectomy and possibly GP IIb/IIIa inhibitors, and impaired reflow should be treated with vasodilators. Although many devices promise better outcomes based on mechanisms that intuitively should enhance patency or decrease complications, extensive trials have shown difficulty in improving results.

REFERENCES

1. Fitzgibbon GM, Kafka HP, Leach AJ, et al. Coronary bypass graft fate and patient outcome: angiographic follow-up of 5,065 grafts related to survival and reoperation in 1,388 patients during 25 years. *J Am Coll Cardiol* 1996;28:616-626.
2. Nwasokwa ON. Coronary artery bypass graft disease. *Ann Intern Med* 1995;123:528-545.
3. Lee MS, Park SJ, Kandzari DE, et al. Saphenous vein graft intervention. *JACC Cardiovasc Interv* 2011;4:831-843.
4. Cox JL, Chiasson DA, Gotlieb AI. Stranger in a strange land: the pathogenesis of saphenous vein graft stenosis with emphasis on structural and functional differences between veins and arteries. *Prog Cardiovasc Dis* 1991;34:45-68.
5. Singh M, Rihal CS, Lennon RJ, et al. Prediction of complications following nonemergency percutaneous coronary interventions. *Am J Cardiol* 2005;96:907-912.
6. Gibbons RJ, Balady GJ, Beasley JW, et al. ACC/AHA guidelines for exercise testing: executive summary. A report of the American College of Cardiology/American Heart Association Task Force on Practice Guidelines (Committee on Exercise Testing). *Circulation* 1997;96:345-354.
7. Ellis SG, Brener SJ, DeLuca S, et al. Late myocardial ischemic events after saphenous vein graft intervention—importance of initially "nonsignificant" vein graft lesions. *Am J Cardiol* 1997; 79:1460-1464.
8. Labinaz M, Kilaru R, Pieper K, et al. Outcomes of patients with acute coronary syndromes and prior coronary artery bypass grafting: results from the platelet glycoprotein IIb/IIIa in unstable angina: receptor suppression using integrilin therapy (PURSUIT) trial. *Circulation* 2002;105:322-327.
9. Shah PJ, Gordon I, Fuller J, et al. Factors affecting saphenous vein graft patency: clinical and angiographic study in 1402 symptomatic patients operated on between 1977 and 1999. *J Thorac Cardiovasc Surg* 2003;126:1972-1977.
10. Smith Jr SC, Feldman TE, Hirshfeld Jr JW, et al. ACC/AHA/SCAI 2005 guideline update for percutaneous coronary intervention: a report of the American College of Cardiology/American Heart Association Task Force on Practice Guidelines (ACC/AHA/SCAI Writing Committee to Update 2001 Guidelines for Percutaneous Coronary Intervention). *Circulation* 2006;113:e166-e286.
11. Price MJ, Housman L, Teirstein PS. Rescue percutaneous coronary intervention early after coronary artery bypass grafting in the drug-eluting stent era. *Am J Cardiol* 2006;97:789-791.
12. Douglas Jr JS, Gruentzig AR, King 3rd SB, et al. Percutaneous transluminal coronary angioplasty in patients with prior coronary bypass surgery. *J Am Coll Cardiol* 1983;2:745-754.
13. de Feyter PJ, van Suylen RJ, de Jaegere PP, et al. Balloon angioplasty for the treatment of lesions in saphenous vein bypass grafts. *J Am Coll Cardiol* 1993;21:1539-1549.
14. Gruberg L, Hong MK, Mehran R, et al. In-hospital and long-term results of stent deployment compared with balloon angioplasty for treatment of narrowing at the saphenous vein graft distal anastomosis site. *Am J Cardiol* 1999;84:1381-1384.
15. Liu MW, Douglas Jr JS, Lembo NJ, et al. Angiographic predictors of a rise in serum creatine kinase (distal embolization) after balloon angioplasty of saphenous vein coronary artery bypass grafts. *Am J Cardiol* 1993;72:514-517.
16. de Jaegere PP, van Domburg RT, Feyter PJ, et al. Long-term clinical outcome after stent implantation in saphenous vein grafts. *J Am Coll Cardiol* 1996;28:89-96.
17. Kahn JK, Rutherford BD, McConahay DR, et al. Initial and long-term outcome of 83 patients after balloon angioplasty of totally occluded bypass grafts. *J Am Coll Cardiol* 1994;23:1038-1042.
18. Levine GN, Bates ER, Blankenship JC, et al. 2011 ACCF/AHA/SCAI Guideline for Percutaneous Coronary Intervention. A report of the American College of Cardiology Foundation/American Heart Association Task Force on Practice Guidelines and the Society for Cardiovascular Angiography and Interventions. *J Am Coll Cardiol* 2011;58:e44-e122.
19. Grüntzig AR, Senning Å, Siegenthaler WE. Nonoperative dilatation of coronary-artery stenosis. *N Engl J Med* 1979;301: 61-68.
20. Plokker HW, Meester BH, Serruys PW. The Dutch experience in percutaneous transluminal angioplasty of narrowed saphenous veins used for aortocoronary arterial bypass. *Am J Cardiol* 1991;67:361-366.
21. Savage MP, Douglas Jr JS, Fischman DL, et al. Stent placement compared with balloon angioplasty for obstructed coronary bypass grafts. Saphenous Vein De Novo Trial Investigators. *N Engl J Med* 1997;337:740-747.
22. Piana RN, Moscucci M, Cohen DJ, et al. Palmaz-Schatz stenting for treatment of focal vein graft stenosis: immediate results and long-term outcome. *J Am Coll Cardiol* 1994;23:1296-1304.
23. Hanekamp CE, Koolen JJ, Den Heijer P, et al. Randomized study to compare balloon angioplasty and elective stent implantation in venous bypass grafts: the Venestent study. *Catheter Cardiovasc Interv* 2003;60:452-457.
24. Vermeersch P, Agostoni P, Verheye S, et al. Randomized double-blind comparison of sirolimus-eluting stent versus bare-metal stent implantation in diseased saphenous vein grafts: six-month angiographic, intravascular ultrasound, and clinical follow-up of the RRISC Trial. *J Am Coll Cardiol* 2006;48:2423-2431.
25. Vermeersch P, Agostoni P, Verheye S, et al. Increased late mortality after sirolimus-eluting stents versus bare-metal stents in diseased saphenous vein grafts: results from the randomized DELAYED RRISC Trial. *J Am Coll Cardiol* 2007;50:261-267.
26. Brilakis ES, Lichtenwalter C, Abdel-karim AR, et al. Continued benefit from paclitaxel-eluting compared with bare-metal stent implantation in saphenous vein graft lesions during long-term follow-up of the SOS (Stenting of Saphenous Vein Grafts) trial. *JACC Cardiovasc Interv* 2011;4:176-182.
27. Brilakis ES, Lichtenwalter C, de Lemos JA, et al. A randomized controlled trial of a paclitaxel-eluting stent versus a similar bare-metal stent in saphenous vein graft lesions the SOS (Stenting of Saphenous Vein Grafts) trial. *J Am Coll Cardiol* 2009;53: 919-928.
28. Mehilli J, Pache J, Abdel-Wahab M, et al. Drug-eluting versus bare-metal stents in saphenous vein graft lesions (ISAR-CABG): a randomised controlled superiority trial. *Lancet* 2011; 378:1071-1078.
29. Lee MS, Yang T, Kandzari DE, et al. Comparison by meta-analysis of drug-eluting stents and bare metal stents for saphenous vein graft intervention. *Am J Cardiol* 2010;105:1076-1082.
30. Shishehbor MH, Hawi R, Singh IM, et al. Drug-eluting versus bare-metal stents for treating saphenous vein grafts. *Am Heart J* 2009;158:637-643.
31. Wiisanen ME, Abdel-Latif A, Mukherjee D, et al. Drug-eluting stents versus bare-metal stents in saphenous vein graft interventions: a systematic review and meta-analysis. *JACC Cardiovasc Interv* 2011;3:1262-1273.
32. Goswami NJ, Gaffigan M, Berrio G, et al. Long-term outcomes of drug-eluting stents versus bare-metal stents in saphenous vein graft disease: results from the Prairie "Real World" Stent Registry. *Catheter Cardiovasc Interv* 2009;75:93-100.
33. Lee MS, Hu PP, Aragon J, et al. Comparison of sirolimus-eluting stents with paclitaxel-eluting stents in saphenous vein graft intervention (from a multicenter Southern California Registry). *Am J Cardiol* 2010;106:337-341.
34. Papayannis AC, Michael T, Yangirova D, et al. Optical coherence tomography analysis of the SOS Xience V study: the use of the everolimus-eluting stent in saphenous vein graft lesions. *J Am Coll Cardiol* 2012;59:E119.
35. Papayannis AC, Michael TT, Yangirova D, et al. Optical coherence tomography analysis of the stenting of saphenous vein graft (SOS) Xience V Study: use of the everolimus-eluting stent in saphenous vein graft lesions. *J Invasive Cardiol* 2012;24:390-394.
36. Leborgne L, Cheneau E, Pichard A, et al. Effect of direct stenting on clinical outcome in patients treated with percutaneous coronary intervention on saphenous vein graft. *Am Heart J* 2003; 146:501-506.
37. Carter LI, Golzar JA, Cavendish JJ, et al. Embolic protection of saphenous vein graft percutaneous interventions. *J Interv Cardiol* 2007;20:351-358.
38. Baim DS, Wahr D, George B, et al. Randomized trial of a distal embolic protection device during percutaneous intervention of saphenous vein aorto-coronary bypass grafts. *Circulation* 2002; 105:1285-1290.
39. Stone GW, Rogers C, Hermiller J, et al. Randomized comparison of distal protection with a filter-based catheter and a balloon occlusion and aspiration system during percutaneous intervention of diseased saphenous vein aorto-coronary bypass grafts. *Circulation* 2003;108:548-553.
40. Dixon SR. Saphenous vein graft protection in a distal embolic protection randomized trial. Presented at the Transcatheter Cardiovascular Therapeutics Meeting, Washington, DC, October 16-21, 2005.
41. Bhatt DL, Topol EJ. Percutaneous coronary intervention for patients with prior bypass surgery: therapy in evolution. *Am J Med* 2000;108:176-177.
42. Grube E, Schofer JJ, Webb J, et al. Evaluation of a balloon occlusion and aspiration system for protection from distal embolization during stenting in saphenous vein grafts. *Am J Cardiol* 2002;89:941-945.
43. Mauri L, Cox D, Hermiller J, et al. The PROXIMAL trial: proximal protection during saphenous vein graft intervention using the Proxis Embolic Protection System: a randomized, prospective, multicenter clinical trial. *J Am Coll Cardiol* 2007; 50:1442-1449.
44. Kuntz RE, Baim DS, Cohen DJ, et al. A trial comparing rheolytic thrombectomy with intracoronary urokinase for coronary and vein graft thrombus (the Vein Graft AngioJet Study [VeGAS 2]). *Am J Cardiol* 2002;89:326-330.
45. Strauss BH, Natarajan MK, Batchelor WB, et al. Early and late quantitative angiographic results of vein graft lesions treated by excimer laser with adjunctive balloon angioplasty. *Circulation* 1995;92:348-356.
46. Bittl JA, Sanborn TA, Yardley DE, et al. Predictors of outcome of percutaneous excimer laser coronary angioplasty of saphenous vein bypass graft lesions. The Percutaneous Excimer Laser Coronary Angioplasty Registry. *Am J Cardiol* 1994;74:144-148.
47. Holmes Jr DR, Topol EJ, Califf RM, et al. A multicenter, randomized trial of coronary angioplasty versus directional atherectomy for patients with saphenous vein bypass graft lesions. CAVEAT-II Investigators. *Circulation* 1995;91:1966-1974.
48. Holmes Jr DR, Teirstein P, Satler L, et al. Sirolimus-eluting stents vs vascular brachytherapy for in-stent restenosis within bare-metal stents: the SISR randomized trial. *JAMA* 2006;295: 1264-1273.
49. Schachinger V, Hamm CW, Munzel T, et al. A randomized trial of polytetrafluoroethylene-membrane-covered stents compared with conventional stents in aortocoronary saphenous vein grafts. *J Am Coll Cardiol* 2003;42:1360-1369.
50. Stankovic G, Colombo A, Presbitero P, et al. Randomized evaluation of polytetrafluoroethylene-covered stent in saphenous vein grafts: the Randomized Evaluation of polytetrafluoroethylene COVERed stent in Saphenous vein grafts (RECOVERS) Trial. *Circulation* 2003;108:37-42.
51. Levine GN, Bates ER, Blankenship JC, et al. 2011 ACCF/AHA/SCAI Guideline for Percutaneous Coronary Intervention: a report of the American College of Cardiology Foundation/American Heart Association Task Force on Practice Guidelines and the Society for Cardiovascular Angiography and Interventions. *Circulation* 2011;124:e574-e651.
52. Kumar D, Dangas G, Mehran R, et al. Comparison of bivalirudin versus bivalirudin plus glycoprotein IIb/IIIa inhibitor versus heparin plus glycoprotein IIb/IIIa inhibitor in patients with acute coronary syndromes having percutaneous intervention for narrowed saphenous vein aorto-coronary grafts (the ACUITY trial investigators). *Am J Cardiol* 2010;106: 941-945.
53. Roffi M, Mukherjee D, Chew DP, et al. Lack of benefit from intravenous platelet glycoprotein IIb/IIIa receptor inhibition as adjunctive treatment for percutaneous interventions of aortocoronary bypass grafts: a pooled analysis of five randomized clinical trials. *Circulation* 2002;106:3063-3067.
54. Rawitscher D, Levin TN, Cohen I, et al. Rapid reversal of no-reflow using abciximab after coronary device intervention. *Cathet Cardiovasc Diagn* 1997;42:187-190.
55. Jneid H, Anderson JL, Wright RS, et al. 2012 ACCF/AHA Focused Update of the Guideline for the Management of Patients With Unstable Angina/Non-ST-Elevation Myocardial Infarction (Updating the 2007 Guideline and Replacing the 2011 Focused Update): a report of the American College of Cardiology Foundation/American Heart Association Task Force on Practice Guidelines. *Circulation* 2012;126:875-910.
56. Abbo KM, Dooris M, Glazier S, et al. Features and outcome of no-reflow after percutaneous coronary intervention. *Am J Cardiol* 1995;75:778-782.

57. Sdringola S, Assali A, Ghani M, et al. Adenosine use during aortocoronary vein graft interventions reverses but does not prevent the slow-no reflow phenomenon. *Catheter Cardiovasc Interv* 2000;51:394-399.
58. Fischell TA, Carter AJ, Foster MT, et al. Reversal of "no reflow" during vein graft stenting using high-velocity boluses of intracoronary adenosine. *Cathet Cardiovasc Diagn* 1998;45: 360-355.
59. Hillegass WB, Dean NA, Liao L, et al. Treatment of no-reflow and impaired flow with the nitric oxide donor nitroprusside following percutaneous coronary interventions: initial human clinical experience. *J Am Coll Cardiol* 2001;37:1335-1343.
60. Michaels AD, Appleby M, Otten MH, et al. Pretreatment with intragraft verapamil prior to percutaneous coronary intervention of saphenous vein graft lesions: results of the randomized, controlled vasodilator prevention on no-reflow (VAPOR) trial. *J Invasive Cardiol* 2002;14:299-302.

61. Kaplan BM, Benzuly KH, Kinn JW, et al. Treatment of no-reflow in degenerated saphenous vein graft interventions: comparison of intracoronary verapamil and nitroglycerin. *Cathet Cardiovasc Diagn* 1996;39:113-118.
62. Fischell TA, Subraya RG, Ashraf K, et al. "Pharmacologic" distal protection using prophylactic, intragraft nicardipine to prevent no-reflow and non-Q-wave myocardial infarction during elective saphenous vein graft intervention. *J Invasive Cardiol* 2007;19: 58-62.
63. Hartmann JR, McKeever LS, Stamato NJ, et al. Recanalization of chronically occluded aortocoronary saphenous vein bypass grafts by extended infusion of urokinase: initial results and short-term clinical follow-up. *J Am Coll Cardiol* 1991;18: 1517-1523.

64. Chapekis AT, George BS, Candela RJ. Rapid thrombus dissolution by continuous infusion of urokinase through an intracoronary perfusion wire prior to and following PTCA: results in native coronaries and patent saphenous vein grafts. *Cathet Cardiovasc Diagn* 1991;23:89-92.
65. Hartmann JR, McKeever LS, O'Neill WW, et al. Recanalization of Chronically Occluded Aortocoronary Saphenous Vein Bypass Grafts With Long-Term, Low Dose Direct Infusion of Urokinase (ROBUST): a serial trial. *J Am Coll Cardiol* 1996;27: 60-66.

CHAPTER 18

Stenting in Acute Myocardial Infarction

MARCO VALGIMIGLI

KEY POINTS

- The use of bare metal stents (BMS) in the setting of patients suffering from ST segment elevation myocardial infarction (STEMI) decreases the need for target vessel reintervention compared with balloon angioplasty but is not associated with a significant reduction in mortality, nor does it affect the rate of reinfarction.

- First-generation sirolimus- or paclitaxel-eluting stents significantly reduce the need for target vessel reintervention compared with BMS in the setting of STEMI.

- Patients with STEMI are at increased risk of stent thrombosis as compared with patients with stable coronary artery disease after both drug-eluting stent (DES) and BMS implantation.

- The overall incidence of stent thrombosis does not differ at up to 5-year follow-up between first-generation DES compared with BMS. However, the temporal distribution of stent thrombosis after first-generation DES differs from that observed after BMS implantation, because it tends to be lower within the first year but occurs more frequently from 1 year onward.

- Newer generation DES, in particular the everolimus-eluting stent and Biolimus A9 eluting-stent, appear to reduce the risk for overall or very late stent thrombosis compared with first-generation DES.

- There is a paucity of randomized clinical trial data regarding the optimal duration of dual antiplatelet therapy with aspirin and an oral P2Y$_{12}$ receptor blocker after BMS or DES implantation for STEMI.

Primary percutaneous coronary intervention (PCI) is noninferior to fibrinolytic therapy in patients presenting early with ST segment elevation myocardial infarction (STEMI) and is the preferred reperfusion strategy when symptom duration is longer than 3 hours.[1] This largely reflects the capability of mechanical intervention to obtain a more successful vessel recanalization with less associated life-threatening bleeding, thus counterbalancing the PCI-related delay under controlled conditions.[2] The overall success of primary PCI is at least partially related to vessel stenting, which makes the mechanical procedure more predictable and provides greater success rates at both short- and long-term follow-up.

Bare Metal Stents

A number of trials have evaluated the efficacy of bare metal stents (BMS) in the setting of STEMI, and these will be described here.

STENT TRIALS

STENT-PAMI Trial

The Stent in Primary Angioplasty in Myocardial Infarction (Stent PAMI) trial was a multicenter study that compared primary percutaneous transluminal coronary angioplasty (PTCA) with PTCA accompanied by implantation of a heparin-coated Palmaz-Schatz stent.

Patients with acute myocardial infarction underwent emergency catheterization and angiography; those with vessels suitable for stenting were randomly assigned to undergo angioplasty with stenting (452 patients) or angioplasty alone (448 patients).[7] The mean (± standard deviation [SD]) minimal luminal diameter was larger after stenting than after angioplasty alone (2.56 ± 0.44 mm vs. 2.12 ± 0.45 mm; P < .001), although fewer patients assigned to stenting had Thrombolysis In Myocardial Infarction (TIMI) grade 3 blood flow (89.4% vs. 92.7%; P = .10). Mortality trended higher in the stent arm (3.5% vs. 1.89%; P = .15). At 6 months, significantly fewer patients assigned to stenting had angina (11.3% vs. 16.9%; P = .02) or needed target vessel revascularization (TVR) because of ischemia (7.7% vs. 17.0%; P < .001). The combined primary endpoint of death, reinfarction, disabling stroke, or TVR because of ischemia occurred in significantly fewer patients in the stent group than in the angioplasty group (12.6% vs. 20.1%; P < .01), driven entirely by the decreased need for TVR. At 6 months, mortality was 4.2% in the stent group compared with 2.7% in the angioplasty group (P = .27). Angiographic follow-up at 6.5 months demonstrated a lower incidence of restenosis in the stent group than in the angioplasty group (20.3% vs. 33.5%; P < .001). This difference in favor of the stent group was explained by significantly greater luminal gain with stenting (2.21 vs. 1.78 mm; P < .001) because late luminal loss was also greater after stenting than balloon angioplasty (0.76 vs. 0.54 mm; P < .001), reflecting in-stent intimal growth of hyperplasia versus vessel recoil and negative remodeling, respectively. Unlike many other studies, patients presenting with a large thrombus burden were not systematically excluded from recruitment, which may at least partially explain the early hazard of stenting on TIMI 3 flow and mortality observed at 30 days.

Given its design, STENT-PAMI could not assess the effect of the heparin coating of the stent relative to that of its metal scaffolding. It is possible that the scaffolding effect of the stent, which enlarges the lumen and seals dissections, accounted for most of the benefit associated with stenting. However, the ability of a heparin coating to reduce platelet deposition and thrombus formation may have also contributed to the low rate of subacute thrombosis observed. Unfortunately, the specific role of a heparin-coated stent in the setting of primary stenting has not been further investigated. In addition, the use of oral P2Y$_{12}$ receptor blockers—in this case ticlopidine—was more frequent in the stent group, which also may have influenced the trial findings.

CADILLAC Trial

The Controlled Abciximab and Device Investigation to Lower Late Angioplasty complications (CADILLAC) trial randomly assigned 2082 patients with acute myocardial infarction using a 2 by 2 factorial design to undergo PTCA alone, PTCA plus abciximab therapy, stenting alone with the MultiLink stent, or stenting plus abciximab therapy.[5] Normal flow was restored in the target vessel in 94.5% to 96.9% of patients and did not differ according to the reperfusion strategy. At 6 months, the primary endpoint—a composite of death, reinfarction, disabling stroke, and ischemia-driven TVR—had occurred in 20.0% of patients after PTCA, 16.5% after PTCA plus abciximab, 11.5% after stenting, and 10.2% after stenting plus

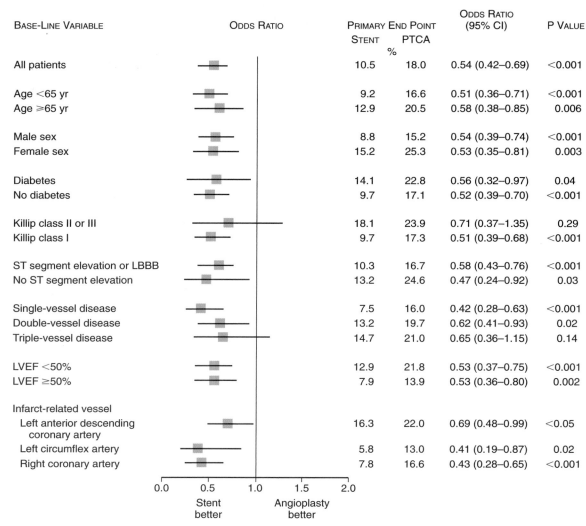

BASE-LINE VARIABLE	ODDS RATIO	PRIMARY END POINT STENT %	PTCA	ODDS RATIO (95% CI)	P VALUE
All patients		10.5	18.0	0.54 (0.42–0.69)	<0.001
Age <65 yr		9.2	16.6	0.51 (0.36–0.71)	<0.001
Age ≥65 yr		12.9	20.5	0.58 (0.38–0.85)	0.006
Male sex		8.8	15.2	0.54 (0.39–0.74)	<0.001
Female sex		15.2	25.3	0.53 (0.35–0.81)	0.003
Diabetes		14.1	22.8	0.56 (0.32–0.97)	0.04
No diabetes		9.7	17.1	0.52 (0.39–0.70)	<0.001
Killip class II or III		18.1	23.9	0.71 (0.37–1.35)	0.29
Killip class I		9.7	17.3	0.51 (0.39–0.68)	<0.001
ST segment elevation or LBBB		10.3	16.7	0.58 (0.43–0.76)	<0.001
No ST segment elevation		13.2	24.6	0.47 (0.24–0.92)	0.03
Single-vessel disease		7.5	16.0	0.42 (0.28–0.63)	<0.001
Double-vessel disease		13.2	19.7	0.62 (0.41–0.93)	0.02
Triple-vessel disease		14.7	21.0	0.65 (0.36–1.15)	0.14
LVEF <50%		12.9	21.8	0.53 (0.37–0.75)	<0.001
LVEF ≥50%		7.9	13.9	0.53 (0.36–0.80)	0.002
Infarct-related vessel					
Left anterior descending coronary artery		16.3	22.0	0.69 (0.48–0.99)	<0.05
Left circumflex artery		5.8	13.0	0.41 (0.19–0.87)	0.02
Right coronary artery		7.8	16.6	0.43 (0.28–0.65)	<0.001

Figure 18-1 Odds ratio plot showing the effect of stenting versus balloon angioplasty according to various subgroups in the CADILLAC trial.[5] The treatment effect of stenting was consistent across the subgroups studied. *CI*, Confidence interval; *LBBB*, left bundle branch block; *LVEF*, left ventricular ejection fraction; *PTCA*, percutaneous transluminal coronary angioplasty.

abciximab (P < .001). The effect of stenting was consistent across many prespecified subgroups (Figure 18-1). There were no significant differences among the groups in the rates of death, stroke, or reinfarction. The difference in the incidence of the primary endpoint was entirely the result of differences in the rates of TVR, ranging from 15.7% after PTCA to 5.2% after stenting plus abciximab (P < .001). The rate of angiographic restenosis was 40.8% after PTCA and 22.2% after stenting (P < .001), and the respective rates of reocclusion of the infarcted-related artery were 11.3% and 5.7% (P = .01), both independent of abciximab use. The findings of this randomized trial support the use of stenting in the setting of ST-elevation myocardial infarction to reduce the risk of early and late restenosis, reocclusion of the infarct-related artery, and the need for TVR.

ZWOLLE II Trial

In this single-center trial, 1,683 consecutive patients with STEMI were randomly assigned before angiography to stenting or balloon angioplasty alone (N = 834)[6]. No exclusion criteria were applied. The primary endpoint was the combination of death or reinfarction at 1 year. A total of 785 patients (92.5%) in the stent group and 763

patients (91.5%) in the balloon angioplasty group actually underwent primary PCI.[6] The two groups were comparable in terms of the angiographic outcomes of postprocedural TIMI flow, myocardial blush grade, and distal embolization. No difference in clinical outcomes between treatments was observed by both intention to treat (14% vs 12.5%; relative risk [RR], 1.21; 95% confidence interval [CI], 0.81-1.62) and actual treatment analyses (12.4% vs. 11.3%; RR, 1.16; 95% CI, 0.84-1.59; Figure 18-2). Unlike previous STEMI studies focusing on highly selected patient population, the reintervention rate did not differ among treatment approaches (19.6% vs. 20.7%; RR, 0.98; 95% CI, 0.78-1.22). Therefore, the authors concluded that in unselected patients presenting with STEMI, stenting does not seem to improve significantly the rates of reinfarction and TVR compared with balloon angioplasty.

Meta-Analyses

Several randomized controlled studies have addressed the additive value of stenting compared with balloon angioplasty alone for the treatment STEMI, and several meta-analyses have considered the cumulative evidence provided by available data.[3,4] In the first

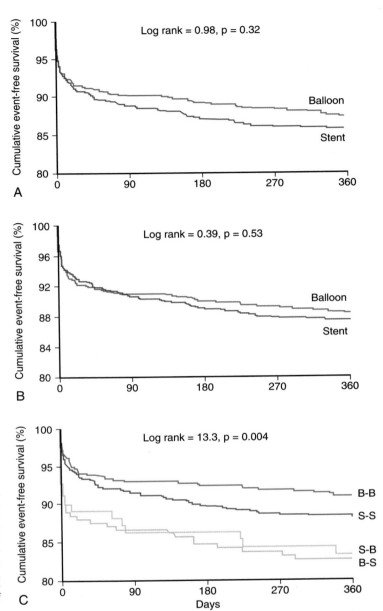

Figure 18-2   ZWOLLE-2 trial. Kaplan-Meier event-free survival curves for combined death or reinfarction according to intention to treat analysis **(A)**, actual treatment analysis **(B)**, and analysis of four subgroups according to initial randomization allocation and final treatment **(C)**. *B-B,* Randomly allocated to balloon and actually treated with balloon; *B-S,* randomly allocated to balloon but treated with stent; *S-B,* randomly allocated to stent but treated with balloon only; *S-S,* randomly allocated to stent and actually treated with stent. (From Suryapranata H, De Luca G, van't Hof AW, et al. Is routine stenting for acute myocardial infarction superior to balloon angioplasty? A randomised comparison in a large cohort of unselected patients. *Heart* 2005;91:641-645.)

systematic review of the literature, primary stenting was compared with primary angioplasty in nine studies, consisting of a total of 4120 patients.[3] When this analysis included all four arms of the CADILLAC trial[5] (i.e., those with or without abciximab infusion), there were no differences in mortality (3.0% vs. 2.8%) or the rate of reinfarction (1.8% vs. 2.1%) between balloon angioplasty and stent implantation. However, major adverse cardiac events were reduced, driven by the reduction in subsequent TVR with stenting. A subanalysis that excluded the two arms of the CADILLAC trial[5] allocated to receive abciximab showed similar results, except that the difference in reinfarction rate between these two reperfusion strategies was greater.

A more recent meta-analysis, including a total of 4433 patients, demonstrated that stenting had no effect on mortality compared with balloon angioplasty, but significantly reduced the rates of reinfarction (odds ratio [OR] at 30 days, 6, and 12 months were, respectively, 0.52, 95% CI, 0.31-0.87; 0.67, 95% CI, 0.45-1.00; and 0.67, 95% CI, 0.45-0.98) and TVR.[4]

The partially discrepant finding between these meta-analyses appears to be driven by differences in the inclusion of eligible trials, which raises a note of caution toward the possibility that existing estimates of the effect of BMS on reinfarction may be subject to considerable bias. Current data should also be interpreted cautiously, bearing in mind that the more potent postinterventional antithrombotic therapies that were systematically present in patients treated with stenting to prevent early reocclusion were frequently omitted in the control group. This hypothesis is also partially supported by the finding that at meta-analysis, stented patients tended to bleed more than those who were treated with balloon angioplasty only (OR,1.34; 95% CI, 0.95-0.88). Therefore, a reasonable unifying hypothesis in reconciling the discrepant findings among studies regarding the effect of stenting on the rate of reinfarction is that because stent deployment requires the addition of an oral $P2Y_{12}$ receptor blocker to prevent acute and subacute stent thrombosis, the intensification of platelet inhibition associated with stent implantation, and not the stent itself, may decrease the risk for reinfarction compared with balloon angioplasty alone, coming at the cost of a slightly higher probability of bleeding. Thus, it remains to be determined whether the lower infarct rate observed in the stent arms of some studies is mainly related to the coronary device itself or to the different antithrombotic regimen used in the study groups.

The present evidence in support of the role of stenting in the setting of STEMI is based mainly on a relatively low-risk cohort of patients, as indicated by the relatively low 30-day mortality (5%) and reinfarction rates (4%) of the pooled data. Patients with cardiogenic shock were generally excluded; in none of these investigations were patients recruited before coronary angiography. Therefore, these trials included patients who were suitable candidates for BMS, whereas patients with a diffusely diseased or small coronary vessel, large thrombus burden, severe coronary calcification or tortuosity, and sometimes bifurcated lesions were mostly excluded. Thus, particular care should be taken in extrapolating these findings to the "real-world" setting, in which an unselected and much higher risk patient population is treated.

A recent meta-analysis of stent versus balloon angioplasty for the treatment of STEMI, encompassing 10 randomized controlled trials and 6192 patients, included the Zwolle II study, which randomly assigned treatment prior to angiography.[8] Details of each of the included trials are shown in Table 18-1. Compared with balloon angioplasty, BMS reduced the rate of reocclusion (6.7% vs. 10.1%; OR, 0.62; 95% CI, 0.40-0.96; $P = .03$), restenosis (23.9% vs. 39.3%; OR, 0.45; 95% CI, 0.34-0.59; $P = .001$), and TVR (12.2% vs. 19.2%; OR, 0.50; 95% CI, 0.37-0.69; $P = .001$) but did not reduce subacute thrombosis (1.7% vs. 1.7%), mortality (5.3% vs. 5.1%), or reinfarction (3.9% vs. 4%) (Figure 18-3).

These meta-analyses show the value of stenting on early and late vessel patency but also emphasize two key messages:

1. After BMS, the need for reintervention remains relatively high, in the range of 20% in unselected patients and/or lesion subsets. Therefore, better-performing coronary devices that can further reduce the lumen loss over time remain desirable.
2. As shown in the Zwolle II study, in unselected patients presenting with STEMI (i.e., those who have not been selected as good stent candidates based on angiographic criteria), clinical outcomes after BMS may remain suboptimal and not much better than those after stand-alone balloon angioplasty.

◆ First-Generation Drug-Eluting Stents

RANDOMIZED TRIALS

Strategy

The Single High-Dose Bolus Tirofiban and Sirolimus-Eluting Stent vs. Abciximab and Bare-Metal Stent in Acute Myocardial Infarction (STRATEGY) trial was the first study to evaluate the value of the sirolimus-eluting stents (SES) in patients undergoing primary PCI. In this trial, a lower-priced glycoprotein IIb/IIIa inhibitor (tirofiban) was used to offset the cost associated with a more expensive stent.[9] A total of 175 patients (80% of the screened population) were randomly allocated to receive tirofiban or abciximab; they were subsequently transferred to the catheterization laboratory to receive an SES or BMS, respectively.

There were no significant differences between the two groups in the incidence of major adverse cardiovascular or cerebrovascular events (MACCE) during the first 30 days, whereas at 8 months the MACCE rate was significantly lower in the tirofiban plus SES compared with the abciximab plus BMS group (18% vs. 32%, respectively; hazard ratio [HR], 0.53; 95% CI, 0.28-0.92; $P = .04$), driven by a reduction in the rate of TVR (7% vs. 20%, respectively; HR, 0.30; 95% CI, 0.12-0.77; $P = .01$). At 5 years, the cumulative incidence of major adverse cardiac events (MACE; death, myocardial infarction, or TVR) trended lower in the tirofiban-SES group (29.9% vs. 43.2%; HR: 0.63; 95% CI, 0.39-1.03; $P = .067$). All-cause mortality (18.4%; 95% CI, 12% to 28%) and the composite of death or myocardial infarction (21.8%; 95% CI, 14% to 32%) were similar in the tirofiban-SES compared with the abciximab-BMS group (15.9%; 95% CI, 10% to 25%; $P = .70$; and 25.0%; 95% CI, 17% to 35%; $P = .58$, respectively), whereas the need for target vessel revascularization remained reduced (10.3% vs. 26.1%; HR, 0.37; 95% CI, 0.17-0.79; $P = .007$) in the tirofiban-SES group (Figure 18-4).[10] The cumulative incidence of definite, probable, or possible stent thrombosis was 6.9% versus 7.9% in the tirofiban-SES group and abciximab-BMS group, respectively (HR, 0.86; 95% CI, 0.29-2.6; $P = .78$). The cumulative incidence of definite and of definite/probable stent thrombosis also did not differ between the two groups.

This trial was underpowered to assess the effect of tirofiban-supported SES implantation on the rate of clinical events because the primary endpoint was a combination of clinical and angiographic

| TABLE 18-1 | Summary of Major Randomized Controlled Trials of Bare Metal Stent Versus Balloon Angioplasty in Patients with ST Segment Elevation Myocardial Infarction |

Trial	Year	No. of Sites	No. of Patients	No. of BMS Patients	No. of Patients, B	Time from SO (hr)	No. of Crossover BMS (%)	Vessel Size (mm)	No. of Crossover B (%)	Follow-up (mo) Clinical	Follow-up (mo) Angiographic
FRESCO[5]	1998	1	150	75	75	<6 (6-24)*	0 (0)	>2.5	0 (0)	6	6
GRAMI[6]	1998	8	104	52	52	<24	0 (0)	>2.5	13 (25)	12	0.24
ZWOLLE I[7]	1998	1	227	112	115	<6 (6-24)*	2 (2)	>3.0	15 (13)	24	6
Stent PAMI[8]	1999	62	900	452	448	<12	7 (2)	3.0-4.5	67 (15)	12	6
PASTA[9]	1999	6	136	67	69	<12	1 (1)	>2.5	7 (10)	12	6
STENTIM-2	2000	17	211	101	110	<12	3 (3)	>3.0	33 (36)	12	6
Psaami[15]	2001	1	88	44	44	<6 (6-24)*	1 (2)	>3.0	12 (27)	24	6
CADILLAC[17]	2002	76	2082	1036	1046	<12	22 (1)	2.5-4.5	168 (18)	6	7
STOPAMI 3[19]	2004	611	611	305	306	<48	14 (5)	All	93 (30)	6	NA
ZWOLLE II[20]	2005	1	1683	849	834	<6 (6-24)*	109 (13)	All	214 (26)	12	6
Total			6192	3093	3099		159 (5.1)		622 (20.1)		

B, Balloon group; *BMS*, bare-metal stent group; *SO*, symptom onset; *NA*, not available; *Year*, year of publication; *Sites*, number of centers involved in trial.
*For continuing myocardial ischemia; *NA*, not available.
From Svilaas T, van der Horst IC, Zijlstra F. A quantitative estimate of bare-metal stenting compared with balloon angioplasty in patients with acute myocardial infarction: angiographic measures in relation to clinical outcome. *Heart* 2007;93:792-800.

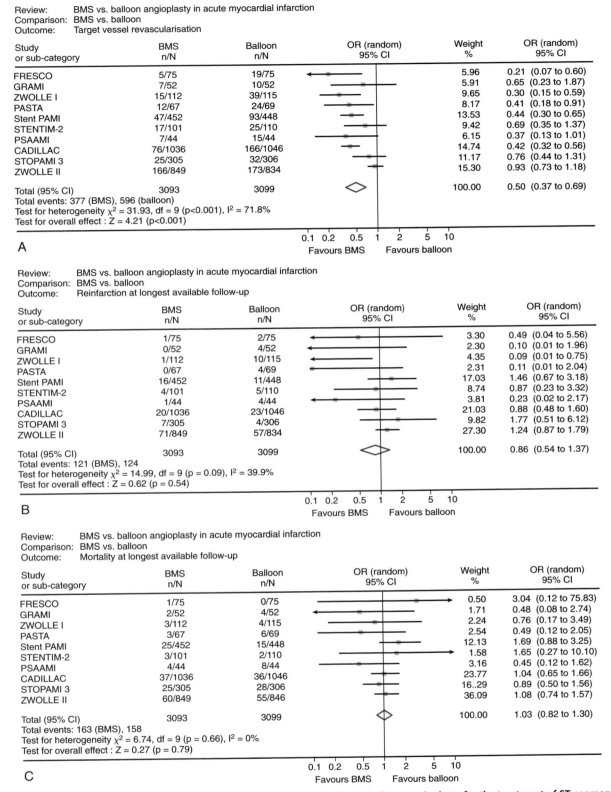

Figure 18-3   Forrest plot showing the pooled effect of stenting *(BMS)* compared with balloon angioplasty for the treatment of ST-segment elevation myocardial infarction (STEMI) in a meta-analysis of stent versus balloon angioplasty for the treatment of STEMI. A, Target vessel revascularization. **B,** Reinfarction. **C,** Mortality. *CI,* Confidence interval; *OR,* odds ratio. (From Svilaas T, van der Horst IC, Zijlstra F. A quantitative estimate of bare-metal stenting compared with balloon angioplasty in patients with acute myocardial infarction: angiographic measures in relation to clinical outcome. *Heart* 2007;93:792-800.)

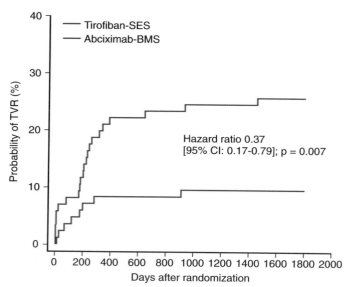

Figure 18-4   The 5-year probability of target vessel revascularization *(TVR)* in patients randomly assigned to tirofiban plus sirolimus-eluting stent *(SES)* or to abciximab infusion plus bare metal stenting (BMS) in the **STRATEGY trial.** *CI,* Confidence interval. (From Valgimigli M, Percoco G, Malagutti P, et al. Tirofiban and sirolimus-eluting stent vs. abciximab and bare-metal stent for acute myocardial infarction: a randomized trial. *JAMA* 2005;293:2109-2117.)

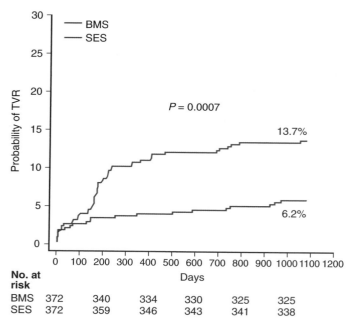

Figure 18-5   Cumulative risk of events at 1080 days for target vessel revascularization *(TVR)* in patients allocated to a bare metal stent *(BMS)* or sirolimus-eluting stent *(SES)* in the MULTISTRATEGY trial. SES was associated with a significant, long-term reduction in TVR compared with BMS. (From Valgimigli M, Campo G, Percoco G, et al. Comparison of angioplasty with infusion of tirofiban or abciximab and with implantation of sirolimus-eluting or uncoated stents for acute myocardial infarction: the MULTISTRATEGY randomized trial. *JAMA* 2008;299:1788-1799.)

outcomes. In addition, no conclusion can be drawn regarding the relative contribution of the specific glycoprotein IIb/IIIa inhibitor or stent type with respect to the other because only their combination was tested. Finally, it remains likely that protocol-mandated angiographic follow-up (performed in 76% of the enrolled population) increased the magnitude of clinical benefit of study treatment over the combination of abciximab plus BMS. Thus, the true clinical benefit of SES implantation in patients with STEMI remains speculative.

TYPHOON Trial

In the industry-sponsored Trial to Assess the Use of the Cypher Sirolimus-eluting Coronary Stent in Acute Myocardial Infarction Treated with Balloon Angioplasty (TYPHOON) study, 712 patients presenting within 12 hours after onset of symptoms of first myocardial infarction requiring primary PCI on a native coronary artery were randomized at 48 sites to receive SES or any BMS.[11] Of these, 210 patients were scheduled to undergo angiographic follow-up. The rate of target vessel failure, defined as TVR, recurrent myocardial infarction, or cardiac death at 1 year, was 7.3% in the SES group versus 14.3% in the BMS group (P = .0036). This reduction was driven entirely by a decrease in the rate of TVR (5.6% vs. 13.4%). Overall, 71% of patients received glycoprotein (GP) IIb/IIIa inhibitors during the procedure. The rate of acute or subacute thrombosis did not differ in the SES group (3.1%) compared with the BMS group (3%), and the incidence of late stent thrombosis (between 30 days and 1 year) was 0.3% in the SES versus 0.6% in the BMS group. The benefit of SES implantation was confirmed at 4-year follow-up; SES implantation was associated with significantly greater freedom from target lesion revascularization, with no signal of a late ischemic hazard, because the overall rate of myocardial infarction or stent thrombosis did not differ.[12] However, because a longer than 1-year follow-up was not prespecified in the original protocol, 4-year follow-up was available in only approximately 70% of the original patient cohort.

MULTISTRATEGY Trial

In the Multicentre evaluation of Single high-dose Bolus Tirofiban vs. Abciximab with Sirolimus-eluting Stent or Bare-Metal Stent in

Acute Myocardial Infarction (MULTISTRATEGY) study, patients were randomly assigned with the use of a 2 by 2 factorial design to one of four interventional strategies of reperfusion—abciximab with a BMS, abciximab with an SES, tirofiban with a BMS, or tirofiban with an SES.[13] Between October 2004 and April 2007, 1030 patients were screened; of these, 745 were enrolled and randomly assigned to the four treatment groups. At 30 days, the incidence of the primary clinical endpoint—composite of death, reinfarction, or revascularization of the target vessel—was 5.9% versus 3.9% (P = .12) in the BMS and SES groups, respectively. At 8 months, the MACCE rate was higher in the BMS group (54 patients, 14.5%) compared with the SES group (29 patients, 7.8%; P = .0039). There was no evidence of heterogeneity among sites (χ^2 = 3.95; P = .18). The composite of death or reinfarction and the incidence of stent thrombosis were similar across the four groups, but reintervention was reduced from 10.2% with the BMS to 3.2% with the SES (P = .0004). In the multivariate analysis, patients in the SES group were approximately half as likely as those in the uncoated stent group to have a major adverse cardiac event (HR, 0.53; P = .006).

At 3 years, the rate of overall mortality did not differ (7.5% with BMS and 7.0% with SES; P = .79) and the cumulative incidence of cardiovascular death was identical (5.65% in each arm; P > 0.99).[14] The composite of all-cause death or myocardial infarction was also similar (13.2% vs. 12.6%; P = .83) but TVR remained more than twice as common with BMS (51 patients, 13.7%; vs. 23 patients, 6.2%; HR, 2.29; 95% CI, 1.4-3.7; P = .0007; Figure 18-5). The use of SES was associated with an almost fivefold decrease of coronary artery bypass grafting (CABG) (0.8% vs. 3.8%; HR, 4.7; 95% CI, 1.4-16.2; P = .007) and a twofold decrease of repeat PCI (5.4% vs. 10%; HR, 1.89; 95% CI, 1.1-3.2; P = .019). Consequently, the MACCE rate remained higher with the BMS (83 patients, 22.3%) compared with the SES (59 patients, 15.9%; HR, 1.45; 95% CI, 1.04-2.03; P = .026; Figure 18-6).

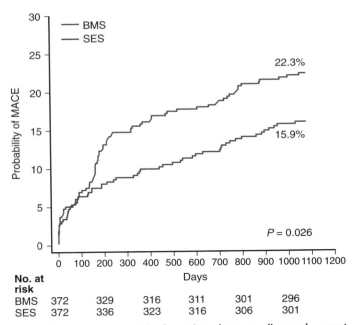

Figure 18-6 Cumulative risk of a major adverse cardiovascular event *(MACE)* in patients allocated to a bare metal stent *(BMS)* or sirolimus-eluting stent *(SES)* over long-term follow-up in the MULTISTRATEGY trial. (From Valgimigli M, Campo G, Gambetti S, et al; MULTISTRATEGY Investigators. Three-year follow-up of the MULTIcentre evaluation of Single high-dose Bolus TiRofiban vs. Abciximab with Sirolimus-eluting STEnt or Bare-Metal Stent in Acute Myocardial Infarction StudY (MULTISTRATEGY). *Int J Cardiol* 2011 Aug 22 (e-pub).)

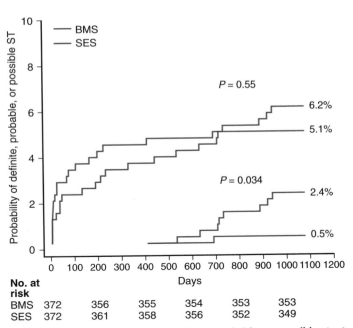

Figure 18-7 Cumulative risk for definite, probable, or possible stent thrombosis *(ST)* over long-term follow-up in the MULTISTRATEGY trial. The landmark analysis of the event rate at 370 days up to 3-year follow-up is also shown. *BMS,* Bare metal stent; *SES,* sirolimus-eluting stent.

Overall, there were 26 cases of definite stent thrombosis, of which 13 events occurred in each stent group, leading to an identical 3-year cumulative incidence of 3.5% in the two treatment groups (P > .99). The rate of Academic Research Consortium (ARC)–defined definite or probable stent thrombosis was also similar (17 patients, 4.6% with BMS and 15 patients, 4.0% with SES; P = .71), as well as the rate of any stent thrombosis (19 patients, 5.1% with BMS vs. 23 patients, 6.2% with SES; P = .52). The rate of definite and definite/probable stent thrombosis did not differ between the two stent groups at any time point during follow-up. Although the cumulative incidence of any stent thrombosis was numerically lower in the SES group within the first year (3.8% vs. 4.6%; P = .57), it was significantly higher in the SES group after the first year (2.4% vs. 0.5%; P = .034; Figure 18-7). After censoring patients in both groups who underwent TVR not related to definite stent thrombosis, the cumulative 3-year incidence of any stent thrombosis was identical (5.7% in the BMS vs. 5.6% in the SES group; P = .92), again reflecting a lower number of observed events in the SES group within the first year (3.1% vs. 5.1%; P = .18) but a higher rate of definite, probable, or possible stent thrombosis thereafter (2.5% vs. 0.6%; P = .044) in the SES arm. Therefore, the long-term follow-up of MULTISTRATEGY is in keeping with the observation that the incidence of very late ST after first-generation DES implantation is higher compared with BMS.[15] However, because very late ST is a relatively rare phenomenon, the absolute excess of events beyond 1 year in the DES arm may be offset by the early avoidance of coronary complications related to intimal hyperplasia. Consistent with this interpretation, patients undergoing TVR not driven by stent thrombosis in both arms of MULTISTRATEGY had a threefold higher incidence of myocardial infarction, which both preceded or followed coronary intervention.

HORIZONS AMI Trial

The Harmonizing Outcomes with RevasculariZatiON and Stents in Acute Myocardial Infarction (HORIZONS-AMI) trial was a prospective, open-label, factorial, randomized, multicenter study comparing bivalirudin monotherapy with heparin plus a GP IIb/IIIa inhibitor and paclitaxel-eluting stents (PESs) with BMS in 3602 patients with STEMI undergoing a primary PCI management strategy.[16,17] Consecutive patients aged 18 years or older with a symptom duration of 20 to 720 minutes and ST segment elevation of 1 mm or more in two or more contiguous leads, new left bundle branch block, or true posterior myocardial infarction were eligible for enrollment. After emergent angiography, the primary management strategy was primary PCI in 3345 patients (93%), deferred PCI in 2 patients (<1%), primary CABG in 62 patients (2%), and medical management in 193 patients (5%).[12] Stenting was performed in 3202 patients, of whom 3006 (93%) were randomly allocated to receive a PES (2257 patients, 75%) or a BMS (749 patients, 25%). PES significantly reduced the 3-year rates of ischemia-driven target lesion revascularization by 5.7% (95% CI, 2.7-8.6) compared with BMS. However, a marked increase in target lesion revascularization procedures occurred in the 1006 patients who underwent protocol-specified routine follow-up angiography at 13 months (Figure 18-8). For the 2000 patients in whom a 13-month routine protocol follow-up angiography was not undertaken, the absolute risk reduction in target lesion revascularization at 3 years with a PES compared with a BMS was 4.6%, resulting in a number needed to treat of 22. Patients who received a PES did not have different 3-year rates of safety from major adverse cardiac events (HR, 1.05; 95% CI, 0.84-1.33), reinfarction (HR, 1.05; 95% CI, 0.76-1.46), or mortality (HR, 0.84; 95% CI, 0.60-1.17) compared with those who received a BMS. Similarly, rates of stent thrombosis did not differ between PES and BMS at the end of the 3-year follow-up (HR, 1.10; 95% CI, 0.74-1.65) or at any other time point (Figure 18-9). However, the rate of stent thrombosis occurring after 1-year follow-up was almost twice as high in the PES group (1.7%) compared with the BMS group (0.9%), which is in keeping with the 3-year results of the MULTISTRATEGY trial.

Meta-Analysis

A meta-analysis to assess the safety and efficacy of drug-eluting stents (DES) compared with BMS for patients with STEMI included 15

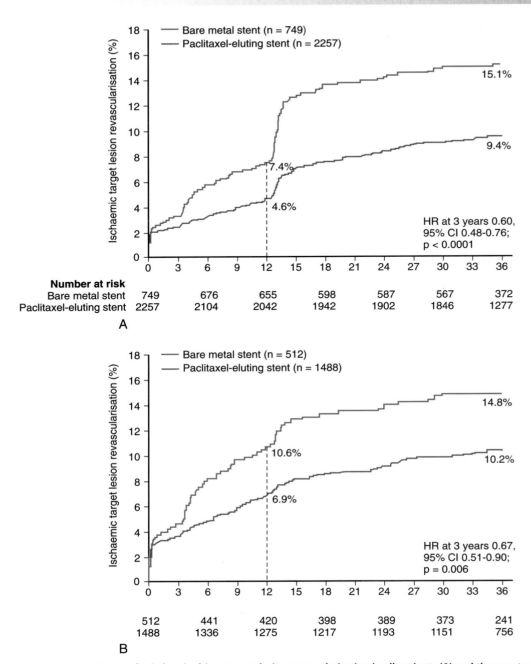

Figure 18-8   **Time to event curves to 3 years for ischemia-driven target lesion revascularization in all patients (A) and those not undergoing routine 13-month angiographic follow-up (B) in the HORIZONS-AMI trial.** Paclitaxel-eluting stents significantly reduced ischemia-driven target lesion revascularization compared with bare metal stents for patients presenting with ST-elevation myocardial infarction, whether or not protocol-mandated follow-up angiography was performed. *CI,* Confidence interval; *HR,* hazard ratio. (From Stone GW, Witzenbichler B, Guagliumi G, et al; HORIZONS-AMI Trial Investigators. Heparin plus a glycoprotein IIb/IIIa inhibitor vs. bivalirudin monotherapy and paclitaxel-eluting stents vs. bare-metal stents in acute myocardial infarction [HORIZONS-AMI]: final 3-year results from a multicentre, randomised controlled trial. *Lancet* 2011;377:2193-2204.)

randomized clinical trials, of which 13 were published as peer-reviewed articles and two were presented at scientific meetings only (see Table 18-2).[18] In sum, these trials randomly allocated 7867 patients undergoing primary PCI in the setting of STEMI to treatment with early-generation DES or BMS. Seven trials allocated patients to SES, five to PES, and three trials used both types. The maximum length of follow-up ranged from 7 months to 6 years, with a duration of follow-up of 3 years or more in 11 trials. The clinical characteristics of included patients are summarized in Table 18-2. The mean age

ranged from 59 to 65 years, the percentage of men from 70% to 83%, the percentage of patients with diabetes from 10% to 28%, and the percentage of patients with multivessel disease from 34% to 53%. The duration of protocol-recommended dual antiplatelet therapy for patients with DES ranged from 3 to 12 months, with identical recommended durations in DES and BMS patients in all but one trial.

During the first year after stent implantation, patients with DES tended to be less likely than patients with BMS to experience definite stent thrombosis (RR, 0.80; 95% CI, 0.58-1.12). Conversely, patients

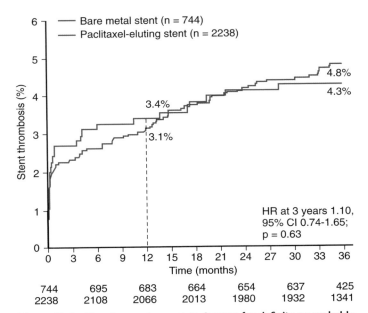

Figure 18-9   Time to event curves to 3 years for definite or probable stent thrombosis in patients randomly allocated to receive paclitaxel-eluting stents or bare metal stents in the HORIZONS-AMI trial. The overall rates of stent thrombosis were similar between groups. *CI,* Confidence interval; *HR,* hazard ratio. (From Stone GW, Witzenbichler B, Guagliumi G, et al; HORIZONS-AMI Trial Investigators. Heparin plus a glycoprotein IIb/IIIa inhibitor vs. bivalirudin monotherapy and paclitaxel-eluting stents vs. bare-metal stents in acute myocardial infarction [HORIZONS-AMI]: final 3-year results from a multicentre, randomised controlled trial. *Lancet* 2011;377:2193-2204.)

with DES were more likely than patients with BMS to experience definite stent thrombosis during subsequent years (RR, 2.10; 95% CI, 1.20-3.69). A test of interaction between the risk of definite ST and time was significant (*P* for interaction = .009; Figure 18-10). A total of 14 trials contributed to the analysis of the risk of TVR, which was the primary efficacy endpoint of the study. TVR occurred in 429 patients treated with DES (9.0%) and 452 patients treated with BMS (14.6%), resulting in a pooled relative risk of 0.51 (95% CI, 0.43-0.61; see Figure 18-10) and no evidence for heterogeneity between trials (I² = 24%; *P* for heterogeneity = .19). The stratified analyses according to methodologic and clinical characteristics indicated a greater benefit from DES in small as compared with large trials, suggesting that small study bias may have contributed to the findings. In the analysis stratified according to time (see Figure 18-10), a more pronounced reduction was found in the relative risk of TVR for DES as compared with BMS during the first year (RR, 0.46; 95% CI, 0.38-0.55) as opposed to subsequent years (RR, 0.75; 95% CI, 0.59-0.94), with a positive test of interaction between the risk of TVR and time (*P* for interaction = .007). Sensitivity analyses of time-dependent effects after restriction to trials of higher methodologic quality showed similar results.

This meta-analysis of 15 randomized trials suggests time-dependent clinical effects of early generation U.S. Food and Drug Administration (FDA)–approved DES compared with BMS for definite stent thrombosis, definite or probable stent thrombosis, TVR, and myocardial infarction. During the first year, there was a safety advantage of DES over BMS in terms of lower rates of stent thrombosis and MI, whereas an opposite pattern emerged during subsequent years, with a safety advantage of BMS over DES. This qualitative interaction between risks and benefits was particularly robust for definite stent thrombosis, with a trend toward a 20% relative risk reduction during the first year, which was offset by a more than 100% relative risk increase during subsequent years (*P* for interaction = .009). For the

primary effectiveness outcome of TVR, a quantitative interaction was observed, with a more than 50% relative risk reduction of TVR during the first year; this decreased to 25% during subsequent years (*P* for interaction = .007). Overall, the effectiveness of DES in reducing the rate of TVR was maintained across the entire duration of follow-up, with an estimated number needed to treat of 15 to prevent one TVR during the first 5 years after stent implantation. No evidence of an increased risk for any safety outcome was observed with DES, with relative risk ratios near 1 for all-cause death, cardiac death, myocardial infarction, stent thrombosis, and the composite of death or myocardial infarction.

TEMPORAL DIFFERENCES IN THROMBOTIC EVENTS

Patients with STEMI are at increased risk of stent thrombosis as compared with patients with stable coronary artery disease after DES and BMS implantation. However, the observed differential in timing of stent thrombosis suggests differences in the underlying pathophysiologic pathways leading to this adverse event after DES implantation. Early stent thrombosis is closely related to the acute phase after the coronary event and procedure, with pronounced activation of platelets and the coagulation cascade. Experimental data have suggested that durable, polymer-based DES may exert antithrombogenic properties, resulting in a lower degree of thrombus adhesion,[19] which may be of particular importance for patients with STEMI. This is consistent with the results noted earlier, which provide preliminary clinical evidence of a somewhat lower risk of definite stent thrombosis after DES as compared with BMS implantation among patients with STEMI. Conversely, stent thromboses occurring later, after PCI, may be related to a chronic process with delayed arterial healing and vessel remodeling caused by chronic local inflammation that is potentially related to the persistence of durable polymers and/or the long-term effects of drug elution. Consistent with this hypothesis, autopsy data have indicated a differential healing response of DES implanted into plaques of patients with STEMI as compared with those with stable coronary artery disease, with evidence of persistent inflammation and a higher proportion of uncovered struts among coronary segments treated with DES than BMS.[20] Among patients treated with DES, incomplete stent apposition has been recognized as an important morphologic substrate associated with the occurrence of very late stent thrombosis.[21] It is more frequently observed in patients with STEMI than in those who undergo DES implantation for stable angina and may be related to incomplete stent apposition at the time of implantation, presence of jailed thrombus with subsequent resolution, or vessel remodeling in response to toxic effects of the drug or polymer. In addition, optical coherence tomography[22] and intravascular ultrasound studies[23] among patients with STEMI have provided evidence for a higher rate of uncovered stent struts and incomplete stent apposition with DES compared with BMS.

All these factors may be of particular relevance to the relative safety of discontinuing dual antiplatelet therapy during long-term follow-up. The higher risk of definite stent thrombosis with early generation DES than BMS more than 1 year after stent implantation directly translated into an increased risk of myocardial infarction, with identical numbers needed to harm of 76 for both stent thrombosis and MI.[18] Whether prolongation of dual antiplatelet therapy beyond 1 year in patients with STEMI who are at a higher risk of very late ST compared with other patient subsets may overcome this disadvantage and, in turn, translate into a lower overall relative risk of stent thrombosis and myocardial infarction with DES compared with BMS remains subject to debate. In addition, the use of newer generation DES with durable polymers of improved biocompatibility,[24] biodegradable polymers that dissolve completely once the drug is eluted,[25] or even fully bioresorbable vascular scaffolds[26] are currently being investigated to address this issue in patients with STEMI.

TABLE 18-2 Randomized Controlled Studies on Drug-Eluting Stents in Acute Myocardial Infarction

Trial Acronym	Stent Types	No. of Patients	Age, Mean (SD)	Males, N (%)	Diabetes, N (%)	Hypertension, N (%)	Smokers, N (%)	MVD, N (%)	RVD, Mean (SD)	No. of Stents, Mean (SD)	Stent Length (mm), Mean (SD)	Stent Diameter (mm), Mean (SD)	Longest FUP (yr)
Pasceri et al	SES vs. BMS	32/33	62 (—)	—	—	—	—	—	—	—	—	—	3
PASSION	PES vs. BMS	310/309	61 (13)	470 (76)	68 (11)	193 (31)	319 (52)‡	278 (45)	3.2 (0.5)	1.3 (0.6)	19 (6)	3.2 (0.3)	5
STRATEGY	SES vs. BMS	87/88	63 (12)*	128 (73)	26 (15)	92 (53)	70 (40)	72 (41)	2.3 (0.5)*		—	—	5
BASKET-AMI	SES vs. PES vs. BMS	75/67/74	—	—	—	—	—	—	—	—	—	—	3
TYPHOON	SES vs. BMS	356/359	59 (12)	558 (78)	116 (16)	289 (41)	356 (50)	336 (47)	2.8 (0.6)	1.1 (0.4)	21 (8)	3.1 (0.4)	4
PASEO	SES vs. PES vs. BMS	90/90/90	62 (16)	190 (70)	69 (26)	71 (26)	68 (25)	—	3.2 (0.5)	1.2 (0.5)	21 (7)	3.1 (0.4)	6
SESAMI	SES vs. BMS	160/160	63 (12)	256 (80)	65 (20)	185 (58)	174 (54)	150 (47)	—	1 (-)	18 (4)	3.1 (0.2)	3
MISSION	SES vs. BMS	158/152	59 (11)	241 (78)	30 (10)	87 (28)	169 (55)	106 (34)	2.8 (0.6)	—	26 (12)	3.3 (0.3)	3
HAAMU-STENT	PES vs. BMS	82/82	63 (13)	118 (72)	24 (15)	75 (46)	70 (43)	—	—	—	—	—	1
Diaz de la Llera et al	SES vs. BMS	60/60	65 (13)	95 (79)	33 (28)	—	82 (68)	56 (47)	—	—	30 (15)	3.2 (0.4)	1
MULTI-STRATEGY	SES vs. BMS	373/372	64 (12)	565 (76)	108 (15)	426 (57)	277 (37)	399 (53)	2.8 (0.4)*	1 (0)	22 (5)	3.1 (0.4)	3
SELECTION	PES vs. BMS	40/40	61 (—)	66 (83)	10 (13)	37 (46)	43 (54)	36 (45)	2.9 (0.4)	—	20 (5)	3.1 (0.3)	7 mo
GRACIA-3	PES vs. BMS	217/216	61 (1)	358 (83)	80 (18)	188 (43)	210 (48)	163 (38)	2.9 (0.04)	—	—	—	1
HORIZONS-AMI	PES vs. BMS	2257/749	60 (—)*	2307 (77)	478 (16)	1544 (51)	1429 (48)	—	2.9 (0.5)†	1.5 (0.8)	30 (16)	—	3
DEDICATION	SES vs. BMS	313/313	62 (—)	458 (73)	65 (10)	207 (33)	336 (54)	235 (38)	—	—	22 (10)	3.5 (0.5)	3

BASKET-AMI, Basel Stent KostenEffektivitäts in Acute Myocardial Infarction Trial; BMS, bare metal stent; DEDICATION, Drug Elution and Distal Protection in ST-Segment-Elevation Myocardial Infarct; FUP, follow-up; GRACIA-3, Grupo de Análisis de la CardiopatíaIsquémicaAguda; HAAMU-STENT, Helsinki Area Acute Myocardial infarction treatment reevalUation—Should The patient get a drug-Eluting or a Normal sTent; HORIZONS-AMI, Harmonizing Outcomes with Revascularization and Stents in Acute Myocardial Infarction; MISSION, A Prospective Randomised Controlled Trial to Evaluate the Efficacy of Drug-Eluting Stents vs. Bare-Metal Stent in Acute Myocardial Infarction Study; MULTI-STRATEGY, Multicenter Evaluation of Single High-Dose Bolus Tirofiban vs. Abciximab with Sirolimus-Eluting Stent or Bare-Metal Stent in Acute Myocardial Infarction Study; MVD, multivessel disease; PASEO, Paclitaxel or Sirolimus-Eluting Stent vs. Bare Metal Stent in Primary Angioplasty; PASSION, Paclitaxel-Eluting Stent vs. Conventional Stent in Myocardial Infarction with ST-Segment Elevation; PES, paclitaxel-eluting stent; RVD, reference vessel diameter; SELECTION, Single-Center Randomized Evaluation of Paclitaxel-Eluting Vs. Conventional Stent in Acute Myocardial Infarction; SES, Sirolimus-eluting stent; SESAMI, Sirolimus-Eluting Stent Vs. Bare-Metal Stent in Acute Myocardial Infarction; STRATEGY, Single High Dose Bolus Tirofiban and Sirolimus Eluting Stent vs. Abciximab and Bare Metal Stent in Myocardial Infarction; TYPHOON, Trial to Assess the Use of the Cypher Stent in Acute Myocardial Infarction Treated with Balloon Angioplasty.

*Estimated mean and SD from median and IQR.

†RVD is procedural, not baseline.

‡Includes all patients with a history of smoking, not just current smokers.

Adapted from Kalesan B, Pilgrim T, Heinimann K, et al. Comparison of drug-eluting stents with bare metal stents in patients with ST-segment elevation myocardial infarction. *Eur Heart J* 2012;33:977-987.

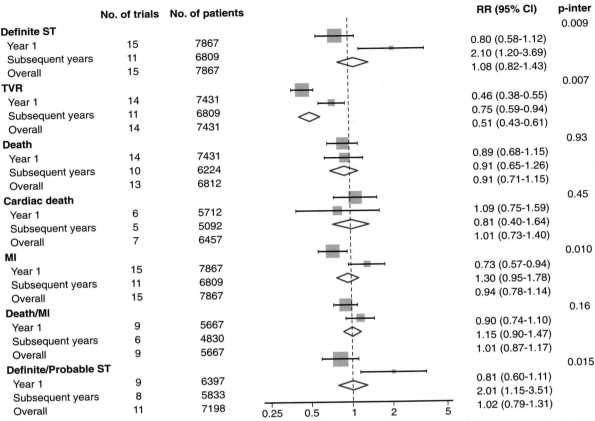

	No. of trials	No. of patients		RR (95% CI)	p-inter
Definite ST					0.009
Year 1	15	7867		0.80 (0.58-1.12)	
Subsequent years	11	6809		2.10 (1.20-3.69)	
Overall	15	7867		1.08 (0.82-1.43)	
TVR					0.007
Year 1	14	7431		0.46 (0.38-0.55)	
Subsequent years	11	6809		0.75 (0.59-0.94)	
Overall	14	7431		0.51 (0.43-0.61)	
Death					0.93
Year 1	14	7431		0.89 (0.68-1.15)	
Subsequent years	10	6224		0.91 (0.65-1.26)	
Overall	13	6812		0.91 (0.71-1.15)	
Cardiac death					0.45
Year 1	6	5712		1.09 (0.75-1.59)	
Subsequent years	5	5092		0.81 (0.40-1.64)	
Overall	7	6457		1.01 (0.73-1.40)	
MI					0.010
Year 1	15	7867		0.73 (0.57-0.94)	
Subsequent years	11	6809		1.30 (0.95-1.78)	
Overall	15	7867		0.94 (0.78-1.14)	
Death/MI					0.16
Year 1	9	5667		0.90 (0.74-1.10)	
Subsequent years	6	4830		1.15 (0.90-1.47)	
Overall	9	5667		1.01 (0.87-1.17)	
Definite/Probable ST					0.015
Year 1	9	6397		0.81 (0.60-1.11)	
Subsequent years	8	5833		2.01 (1.15-3.51)	
Overall	11	7198		1.02 (0.79-1.31)	

0.25   0.5   1   2   5

Figure 18-10   Risk of clinical outcomes after drug-eluting stent *(DES)* compared with bare metal stent *(BMS)* for the treatment of ST-elevation myocardial infarction, stratified according to time. Significant quantitative interactions between the effect of DES and time were observed for the endpoints of stent thrombosis and myocardial infarction, with a potential safety benefit for BMS after 1 year follow-up. *CI,* Confidence interval; *MI,* myocardial infarction; *p-inter, P* for interaction between year 1 and subsequent years using metaregression; *ST,* stent thrombosis; *TVR,* target vessel revascularization. (From Kalesan B, Pilgrim T, Heinimann K, et al. Comparison of drug-eluting stents with bare metal stents in patients with ST-segment elevation myocardial infarction. *Eur Heart J* 2012;33:977-87.)

⬛ Newer Generation Drug-Eluting Stents

Compared with early-generation DES, data regarding the safety and efficacy of newer generation DES in patients with STEMI are more limited because very long-term follow-up for these stents is comparatively lacking.

EVEROLIMUS-ELUTING STENTS

This newer generation DES has been studied in the Evaluation of the Xience-V stent in Acute Myocardial INfArcTION (EXAMINATION) trial.[27] This was a multicenter, prospective, randomized, single-blind, all-comer trial, which compared the performance of an everolimus-eluting stent with BMS in patients presenting up to 48 hours after STEMI requiring emergent PCI.[28] A total of 1504 patients were randomized at 12 medical centers. The primary endpoint was the composite of all-cause death, any recurrent myocardial infarction, and any revascularization at 1 year. Main secondary endpoints included the device-oriented combination of cardiac death, target vessel–related myocardial infarction, or target lesion revascularization. The safety endpoint was definite or probable stent thrombosis at 1 year. The primary endpoint occurred in 89 patients (11.9%) of the everolimus-eluting stent (EES) group and in 106 patients (14.2%) in the BMS group (*P* = .16). The device-oriented secondary endpoint occurred in 48 patients (6.4%) of the everolimus-eluting stent group and in 73 patients (9.8%) of the BMS group as a result of a reduction in target lesion revascularization (2.1% vs. 5.0%). Both

the rates of definite and definite or probable stent thrombosis were significantly lower in the everolimus-eluting stent group (0.5% and 0.9% vs. 1.9% and 2.5%, respectively; both *P* = .01). Clinical and procedural features were comparable between groups, compliance to dual antiplatelet therapy was high (almost 100%) in acute and subacute phase after STEMI in both groups, and both Xience V and Multilink Vision shared the same stent platform. Longer follow-up of the EXAMINATION trial is needed to determine whether the efficacy and safety performance of this newer generation DES is maintained beyond 12 months, unlike the results of many previous randomized controlled studies comparing first-generation DES with BMS.

Supportive data with respect to this important issue has come from the COMPARE study, which included patients on an all-comer basis who were randomly allocated to an everolimus-eluting stent or PES. Patients with STEMI represented as much as 25% of the overall patient population. The 2-year results of this specific STEMI cohort were recently reported and showed that the primary composite of all death, nonfatal myocardial infarction, and target vessel revascularization occurred in 9.0% of EES patients and 13.7% of PES patients (RR, 0.66; 95% CI, 0.50-0.86) driven by a lower rate of myocardial infarction (3.9% vs. 7.5%; RR, 0.52; 95% CI, 0.35-0.77) and target vessel revascularization (3.2% vs. 8.0%; RR, 0.41; 95% CI, 0.27-0.62), in parallel with a lower rate of definite or probable stent thrombosis (0.9% vs. 3.9%; RR, 0.23; 95% CI, 0.11-0.49; Figure 18-11). Differences significantly increased between 1- and 2-year follow-up for the primary composite endpoint (*P* = .04), target vessel

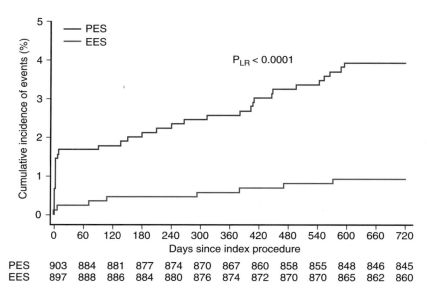

Figure 18-11 Kaplan-Meier cumulative event curves for definite and probable stent thrombosis (ST) at 2-year follow-up in the COMPARE trial. The absolute difference in rates of Academic Research Consortium–defined definite and probable ST between stent groups was 1.9% at 1 year, which significantly increased to 3.9% at 2 years. The *red line* indicates paclitaxel-eluting stent *(PES)*; the *blue line* indicates everolimus-eluting stent *(EES)*. (From Smits PC, Kedhi E, Royaards KJ, et al. 2-year follow-up of a randomized controlled trial of everolimus- and paclitaxel-eluting stents for coronary revascularization in daily practice. COMPARE [Comparison of the everolimus eluting XIENCE-V stent with the paclitaxel eluting TAXUS LIBERTE stent in all-comers: a randomized open label trial]. *J Am Coll Cardiol* 2011;58:11-18.)

revascularization ($P = .02$), and definite or probable stent thrombosis ($P = .02$).

BIOLIMUS-ELUTING STENTS

Experimental data, autopsy findings, and in vivo intravascular ultrasound studies of patients with very late stent thrombosis have shown evidence of incomplete endothelialization, delayed arterial healing, and vessel remodeling caused by chronic inflammation. The persistence of durable polymer material on the stent surface after completion of drug release has been suggested as a potential trigger for the chronic inflammatory response that leads to very late stent thrombosis. Biodegradable polymer DES aim to overcome this limitation by providing controlled drug release, with subsequent degradation of the polymer material, thereby eliminating the inflammatory stimulus. Specifically, biolimus-eluting stents (BES) were designed with a biodegradable polymer applied to the stent's abluminal surface, which is metabolized to water and carbon dioxide within 6 to 9 months. Biolimus is a highly lipophilic sirolimus analogue that inhibits proliferation of smooth muscle cells by causing an arrest of the cell cycle at G0 with similar potency to sirolimus. The primary results of the LEADERS (Limus Eluted from A Durable vs. ERodable Stent coating) trial have shown that similar biodegradable polymer BES is noninferior to durable polymer sirolimus-eluting stent (SES) for the endpoint of cardiac death, myocardial infarction, or clinically indicated TVR at 9 months.[29] At 4-year follow-up, this endpoint occurred in 160 patients (19%) with biodegradable polymer BES and 192 patients (23%) with durable polymer SES, with an absolute risk difference of −0.039, a one-sided *P* value for noninferiority of <.0001, and a trend toward superiority (RR, 0.81. 95% CI, 0.66-1.00; $P = .05$; Figure 18-12).[19] In stratified analyses of the primary endpoint according to prespecified patient characteristics, similar results were observed across most subgroups. However, the biodegradable polymer BES seemed superior to the durable polymer SES in patients with STEMI at baseline (RR, 0.45; 95% CI, 0.24-0.83) compared with patients without (RR, 0.88; 95% CI, 0.70-1.10; *P* interaction = .043), and appeared to reduce the risk of cardiovascular events caused by very late stent thrombosis.

DURATION OF DUAL ANTIPLATELET THERAPY AFTER CORONARY STENTING

Clopidogrel therapy lasting 9 to 12 months after BMS was shown to reduce the composite of death, myocardial infarction, or stroke by almost 30% in patients with non–ST segment elevation acute coronary syndrome compared with a 1-month duration of treatment.[30,31] Long-term therapy with clopidogrel is also recommended for patients with STEMI,[32,33] and this recommendation has been recently extended to newer oral $P2Y_{12}$ receptor blockers, including prasugrel and ticagrelor. Of note, no dedicated randomized STEMI trial has ever assessed the optimal duration of dual antiplatelet therapy after bare metal or drug-eluting stenting.

Recently, the Prolonging Dual Antiplatelet Treatment after Grading Stent-Induced Intimal Hyperplasia study (PRODIGY) randomized 2013 patients to receive one of the four stent types, including EES, PES, Endeavor zotarolimus-eluting stent, or a third-generation, thin-strut BMS.[34] At 30 days, patients in each stent group were randomized in a balanced fashion to 6 or 24 months of dual antiplatelet treatment consisting of aspirin and clopidogrel. Patients with STEMI comprised 33% of the overall patient population. There was no significant difference in the incidence of death from any cause, myocardial infarction, or cerebrovascular accident at 2 years with clopidogrel continuation (use of clopidogrel plus aspirin) as compared with clopidogrel discontinuation (use of aspirin alone) after 6 months, whereas 2-year clopidogrel therapy resulted in a significant increase of bleeding episodes that required medical or surgical treatment or red blood cell transfusion, or were life-threatening (Figure 18-13). These findings support the concept that the clinical benefit of prolonged dual antiplatelet therapy after PCI for STEMI deserves further evaluation through an adequately powered, randomized clinical trial.

Conclusion

The use of BMS in the setting of patients with STEMI reduces the need for repeat target vessel intervention compared with stand-alone balloon angioplasty but fails to affect mortality or reinfarction rates. First-generation sirolimus-eluting stents or PES reduce the need for reintervention even further compared with BMS but increase the risk of very late stent thrombosis, resulting in a late hazard for reinfarction. Newer generation DES, particularly the durable polymer everolimus-eluting and biodegradable polymer biolimus-eluting stents, may have an improved safety profile compared with first-generation DES, and this requires further study. A 12-month duration of dual antiplatelet therapy is recommended by current American and European guidelines, although there is a lack of definitive evidence regarding the optimal duration of dual antiplatelet therapy after stenting; additional studies are needed to elucidate the potential benefits versus the risks of prolonged duration of concomitant therapy with aspirin and oral $P2Y_{12}$ receptor blockers in these patients.

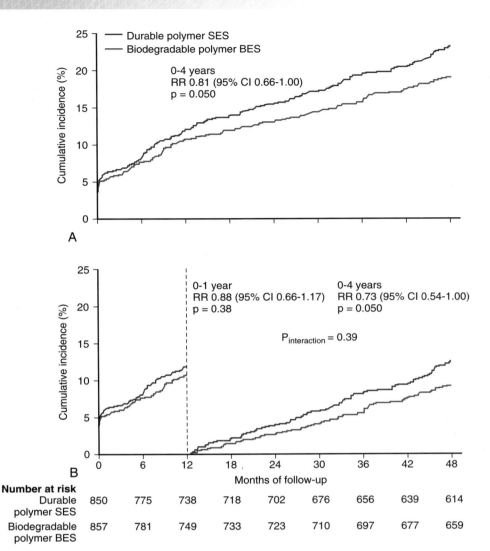

Figure 18-12 Cumulative incidence for 4 years (A) and for year 1 and years 1 to 4 separately (B) of the primary endpoint consisting in the composite of cardiac death, myocardial infarction, or clinically indicated target vessel revascularization of the LEADERS trial. The biolimus-eluting stent *(BES)* fulfilled the criteria for noninferiority and strongly tended to superiority at 4 years. *CI,* Confidence interval; *RR,* relative risk; *SES,* sirolimus-eluting stent. (From Windecker S, Serruys PW, Wandel S, et al. Biolimus-eluting stent with biodegradable polymer vs. sirolimus-eluting stent with durable polymer for coronary revascularisation [LEADERS]: a randomized non-inferiority trial. *Lancet* 2008; 372:1163-1173.)

Figure 18-13 Cumulative rates of bleeding in the PRODIGY trial, which randomly assigned patients with acute coronary syndrome treated with PCI to either a 24- or a 6-month duration of dual antiplatelet therapy. Bleeding was more frequent with the prolonged duration of antiplatelet therapy, irrespective of definition. *RBC,* Red blood cell; *TIMI,* Thrombolysis In Myocardial Infarction. (Adapted from Valgimigli M, Campo G, Monti M, et al. Short- versus long-term duration of dual-antiplatelet therapy after coronary stenting: a randomized multicenter trial. *Circulation* 2012;125:2015-2026.)

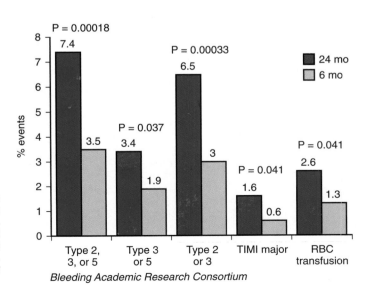

REFERENCES

1. Antman EM, Anbe DT, Armstrong PW, et al. ACC/AHA guidelines for the management of patients with ST-elevation myocardial infarction: a report of the American College of Cardiology/American Heart Association Task Force on Practice Guidelines (Committee to Revise the 1999 Guidelines for the Management of Patients with Acute Myocardial Infarction). *Circulation* 2004;110:e82-e292.

2. Boersma E. Does time matter? A pooled analysis of randomized clinical trials comparing primary percutaneous coronary intervention and in-hospital fibrinolysis in acute myocardial infarction patients. *Eur Heart J* 2006;27(7):779-788.

3. Zhu MM, Feit A, Chadow H, et al. Primary stent implantation compared with primary balloon angioplasty for acute myocardial infarction: a meta-analysis of randomized clinical trials. *Am J Cardiol* 2001;88:297-301.

4. Nordmann AJ, Bucher H, Hengstler P, et al. Primary stenting vs. primary balloon angioplasty for treating acute myocardial infarction. *Cochrane Database Syst Rev* 2005(2):CD005313.

5. Stone GW, Grines CL, Cox DA, et al. Comparison of angioplasty with stenting, with or without abciximab, in acute myocardial infarction. *N Engl J Med* 2002;346:957-966.

6. Suryapranata H, De Luca G, van 't Hof AW, et al. Is routine stenting for acute myocardial infarction superior to balloon angioplasty? A randomised comparison in a large cohort of unselected patients. *Heart* 2005;(5):641-645.

7. Grines CL, Cox DA, Stone GW, et al. Coronary angioplasty with or without stent implantation for acute myocardial infarction. Stent Primary Angioplasty in Myocardial Infarction Study Group. *N Engl J Med* 1999;341:1949-1955

8. Svilaas T, van der Horst IC, Zijlstra F. A quantitative estimate of bare-metal stenting compared with balloon angioplasty in patients with acute myocardial infarction: angiographic measures in relation to clinical outcome. *Heart* 2007;93:792-800.

9. Valgimigli M, Percoco G, Malagutti P, et al. Tirofiban and sirolimus-eluting stent vs abciximab and bare-metal stent for acute myocardial infarction: a randomized trial. *Jama* 2005;293:2109-2117.

10. Tebaldi M, Arcozzi C, Campo G, et al. The 5-year clinical outcomes after a randomized comparison of sirolimus-eluting vs. bare-metal stent implantation in patients with ST-segment elevation myocardial infarction. *J Am Coll Cardiol* 2009;54:1900-1901.

11. Spaulding C, Henry P, Teiger E, et al. Sirolimus-eluting vs. uncoated stents in acute myocardial infarction. *N Engl J Med* 2006;355:1093-1104.

12. Spaulding C, Teiger E, Commeau P, et al. Four-year follow-up of TYPHOON (trial to assess the use of the CYPHer sirolimus-eluting coronary stent in acute myocardial infarction treated with BallOON angioplasty). *JACC Cardiovasc Interv* 2011;4:14-23.

13. Valgimigli M, Campo G, Percoco G, et al. Comparison of angioplasty with infusion of tirofiban or abciximab and with implantation of sirolimus-eluting or uncoated stents for acute myocardial infarction: the MULTISTRATEGY randomized trial. *JAMA* 2008;299:1788-1799

14. Valglimigli M, Campo G, Gambetti S, et al; MULTISTRATEGY Investigators. Three-year follow-up of the MULTIcentre evaluation of Single high-dose Bolus TiRofiban vs. Abciximab with Sirolimus-eluting STEnt or Bare-Metal Stent in Acute Myocardial Infarction StudY (MULTISTRATEGY). *Int J Cardiol* 2011; Aug 22 (e-pub).

15. Roukoz H, Bavry AA, Sarkees ML, et al. Comprehensive meta-analysis on drug-eluting stents vs. bare-metal stents during extended follow-up. *Am J Med* 2009;122:581 e581-e510.

16. Stone GW, Lansky AJ, Pocock SJ, et al. Paclitaxel-eluting stents vs. bare-metal stents in acute myocardial infarction. *N Engl J Med* 2009;360:1946-1959.

17. Stone GW, Witzenbichler B, Guagliumi G, et al. Heparin plus a glycoprotein IIb/IIIa inhibitor vs. bivalirudin monotherapy and paclitaxel-eluting stents in acute myocardial infarction (HORIZONS-AMI): final 3-year results from a multicentre, randomised controlled trial. *Lancet* 2011;377:2193-2204. DUPLICATE OF 11B

18. Kalesan B, Pilgrim T, Heinimann K, et al. Comparison of drug-eluting stents with bare metal stents in patients with ST-segment elevation myocardial infarction. *Eur Heart J* 2012;33:977-987.

19. Kolandaivelu K, Swaminathan R, Gibson WJ, et al. Stent thrombogenicity early in high-risk interventional settings is driven by stent design and deployment and protected by polymer-drug coatings. *Circulation* 2011;123:1400-1409.

20. Nakazawa G, Finn AV, Joner M, et al. Delayed arterial healing and increased late stent thrombosis at culprit sites after drug-eluting stent placement for acute myocardial infarction patients: an autopsy study. *Circulation* 2008;118:1138-1145.

21. Cook S, Wenaweser P, Togni M, et al. Incomplete stent apposition and very late stent thrombosis after drug-eluting stent implantation. *Circulation* 2007;115:2426-2434.

22. Guagliumi G, Costa MA, Sirbu V, et al. Strut coverage and late malapposition with paclitaxel-eluting stents compared with bare metal stents in acute myocardial infarction: optical coherence tomography substudy of the Harmonizing Outcomes with Revascularization and Stents in Acute Myocardial Infarction (HORIZONS-AMI) Trial. *Circulation* 2011;123:274-281.

23. Maehara A, Mintz GS, Lansky AJ, et al. Volumetric intravascular ultrasound analysis of paclitaxel-eluting and bare metal stents in acute myocardial infarction: the harmonizing outcomes with revascularization and stents in acute myocardial infarction intravascular ultrasound substudy. *Circulation* 2009; 120:1875-1882.

24. Smits PC, Kedhi E, Royaards KJ, et al. 2-year follow-up of a randomized controlled trial of everolimus- and paclitaxel-eluting stents for coronary revascularization in daily practice. COMPARE (Comparison of the everolimus eluting XIENCE-V stent with the paclitaxel eluting TAXUS LIBERTE stent in all-comers: a randomized open label trial). *J Am Coll Cardiol* 2011;58:11-18.

25. Stefanini G, Kalesan B, Serruys P, et al. Long-term clinical outcomes of biodegradable polymer sirolimus-eluting stents vs. durable polymer sirolimus-eluting stents in patients with coronary artery disease (LEADERS): 4 year follow-up of a randomised non-inferiority trial. *Lancet* 2011;378:1940-1948.

26. Onuma Y, Serruys PW. Bioresorbable scaffold: the advent of a new era in percutaneous coronary and peripheral revascularization? *Circulation* 2011;123:779-797.

27. Sabate M. *Results of the evaluation of the Xience-V stent in Acute Myocardial INFArcTION (EXAMINATION) trial.* Presented at the European Society of Cardiology (ESC) Congress. Paris, August 30th. 2011.

28. Sabaté M, Cequier A, Iñiguez A, et al. Rationale and design of the EXAMINATION trial: a randomised comparison between everolimus-eluting stents and cobalt-chromium bare-metal stents in ST-elevation myocardial infarction. *EuroIntervention* 2011;7:977-984.

29. Windecker S, Serruys PW, Wandel S, et al. Biolimus-eluting stent with biodegradable polymer vs. sirolimus-eluting stent with durable polymer for coronary revascularisation (LEADERS): a randomized non-inferiority trial. *Lancet* 2008;372:1163-1173.

30. Mehta SR, Yusuf S, Peters RJ, et al. Effects of pretreatment with clopidogrel and aspirin followed by long-term therapy in patients undergoing percutaneous coronary intervention: the PCI-CURE study. *Lancet* 2001;358:527-533.

31. Steinhubl SR, Berger PB, Mann 3rd JT, et al. Early and sustained dual oral antiplatelet therapy following percutaneous coronary intervention: a randomized controlled trial. *Jama* 2002;288:2411-2420.

32. Kushner FG, Hand M, Smith Jr SC, et al. 2009 Focused Updates: ACC/AHA Guidelines for the Management of Patients With ST-Elevation Myocardial Infarction (updating the 2004 Guideline and 2007 Focused Update) and ACC/AHA/SCAI Guidelines on Percutaneous Coronary Intervention (updating the 2005 Guideline and 2007 Focused Update): a report of the American College of Cardiology Foundation/American Heart Association Task Force on Practice Guidelines. *Circulation* 2009;120:2271-2306.

33. Van de Werf F, Bax J, Betriu A, et al. Management of acute myocardial infarction in patients presenting with persistent ST-segment elevation: the Task Force on the Management of ST-Segment Elevation Acute Myocardial Infarction of the European Society of Cardiology. *Eur Heart J* 2008;29:2909-2945.

34. Valgimigli M, Campo G, Monti M, et al. Short- versus long-term duration of dual-antiplatelet therapy after coronary stenting: A randomized multicenter trial. *Circulation* 2012;125:2015-2026.

INDEX

Page numbers followed by "f" indicate figures, "t" indicate tables, and "b" indicate boxes.